Ju[illegible]TH [illegible]7

To Gregory

with many greetings
and thanks from

Gunnar

THE SHAPING OF A PROFESSION

THE SHAPING OF A PROFESSION

Physicians in Norway, Past and Present

ØIVIND LARSEN
Editor

Bent Olav Olsen
Associate editor

Science History Publications/USA
1996

Published in the United States of America by
Watson Publishing International
a division of
Science History Publications/USA
P.O. Box 493, Canton, MA 02021
1996

Library of Congress Cataloging-in-Publication Data

The shaping of a profession: physicians in Norway, past and present/
Øivind Larsen, editor; Bent Olav Olsen, associate editor.
p. cm.
Includes bibliographical references and index.
ISBN 0-88135-168-7
1. Physicians–Norway–History. 2. Medicine–Norway–History.
I. Larsen, Øivind, 1938–. II. Olsen, Bent Olav, 1965–.
[DNLM: 1. Physicians–history–Norway. 2. History of Medicine,
Modern–Norway. WZ 70 GN6 S5 1996]
R647.S53 1996
610.69'52'09481--dc21
DNLM/DLC
for Library of Congress 96-46645
CIP

Typeset with Garamond 10/11 points and printed in Norway by
a.s. Joh. Nordahls Trykkeri
Strømsveien 102, N-0663 Oslo;
text on 90 g G-print matte paper,
and photographs in duotone on 115 g G-print glossy paper

Binding: AiT Norbok, N-2800 Gjøvik

Contents

Preface

The survey of the development of the Norwegian medical profession presented here is a description of a medical historical project carried out in the Department of Medical History, Institute of General Practice and Community Health at the University of Oslo, Norway.

This work was planned as a parallel to another project, which aimed at compiling a complete encyclopaedia of biographies for all the slightly more than 21,500 physicians who are considered to have lived and worked in Norway from ancient times and up to now (Larsen Ø. ed., *Norges Leger I–V.* (The Physicians of Norway) Oslo: Den norske lægeforening, 1996), and information from this database of course has been an important source for the present study.

Initially, it had been decided to combine the collection of biographical data from the Norwegian physicians with a postal survey, using an overlapping questionnaire design, in order to obtain research material for this study of the profession. However, as a more comprehensive questionnaire study on doctors' living conditions already was under consideration in The Norwegian Medical Association, the two projects were coordinated. The questionnaire survey was arranged separately, and extended to a large-scale investigation named Legekårsundersøkelsen (the investigation on physicians' living and working conditions). Some results are mentioned in this book, especially in chapters 27 and 28, but for details the reader is referred to the original publications.

To write the history of a profession is a task which may be approached in different ways. What has been our objective here is to select topics which are general in nature, and which may be of interest to other professions and vocational groups, and to those outside the borders of Norway as well.

The preparation of this book has been an interesting and stimulating teamwork process. Many persons have contributed, not only those who were committed to write chapters of their own, but also many others who have engaged in lively discussions and exchanges of points of view.

As the editor and the person mostly responsible for the project, I am the one who has had the most rewarding time, and I want to express my sincere thanks to everyone, from young students to senior professors, for their eagerness and efforts.

But also colleagues outside our own

group have contributed with criticism and comments of extreme value. My thanks go to Professor John C. Burnham of the Ohio State University, Columbus, Ohio, for his encouragement and careful comments on most of the chapters of this book. Likewise, my thanks are due to Professor Jan Sundin from the University of Linköping, Sweden, for his constructive criticism. In December 1995 these two consultants and most of the authors gathered in Oslo for a seminar on the project. I do not need to describe in more detail how useful such days of intensive discussions can be.

A special thanks should be directed to Mr. Magne Nylenna MD, the editor of The Journal of the Norwegian Medical Association, for his comments on my manuscripts. His trained editor's eye instantly caught both unclear language and unclear argumentation.

In the spring of 1995, I had the opportunity to present some parts of the project in a guest lecture at the Free University of Berlin, Germany. The discussion afterwards left me with several good ideas which I hope have been a benefit to the result.

For those parts of the book which rely on original research work performed within the framework of the project, many persons have contributed with practical assistance. The staff at my home base, the Institute of General Practice and Community Medicine at the University of Oslo, Norway, should be mentioned for their willingness to assist, and not least for their patience with those of us who were engaged in the project. Among them, Mrs. Elin Olaug Rosvold MD, also active as a researcher in the project, has to be duly acknowledged for her most valuable assistance in the editorial work. Mrs. Anne Sofie Frøyshov Larsen MD sampled and surveyed the veterinarians for the comparisons presented in Chapter 26.2.

In addition to the other names appearing in the table of contents, I want to mention Mr. Bent Olav Olsen MA, who has been my associate editor, and has been in charge of the management of most of the numerous details inherent in a project like this, besides his participation as a researcher and an author. Likewise, Miss Naidi Engelskjøn MA contributed with research assistance in the work with other chapters than her own.

Mrs. Tran Thi Tuyet Hoa and Mr. Nguyen Doan Ba Phuc MD deserve a special thanks for their meticulous and timeconsuming preparation of huge amounts of material from one of our most important information sources: the annual reports submitted by the district physicians to the health authorities in the nineteenth century. Thanks also go to Mr. Jo Eidet and Miss Anita Sørheim for their research assistance.

Thanks are due to Mrs. Linda Grytten and to Mrs. Toula Aastorp for their translation of texts which were not initially prepared in English. In the final stages of the project, much of the polishing of the manuscripts relied on Mr. Are Martin Berntzen, Miss Irene Burazer, Mr. Annar Bøhn, Miss Eugenie E. Larson, Mr. Espen Evjenth Lindbäck, Miss Teresa Victoria Løvold, Miss Jorunn Pettersen, and Miss Camilla Wiig. The managing skills of Mr. Njål Engløk proved to be an indispensable asset to the project in its last, rather hectic phases.

My sincere thanks are also due to Mr. Neale Watson, president of Watson Publishing International. His enthusiastic engagement in the project, including two visits in Norway to clear up problems and give us advice, provided stimulating encouragement.

A grant from The Ella and Kaare Nygaard Foundation, St. Olaf College, Northfield, Minnesota, allowed me to visit the U.S. Mid-West in the winter of 1996, in order to collect information on the Norwegian emigrant physicians of Norse America. The staff at the archives of the Norwegian-American Historical Association in Northfield was very helpful to me during my stay, and so were colleagues at the Gundersen Clinic in La Crosse, Wisconsin. Also, at the Mayo Clinic in Rochester, Minnesota, and at the Westerheim Museum in Decorah, Iowa, I was met with the same warmth and enthusiasm.

The main financial burden of the project was carried by The Norwegian Medical Association. It goes without saying that the whole process could not have been carried through without the generosity of the Association. The Norwegian Medical Society contributed to the covering of the expenses of the 1995 coordinating seminar, and our thanks are due to the Board of the society.

At the end of a project like this one, I feel a little bit uncomfortable: A large number of collaborators have done a substantial amount of work, and have invested their time and efforts. But it is the responsibility of the project management, and of the editor, to ensure that a reasonably acceptable entity is the result. And for a large topic like the emergence of a profession, perhaps quite different aspects should have been covered? Or perhaps the aspects covered should have been looked upon from quite different angles?

Anyhow, by now it is too late to make any changes which could possibly alleviate such depressing thoughts. The book is presented to the readership in the hope that it will inspire or provoke further studies in profession history.

Oslo, November 1996,

Øivind Larsen

C H A P T E R 1

Introduction

ØIVIND LARSEN

1.1. An Intriguing History

Medical history contains many elements that may make you pause and reflect. One of them is the fact that the history of medicine as a science and the history of health services are very short, when a quantitative perspective is applied. Of course substantial scientific achievements had taken place through the centuries, but they did not have so many practical consequences. Even two hundred years ago, in the Age of Enlightenment, when culture and science flourished in European cities, and the United States of America had been settled as a new, modern world on the other side of the Atlantic, effective medical services that could be offered when needed were still scarce. The prevailing health conditions for the general population, even in the most developed regions, still were rather unchanged from the centuries before. And public concern about health, the thought of introducing medical considerations on a larger scale into the political setup of a state, was still a novelty.

Another point to consider is the widening of the scope and impact of medical work. The practice of medicine in cases of disease was primarily confined to a relationship between the patient and the doctor, and included only a few others. The extensive development within medicine in the two centuries to follow has also led to a situation where a professional action, for example the decision by a doctor to carry out a certain set of physical examinations or to implement a certain medical treatment, puts a large-scale system into motion: laboratory people, hospital staff, health insurance clerks, and so on. This complexity has evolved at an accelerating pace. However, it was not until the twentieth century that medicine really went public, with changes in the social attitudes of all parties that were involved following as an inevitable consequence.

With some outstanding exceptions, such as the dietary prevention of scurvy and the smallpox vaccination, only a few results from eighteenth-century medical science had a direct influence on the health conditions of the masses. Emerging social thinking, supported by the needs of a mercantilistic economy, had stimulated theoretical work in social medicine. Johann Peter Frank (1745–1821), the builder of social medical theory in the Austrian absolutistic empire, had launched an outline for a comprehensive health policy, but it was not implemented as a whole as he intended. It was only for specific minor groups that the new principles of public health and public responsibility could be put into force. And in a world where poverty was a main problem for large parts of the population, much would have to change before any significant impact by medicine could be expected.

But in the later half of the eighteenth century the health of the population emerged as a growing public concern. New statistics revealed the health conditions in more detail than before and rendered a better background for assessment of the demands (Imhof and Larsen 1975).

New training programs for health personnel, primarily for surgeons and physicians, were established. The surgeons had been craftsmen and had had only a little, if any, theoretical background. Some of them belonged to guilds that functioned like professional associations, but there were also people who presented themselves as oculists or bonesetters, often traveling around and offering their services. On the other hand, the academic physicians were few in number, and their proficiency had mainly a theoretical character. These traditional types of medical professionals were soon replaced, when a new sort of medical school was introduced at the end of the eighteenth century. The new surgical academies educated a new medical hybride: the academic physician who also had the practical skills of a surgeon. But even in spite of the new initiatives, little happened that could be measured in terms of reduced morbidity and mortality in the population.

There obviously also existed an attitude towards suffering and disease that was profoundly different, not only from those of the twentieth century, but also from the attitudes found only decades later. A fatalistic view, that primarily attributed disease and death to the inevitable evils of nature might have contributed to the fact that in most European countries health problems were not a main issue in politics at the beginning of the eighteenth century, even though the statistics at hand and new political situations in several countries should have provided opportunities to put health on the political agenda.

Therefore, in the 1990s, when health problems claim a lion's share of both public interest and public expenditures, one might reflect that the lesson taught by medical history is ambiguous: On the one hand, a long life, free of impairments, pains and complaints has been accepted as normal, and as a valid political objective of a modern society. Ethics, a new assessment of the value of the individual, and increasing standards for humanity have come to stay.

On the other hand, where are the limits, where does the responsibility of health care end? A cynical politician might be attracted by this way of thinking and draw other conclusions from reading medical history: In the eighteenth century, only a few generations ago, nations were prospering with an almost non-existent concern about health. Where is the lowest level of balance, what are the lowest acceptable levels for health and health services that the population must endure? Which constraints may be laid on the development of health care for financial reasons? In a developed country the answers to such questions might lead to considerable setbacks. And in lesser-favored countries with obvious demands, medical and social progress might be hampered and preference given to other fields.

Truly, medical history is an intriguing discipline, teaching progress and prospects, but also the consequences of choices.

1.2. The Medical Profession

Taking Norway as an example, a medical profession in the modern sense of the expression was almost non-existent at the beginning of the nineteenth century. Some one hundred persons could be counted as medical men. There were no women practicing medicine in a formal position at this time, but in folk medicine there were also women with healing skills who met the needs of the population for medical assistance. The number of one hundred depends somewhat on what the definition of a doctor is, and this group was in no way homogeneous.

To make a living as a doctor among people who generally were used to some sort of self-containing or barter economy was not easy, and the official posts as district medical officers, military surgeons, or doctors employed by the early industries, mainly mining enterprises, were few and scattered all over the country. No activity of a medical professional body can be traced at this stage.

At the end of the century, however, the situation had totally changed. By then, Norway had a strong and united staff of physicians numbering more than one thousand. With almost no exceptions all of them had attended the same medical school, the medical faculty at the Royal Frederiks University in the Norwegian capital then named Christiania (from 1877: Kristiania, from 1924: Oslo).

The Norwegian Medical Association, founded in 1886, had a considerable impact. From 1833 on The Norwegian Medical Society, an organization devoted to medical science and health policy, had exerted a substantial influence on the development of a modern health care system. With predecessors dating back to the 1820s, scientific medical periodicals gave their support to a national medicine.

During the course of the nineteenth century, freed from its linkage to Denmark in 1814, but in a looser union with Sweden until 1905, Norway underwent a thorough transformation in nearly all fields, including the stirring up of the population caused by the demographic transition. A series of new occupational groups appeared, the growing group of physicians being only one of them.

The physicians made up a group that had the features of a profession. Among these markers were relative autonomy in relation to others and also to the authorities. Furthermore, the physicians' group met the definition of a profession that implies that the individual members themselves should govern the continuous development and reformulation of the contents and objectives of their work.

Seen through the eyes of a medical historian, this process might be interpreted in two ways. One of them is rather harsh on the physicians: The members of the profession depicted and developed a demand for services that could be supplied by themselves. The medical profession was a new vocational group, clearing its way and assessing its place in the market. Reference to special ethical standards, exclusive for the profession, might be seen as a reinforcement of the autonomy. Physicians who hailed the Hippocratical heritage might be accused of promoting their own superiority in medical matters, defining their market in the open society and securing their hegemony in hospitals and institutions. Professionalism contains explicit elements of inclusiveness, but also has strong elements of exclusion, a fact that special relevance in Norway, where the population had a long tradition of relying on local knowledge, quacks, and folk medicine.

An opposite interpretation would be an altruistic one: Faced with the medical and social demands in a rapidly developing nation, young people trained in medicine to implement scientific knowledge and innovation to the benefit of the population, and to fight superstition, nihilism and negligence when health was at stake. We may also add the emerging and increasingly politically loaded moral obligation to fight misery and disease caused by social injustice and inequality.

The forces and motives creating a medical profession obviously are multiple, suspended between the extremes.

But where?

1.3. *The Process of Shaping*

The people who have constituted the Norwegian medical profession through the last two hundred years, together with some colleagues from earlier centuries, present themselves through the biographical data that are available (Larsen 1996). The biographies indicate social background, professional career, demographic behavior, and to a certain degree achievements in life.

The biographies sketch a socialization of the individuals into a professional pattern. But what is this pattern like? How do the norms and standards of a profession evolve? And to what extent is this process of delineation of a profession and the formation of a social role a national one, a process that can be described as specific for Norway? To what extent is the socialization of the new professional group influenced from abroad, and to what extent has it been actively tailored according to international models? In short, how was the Norwegian medical profession shaped?

A historical approach based on biographies can only render a partial picture of what has happened. Neither the condensed facts of a biographical encyclopedia nor the more narrative texts in interviews, autobiographies, or obituaries reveal in sufficient detail the reasons behind the thousands of personal decisions made during the life of every single member of the profession. But these single decisions, when added to each other and considered on the aggregated level, make up the behavior of the profession as such, and call for historical interest.

This point can be clarified by means of an example: The decision made by a doctor to move to an outskirt in the north of Norway may be interpreted in different ways. The decision might be a sign of a commitment to medicine and a devotion to a population in need of health services. However, the doctor may also have moved up north for more prosaic reasons: a post was available just there; economic prospects seemed tempting; there were family ties to just that district; a sense of adventure played its part – or the doctor simply looked forward to pursue his or her favorite pastimes: fishing and hunting.

The decision to move back again, for example, to the city where she or he graduated from medical school, and to take up a post in a hospital, may be regarded from outside as a move up or down the professional ladder. However, some factors that affect the decision only rarely appear on the surface. Perhaps the spouse could no longer stand the ever-ringing phone in the bedroom of the district physician's home. Or did the spouse want to take up an independent, personal professional career? Or was it that the physician had gotten tired of the lack of an accompanying person to share the medical duties? Perhaps the time had come to move to a place where relevant schools for the children were at hand.

Obituaries and life stories presented at festive occasions often emphasize the professional part. Reference is often made to the person's social commitment. But the real weight of the non-professional elements that influence a career is left to the judgment of the reader.

Circumstances regulating careers as well as private lives may also be sought inside the professional group and in the interface between profession and society. In the case of migration, specialization rules set up by the authorities, or – as in Norway – delegated to the professional association, gain in weight as history passes on. Invisible rules and unwritten practice may require some years of service in a faraway district for the candidate to be eligible for a more attractive post elsewhere in the country, or for an advancement, for example, in the public health services. At least in certain periods, economy may also be an important factor. When prospects for a good income as a district physician, or in a private practice, twinkle ahead, to spend some years in such activities just after graduation in order to pay back mortgages and settle the personal economy, may seem sensible and has to be judged separatly from the doctor's primary plans for a career.

And what were the shifts in attitudes towards the career in the course of time? We know that up to, say, World War II, the image of the Norwegian doctor, in the doctor's own eyes, and in the eyes of the population as well, was the role of the doctor in primary care: the private practitioner or the district physician. For a long time, a career aiming at a practice in primary or specialist care as the ending point was a wide-spread pattern. After the war, the situation changed. In somewhat oversimplified terms, one might say that the situation was turned upside down: For many physicians the period in primary practice became a prelude to hospital or academic life.

And in what periods did achievement of prosperity outweigh professional success?

1.4. The History of the Profession

In Norway, the development of the medical profession has been touched on by several authors. A rather penetrating review of the early years of a national medicine was given by Laache in 1911 in connection with the one hundreth anniversary of the Royal Frederiks University in Kristiania (Laache 1911). When the time had arrived for a comprehensive compilation of a medical history of Norway, Reichborn-Kjennerud, Grøn and Kobro described the development with joint efforts, based on different types of research and seen from different angles in 1936 (Reichborn-Kjennerud et al. 1936). In the same year the first fifty years of existence of the Norwegian Medical Association was reviewed (Berner 1936). More recently interest in professions as such has increased, and in Norway classical works were published by Lindbekk (1967) and (Torgersen 1972). Here, the medical profession is discussed within a theoretical framework.

Are explanatory factors for the development of the medical profession to be found by looking at the situation of morbidity and mortality patterns in the different parts of the country? And, pertaining to the society in general, perhaps geographical differences and changes over time might also be revealed in the perception of disease, in the psychological and emotional bases for the emergence of demands. Our own inquiry into the period 1868 to 1900 (Larsen et al. 1980, Larsen 1991) concentrated on a time that was the heyday of urbanization, internal migration, and societal change in Norway. The society at that time was at the height of the process of demographic transition.

Infectious diseases constituted the dominant part of the health problems. We therefore found this threat to health suitable as an indicator for morbidity – and for the perception of morbidity by the different parties afflicted. The available source material of local medical reports contained statistical and narrative information from different levels in the public health system. As could be expected, morbidity and mortality increased with the degree of urbanization and demographical unrest.

More interesting, however, was the finding of a gradient in the perception of disease. Being sure to exercise due caution in making the interpretation, there seemed to be a higher degree of acceptance for disease in the urban regions than in the countryside in the last decades of the nineteenth century; a shift in this tendency was at first observed around 1890. Obviously the perception of disease as a cost of social progress waned at this point. This finding indicates an increasing demand for health services and doctors, but nevertheless does not prove anything pertaining to the development of the medical profession. Later chapters in this book supplement the 1980 study and describe in more detail the tasks and the working conditions that met the district physicians in this period.

Another approach follows the lines of reasoning introduced by McKeown (1976) in his book The Modern Rise of Population. Here, economy is placed in the forefront. The development of social welfare is given priority in the interpretation of the changing morbidity and mortality patterns, and of the development of medicine and health care as well. These and other hypotheses and theories were discussed by the historian Fritz Hodne in our project of 1983–1986 (Larsen, Berg, Hodne 1986), which was set up by the Norwegian Medical Association in connection with its one hundreth anniversary in 1986.

The financial funding for a national health system and for the activities of a medical profession within its framework developed continuously from a very low level at the beginning of the nineteenth century to such a high level in the later half of the twentieth century that brakes had to be put on, and constraints applied. Within this setting, a discussion of the theory of supplier-induced demand in the health care system is highly relevant, and may add important clues to the understanding of the forces forming the medical profession (Vallgårda 1989).

Also in Norway the increased interest in the concept of welfare and the historical process towards a welfare state has stimulated activity in various research groups (Seip 1994a, 1994b, Falkum and Larsen 1981).

The political scientist Ole Berg, however, as part of the anniversary project of 1986, studied the life and function of the physicians' professional body, the Norwegian Medical Association, as an organization. From its foundation in 1886, this association rapidly developed into a stronghold for a unified medical profession. Throughout its existence, nearly all Norwegian doctors have enrolled as members of the association, and the association has exerted a strong discipline within its ranks. This supremacy has been underscored and reinforced by the authorities, who have delegated to the association such privileges as issuing specialist certificates and setting up programs for postgraduate training in order to develop, maintain, and update the base of knowledge of the members of the profession.

In itself, the role of the association is an interesting phenomenon calling for thorough scientific scrutinization, both from the viewpoint of strategy and leadership, but also as seen from the perspective of the individual members of the profession. Their obvious need for joining a strong community is striking – and their acceptance of its dominance as well. The study by Berg confirms that the Norwegian Medical Association has been, and still is, instrumental for the development of the medical profession as a group and for the attitudes of society towards it. But the socialization of individuals into a professional role takes place prior to entering the fellowship of colleagues; it occurs when they are students, but also even before that, when they are deciding to enter medicine. The third aspect covered by the 1986 study, in addition to presenting a chronological history of the Norwegian physicians, was based on an examination of expectations and experiences in a sample of the medical profession. Certain differences and developmental lines over time were observed, which in themselves were interesting. But one question remained to be answered: To what extent were some of the trends universal, and also part of the effect of time in other types of occupations, for example the variations in devotion to work compared to giving priority to leisure and other activities (Larsen et al. 1986)?

The establishing of a national medicine on the academic level, of course took place under the auspices of the universities. The medical faculty in Oslo, which by far is the oldest one in Norway, celebrated its 175th year of existence in 1989 (Larsen 1990). One of the prominent traits that emerged from an overview of the activities of the faculty was the fact that strong personalities and outstanding scientists achieved a substantial influence, even beyond their own discipline, not only in times when the faculty was only a small circle of colleagues, but also later on, when the faculty had multiplied its size and complexity.

The importance of scientifically outstanding research groups for the development of a reputation is also remarkable at the other universities, for example, in Bergen (Universitetet i Bergens historie 1996) and in Tromsø (Fulsås 1993).

Public opinion about the historical development of the medical profession has not been heard in a sufficient way in regard to the present time. Firsthand knowledge, of course, cannot be obtained from the generations that have passed away. That is a weakness, if one aims at obtaining a comprehensive view on how the corps of physicians found its form, or was given its form through tasks and expectations. However, some indirect information is at hand, thanks to the more general historical descriptions of medicine in society. This does in no way preclude the need for modern studies of the negative attitudes towards physicians and the practical consequences of such more general trends in public opinion.

No doubt that opposition and negative attitudes towards doctors in general in certain periods have been factors of practical importance for the physicians and for the profession as such, independent of what reasons were hidden behind the sentiments.

The nature of health care is probably responsible for at least a part of the resentment that sometimes comes to surface. The paternalistic elements of a physician's work may be questioned, even when unjustified, simply because society has changed. In addition to, say, the antiauthoritarian traits of the 1970s and the years that followed, it might be assumed that a general rejection of ill-health and disease – now more than before perceived as a right and a matter of course – selected physicians as its main target. The increasing volume and complexity of the health care system – which, among other things, includes a growing number of separate professional groups pursuing their own interests – of course has an inherent potential for strain. And so also has the substantial financial aspects of a modern health care system in a society where local democracy has become a main management principle and where, for example, the gate-keeping functions of the physicians do not necessarily automatically fit in anymore.

In 1976 professor Peter F. Hjort (1924 –) became leader of a new research group which was established at the National Institute of Public Health in Oslo. The objective of the group was to study the function of the Norwegian health care system, its services to the individual and to society, its use of resources, and its quality. From 1978 onwards a series of reports has been published. As central decision makers in the health care system, the physicians now experienced a new public interest in their work. Medicine was put into a framework of economy and sociology that was new, could be perceived as strange, and felt as a threat to old values.

When behavioral sciences in medicine were introduced as an academic discipline in the 1970s, a new focus was set on the physician-patient relationship, a topic which also deserves historical research.

The approach chosen for this volume, however, has been to look at the development of the medical profession through the eyes of those involved in it: inside, outside, or at the rim of the profession. This explains why the volume is given the format of an anthology.

It is impossible to cover all angles of interest within one single volume. Therefore a selection of topics has been carried out. The emphasis has been steered towards certain core themes, which have been chosen for the following reasons: Although mathematicians probably will object to the assumption, in profession history the difference between zero and one is larger and more interesting than the difference between one and two. In the two hundred years that have elapsed in the modern development of the Norwegian medical profession, the first century contains the period when the profession evolved from being practically non-existent and without a clear definition to achieving a status in line with professional standards abroad. It was as though Norwegian physicians had dressed in an invisible uniform. The next century is more of a period of growth and adjustment. The shaping of the profession primarily takes place in the nineteenth century. This fact makes it sensible to pay special attention to what happened in those remote, but historically recent years – the first one out of two interesting centuries.

The shaping of the profession consists of several elements. Some of them seem more important than others, and some have been discussed previously in literature and in our own studies. It has also been our policy not to repeat findings and discussions that we have presented before, unless there are special reasons, or because it is necessary to link chapters together and to give a balanced basis for discussion.

In this volume, the diffusion of knowledge has been intentionally highlighted. How were the new national medicine and the new national health services influenced from abroad, through medical training of students, study travels by Norwegian physicians, books, periodicals?

The different entries call for a general interpretation, and this discussion preferably should pursue the lines of some hypothesis, which the reader should have in mind when reading the chapters. Therefore, the following framework is suggested for the considerations presented in the text.

1.5. Images and Objectives

In our 1986 study (Larsen et al. 1986) we argued that the role of the physician might be divided into three parts. The first part of the physician's role is to be the life saver, the man or woman with skills and competence to save you when life is at stake. The second part of the role is to be the caring supporter, mothering you and giving you the comfort you need during the hardship of disease. The third part of the role is to be the gate-keeper. The physician has the authority to give access to public support and public money, or speaking more generally in sociological terms: to legitimate the sick role of the patient so that the practical consequences of this new role setting can be implemented.

A hypothesis to be further verified is that the attitudes unfavorable to the physicians are dependent on how these three role parts are perceived by the public and by the professionals themselves. The development over time should be discussed according to this.

However, this model will profit from being somewhat refined: The roles of the physician, as mentioned above, are mainly based on attitudes held by the outside world. They are *images* of the doctor that have been culturally determined. The socialization into the role of a doctor is primarily a question of acceptance of expectations, and success will depend on how well the physician can live up to them. Another hypothesis is that the variations in expectations constitute one of the most important denominators for the development of the medical profession.

This, however, needs a supplement. The profession as a body defends some ideological principles, partly worded in codes of ethics, but also settled in common attitudes, of course underlying historical variations. The professional *objectives* may be sorted into a list with different practical consequences for the members of the group:

1. Serve the sick. This objective is central to all considerations about what a physician should do, and is morally rooted and legitimated. In periods and situations when this objective has priority, the patient-doctor relationship is the most important issue.

2. Serve the society. This was the objective of the district physicians and medical officers of the past. At the time when strong personalities from the medical corps established the Norwegian public health system, this objective was their dominating and leading star. Medical knowledge was to be implemented through active shaping of the society and by means of health administration. In periods of a medical policy of this kind, ideas of public health, health education, preventive measures, and community medicine may experience a flourishing time.

3. Serve the science. The medical professionals of the nineteenth century who spared no costs and efforts to learn more; the many physicians of the twentieth century who collected material for research in addition to their hospital work, and wrote their dissertations in late evenings and nights, often sacrificing both spouses and personal economy, fulfilled one of the basic requirements of the definition of a profession: to take an active part in the development and reformulation of the basis of knowledge behind their work. A general interest in research by the profession as such will contribute to scientific progress and strengthen the esteem of medicine in general.

4. Serve yourself. In most societies it is legitimate to strive for personal success. Success may be sought for its own sake – and it may be showed off, for example, by conspicuous consumption, as discussed by the Norse-American sociologist Thorstein Veblen in his famous book *The Theory of the Leisure Class* (Veblen 1899). It is a socially accepted behavior to educate oneself to enter a professional career that gives returns according to preferences and expectations: material possessions, living standards, and so on. It lies within the codes of behavior in any modern society to chose your career from among those available and to pursue it on the basis of such considerations. But in that perspective medicine is only one of several possible paths to the goal. Likewise, under such circumstances your choice of activity within medicine will have other motives than if you have some of the previously mentioned objectives in mind. Historical variations will obviously occur as to the importance of this type of objective, weighed against the others, but also as to what kind of reward is the most attractive at the time in question: money, esteem, gratitude, power, and so on.

Images and objectives do not necessarily develop identically within the different branches of medicine. Patient orientation, public responsibility, scientific commitment, and the interest in pursuing personal goals vary.

The professionalization within the profession is also an interesting topic. To the leaders of the profession as a whole in Norway, the Norwegian Medical Association it is a constant challenge to harmonize and coordinate the interests of its subgroups.

The setup for a general discussion of the shaping of the medical profession in Norway could be a framework which is indeed a framework: A grid where the three images and the four objectives make up the boxes that have to be considered in time and space.

The images pass over steps of history

where the pursuit of personal objectives is severely hampered. Some examples: To become wealthy through medicine is not easy when the prevalent role for the physician is as a gate-keeper civil servant, paid and esteemed by the authorities according to how this function is performed. Alternatively, to acquire scientific credit is not easy when the caring function is the only one that is expected from you by your employer, the hospital owner.

But, on the other hand, the further development of a strong and united profession, maintaining its difference from other vocational groups, is hardly possible in a society where the physicians mainly are found as ordinary employees in the civil services, with caring for individual patients as the strongest of their internalized reasons for being doctors.

These considerations serve as an approach to an underlying, general hypothesis which perhaps could be verified, rejected, or at least illuminated by means of a look at the history: The professionalization of the physicians, in spite of attacks and criticisms launched against it from time to time, may be regarded as an important element in meeting the external expectations about the role of the physician. Professionalization may simply be seen as a tool to do the job.

Norway is a country in a quite special situation, because the source material at hand makes the medical profession and its individual members over the years rather readily surveyable. If the history of the profession should support the hypothesis that professionalization has a practical value of its own, this might have a significant bearing on the time to follow. On the contrary, if there are clues that professionalization has hampered the integration of the physicians into a comprehensive health care system, other conclusions have to be drawn. And if the historical findings are inconclusive, there is a definite need for more research.

Curiosity and concerns about the social role of the professionalization of physicians were the reasons for writing this book, and also for naming it *The Shaping of a Profession.*

References

Berner, J. *Den norske lægeforening 1886–1936.* Oslo: Centraltrykkeriet, 1936.

Falkum, E., and Ø Larsen. *Helseomsorgens vilkår.* Oslo: Universitetsforlaget, 1981.

Fulsås, N. *Universitetet i Tromsø 25 år.* Tromsø: Universitetet i Tromsø, 1993.

Imhof, A.E., and Ø Larsen. *Sozialgeschicte und Medizin.* Oslo/Stuttgart: Universitetsforlaget/Fischer, 1975.

Laache, S.B. *Norsk medicin i hundrede aar.* Kristiania: Steenske bogtrykkeri, 1911.

Larsen, Ø, O. Berg, and F. Hodne. *Legene og samfunnet.* Oslo: Den norske lægeforening, 1986.

Larsen, Ø, ed. *Norges Leger I–V.* Oslo: Den norske lægeforening, 1996.

Larsen, Ø, H. Haugtomt, and W. Platou. *Sykdomsoppfatning og epidemiologi 1860-1900.* Oslo: Seksjon for medisinsk historie, Universitetet i Oslo, 1980.

Larsen, Ø *Mangfoldig medisin.* Oslo: Det medisinske fakultet, Universitetet i Oslo, 1989, 2. ed., 1990.

Larsen, Ø "Vekst i byen og helse på landet – noen trekk ved folkehelse og befolkningsutvikling på slutten av 1800-tallet." Jord og gjerning 5(1991):66–78.

Lindbekk, T. *Mobilitets- og stillingsstrukturer innenfor tre akademiske profesjoner 1910–63.* Oslo: Universitetsforlaget, 1967.

McKeown, T. *The modern rise of population.* London: Arnold, 1976.

Reichborn-Kjennerud, I., E. Grøn, and I. Kobro. *Medisinens historie i Norge.* Oslo: Grøndahl, 1936.

Seip, A.L. *Sosialhjelpstaten blir til. Norsk Sosialpolitikk 1740–1920.* Oslo: Gyldendal, 1984, 2. ed., 1994a.

Seip, A.L. *Veiene til velferdsstaten. Norsk*

Sosialpolitikk 1920–75. Oslo: Gyldendal, 1994b.

Torgersen, U. *Profesjonssosiologi.* Oslo/Bergen/ Tromsø: Universitetsforlaget, 1972.

Universitetet i Bergens historie I–II. Bergen: Universitetet i Bergen, 1996.

Vallgårda, S. "The increased obstetric activity: a new meaning to induced labour?" *Journal of Epidemiology and Community Health 43(*1989):48–52.

Veblen, T. The Theory of the Leisure Class (1899). London: Unwin, 1970.

CHAPTER 2

What Is Norway Like?

ØIVIND LARSEN

2.1. Geography and Population

Foreign readers who are unfamiliar with the country of Norway and its population, perhaps would want some reference made to information on what the country is like, in order to be able to set the development of its medical profession within a proper context.

But native-born Norwegians may also feel a need from time to time to reflect on how nature and society make up the stage for the activities of its inhabitants, and so also for the medical profession. Sociologists and historians discuss similarities and differences in the development, but often conclusions that at first glance may seem to be of theoretical importance in the real world were based on trivialities only known to those acquainted with the local conditions.

Literature on Norwegian conditions is readily available. One example that can be recommended is the yearly updated series of Statistical Yearbooks published by the Central Bureau of Statistics. There is also a series named Historical Statistics, which is published at intervals and in which the development over time is reviewed. Norway has a well-earned reputation for its national statistics. An early example of advanced statistical methodology was a punch card technique introduced for making calculations during the census of 1900. The Norwegian Cancer Registry, established in 1952, and the Medical Birth Registry (1967) serve as examples of important source material for medical studies. A number of health surveys from Norway have been presented in the medical literature; most of these studies were performed since the 1960s, but even earlier studies are also available (Natvig & Thiis-Evensen sen. 1983). The central population register from 1964 and a system for household surveys from 1966 are other examples of why the Norwegian population is rather translucent to the researcher.

For a contemporary account of the land and the society in the nineteenth century, a period of special interest in connection with the shaping of the Norwegian medical profession, our readers are referred to a report that was written in French and published in connection with the Universal Fair in Paris in 1878 (Broch 1878). Here, a condensed but comprehensive survey of the nation and its activities is presented to the public. As examples of sources for the general history of Norway, foreign readers are referred to the books in English by T.K. Derry (e.g., 1968) and the review of the economic history of Norway by F. Hodne (1975). Norway as an arena for a modern health care system has

DIAGRAM 2.1.
This map of Norway illustrates the country and its counties. The old names of the counties are shown in table 2.1

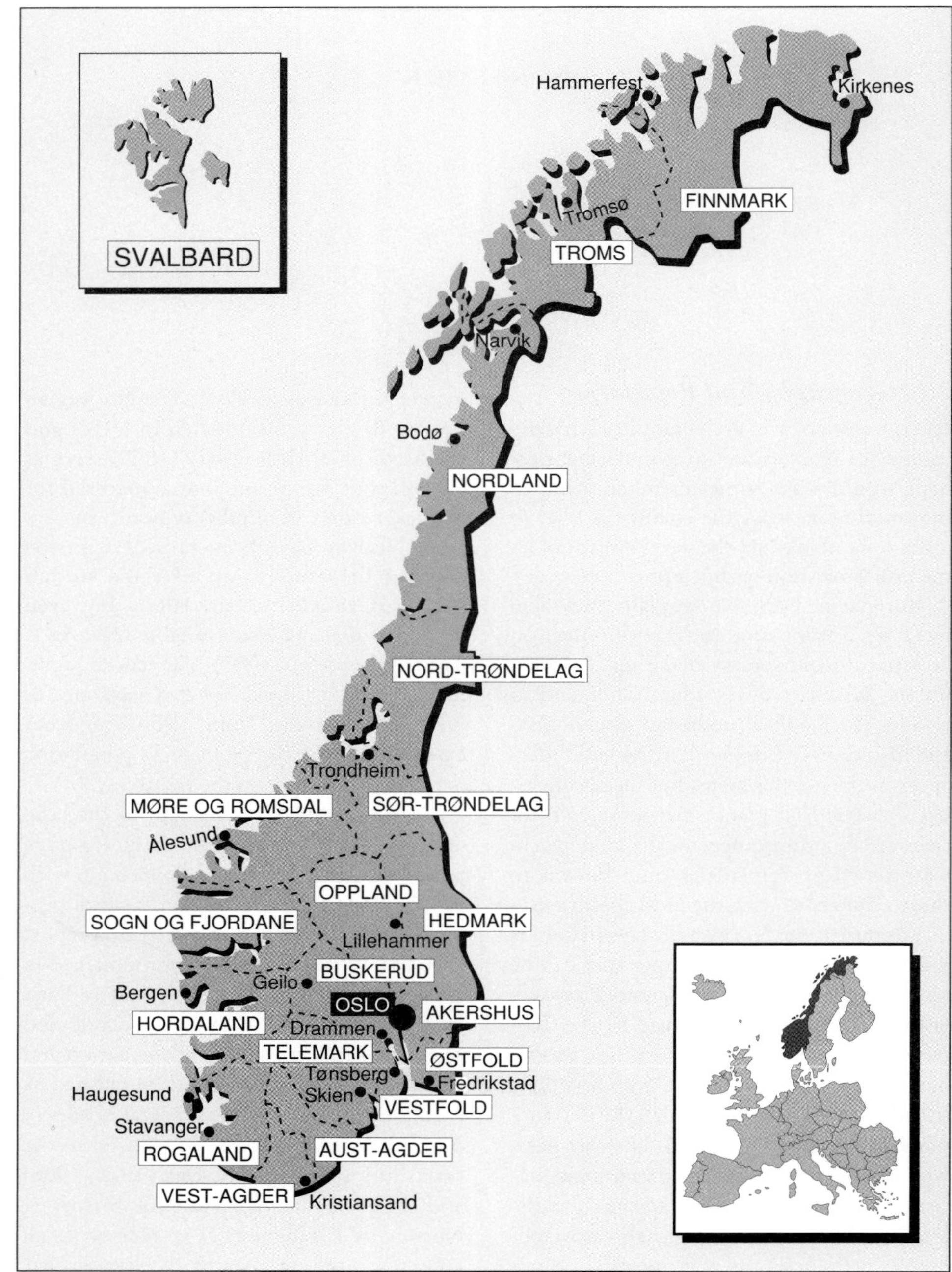

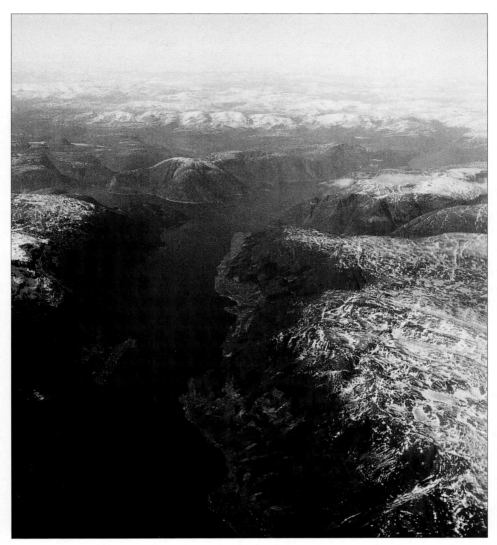

Figure 1: The fiords of Norway usually have room for settlements at the shores. When roads were more scarce, traffic across the fiord was more convenient than along the shores or across mountains or through dense forests. Therefore, many municipalities, as well as the districts of the physicians, were distributed on both sides of a fiord. This pattern has changed in modern times, but it is one of the explanations why formely so many of the district physicians had to use a boat in their house calls (Sørfjorden, Hardanger. Photo: Øivind Larsen 1996).

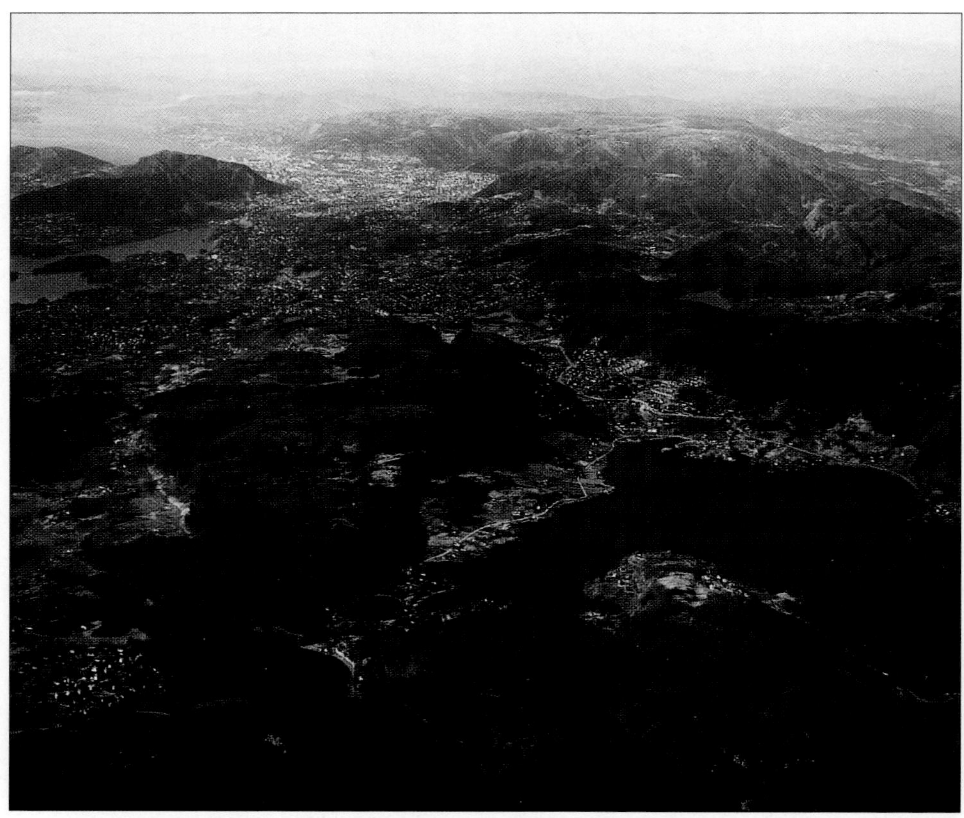

Figure 2: The coastal districts of Western and Northern Norway are well suited for variation in industry, occupations and settlement (Hordaland, from the south towards the city of Bergen. Photo:Øivind Larsen 1996).

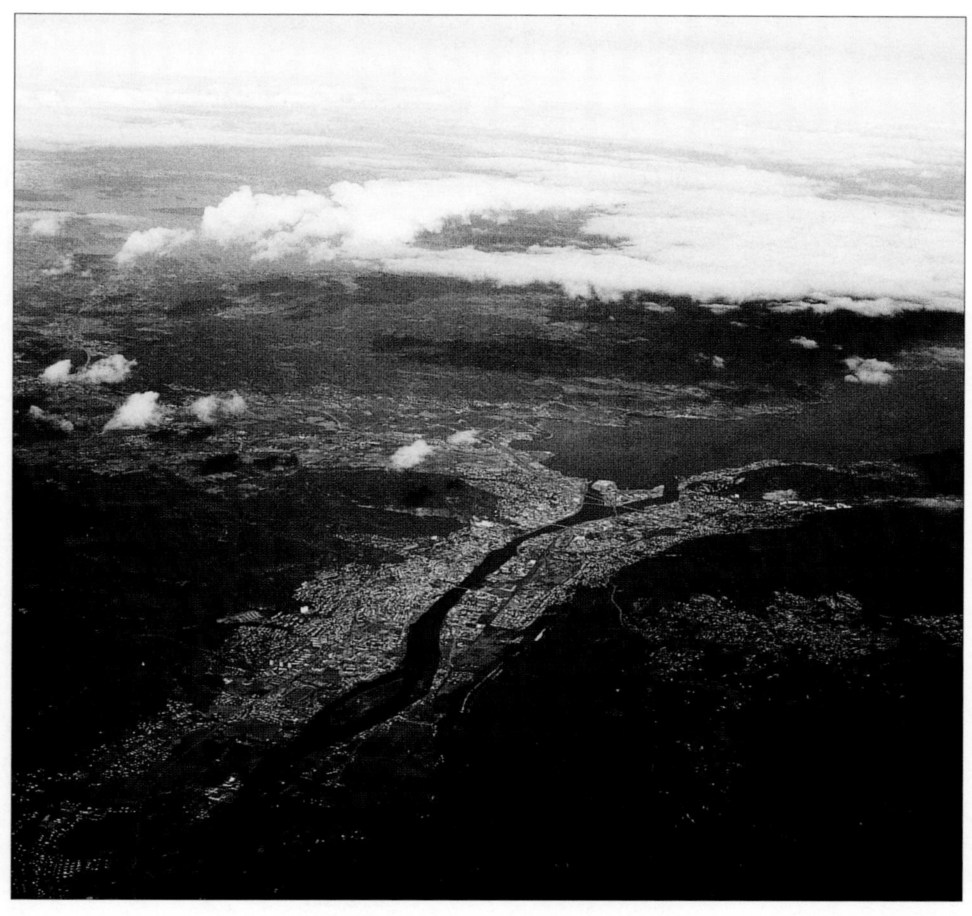

Figure 3: The outlets of the big rivers often gave rise to industry and commerce (Drammen, Eastern Norway. Photo:Øivind Larsen 1996).

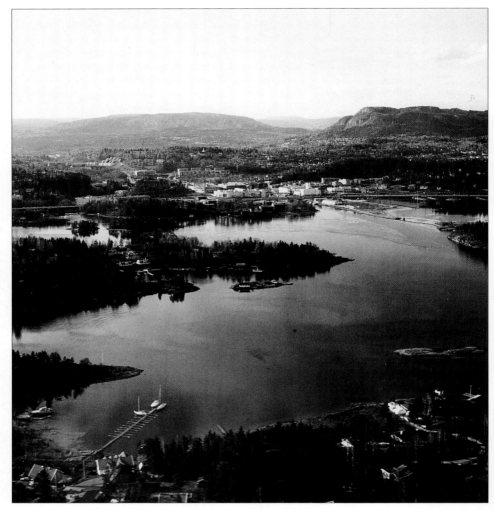

Figure 4: Even the urban settlement around Oslo is dominated by sea, lakes, and forests (Sandvika. Photo: Øivind Larsen 1996).

been surveyed by Nylenna in 1995. And for a general overview of Norway as part of the international community, the comparative statistics, as published in the World Data series of *Encyclopaedia Britannica*, are a useful tool.

By many foreigners, Norway has been labeled the land of the midnight sun, one of its several stereotypes. Situated at the top of Europe (Diagram 2.1), half of its elongated mainland stretches beyond the Arctic Circle and leaves the inhabitants there with dark winters and the special around-the-clock light of the Nordic summers, which attracts scores of tourists from all over the world.

Foreigners are often impressed by the distances in Norway, at least as compared to other countries in Western Europe; a journey from the south to the northernmost parts may be equal to taking a trip southward to the Mediterranean region.

In spite of the latitude, the climate is reasonably favorable in most of the 323,752 square kilometers that make up the Norwegian mainland. Mountains, more or less deserted plains, forests, mires, and lakes often make the view from the window of your domestic flight airliner rather astonishing, and you may ask: Where are the 4,381,441 (Figures from The Central Bureau of Statistics 1 July 1996) inhabitants who were supposed to live here in 1996 to be found? And where are the 15,368 physicians (1996)? The answer lies in the skewed distribution: More than 700,000 of the Norwegians are living in the urban agglomeration which is composed of the capital of Oslo in the south and its surroundings.

In the southeastern parts of the country, you find a friendly landscape with farmland and townships, separated by rolling hills with forests. Long valleys with settlements in the bottom and on the slopes cut into the more mountainous areas to the north and west.

Across the mountains with their peaks and glaciers, steep-sided fjords break up the coastline, mostly leaving space for people to settle along the shores or in the short valleys inside. Islands and a landscape with lower hills are found nearer to the ocean, where farmland, townships, fishing villages, and cities alternate with one another along the coast.

The urban settlements in Norway all have less than 60,000 inhabitants, except for the capital of Oslo and the cities of Bergen, Trondheim, and Stavanger, whose populations are in the range of 200,000 to 100,000.

Norway is subdivided into 19 counties; three of them have less than 100,000 inhabitants (Aust-Agder, Sogn og Fjordane, Finnmark) (Table 2.1). Somewhat less than 10 percent of the Norwegians live in Northern Norway, which contains the three northernmost counties. These counties cover more than half the length of mainland Norway. The combination of a sparsely populated countryside with an active policy to preserve the old pattern of a dispersed settlement of people leaves the health services with special challenges.

Cultural and commercial centers are distributed all over Norway. In addition to the Oslo region, Bergen and its surroundings in the west, Trondheim in the middle, and Tromsø in the north play important roles. For example, all these cities have their own universities and, from the point of view of this book, it is of interest that all of them also have medical schools. Stavanger in the southwest is the largest base for the Norwegian oil industry, which is of crucial importance to the general economy.

Politically, Norway is an independent kingdom governed according to democratic principles. However, the traditions of sovereignity have not existed as long as many Norwegians like to think. Even long before the Union Treaty with Denmark in 1450, Norway was under foreign rule; after 1814

TABLE 2.1. *Population density in The Norwegian counties. From Statistical Yearbook 1995.*

Counties	Old names	Population 1994	Sq.km	Pop.density per sq. km
Østfold	Smaalenenes amt	239,371	4,183	61.5
Akershus	Akershus amt	434,544	4,917	94.7
Oslo	Christiania by	482,555	454	1,130.1
Hedmark	Hedemarkens amt	186,657	27,388	7.1
Oppland	Christians amt	183,194	25,174	7.6
Buskerud	Buskeruds amt	228,506	14,927	16.5
Vestfold	Jarlsberg og Laurviks amt	203,231	2,216	95.0
Telemark	Bratsbergs amt	163,143	15,315	11.5
Aust-Agder	Nedenæs amt	99,585	9,212	11.7
Vest-Agder	Lister og Mandals amt	149,563	7,281	21.9
Rogaland	Stavanger amt	354,418	9,141	41.4
Hordaland	Søndre Bergenhus amt	422,581	15,634	28.2
Sogn og Fjordane	Nordre Bergenhus amt	107,612	18,634	6.0
Møre og Romsdal	Romsdals amt	240,215	15,104	16.5
Sør-Trøndelag	Søndre Trondhjems amt	256,266	18,831	14.4
Nord-Trøndelag	Nordre Trondhjems amt	127,560	22,396	6.1
Nordland	Nordlands amt	241,420	38,327	6.7
Troms	Tromsø amt	150,606	25,981	6.0
Finnmark	Finmarkens amt	76,668	48,637	1.7
Total mainland Norway		4,347,695	323,752	14.2

Bergen is included in Hordaland from 1972

there existed a so-called personal union with Sweden until 1905. Norway's independence was violated when the country was occupied by the Germans from 1940 until 1945. Proposals by the government to enter the European Union were rejected by the population in referendums held in 1972 and 1994.

2.2. Diversity and Equality

Since the time of King Olav (995-1030) (later named Saint Olav) at the beginning of the eleventh century, Christianity has been the religion of Norway, and since the Church Reformation in 1536 Protestantism has been the official religion. Medieval stone churches and the special Norwegian stave churches from the same time are still found in most of the country, along with large churches such as the medieval cathedrals of Stavanger and Trondheim.

The engagement in religious activities has been somewhat different in the various parts of the country, resulting in some geographical variations in attitudes and life style. In some districts lay religious communities also have had a dominant influence. However, these differences seem to be rapidly diminishing.

For a long time, great distances and relative isolation often led to distinctive differences between settlements and districts of the country, with a great variation in dialects and in cultural features. However, the small group of lapps, mostly situated in Finnmark, the northernmost county, is a separate ethnic group. The cultural differences are diminishing. A considerable factor in this respect has been the introduction of a national television, which gradually took place beginning in the 1960s.

Norway is divided into municipalities; in 1988 there were 448 of them, in 1996 there are 435. The number of municipalities was even higher in earlier times (746 in 1930), but since then the number has been reduced for practical reasons. Joining together of municipalities very often causes strong local resistance when imposed by the central authorities; the deeply rooted sense of independence and local democracy is felt to be violated. On the other hand, the city of Oslo has been subdivided into municipality-like parts that have a certain autonomy. This illustrates how Norway after all nurses its long traditions for decentralization and local administration.

Local democracy has a high standing in Norway, and the rate of participation as well as commitment and concern in upcoming matters is usually high among the population. This is an important feature to have in mind when interpreting Norwegian politics, and this fact also has considerable interest when looking at the history of the health services. The country was divided into health districts which, at least in the twentieth century, often were almost identical with the municipalities. The sanitation boards, chaired by district physicians, were manned by local politicians and administrators. This linked health and politics closely together, but as a rule left the doctor with the upper hand in medical matters. Beginning in 1984, new legislation made purely political influence on health matters more important, and changed the role and position of the local district physician.

From ancient times, social differences between the layers of the population in Norway have been less important than in other European societies. Especially in the eastern parts of Norway, there formerly were obvious class differences between farm owners and cottagers, and between the forest owners and their workers, but the typical inhabitant of rural Norway was the free farmer, who as a rule had a self-supporting activity based on agriculture, forestry, fishing and hunting. The emerging industry and service trades had to develop on this basis. Nobility or other individuals or institutions who controlled larger shares of capital and resources never had the same importance for the society in Norway as even in the neighboring Nordic countries.

Especially in the years after the Second World War, the social democratic ideology of equality attained a strong position in Norway. That means that the population has a rather even distribution of wealth – and, at least at the present stage of Norwegian history, there is a fairly good and evenly distributed standard of living, compared to other parts of the world, and even to the other affluent European countries. Unemployment is low (1994: 5.4%), and female participation in the workforce is high (1987: 63.7%, 1991: 62.3%).

The special sense of social equality in Norway is important when studying a profession, as it makes up a part of the framework and setting for the development. In large parts of rural Norway of the nineteenth century, a sort of protestant puritanism was a widespread virtue, and many of the traditions of austerity and rejection of conspicuous behavior have persisted, albeit on a higher level. In combination with the newer social democratic political thinking, this has led up to a general internalization of strong feelings for social justice, where equality is an important element.

A consequence is a relatively broad political agreement on supporting the weaker groups through wage policy and social measures. But on the other hand, a certain general skepticism toward those too far above the average living standard is a matter of reality in Norway, a fact which clearly appears, for example, in the taxation system. To a profession such as that of the physicians, this means that success, esteem, and authority mostly have to rely on other personal characteristics and skills than those that are achieved by means of personal wealth.

In all municipalities there is a community center, often a tiny township, but its importance on a local and national level as a rule is far larger than its numbers of inhabitants whould indicate.

Infrastructure in modern times is mostly good. Since the 1960s air travel has become the normal way of commuting over long distances, of which there are several. Formerly, sea transportation had a larger share of the traffic than today. Nowadays an efficient network of highways link the municipalities and the counties together. In the south the railway system has been in existence more than 140 years, and in the north heavily loaded ore transportation trains roll across the border from neighboring Sweden to the ice-free harbor of Narvik.

DIAGRAM 2.2
Gross domestic product by kind of activity. 1930, 1960, and 1990. Percentages. (From Historical Statistics 1994)

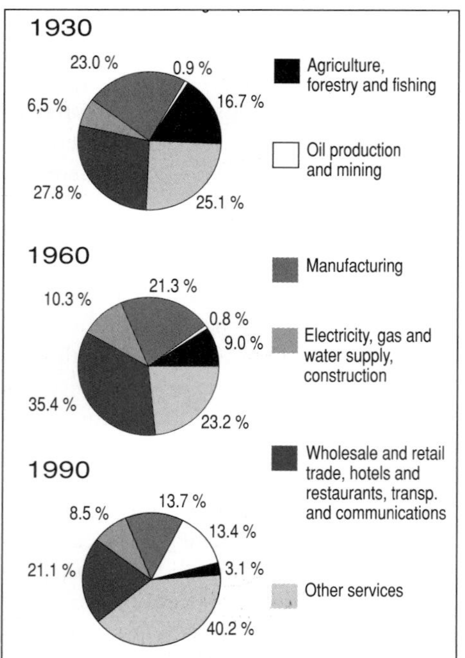

For many years after the Second World War, automobiles could not be bought freely for reasons of national finance. Not until the early 1960s did a modern traffic pattern develop, in which road traffic is very important.

The decentralized settlement of Norway has been aided by the government. Industry has been subsidized in remote parts to keep society running there for political and strategic reasons; the coal mining at the arctic islands of Svalbard is a good example. But other activities have been stimulated, too: the University of Tromsø, established in 1968, has shown itself to be instrumental for the development of the region. So also has military activity, which has kept many a small municipality going.

The importance of the health care system for the economy and the employment situation in the municipalities must also be emphasized, not only because it takes care of the population, but also because health centers, institutions, and hospitals are important employers, not least for the female segment of the inhabitants.

Oil from the North Sea and electricity from the water plants contribute substantially toward making Norway competitive in the international market, both in terms of direct exportation and through its own energy-based industry and other activities (Diagram 2.2). The traditional shipping industry, as well as the fisheries, are still important ways of earning income.

2.3. Norway, Health, and Medicine

Health conditions in the 1990s, as mea-

TABLE 2.2
Vital statistics Norway.

	Average	World Average
Birth rate per 1,000 population (1993) (legitimate 55.6 %; illegitimate 44.4%)	13.8	25.0
Death rate per 1,000 population (1993)	10.9	9.3
Natural increase rate per 1,000 population (1993)	2.9	15.7
Total fertility rate (avg. births per childbearing woman; 1994)	1.9	
Marriage rate per 1,000 population (1993)	4.5	
Divorce rate per 1,000 population (1993)	2.5	
Life expectancy at birth (1993):	male 74.2 years female 80.3 years	
Major causes of death per 100,000 population (1992):	ischemic heart disease 242.6 malignant neoplasms (cancers) 224.5 cerebrovascular disease 126.1	

From: *Britannica Book of the Year 1996,* Encyclopœdia Britannica Inc. 1996

DIAGRAM 2.3
Public and private health expenditures as percentages of gross domestic product (GDP) in 1991 in selected countries, according to Organization for Economic Cooperation and Development data. (From Nylenna 1995.)

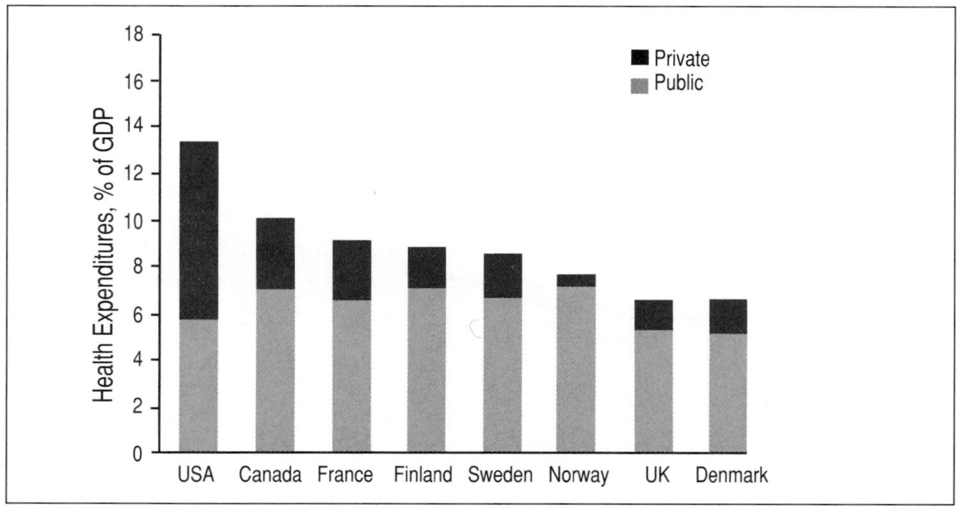

DIAGRAM 2.4.
Physicians and nurses 1950–1985. (From Historical Statistics 1994)

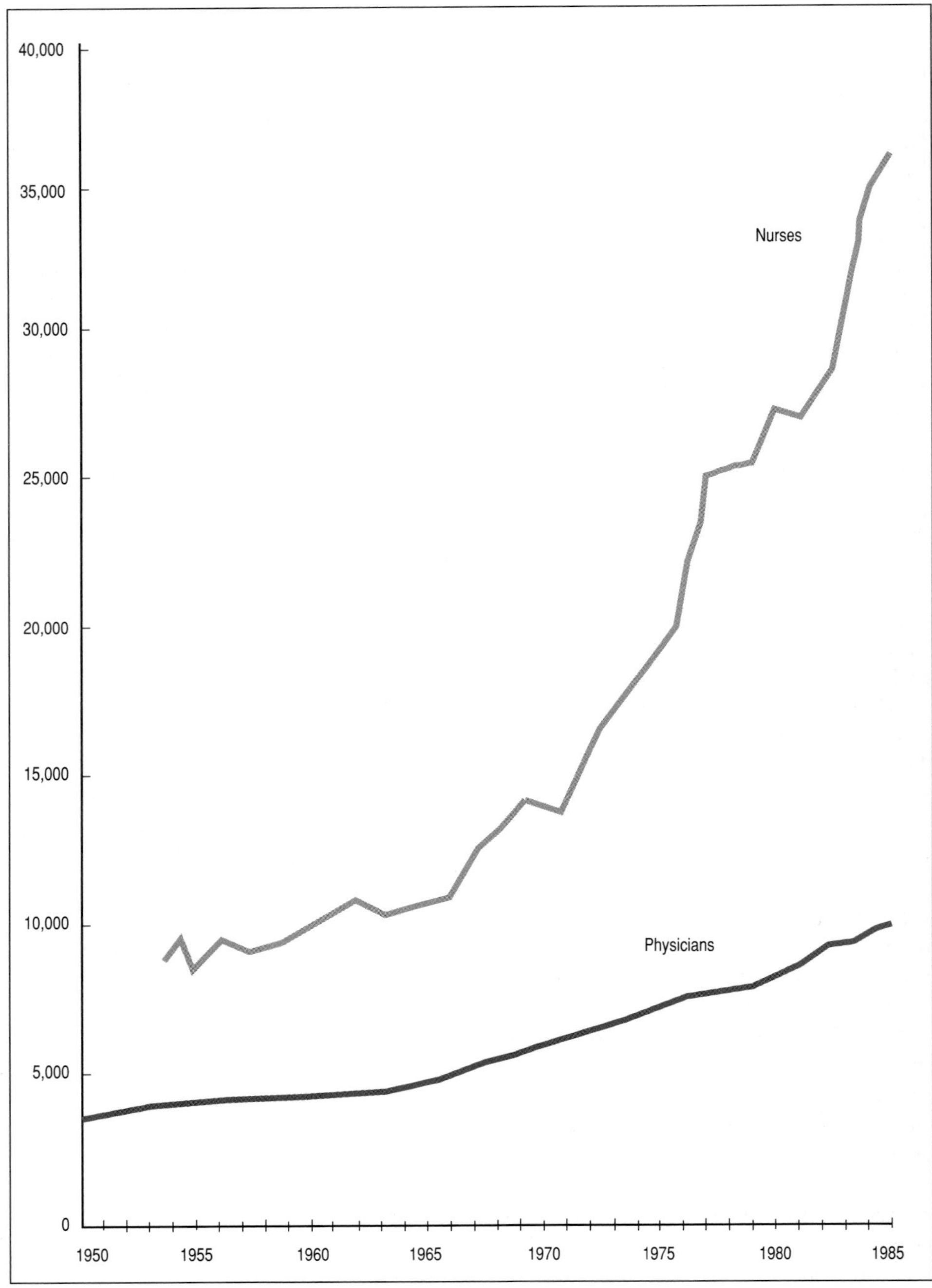

sured in morbidity and mortality, and health services, as measured in quality and universal availability, must be regarded as very favorable in Norway if an international comparison is made (Table 2.2). Of course, deficits exist, but the development and the present state of the Norwegian medical profession has to be discussed in this perspective. In Norway 7.6 percent of the gross domestic product was spent on health in 1991 (Diagram 2.3), a figure inline with the other countries of the West, but lower than the 13.9 percent spent in the United States (Nylenna 1995).

In his survey, Nylenna (1995) has reviewed the principles of the current health care system with its three levels: national, county, and municipal. Norwegian health care at the end of the twentieth century emphasizes giving health services through primary, first line care. This means that the municipal level has a special importance. The number of hospital beds have been reduced, of course, because of shorter stays in hospital, but also because of more outpatient services.

Almost all health expenditures are covered through the national health insurance. This gives a comprehensive coverage to the population, but also constitutes an important political steering instrument that also influences the development of the medical profession. The universal coverage also blurs the real costs of the services, at least on the individual level. Combined with the widening concept of health, this has become an important political issue.

Since World War II the health services have involved more and more groups of personnel in addition to the physicians. Some of these groups are profession-like and profession builders, for example, the nurses. The numerus clausus-system in Norway and other factors limiting the education of physicians have reduced the relative growth of the medical profession in relation to other groups, for example, the nurses (Diagram 2.4). This fact gradually alters the professional climate for the physicians to pursue independent goals. Because so many people are engaged in the health services in some way, and of course because most Norwegians at some time during their life become patients, it is no wonder that health is a top political topic in a country where people are used to having opinions of their own and are used to making them known.

However, an interesting trait has important bearings for the profession of physicians: A recent study based on a population survey (Berg & Hjortdahl 1994) concluded that the general satisfaction with the doctors and the loyality towards them was very high, in spite of the noise and complaints about health matters that often appear in the media. Nylenna also reports that fewer than 0.1 percent of the physicians were sued by patients in 1992; the corresponding number for the United States was 7.7 percent.

References

Berg, O. and P. Hjortdahl, *Medisinen som pedagogikk*. Oslo: Universitetsforlaget, 1994.

Britannica Book of the Year 1996. Chicago: Encyclopædia Britannica Inc., 1996.

Broch, O.J. *Le Royaume de Norvége et le peuple Norvegien*. Christiania: Steen, 1878.

Derry, T.K. *A short history of Norway.* London, Allen & Unwin, 1968.

Historisk statistikk 1994/Historical Statistics 1994. Oslo/Kongsvinger: Statistisk Sentralbyrå, 1995.

Hodne, F. A*n economic history of Norway 1815-1970.* Bergen: Tapir, 1975.

Larsen, Ø. ed. *Berglege Henrik Rosted og levekårene på Kongsberg ved slutten av 1700-tallet.* Kongsberg: Sølvverkets Venner, 1994.

Larsen, Ø. et al.(eds). *Samfunnsmedisin i Norge – teori og anvendelse.* Oslo: Universitetsforlaget, 1992.

Natvig, H. and E. Thiis-Evensen sen. "Arbeidsmiljø og helse". *Norsk bedr.h.tj.* 1983;4:1–333.

Nylenna, M. "Norway's Decentralized, Single-Payer Health System Faces Great Challenges". *JAMA* 274(1995):120-4.

Statistisk Årbok 1995/ Statistical Yearbook 1995. Oslo/Kongsvinger: Statistisk Sentralbyrå, 1995

C H A P T E R 3

The Very Beginning: Folk Medicine, Doctors, and Medical Services

PER HOLCK

3.1. Medicine and Health – What is it all About?

In the study of folk medicine, striking similarities in both concepts of disease and methods of treatment, independent of culture, time and place, become apparent. The same interpretation of a health problem is often found throughout large parts of the world, making it difficult to decide to what extent the different cultures have influenced each other. With regard to Norway, we often think that the oldest remedies have their roots in ancient Greece. There is, however, reason to believe that many of the basic medical principles could have arisen spontaneously, even within our own geographical area.

The concrete knowledge that we have about health conditions in Norway in ancient times derives from archaeological and anthropological studies. Graves from the past containing human bones have given us an insight into some of the diseases that existed in the population, as far back as five to six thousand years ago. Such findings sometimes also prove that attempts at treatment were made.

Written sources may provide indirect information on the understanding of disease and the concept of health. Some of the oldest runes from about 200 AD constitute formulations that lead us to believe that they were magical remedies against the powers of disease. In fact the old Norwegian word "runa" actually means "to practice sorcery."

The Norse concept of disease was based on what many people today would call superstition, with magic as the strongest remedy. Thus, treatment came to play a role completely different from that which we are used to today. Today, the therapeutic measures are the mainstay of medical thinking. In olden times it was more important to find out who or what had caused the patient's pains – because a strong principle in medical thinking was the interpretation of sickness as a result of the work of evil powers. By disclosing and subduing those powers, it was believed that most diseases would go away by themselves. In such cases, the revealing of the "diagnosis" was closely connected to the "treatment."

The three main principles of early medical thinking often encountered in folk medicine were also mixed up in ancient Norway: the animistic ideas of disease as an intruding organism which had to be forced out of the patient again, disease as a consequence of the ill-will of hostile persons and forces, and disease as a consequence of violated norms. And all this was seasoned by an overlay of empirical medical knowledge.

Healing, especially the handling of the evil forces, was not a matter for ordinary people. Special skills and special insights were required for a successful cure. For example a necessary condition was to have experience with the complex world of herbal medicine, and at the same time to be well-informed about the intricate system of sorcery and magic. One had to master what "the evil powers" could do and be able to put oneself in their place, in order to be able to turn the tide to the advantage of the sick person. Knowledge of remedies and procedures were passed on from one person to another in an oral tradition, as we learn from the medieval Sagas and the Edda poems and from the fairy tales.

It is well known that there were people who were specialists in curing disease and who therefore functioned as "doctors." The word "læknir" was used to describe a person who could stop bleeding, in other words a "wound doctor" who knew how to patch people up.

Runes, spells, and invocation of the gods were the remedies at the ordinary man's disposal. Indeed, the "doctor" often had little else to choose from. Some of the more rational herbal remedies that we know of can be traced back to medicine in central Europe and provide evidence of communication with the south, even as long ago as before the Viking times.

3.2. Early Clues of Medical Practice

When a cure has been shown to be effective, it becomes a "force" or a "power," according to superstition. This concept of power was of importance. It was not unusual that the chief or the king was supposed to have such powers, and in the sagas we hear that the kings were able to cure sickness and heal wounds. According to the sagas by Snorre, King Olav (995–1030) helped people who had tumors and throat infections by laying his hands upon them. King Magnus den Gode (1024–1047) went around among his men after the battle of Lyrskog Hede in 1043, examined their hands, and selected twelve men who had the softest hands. We read that none of them had dressed wounds before, but all of them became doctors "who were as good as any others" and that many doctors descended from them. It seems that it was believed that the king's own "healing powers" could be transferred to the men, and that the medical skills – in other words, the magic – were handed down from generation to generation. King Harald Hårdråde (1015–1066) cured an insane woman, and also healed the wounds of his men after the battle of Niså in 1062. In the same battle, Håkon Jarl Ivarsson (d. 1065) stopped a man from bleeding to death.

But even ordinary men and women, at the time of the sagas, seem to have been engaged in acts of healing. Again, the Icelandic author and historian Snorre Sturlason (1178/79–1241) gives us an interesting account, this time about wound healing in the year 1030. During the battle of Stiklestad (1030), Tormod Kolbrunarskald was struck by an arrow in his chest. He went to a house where several wounded men sat. A woman there was attending them. Then the woman asked him to see his wounds so that she could bandage them. He sat down and took his clothes off. When the woman saw his wounds, she carefully felt the wound he had in his side and noticed that there was an arrowhead in it, but she could not find out which way the arrowhead had entered. She had made something in a pot; crushed onion and other herbs, stewed together and she gave the wounded men some of this to eat: in this way she tried to find out if they had wounds in the abdominal cavity, because if they did she could smell the onion from the wounds that were penetrating it. Bringing some of this stew to Tormod, she told him to eat it. He refused and argued that he did not suffer from a stew disease. She then took pliers and tried to remove the arrowhead; but it held firm and could not be moved. There also was little that protruded, because the wound had swelled up. Then Tormod asked her to cut through to the arrowhead so he could get a good hold of it himself and pull it out with the pliers. She did as he said. Then Tormod took the pliers and pulled out the arrow. There were hooks on it, on which fibers from his heart had fastened, some of them red, some of them white, obviously fat, according to the saga. "We have been well fed by the King", Tormod remarked, and died. In their own way, tell-tale stories like this one propagated a toughness against pain and disease.

3.3. Folk Medicine and Christianity

In Viking times (ca. 800–1050), apart from the scattered influence of ancient Greek medicine, the art of medicine was mainly folk medicine, with a strong element of magic. This picture was not significantly altered when Christianity was introduced in Norway, mainly in the first decades of the eleventh century. In fact, just the opposite occurred. Christian symbols predominated and were used as powerful, protective remedies in folk medicine: the church, earth from the churchyard, the sign of the Holy Cross, the name of Jesus, the Bible, and soon all were used as important elements in the complicated pattern of treatment that was supposed to heal both people and animals.

With the books that came with the introduction of Christianity, the country was introduced to the influence of contemporary European scientific medicine; both the Sagas and the so-called diplomas bear witness to this. Sometimes, foreign possibly university-educated doctors visited Norway. Thus, Duke Skule (1189–1240) had a Belgian – Master Sigar from Brabant – as his personal physician. When a Spanish messenger visited Tønsberg in connection with the wedding of Kristin (1234–1262), the daughter of King Håkon Håkonssøn (1204–1263), a Spanish doctor looked after her brother, Håkon the Younger (born 1243), who was ill and died in 1257. King Håkon 5th Magnussøn (1270–1319) also had a foreign doctor, Raimund Calmeta, who was mentioned in 1313.

We know of no prominent Norwegian doctor from this time, but in Denmark there was the famous canon from Roskilde, Henrik Harpestreng (1164–1244), and Iceland had the famous doctor Hrafn Sveinbjørnsson who died in 1213 and even became the subject of his own saga. Hrafn had also been in Norway, and had made extensive travels abroad, to Santiago de Compostela and to Rome (Tjomsland 1951).

Mostly the Norwegians had to make do with more or less self-taught practitioners of folk medicine, in addition to some barbers who also ran their own surgical practices. Surgery had been separated from medicine since the Council of Tours in 1163. External treatment of the body was taken care of by barbers, as a pure handicraft. In Bergen their fee for blood-letting was laid down by a royal decree in 1282 (Scharffenberg 1902). A specific "doctors' pay" is indeed mentioned in the old Norwegian law texts, but it seems that this only covered the fee for the treatment of wounds.

The Council of Tours in 1163 stated that the church does not shed blood, practically forbidding the clergy to occupy themselves with medicine. However, after the decree of Pope Coelestin 5th (1214–1296) in 1294, the range of medical help that priests could give with regard to internal diseases was extended to include the poor, in addition to relatives and friends (Reichborn-Kjennerud 1925). Thus general care of sick people in cloisters and infirmaries was permitted and probably also included care of people other than the poor.

The infirmary service was a result of medieval Christian views on charity and health. We know of only a few such infirmaries in Norway. Besides, most of them were closed down, or changed, as a result of the Reformation. Medical treatment, as we know it, was probably not offered. In reality, they were closer to being institutions for old and frail people and travelers. Some were isolation hospitals for lepers. Covering costs usually depended on the receipt of alms. As early as the end of the twelfth century, an infirmary under the auspices of the cathedral existed in Trondheim. A century later, a Maria Infirmary is also mentioned there. A separate infirmary for lepers supposedly also existed.

In Bergen – at that time Norway's largest city – an "All Saints Infirmary" was founded in 1248. At about the same time, an infirmary for female lepers is mentioned. During the fifteenth century an infirmary at Nonneseter Monastery is also mentioned, in addition to a separate "ward" for people suffering from ergot poisoning. The brothers of Saint Antonius were given permission to run this ward until the beginning of the sixteenth century. In Oslo, a Laurentius Infirmary for lepers is mentioned, in addition to another institution for care of the sick at Hovin, outside the city, around 1300. These two institutions were amalgamated during the Reformation and became an ordinary hospital, which is still in existence (Oslo Hospital). Infirmaries also existed in the Middle Ages in Hamar, Tønsberg and Stavanger. In addition, we know of several monasteries outside the towns where sick people were cared for (Halsnøy, Værne, and Fana, for example).

3.4. Medical Literature

Medieval medical books were transcripts of various texts, some by named authors such as Henrik Harpestreng; others were anonymous collections of variable content, mainly on herbal medicine. A common trait for all of them was that they originated from the European Continent. More or less complete copies were disseminated for private use, and these were in widespread use even up until modern times.

Through the art of printing, such herbals became widely distributed. Most of them were written in German. However in 1533, Christiern Pedersen (circa 1480–1544), a Dane who also translated the works of Saxo Grammaticus (circa 1150–1220), published in Danish "A useful medical book for rich and poor, young and old." His compatriot and citizen of Malmö (which was then Danish), Henrik Smid (circa 1495–1563), obtained a wide distribution for his Danish book entitled "A beautiful, merry new herb garden." The first medical book in Sweden, written by Bengt Olofson, was printed in 1578.

Such books rapidly gained popularity, and the works of Henrik Smid were even recommended by the Medical Faculty of the University of Copenhagen. But they were not for all and sundry, even though the foreword to Smid's book could lead us to believe this. For Henrik Smid, the art of medicine was a revelation from God, and each doctor was a kind of prophet. He also complained about the standard of medicine at the time, stating that learned and faithful doctors were scarce in many places. In their place he found lewd monks, nuns, unlearned priests, depraved tradesmen, old wives, yes, even cobblers and blacksmiths, wizards and witches, and other idle folk who would not work, but would rather make a living from the art of medicine.

Knowledge of "advanced" medicine from the books on herbal medicine certainly led to some reduction in the therapeutic use of magic. However, magic was widely used and traditions were still kept by the Lapps. In fact, well into the nineteenth century, being a Laplander was almost synonymous with being a witch in the eyes of many predjudice Norwegians.

3.5. Early Pharmacies

People generally had to rely on themselves and their own knowledge when they were sick, because pharmacies did not exist in Norway in olden days. Sometimes, rich people were sent medicines for their own use as costly gifts from abroad. In 1594, a Dutch merchant living in Bergen, Nicolas de Freundt, who died in 1618, applied for a general permition to trade in drugs, and the next year he obtained Royal consent to open the "Svaneapotek" there. In 1626, a pharmacy was also opened in Christiania, just two years after the city was founded. Later, other Norwegian towns followed, one after the other: Stavanger in 1650, Kristiansand in 1651, Trondheim in 1661, Drammen in 1686, and so on.

3.6. Pharmacists and Medical Officers

That Norway got its first pharmacy almost one hundred years after Denmark was seen as only right and proper at that time, since the establishment of a pharmacy demanded the presence of qualified doctors. It was not until 1593 that Norway got its first medically trained doctor, Henrik Høyer (died 1615), from the Baltic town of Stralsund. He settled in Bergen, where he ran a private practice for a while. Ten years later, the town of Bergen employed the Dane, Willads Nielsen Adamius (circa 1564–1616), as public medical officer (Scharffenberg 1904).

Oslo was worse off in this respect. There was no doctor there at all before the great fire in 1624, when the town was rebuilt near the walls of the fortress of Akershus and renamed Christiania. But we can assume that barbers in the town, and to some degree helpers in the infirmary for lepers, must have had some medical skills. In any case, we are told that in 1611 two barbers certified that a man had brought upon his wife "a terrible sickness" (syphilis?). It was not until 1626 that Christiania got his first public medical officer, Peder Alfsen (circa 1581–1663). He had previously run a practice in Bergen. In contrast to the majority of the first doctors in Norway, who were nearly all Danish or German, Peder Alfsen was a Norwegian (Scharffenberg 1904).

Alfsen did not stay long in Christiania, because he could not earn a living from his practice. There were simply not enough patients for running a practice, even though he was the town's only doctor. His successor, the German Otto Sperling (1602–1681), who was appointed in 1632, does not seem to have done particularly well there, either. Sperling had first thought of settling in Trondheim, but instead he was enticed by the governor himself, Jens Juel (1580–1634), to accept the post of chief medical officer in Christiania. "What will you do in Trondheim?" he is said to have asked. "They have never had a physician there, know also nothing about medicine, but cure themselves with beer from Rostock and Lübeck, with mead and cloudberries, when they have scurvy." But Dr. Sperling also experienced a lack of patients, and he left the country after only five years (Holck 1976).

After Peder Alfsen moved to Trondheim in 1631, one would think that the town was well supplied with doctors. However, Dr. Alfsen became the presiding judge in the town, instead. He obviously did not want a repetition of his experiences from Christiania, even though we cannot exclude the possibility that he practiced to some extent in the town. Not until 1661 did Trondheim get a public medical officer, Dr. Jens Nicolaisen (1619–1662). He ensured that an pharmacy was established there (Scharffenberg 1905).

In Kristiansand, the first doctor was appointed in 1651. He was also a pharmacist and a wine merchant. Later, the post of "physician to the mines" was established in the silver mining town of Kongsberg in 1656 (Larsen 1994).

It was not easy to practice as a doctor and make a living from it. Part of the explanation for this is found in a note though it was written 150 years later, by the doctor and deputy of the first Norwegian national assembly at Eidsvoll in 1814, Alexander Møller (1762–1847), who practiced in Arendal. Regarding his patients' attitudes toward disease, he wrote that they saw disease as divine retribution for their sins, which could not be cured without their own and the priest's prayers and supplications. He saw this attitude as an explanation of why only one doctor could make a living from thirty to forty thousand people (Chancellary report 1803). Being healed with the help of doctors was seen as a kind of interference with God's divine providence. Even in the larger towns, the situation was the same. In a book of memoirs from Bergen in the first half of the nineteenth century, we can read that most people ordinary people as well as minor merchants, craftsmen and traders never or at least very seldom make use of expert medical help. There are several reasons for this. In many cases it is worship of fatalism, or else more faith in quacks and old women. Sometimes it can simply be ascribed to apathy and the power of habit, or else in some cases to economic considerations (Gran 1873).

This was certainly the general opinion of people throughout the country. To consult a doctor was almost impossible, and the chance that he would really achieve anything was not very great. It was certainly also an economic matter for most people, because consulting a doctor was very expensive. For example, at the end of the nineteenth century a man on a mountain farm in Hallingdal sent for the district physician, who lived in Nes, about 60-70 kilometers away. For the doctor's visit the farmer had to pay 60 kroner, about one-third of what he could expect to earn from the farm in a whole year (Norsk Etnografisk Samling 1960).

3.7. Medicine and the Clergy

It can be seen from the Norwegian laws of King Christian 5th (1646–1699) from 1687 on that ministers had the duty of visiting and treating the sick in the parish at that time. Doctors are not mentioned in the law at all. It was the clergy who were supposed to visit the sick and disabled, and conscientiously, when there was reason, remind folk that they should, in good time, when they are sick, send for him, so that he could come to them and give them a reminder and good advice, and that they should not wait until they are desperately ill. The ministers should even teach midwives how they should conduct themselves in their work and at the same time exhort the confined women to pray for their unborn baby.

It can not have been easy to be a minister in those days, when they obviously were also expected to have a certain command of the medical literature. Some ministers gained reputation as clever "doctors." Niels Schytte (1692–1739), who was minister in Lindås in the county of Hordaland, was of this type, and he made tangible efforts to eradicate superstition in his parish. Dressed in disguise and pretending to be sick, he let himself be taken to "wise" women. But as soon as he had come inside, it is said that he struck them with his walking stick, so that they had to use all of their healing words afterwards to cure themselves (Sandvik 1993).

His son, Erik Gerhard Schytte (1729–1808), was certainly of a less choleric temperament. As a student in Copenhagen, he read medicine and became equally educated both in medical matters and as a minister. He settled in Bodø and turned the vicarage into a kind of hospital, where his wife Anna also helped and cared for the sick. For his contribution there, and also for his work in improving the supply of doctors in Northern Norway, he was the "Æsculap of the North."

Jacob Lund (1724–1785), who was minister in Kragerø from 1766 on, should also be mentioned. In his youth he had studied medicine in Copenhagen, but he gave up his studies at the request of his friends in order to dedicate himself to theology, instead. He is said to have been the first to give inoculation against smallpox in Norway.

Another such "minister-doctor" was the well-known Niels Hertzberg (1759–1841) in Kvinnherad and Ullensvang in Western Norway, who strongly believed in giving health education to his parishioners. He had also learned from his father, the priest and propagator of potato growing, Peder Harboe Hertzberg (1728–1802). During the nearly three years he was assistant to his father, he was taught by him a good, practical knowledge of medicine that could be used to help people in their isolated living. But Niels Hertzberg himself was surprised that he never was accused and charged in the Law Courts with quackery or with being an unqualified doctor. According to information from that time, Niels Herzberg not only functioned as a doctor and a surgeon, but also assisted with childbirth. He saw to it that people were vaccinated against smallpox in his parish as early as 1803, just seven years after the English doctor, Edward Jenner (1749–1823) had published his paper on smallpox vaccination.

That ministers functioned as doctors may be seen as a direct continuation of the Catholic tradition that began when the learned clergy, who possibly also possessed knowledge of monastic medicine, were among the only ones who had any real knowledge of such matters.

3.8. Surviving Folk Medicine

Folk medicine has always existed in a parallel relationship with authorized and scholary medicine. However, folk medicine has also changed and in a way adapted itself to the level at which learned medicine functioned at any given time. It has developed as a synthesis of empirical knowledge and ancient traditions, mixed up with medieval sorcery and Christian ideals of piety, brought together in a mythical-magical health faith. At the same time, folk medicine has absorbed such a large part of the basic principles of the faith of the people that the two concepts cannot be separated. Therefore, a review of some principles from folk medicine is necessary, both as part of the general medical history of the country, and as a means of understanding still-existing folk medicine and even modern alternative medicine.

Folk medicine in Norway has been and still is partly based on belief in the supernatural, and partly on a considerable amount of rational knowledge about the healing qualities of herbs. Thus, the healing process often consisted of elements of quite different origins. It was not unusual that it was regarded as a battle, a driving out of the diseases by power, an exorcism of demons by the means of spells and magic. Sometimes the disease was addressed with flattering words, in order to make the evil powers leave voluntarily. The name of the sick person had to be mentioned so that the act could be precisely placed. Often the disease was given a place of exile, where it could do no damage. The formula that was read became a command directed toward the power that was to be driven out.

An important principle in folk medicine was that "the doctor" could not treat himself or his relatives. The background for this lies in the concept of disease, which claims that deceased members of the family, wishing to take living family members with them into the kingdom of the dead, could cause disease. It was an old belief that death led to disease, and not necessarily the other way around.

Even in the nineteenth century, many doctors were called to the village's "wise" woman or man, who, on their deathbed, had realized the limitations of their powers, and now, as a last resort, wished to challenge fate with the help of their professional opponent.

Darkness has always been associated with eeriness, a time when evil powers freely could play their evil tricks on people. Thus, folk medicine remedies worked best in the time between sunset and sunrise. This applied both to collecting healing herbs or preparing lotions and medications.

Not only the time of day, but also the choice of day, has been of great importance in folk medicine beliefs. Thursday was regarded as an important day on which to carry out treatment, and treatment carried out on three Thursdays in a row was supposed to be especially effective.

Naturally, the North was the place where darkness and evil powers belonged. Thus, it was believed that diseases were sent from the North, and treatment could then involve sending them back to where they came from, for example, by using north-flowing water or the moss from the north side of a tree trunk.

In folk medicine, the rare and unusual have always been regarded as a more powerful and effective medication than that which can be found everywhere. Thus, the place where the medication was found was also important. Soil, or the objects found there, especially metal objects, had, as a rule, a wide range of use, undoubtedly because one perceived a direct connection between earth and the dead. For example, in heathen times, soil from gravemounds had the same significance as soil from churchyards later in the Christian times. Objects found at crossroads, objects that were untouched by human hands, and so on have also been regarded as unusual, and this was therefore of significance in interpreting the healing power of the remedy.

One thought of the evil, disease-creating world as an opposite to the world of man. Magic cures should therefore be carried out in the opposite direction to that which was normal, for example, in the opposite direction to the path of the sun, with the left hand, and so on. The Lord's Prayer, read backwards, was regarded as a particularly powerful remedy. These are all examples of how things that people regarded as deviant from everyday acts could be exalted and given magical qualities and powers, and could thus, in the past, be regarded as useful remedies in the fight against disease, pain, and death.

However, the differences between folk medicine and "learned" medicine were not always so great. When the first pharmacopoeia for Denmark and Norway was published in 1658, it gave a description of medicaments that were more than equal to any witch or sorcerer's home-brew. Ingredients such as pulverized skull, human fat, urine, mummies, and dried snake meat were mentioned. The first pharmacopoeia published in Sweden in 1686 was of the same kind. Even in the first Norwegian medical journal "Eyr", at the end of the 1820s, we can come across articles with titles such as "On the storage of leeches," "Warm animal blood as an internal medication," and "Drunkenness cured with a mixture of sulfuric acid and spirits." It is therefore not surprising that people who relyied on folk medicine sometimes perceived authorized medical science as a confirmation of their own theories and methods.

Folk medicine in its traditional form has

existed right up until the twentieth century, with certain offshoots surviving right up until, say, around 1950, and then later fading and blending in with modern alternative medicine. There can be several reasons for this. Contrary to "learned" medicine, which carried out bloody and painful operations as a part of treatment, we never see folk medicine using such frightening and dramatic procedures, perhaps with the exception of blood-letting. The skepticism with which medical officers were met was not only the result of the old antagonism between government officials and the rural population. An important, contributory factor was simply the fact that people in the past had no more wish to have pain than we have today, if it could be avoided. In addition, the curative effect and the prospects of professional medicine in the past was, in many cases, dubious. Also, the cost of treatment often took a big share of the patient's financial resources. Such factors may explain why folk medicine kept its strong position right up until the middle of this century.

3.9. Doctors, Diseases, and Competition

The post of chief medical officer in Norwegian towns was generally maintained as a permanent institution, despite the fact that it was often difficult to fill the post, partly because of the poor, and at times uncertain, pay. No public medical officer was employed at all in Christiania from 1689 to 1729, because of lack of money. When the post was re-established, it was unpaid up until 1792. From 1729 on, public medical officers were also employed in country districts.

In addition there were, quite early, several military surgeons in the country, and they probably carried out some civil duties when it was required (Reichborn-Kjennerud 1936). These surgeons were much lower down the social ladder than the university-educated doctors and "minister-priests," but ranked somewhat higher than farmers and farmer's wives with medical skills and "wise" people of different types.

Even though there were various doubtful elements among these surgeons, there were also some individuals who practiced their craft in an outstanding manner. It is not surprising that there were constant conflicts between the surgeons and the university-educated doctors with regard to who had the right to provide treatment. The social standing of the surgeons vastly improved when formal training for surgeons was established in Copenhagen in 1736, and when the Surgical Academy, founded in 1785, united surgical training with the theoretical background of physicians. In fact, the curriculum at the Royal Academy of Surgeons in Copenhagen set standards for the modern medical education of doctors, so that the earlier, university-educated physicians without surgical skills soon disappeared along with the non-academic surgeons. This was part of an international trend during the Age of Enlightenment.

Some other groups of people without any special education also practiced in Norway. Bone-setters were among them. The so-called ocultists or "cataract stickers," who can in a way be seen as the predecessors of our present-day ophthalmologists, had an even lower social status than the barber surgeons. Their specialty seems to have been cataract operations. It was not possible for such people to settle down and run a practice in one place in Norway. They therefore became a traveling professional group, with all that such a status entails.

Educated doctors in public posts and in private practice as a rule had a solid educational background. But many of them still were foreigners until the nineteenth century. They came from a variety of European universities, and usually they held a doctorate from one of them, as the custom was. Some of them brought new ideas with them, though Norwegian conservatism and skepticism to everything that was new was also apparent in the field of medicine.

In the second half of the eighteenth century and well into the nineteenth century, the "radesyge"-disease was a health problem in Norway. This is regarded as a chronic disease related to syphilis. To curb the disease, a series of new infirmaries were built throughout the country, a welcome supplement to those few medieval leper infirmaries which still existed. At that time, separate wards for internment of the insane were also built. However, medical treatment for ordinary people was still a rarity. People often died at home after being cared for by their relatives. It was these relatives who gathered at the patient's deathbed, settled on the "diagnosis," and later on reported it to the minister. As late as 1880, a doctor from Nordfjord records that only two out of 117 persons who had died in his district had been attended by a doctor during their last illness.

3.10. Setting Standards

The establishment of the university in Christiania in 1811 – the first in Norway – paved the way for an improvement in the education of doctors. But things went slowly in the beginning, and there were only three people who registered to study medicine in 1814, the first year when the new faculty of medicine was operative. There were approximately 900,000 inhabitants in Norway in 1814. There is no standard definition of what a doctor was, but there were probably no more than about 50 qualified doctors and about double that number of lesser qualified military surgeons. Thus, it did not take long before a proposal for a more developed public health service was put forward.

But there was still a strong opposition. It was the countrymen representatives in the Norwegian Parliament in the 1830s who turned out to be most opposed to the plans to better the health services. The plans, they thought, were too costly. The opposition must certainly also be seen in the light of the deep-rooted suspicion that peasants felt toward officials, and a suspicion toward everything that was strange to them.

References

Gran, J. *Skizzer af Bergenske Forholde fra ældre og yngre Tid*. Bergen: 1873.

Holck P. "Leger og sykdommer i 1600-årene," *St. Halvard* (1976): 130–136.

Kancelli-innlegg av 3. desember 1803.

Kolsrud, O (ed.). *Oslo kapitels forhandlinger 1609–1616*. Kristiania/Oslo: 1913–49.

Larsen, Ø. (ed.) *Berglege Henrik Rosted og leverkårene på Kongsberg på slutten av 1700-tallet*. Kongsberg: Sølvverkets venner, 1994.

Larsen, Ø. *Mangfoldig medisin*. Oslo: Det medisinske fakultet, Universitetet i Oslo, 1989.

Norsk Etnografisk Samlings spørreskjemaer: "Folkemedisin" (emnenr. 80, 1960). Questionnaires.

Reichborn-Kjennerud, I., F. Grøn and I. Korbo. *Medisinens historie i Norge*. Oslo: Grøndahl og Søns Forlag, 1936.

Reichborn-Kjennerud, I. "Medicinske forhold i Norge i 1300-aarene," *Norsk Magazin for Lægevidenskaben,* 86(1925): 637–653.

Sandvik, H. "Dei Vise forvidle Væræ!". En distriktsleges kamp mot overtro og trolldom på 1800-tallet. *Tidsskrift for Den norske lægeforening*, 113(1993):3572–74.

Scharffenberg, J. "Havde de priviligerede Kirurger Eneret til at utøvve Kirurgi?" *Ugeskrift for læger* 31(1902):721–723.

Scharffenberg, J. "Bidrag til de norske lægestillingers historie før 1800. I.," *Bergens stadsfysikat. Norsk Magazin for Lægevidenskaben,* 65 (1904):225–295.

Scharffenberg, J. "Bidrag til de norske lægestillingers historie før 1800. II.," *Kristianias stadsfysikat. Norsk Magazin for Lægevidenskaben,* 65(1904):1329–1384.

Scharffenberg, J. "Bidrag til de norske lægestillingers historie før 1800. III.," *Kristianias stadsfysikat. Norsk Magazin for Lægevidenskaben,* 66(1905):825–872.

Smith, H. *Lægebog, inholdenis Mange skøne oc udvalde Lægedoms stycker 1577.* Köbenhavn, Rosenkilde og Bagger: Faksimile-utgave, 1976.

Sverre, NA. *Et studium av farmasiernes historie. 2.ed.* Oslo: Norges Apotekerforening, 1982.

Tjomsland, A. (ed.) *The Saga of Hrafn Sveinbjarnarson.* Ithaca, New York: Cornell University Press, 1951.

CHAPTER 4

National Doctors – The Establishing of a Medical Faculty

ØIVIND LARSEN

Science might be threatening when seen from certain viewpoints. In the twin kingdom of Denmark-Norway, heated discussions on the possiblity of establishing a national university in Norway took place in the eighteenth century. This issue had already been put forward in the seventeenth century, and the founding of a school of higher education for mining (Bergseminaret) in the silver mine city of Kongsberg in 1757 was a beginning. Det Kongelige Norske Videnskabers Selskab, the Royal Norwegian Society of Sciences in Trondheim (1767) dated its origins back to an initiative taken by the prominent scholars Johan Ernst Gunnerus (1718–1773), Gerhard Schøning (1722–1780), and Peter Fredrik Suhm (1728–1798) in 1760. An interest in building up a national science program was definitely at hand.

But the authorities in remote Denmark were reluctant. Several attempts and proposals failed. Were the authorities simply afraid that a national development in the field of science might loosen the ties to the center of power, Copenhagen? Even when money was raised locally in Norway, obstacles remained.

In the light of history, this process may be looked upon not so much as the history of the planning of a university, but as the history of an emerging nationalism and the attempts by the authorities to curb it.

At the turn of the century, during the time of the Napoleonic Wars, the political situation became extremely tense. Communication between Denmark and Norway was severely hampered, because the allied enemies Sweden and England seriously disrupted communication between the two parts of the twin kingdom. Naval forces blocked the seas between Norway and Denmark.

Reinforced by the difficult economic and social situation which these circumstances forced upon Norway, Norwegian discontent with Denmark continually grew, and the university question was part of it. The quest for a national university had gained symbolic value; perhaps volatile explosives were concealed behind the polite phrases and the obsequious wording of the Norwegians?

Something happened on March 1, 1811.

A short time before, a local governor in a part of southern Norway, the mighty count Herman Wedel Jarlsberg (1779-1840), while out traveling on duty in the countryside, received a message that he had to call at the Royal Palace in Copenhagen immediately. The count had good relationships with high-ranking Swedes, and King Frederik VI (1768–1839, King of Norway 1808-1814 and King of Denmark 1808-1839) obviously regarded a conference with this influential Norwegian essential as he planned his next move in the delicate political situation.

We do not know the details of the conversation at the meeting. However, that the establishing of a university was the issue, and that the tide had turned in this matter, is proven by the fact that the count returned home with definite orders to work out detailed plans for a new university.

A few months later, on September 2, 1811, the King signed the document establishing a university in Christiania in Norway, bearing his own name, Det Kongelige Fredriks Universitet, an event that was celebrated all over Norway.

If this concession to Norwegian demands was intended to calm down the waves and secure the relationship between Norway and Denmark, it failed. On January 14, 1814, the linkage between Denmark and Norway fractured when the peace treaty of Kiel was signed. Norway got its own constitution and entered a new era, not as a completely independent state, but in a looser union with Sweden, a situation which lasted until 1905.

The new university was a visible sign that a new and independent nation was emerging. The issue of building up a university had proved its importance. The stage was set for a national science, and for the establishing of a national, learned elite.

So, too, the story of the medical faculty at the new national university in the Norwegian capital has cultural overtones that are equally as interesting as the mere history of the emergence of a medical school.

At the turn of the eighteenth century, the Age of Enlightenment had added new dimensions to science and arts. Philosophers had scrutinized human thinking and behavior, and opened up for a new assessment of the value of human life as such. Mercantilistic economics focused on the value of human labor and subsequently took an interest in the preservation of health and the maintenance of a healthy workforce

But at the same time human suffering was widespread. Growing European cities contained large numbers of sick inhabitants, and the death toll was remarkable. Poverty was a general problem. The cruelties of the French revolution had replaced normal feelings of humanity, and the waves of war in the Napoleonic era put new evidence forward supporting the principles launched by Thomas Robert Malthus (1766–1834); war, famine, and epidemics were the scourges that limited the growth of the human population. But did the suffering appeal to the medical world? Did political forces put health issues forward?

The medical history of the outgoing eighteenth century is an intriguing chapter of the development of welfare. Countries experienced progress and refinement in culture and commerce, but public expenditures for health care were often only diminutive. But was this phenomenon based on defeatism or ignorance? Probably on neither of these two options. As far as can be seen, disease and death to a large extent were regarded as part of life, as inherent in human existence. Freedom from pain, impairment and threats to life were still not thought of as a basic requirement for a full life, nor were they regarded as a human right.

The rather weak demands for medical help and health services also have to be seen in this perspective, even though large hospitals had been built in many European cities in the eighteenth century, and the training of doctors had been improved. The health education policy of the time, which in Denmark had especially been pursued by the influential medical professor Johann Clemens Tode (1736–1806) through his many popular periodicals and journals dealing with medical matters in a popular form,

TABLE 4.1

Academics in Norway 1720 – 1962. The table shows the mean annual number of graduates. Until 1940 only physicians who graduated in Norway are included; after 1940 also physicians trained abroad who had received a Norwegian license.*(Larsen et al 1986 after Lindbekk 1967)*

	Year of graduation											
	1720-59	1760-99	1800-14	1815-29	1830-49	1850-69	1870-89	1890-09	1910-29	1930-49	1950-59	1960-62
Theology	22	22	15	17	23	19	32	22	30	49	33	27
Law	6	18	18	17	39	35	52	81	79	155	156	96
Officers	1	7	21	18	15	15	20	28	26	28	57	38
Medicine				6	14	12	23	45	53	99	117	146
Humanities				1	2	4	8	10	22	69	90	74
Natural Sciences						1	4	6	12	39	82	86
Engineering					1	1	23	79	156	179	437	541
Agriculture								15	53	50	71	84
Economics								2	23	51	87	60
Social Sciences										1	29	29
Dentistry, Pharmacology, Veterinarians									30	51	58	148
Sum	29	47	54	59	94	87	162	288	484	771	1,217	1,329
% Physicians				10.2	14.9	13.8	14.2	15.6	11.0	12.8	9.6	11.0

of course was important in forming general attitudes, but, in a way, it also claimed that responsibility for health was a personal matter.

When it became known that the new university would provide Norway with national scholars and learned men, the priorities of the authorities and those of the population were expressed. Law and theology of course were taken up, because the candidates in these disciplines were required for the running of the country. Nevertheless, the medical faculty was able to start its activity as soon as 1814. The real flourishing of medicine as an academic discipline, however, could only take place after the needs for medical services had been settled and accepted, which was a process that needed time (Table 4.1).

Medical pioneers, such as the first professor of hygiene (from 1824) Frederik Holst (1791–1871), considered it a prime task to describe and to inform about diseases and social misery that a modern state should pay attention to and take responsibility for. The conditions for psychiatric patients may serve as a striking example: institutions designed for treatment of the insane did not exist at the end of the eighteenth century; confinement under jail-like circumstances was the fate of those who could not be handled by the local community. A report on the conditions endured by the insane was presented to the authorities by Holst in 1828 and became the basis for the introduction of psychiatric care consistent with contemporary, international standars.

Premises and facilities were almost totally lacking when the faculty started its teaching with three professors and three regular medical students. A military hospital served as the first university clinic, until a Nation-

DIAGRAM 4.1.
Medical students and population in Norway 1814–1909 (redrawn after Laache 1911).

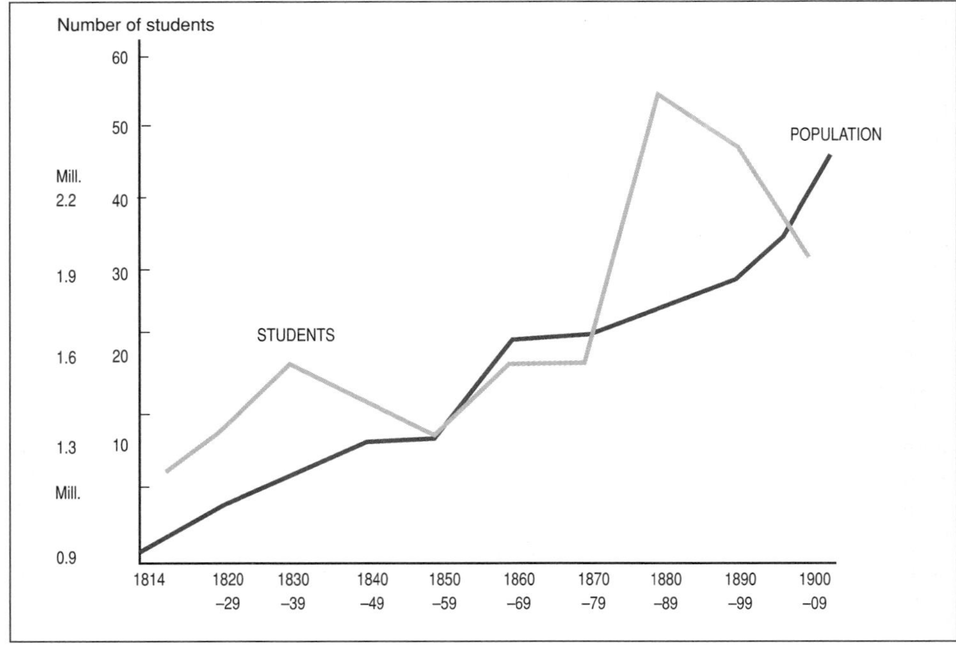

al hospital with teaching obligations was opened in 1826. It was replaced by a new and more suitable hospital in 1883.

Preclinical teaching had only provisional premises until the central building of the university was completed in 1852.

The first regular student to graduate from the new university was Johan Keyser (1795–1839) in 1820. However, there existed some transitional arrangements for students without full qualifications for admittance to academic studies. In 1817 Carl Schultz (1789-1861), the first one in this group, qualified as a physician. The last medical examination of this type took place as late as 1850 (Diagram 4.1).

In the course of the nineteenth century, the curriculum gradually developed. There are many details in this adjustment to medicine and society, but a main concern seems to have been to find the balance between theoretical knowledge and practical skills. The Faculty defended a strong theory, while many physicians favored practice. Discussions were heated, but the objective was clear: the new doctors were expected to have a solid scientific background, paired with skills as practitioners. They were expected to have learned methodological thinking, to have learned to work independently, and to be able to maintain and update their knowledge and proficiency. It seems that the development over time transformed the curriculum and structured it into a more specific preparation for the future practical work of the physicians. The training also became more and more homogenous because of an increasing number of obligatory courses.

This broad interest in medical education among the members of the profession may be taken as proof of their interest in the professional formation of their future colleagues; in the influential Norwegian Medical Society in Kristiania, the curriculum was discussed at every meeting from May 7 1902, until March 25 1903. This engagement also proves that there existed a strong interest in what we here have called professionalization by means of structuring the basic training of the physicians.

It is one thing to build up a national medical school to train new physicians for the country. But it is quite another thing to establish a national medical science; to create a research program that is able to produce original contributions to medical knowledge. The theses defended for the doctoral degree may be regarded as a measure of the scientific activity. The first one was presented by Frederik Holst in 1817. He defended a paper on the Radesyge, the syphilis-like disease that was widespread in Norway in the eighteenth century. The next dissertation took place in 1829, when Christen Heiberg (1799–1872) defended his thesis entitled *De coremorphosi*, on the artifical pupil of the eye. Jens Johan Hjort (1789–1873) followed in 1830 with a thesis on the function of the retina, and Frantz Christian Faye (1806-1890) in 1842 on the seminal vesicles. Thereafter no dissertations were presented until 1875, after which a series followed suit, so that 41 theses had been presented by the turn of the century.

However, to whom were the scientific results presented? The first four theses were written in Latin, and the dissertations and ceremonies were also held in Latin, which was a line with current and established academic traditions (Nordhagen 1995). After 1845 Latin was no longer a requirement. Almost all of th theses were written in Norwegian until publication in German or English gradually took over well into the twentieth century.

For the place of science in the self-image of the new national medicine, this may be a point worthy of reflection. Theses in Latin of course could be read in the contemporary international scientific community. The decision to use the Latin language, however, was probably more an adhesion to traditions than a specific desire to approach a wider audience. The habit of presenting science in Norwegian in the nineteenth century might have set up some barriers to the international world, and the new trend in the twentieth century is a clear sign by the researchers that they also wanted to address international readers.

The long interval between 1842 and 1875, 33 years without any dissertations, calls also for attention. As described in other chapters of this book, Norwegian medical activity and international orientation in the nineteenth century was quite substantial. The explanation may be quite simple: probably the doctorate institution did not have the same standing and importance in the eyes of the profession and in contemporary academic life as in the years to come.

References

Larsen, Ø., O. Berg, F. Hodne. *Legene og samfunnet*. Oslo: Den norske lægeforening, 1986.

Larsen, Ø. *Mangfoldig medisin*. Oslo: Det medisinske fakultet, Universitetet i Oslo, 2. ed., 1990. (The history of the medical faculty of Oslo.)

Nordhagen, R. "Akademiske grader og skiftende sans for seremonier". *Tidsskrift for Den norske lægeforening*,115(1995):3753–6.

CHAPTER 5

Towards a New Demographic Pattern

ØIVIND LARSEN

5.1 A New Nation?

At the beginning and at the end of the nineteenth century, Norway was not the same country.

Of course the mountains, the forests, the rivers, and lakes were there as ever before. But, in less than a century, the social setup had changed profoundly. The political situation had changed dramatically, the economy had expanded, and trade had gained in volume and independence. In culture and in science, a national identity had emerged.

Most important, however, were the extreme changes in the demographic composition of the population. Tables 5.1 and 5.2 give a short impression of what happened: As indicators of a complicated process, the substantial population increase, and the shift from a predominantly young population to a more elderly one have been selected.

At the time of the Napoleonic wars, most of the inhabitants in Norway lived as they had for generations, following traditional patterns in their daily lifes. One hundred years later the Norwegian population had the characteristics of a modern society in rapid development.

Thus, the development of new social

TABLE 5.1
Resident Population, Norway (after Historical Statistics, 1994)

	Total	Percentage population in densely populated areas
1964–66	440,000	6.8
1701	504,000	7.9
1735	616,109	..
1769	723,618	8.9
1801	883,603	8.8
1815	885,431	9.8
1825	1,051,318	10.9
1835	1,194,827	10.8
1845	1,318,471	15.6
1855	1,490,047	16.9
1865	1,701,756	19.6
1875	1,813,424	24.4
1890	2,000,917	31.3
1900	2,240,032	35.7
1910	2,391,782	38.5
1920	2,649,775	45.3
1930	2,814,194	47.3
1946	3,156,950	50.1
1950	3,278,546	52.2
1960	3,591,234	57.2
1970	3,874,133	65.9
1980	4,091,132	70.3
1990	4,247,546	72.4

TABLE 5.2
Percentages of the Norwegian population in different age groups (Historical Statistics 1994)

Year	0–6	7–15	16–44	45–66	67–79	80+
1845	17.0	18.6	42.7	17.0	3.8	0.9
1850	17.4	18.2	43.0	16.9	3.7	0.8
1855	18.3	18.4	42.3	16.3	3.8	0.8
1860	19.1	18.9	41.8	15.2	4.2	0.8
1865	18.6	19.4	41.2	15.6	4.3	0.8
1870	17.4	20.0	41.0	16.4	4.3	0.9
1875	17.0	19.4	40.7	17.6	4.2	1.1
1880	18.0	18.4	40.6	17.8	4.1	1.1
1885	17.9	18.9	40.0	17.6	4.5	1.1
1890	18.0	19.6	39.0	17.2	5.2	1.0
1895	17.6	19.8	39.3	16.7	5.6	1.1
1900	17.7	19.6	39.5	16.5	5.4	1.2
1905	17.5	20.0	39.0	16.9	5.2	1.4
1910	16.5	20.5	39.2	17.3	5.1	1.5
1915	15.8	19.7	40.9	17.2	5.0	1.4
1920	15.3	18.8	42.4	17.1	5.2	1.3
1925	14.5	18.2	43.1	17.5	5.4	1.3
1930	12.2	18.2	44.5	18.1	5.6	1.4
1935	10.2	16.7	46.7	19.1	5.7	1.5
1940	9.9	13.7	48.2	20.8	5.8	1.5
1945	11.5	11.9	46.5	22.1	6.3	1.6
1950	13.5	12.2	42.8	23.4	6.5	1.7
1955	12.4	14.7	39.7	24.5	6.9	1.8
1960	12.0	15.6	37.5	25.6	7.4	2.0
1965	11.7	14.7	37.4	26.1	8.2	2.0
1970	11.8	14.2	37.0	26.0	8.8	2.2
1975	10.9	14.3	38.1	24.9	9.3	2.5
1980	9.2	14.4	40.3	23.3	9.9	3.0
1985	8.6	12.8	42.9	22.0	10.3	3.4
1990	9.1	11.2	43.7	21.6	10.6	3.8

groups and structures, for examples, the establishment of health services and the corresponding formation of a medical profession has to be regarded as a new entity. The society, which had to be served by the new medical profession, was changing all the time. The economic basis for the development of public services, such as health care, was present, but was still not robust at the end of the nineteenth century. Urbanization and a new and more differentiated structure of the workforce had increased the need for medical services, and made it possible to establish them. The medical services were supported by domestic scientific activity and important medical innovations, which came in from abroad and widened the scope of practical medicine, which in turn increased the possibilities and prospects of the members of the profession.

5.2. The Demographic Transition

At some stage in their development, populations seem to undergo the so-called demographic transition. When studying populations from all over the world, one discovers that this quite amazing process starts at different times. In the course of a time span of various lengths some profound changes occur: The rates of deaths and births fall down from a stable level and stabilize on a new and lower level. In Norway, this transition took place in a period which by and large is covered by the nineteenth and the first of the twentieth century (Diagram 5.1).

As a rule, the rates for birth and deaths before the transition fluctuate with sharp peaks and pits around a reasonably stable mean value. After the transition, this oscillation is less obvious or even disappears. A social interpretation of this fact lies at hand: In the old society the hazards of life were so strong that their effects, far more directly than in the time to come, could be visibly deduced the vital statistics because the population was living on the margins of subsistence. A year with meager crops, epidemics, or a bad climate could be reflected in death tolls and birth rates in a way which was not the case when social conditions had improved.

But the demographic changes include another important element, the one which makes the word transition apply: The decline in death and birth rates does not occur at the same time.

The first sign of the demographic transition is a stable and lasting fall in mortality figures. The birth rate, however, remains at a high level for a longer period of time, usually some decades, before a pattern of decline

DIAGRAM 5.1

Births, deaths and emigration per 1,000 inhabitants in Norway 1740–1990

Before 1951 emigration to other continents, later net out-migration (emigration minus immigration) to all countries.

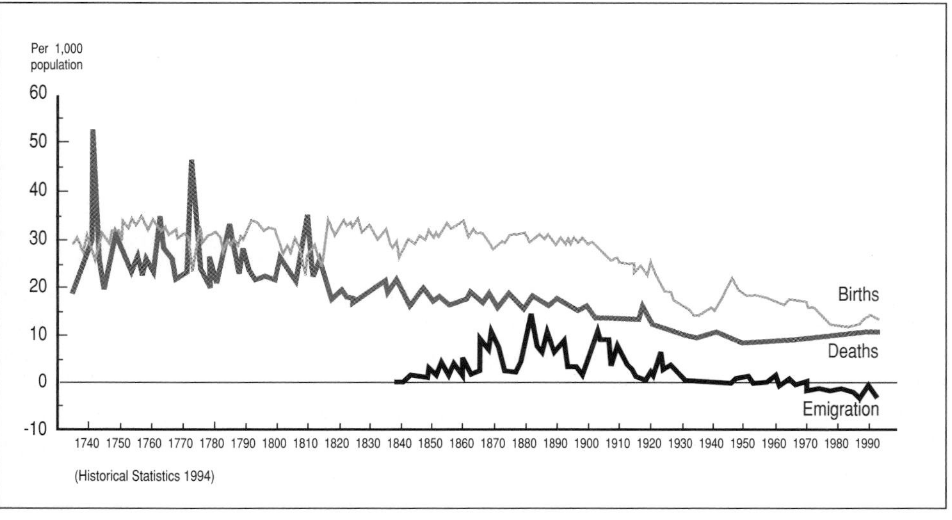

appears. Diagram 5.1 shows clearly how this phenomenon applies for Norway. The demographic effects of this time lag are obvious: The population increased sharply.

Infant mortality has proved to be a sensitive social indicator. If the declining mortality is interpreted as a sign of better living conditions, a fall in infant mortality should be expected, and that is just the case in Norway as well. As a consequence, larger and larger cohorts of young people emerge in the course of the demographic transition, challenge the structures of society, and spark secondary demographic processes such as internal migration, urbanization, development of new occupations, growth in economic sectors and so on.

In Norway, the decline in mortality started rather abruptly in 1815. The birth rates fell gradually from approximately 1890 and reached the new level around 1930. The turnover of people in the old society can be calculated from death and birth rates at around an average value of thirty per thousand. The new level is about one third, or ten per thousand. However, birth rates showed a new increase after World War II, and the population growth continued (Diagram 5.2).

DIAGRAM 5.2
Population in Norway 1665–1993

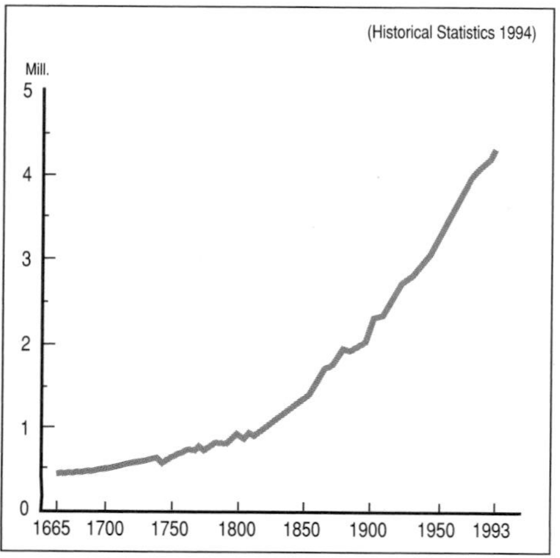

The Danish population, not being so severely affected by wartime at the beginning of the nineteenth century, had a smoother start of the same process some years prior to Norway. Sweden, on the other hand, followed suit only some years later. Finland and Iceland had a development which was strikingly different: The demographic transition in these countries did not start until the second half of the nineteenth century.

5.3. *Stirring Up the Society*

Following the standard transition model, the population of Europe virtually exploded during the nineteenth century. The population of Great Britain more than tripled in one hundred years, increasing from 11 to 38 million people. At the end of the century, Germany had 56 million inhabitants, starting out with only 23. The doubling of the Norwegian population, even as dramatic as it was felt to be here, was indeed a population growth at only a moderate pace, compared to what was going on elsewhere.

However, the social implications were immense in Norway as well. Since the population growth was a result of a decline in mortality, not of an increased birth rate, the increase in population numbers was clearly related to a rise in standard of living, which had forced back important causes of death. In the regions of the country and in the social layers where living conditions were marginal, and touching on the lowest subsistence level, even a slight amelioration would have an effect on the most vulnerable individuals, such as infants, people with chronic diseases, patients suffering from tuberculosis and nutritional diseases, and so on. But, this effect is obvious in, at least, part of what happened in the wake of the demographic transition, but less clear in other segments of the society, where an improved economy also might be accompanied by a less favorable health situation. Some words on migration may explain this point:

The breakup of people in rural districts as a consequence of population pressure was propagated by certain push factors. A pressure was present, based on the fact that in many local communities the prospects of making a living were unfavorable and limited, with few possibilities of absorbing an increasing number of inhabitants. Ninety percent of the Norwegians were living in rural areas in 1815. The units in agriculture were mostly small. Although cottagers were a significant group, social differences were not so marked, and the society was stable. A large increase in the population would disturb this stability and adaption to the available resources. There is, however, no reason to believe that famine and other extremities played any significant role in Norway; the conditions differed in this respect from those in countries where migration waves started because of such dramatic reasons.

In order to assess the impact of push factors on traditional society, it is necessary to consider the effect of the material and immaterial improvement on the standard of living. The agricultural region or the fishing village were perhaps still able to feed some more mouths under the old conditions, but they could not cope with the new expectations.

So the pull factors also had a considerable strength. During the period of modernization of the society, it was easy to observe that the potentials for economic growth were linked to urbanization and to activities in the cities and townships.

A Norwegian peculiarity, in this respect, was the shipping business, especially in the last half of the nineteenth century. The Norwegians had for a long time specialized in carrying freight by sailing ships, even at a time when steamers ploughed the seven seas at higher speed and with better regularity. As discussed by Hodne (Larsen, Berg Hodne 1986), this strategy, which exploited and stimulated local economy, proved to be a success for a considerable period. Sailing ships were relatively cheap to build and equip. They would be financed by capital which could be raised locally. Low personnel costs, with crews recruited in the home district, combined with a market that asked for low-cost transportation of goods and merchandise for which speed was not crucial, secured a solid economy for many smaller cities along the Norwegian coast for some decades. There was still a profit to be made, even from a delayed development.

Norwegian shipping not only stimulated the economy, but it turned the mind of the population towards the outside world. Many Norwegians in the past had tried out the sailor's life before entering another vocational career ashore.

When the clippers and the barques finally became outdated, and steamers took over in the Norwegian merchant fleet, problems arose in local economy. The building and running of a steamer mostly lay beyond the possibilities of small-scale shipowners in local communities. Shipping became centralized, cities prospered and townships suffered.

Compared to other countries in central Europe, Norway experienced a somewhat delayed industrial revolution. At the end of the nineteenth century, the structure of a modern, industrialized state was established. However, the transformation from a mainly rural old-style society also required a more diversified population. The need for educated people to run an administrative and social infrastructure increased; industry and crafts required skilled recruitment, and new vocations and professions emerged: Postal services, telephone and telegraph, railway and seaborn communications created new opportunities for making a career as a civil servant. Here, new possibilities also emerged for women to enter the workforce.

The need for education had at least two sets of social implications: On the one hand, when institutions for education were established, migration was stimulated. An example: Some vocational schools enrolled both sexes, for example, the so-called seminaries that educated primary school teachers. The result of this was often sweet music and subsequent marriage among the students. This illustrates how the development in general expanded the range for making contacts and consequently widening the geographical and social horizons of many Norwegians. On the other hand, to work as a school teacher, a nurse, an engineer or an official, a person usually had to settle in a district other than the one where he or she was born. Internal migration was stimulated.

The waves of internal migration rolled mostly from the countryside to the cities. But the migration of the largest quantitative significance went to the Christiania (Oslo) region. During the last quarter of the century, this city experienced a growth rate unprecedented in Norway: A small city on the northern shores of the Kristiania Fjord, slumbering beneath the walls of the Akershus fortress at the beginning of the century, had gained a respectable population of approximately 120,000 by 1875. In the years to come, urbanization accelerated at an even higher pace. At the turn of the century, 25 years later, the population had doubled, arriving at a remarkable 240,000.

The capital experienced a fever-like construction period. Workers were recruited from the surrounding regions, and so were horses, sleighs and carriages for transportation purposes. Quarries and tile companies were established to meet the requirements for heavy construction materials locally. Public sanitation and infrastructure, like the building of roads and streets, tramways, electricity plants, and distribution systems had to be established. To the new city, Berlin-like in its architecture, people moved in from the countryside. Second-generation city-dwellers were rare specimens in the capital those days; most of the citizens were young people, coming to seek work or education.

The housing had a standard which, at the outset, met the prevailing needs of a modern city. However, flats were expensive. The monthly rent was high. To supplement the family's finances, rooms were hired out. The apartment houses then could be simply overcrowded. Such overcrowding strained the urban infrastructure and was also of medical interest: Contagious diseases could spread very easily, and the possibility of being sick in bed at home became limited for large parts of the population. This fact prompted a development similar to other large cities hospitals with a large capacity had to be established. Ullevål Sykehus in Kristiania, at the time of the opening in 1887, was designed to care for patients with infectious diseases. It was constructed in accordance with the so-called pavilion system for avoiding and eliminating contagious vapors, the miasmas; and it became in the early twentieth century one of the largest hospitals in the Nordic countries.

At the end of the twentieth century, class differences in Norway took on a new dimension. Of course there existed social distinctions between the rich and the poor, but now also between the not-so-rich layers of civil servants, doctors, clergy, school teachers and so on and the less-educated classes. In the countryside, the strong social position of the Norwegian farmer was a fact that even had a political impact on a national level. Over the years the independent Norwegian farmer has maintained a certain status that can not be measured simply in terms of economy.

The social barriers were reflected in the capital even in its architecture. Posh bourgeois palaces in the west of the city contrast-

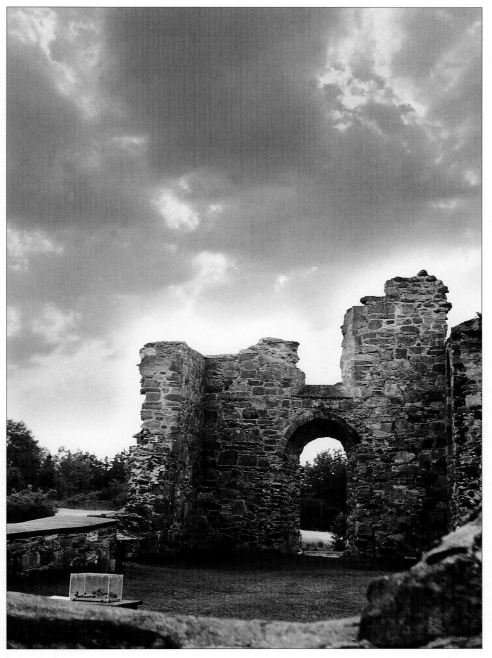

Figure 5: In medieval times, medical activity in the monasteries also played a significant role in Norway. Remnants of the church on Tautra, an island in the Trondheim fiord (Photo: Øivind Larsen 1996).

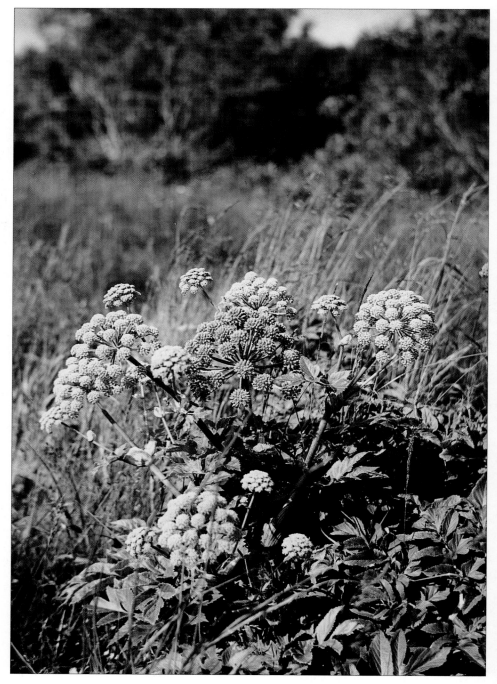

Figure 6: In Norway, as elsewhere, local plants were widely used in folk medicine, both for prevention and cure. The beautiful "kvann" (angelica officinalis) is a prime example: it could be used for many purposes. Its effectiveness against scurvy was especially well known. The specimen shown here was photographed on a shore in the county of Nordland (Photo: Øivind Larsen 1996).

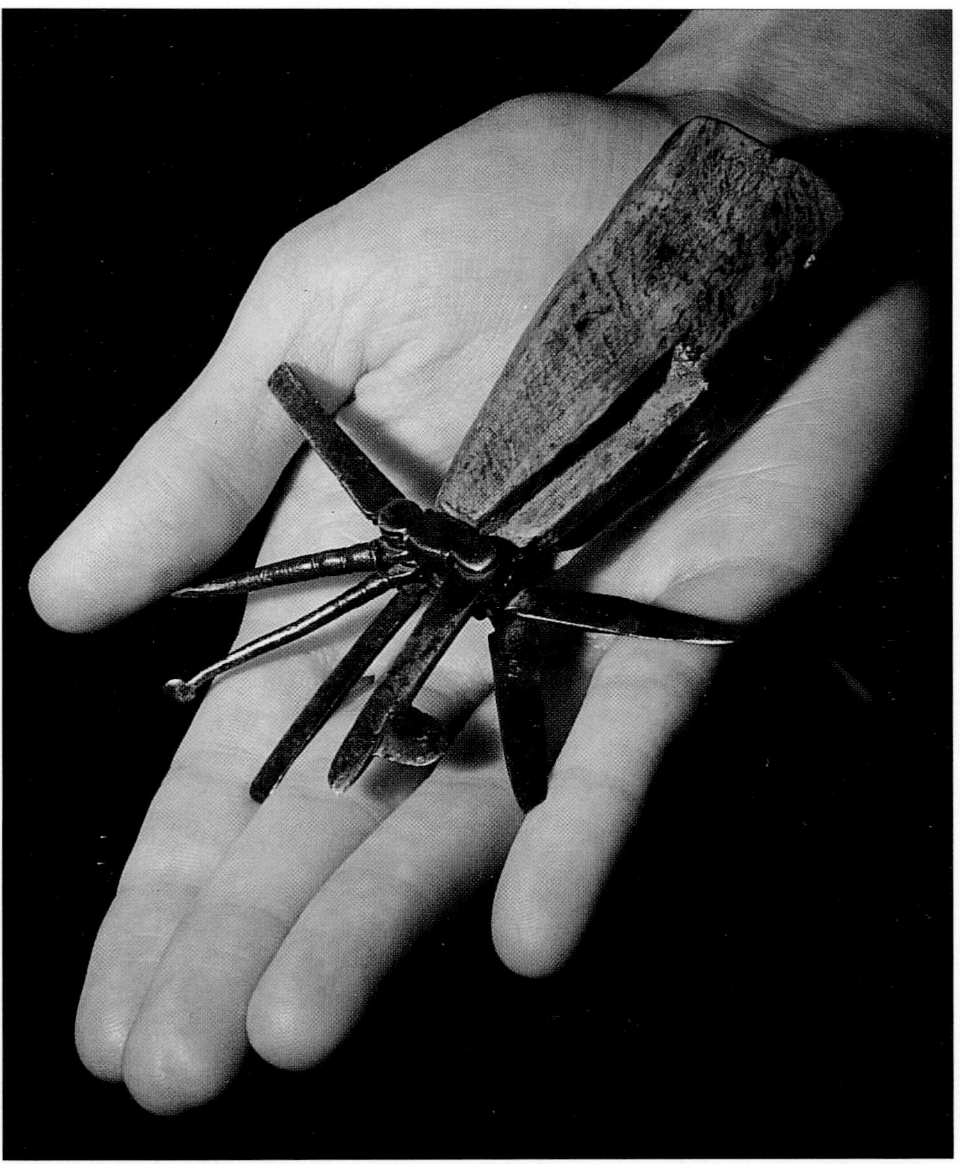

Figure 7: A homemade instrument, kept for generations on a farm in Øvre Eiker, Eastern Norway. The bloodletting iron is clearly visible (Photo: Øivind Larsen 1995).

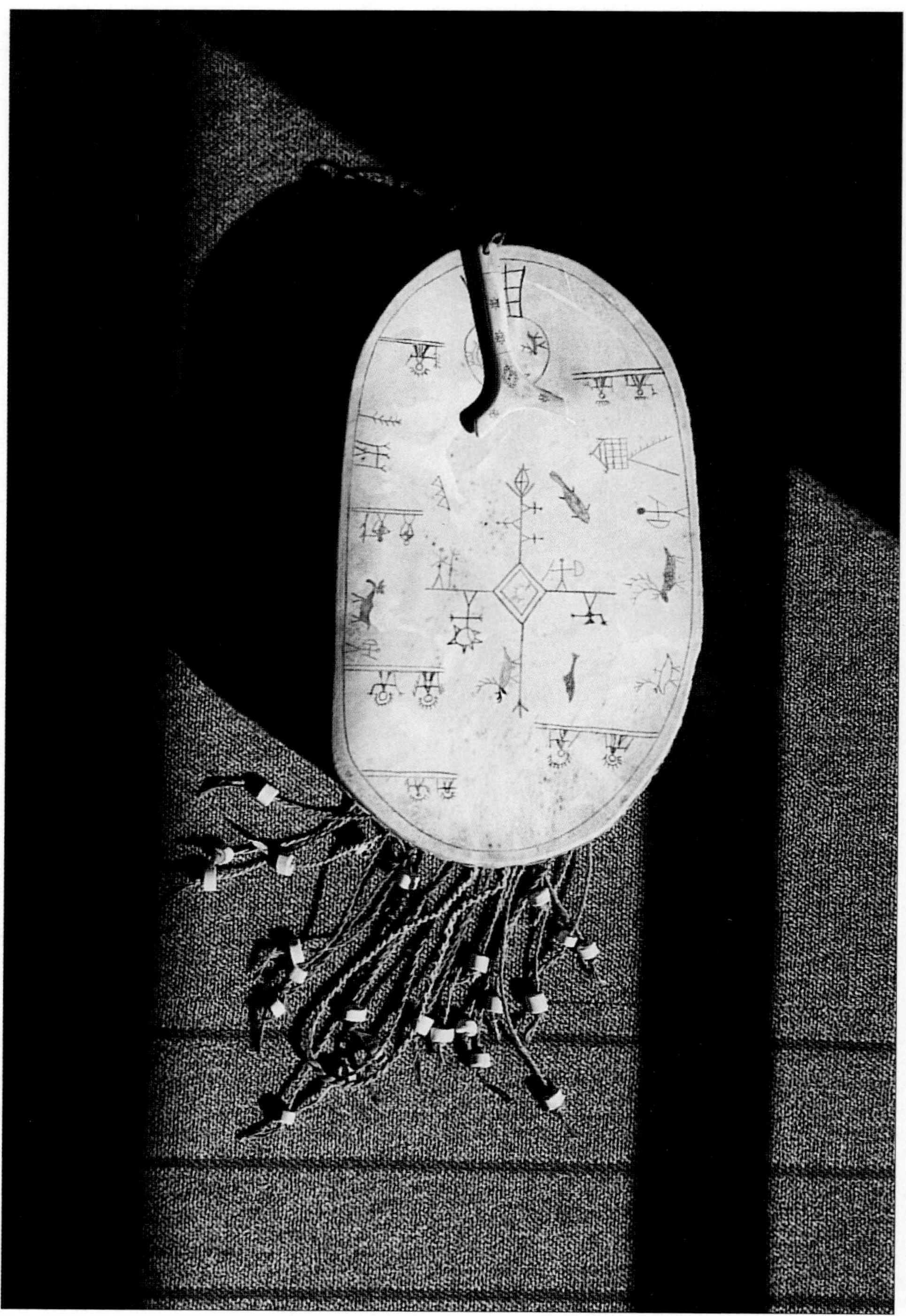

Figure 8: The magic drum of the Lapps (runebommen) was also used in the local folk medicine. The drum shown here belongs to the museum in Kautokeino in Finnmark (Photo: Øivind Larsen 1989).

ed with more modest and humble dwellings in the east.

Still, the position of a housemaid became an important category of jobs for young females from the countryside, even a post with one of the less-well-off families of the urban society. For a young girl to leave home and become a housemaid in Kristiania was an important way of entering the labor market, or achieving vocational training for a future life as a housewife.

The history of the Norwegian population during the nineteenth century, decades of combining a demographic transition with a social modernization, is not complete without a consideration of the migration waves reaching abroad. The emigration went mainly to the United States of America. The numbers of people who packed their belongings and left were remarkably large. In the light of a situation in which a population of one million in 1823 passed the second million in 1891, an emigration of about 800,000 people during the period between 1840 and 1930 is quite impressive. The emigration rate was so large that it touched on the rates of mortality: the number of mostly young people leaving the country was nearly the same as the yearly number of deaths. In the emigration wave of 1866 to 1873, 111,000 persons embarked on emigrant ships bound for overseas. This amounted to 59 percent of the birth surplus. The fourth emigration period after World War I was also heavy. Only Ireland experienced more emigration than Norway during the years 1851 to 1935.

The impact of the demographic processes is an important issue in social research. Life expectancy increased, a fact on the positive side. Locally and nationally it is more concerning to note that much of the internal migration and emigration caused just young people to leave. And what were the differences between the various parts of the country, and between the social layers? Just one example: the decline of the birth rates around 1890 started in urban areas and in the higher classes, with a delay for rural districts and working-class families. What did this mean for the social composition of the population?

The social dimensions of migration are also of importance. Who left? Who stayed? The medical profession had to care for the remaining population in the countryside and for the newly settled, young, and unstable population in the cities as well. It was mandatory for the doctors of the nineteenth century to understand the processes at work, in order to be able to handle the medical problems. The same knowledge is required today in order to get the right historical impressions of the past. The number of physicians increased, and the population\physician rate was more and more favorable, but the medical and social realities had also changed.

5.4. *Health or Prosperity?*

The so-called epidemiological transition is a process that belongs to the twentieth century. In the latter half of the nineteenth centu-

DIAGRAM 5.3
Expected lifespan 1820–1980

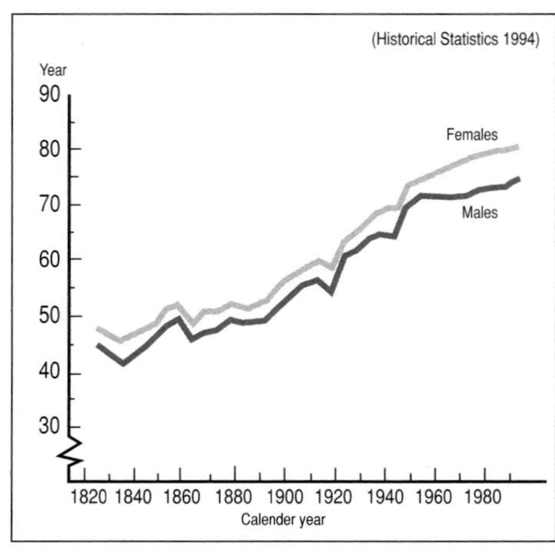

DIAGRAM 5.4
Survivors for different birth cohorts at different ages, Norwegian men. (Redrawn after Borgan 1982 in Larsen and Heiberg 1983)

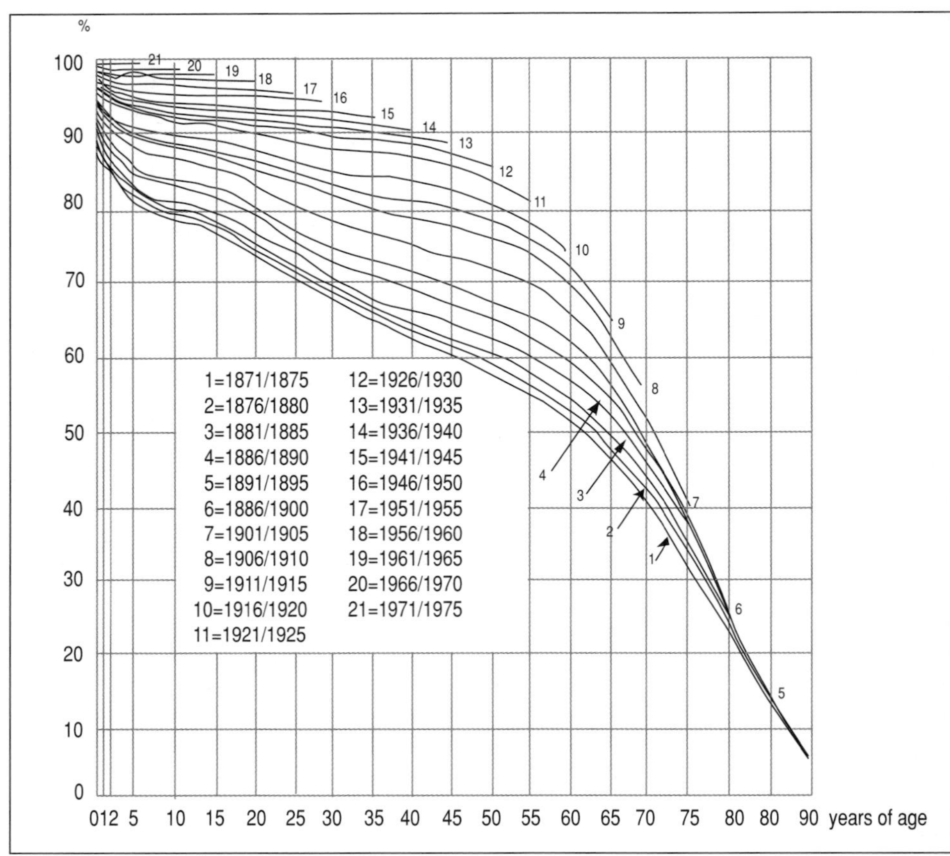

ry, microorganisms were identified as the agents responsible for most of the important diseases and health problems of the population. A series of innovations within the biological sciences, shifting paradigms in medical thinking, and new epidemiological experience gathered during epidemics which were obviously prompted and worsened through demographic processes, made up the scientific basis for numerous promising discoveries within microbiology.

However, medical history tells us that it took more than half a century, until after World War II, before effective therapeutics that specifically killed bacteria became generally available and made the conquest of infectious diseases possible.

The immediate effect of these discoveries was to establish a better understanding of how to prevent infectious diseases. So the decline of the infections gradually proceeded from the turn of the nineteenth century onward, as a combined result of applied medical knowledge and a qualitative increase in welfare and living conditions. Diseases did not disappear from the society. Although the health of the young generally improved, new diseases appeared in the older population,

DIAGRAM 5.5
Schoolgirls in Oslo, mean body weight (From Statistical yearbook for the city of Oslo 1956 and Liestøl 1981, here reproduced after Falkum and Larsen 1981.)

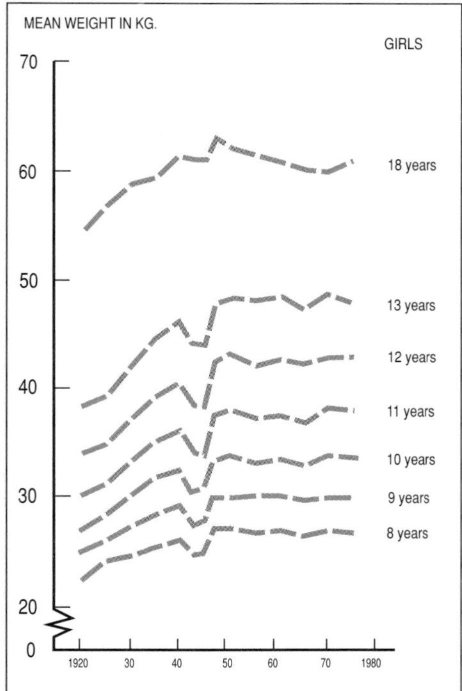

posing new medical problems. Heart disease, cancer, and chronic diseases caused by the wear and tear of a long life were not new to the medical profession, but the new demographic situation resulted in a steady increase in the numbers of this type of patient. This transition has been observed in different societies with the regularity of a biological law.

The changes reflect themselves in several demografic variables. For example, the survival prospects (Diagram 5.3 and 5.4) and the weight curves of children (Diagram 5.5) show that Norway gradually becomes another country. And the health services change profoundly (Diagram 5.6).

The epidemiological statistics, suggest that another regularity exists as well, a sort of transition that might be called the medical urbanization transition, a transition that links the two others together: When migration starts, incidence and prevalence of infectious diseases increase among the mobile and newly settled groups of the population (Larsen, Haugtomt, Platou, 1980). A transition from one type of economic situation to another also is a transition from one sort of health sitation to another. Mapping of morbidity and mortality figures clearly shows how infections ravage the demographically most unstable regions. In the year 1882, for example, 51.8 cases per 1000 of acute diarrhea were registered in Kristiania, against only 3.9 cases in the county of Nordre Bergenhus (today: Sogn og Fjordane). Possible differences in registration cannot outweigh this immense difference and a large number of similar observations for a series of infectious diseases.

The interest in contagious venereal diseases was obviously increasing in the nineteenth century. Did sexual morality undergo a profound transition? To discuss this, it is necessary to have the demographic processes in mind. For example, Kristiania, the most attractive region to move to, at the end of the century was filled with young people, many of them unmarried and without partners at the time of arrival. Given the prosperous economy, at least for some people, and the desperate need for money among others, why question that promiscuity flourished?

And when, generally speaking, no effective treatment was at hand for the sexually transmitted diseases, and the contagiousness of a patient could last for years, no wonder that the danger of inherited syphilis or the hygienic and moral problems of prostitution were taken up in public discussion, in literature, and in the visual arts.

Linked to the demographic processes and to the forces behind them, this medical urbanization transition put forward basic sociohistorical questions: To what extent

DIAGRAM 5.6
Physicians and Population per physician 1860–1985

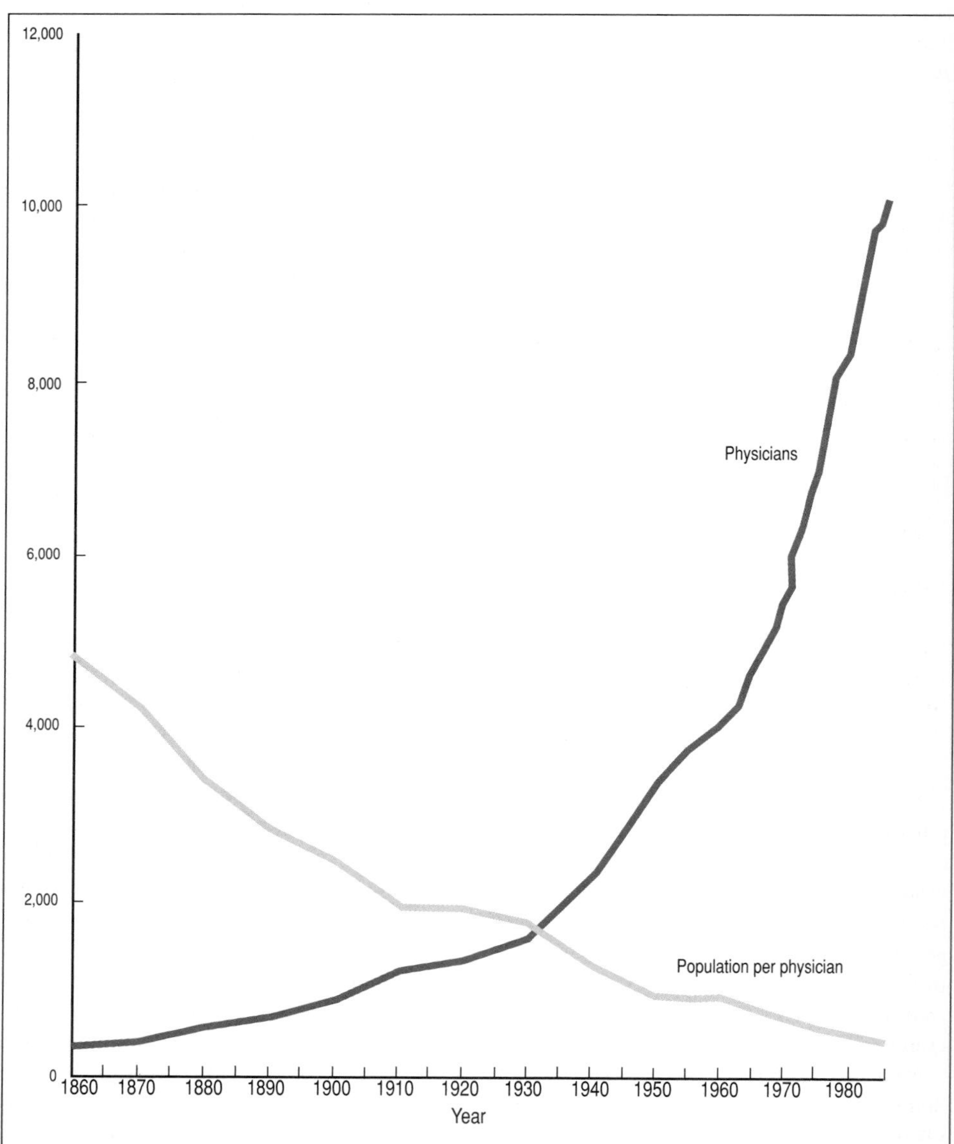

was the move up to and the choice of a new place to live in, a calculated risk? How much did the search for welfare, education, and prosperity sacrifice in terms of diseases and health risks? To what extent was the decision to break up a compromise between conflicting interests, where health for the family was the losing part? To what extent was the higher infant mortality in urban areas, the crowded housing, and the greater risk of attracting infectious diseases something regarded as inevitable in the development of the society? And to what extent was the first generation of urban migrants made up of guest workers who endured hardship because they felt that their real home was elsewhere, and nurtured plans or dreams of moving back home again?

Studies indicate that such risk considerations really existed. A content analysis (Larsen & al. 1980; see chapter 9.0) of the verbal evaluation of the health situation in rural and urbanized counties, as compared to the figures of the health statistics for the period 1868 to 1900, based on the reports of the district health physicians, shows that for a period much more disease seems to have been accepted in urban areas than in the countryside. The closest interpretation of this phenomenon is very simple: Disease was accepted as a price to pay for the economic growth. But did the people know?

There is a turning point. Around 1890, at the same time as fertility rates started to decline, the incidence of infectious diseases in the densely populated areas of the country follows a similar pattern of decline. Was there a shift in the general assessment of contagious diseases and the attitudes toward them?

It is interesting to observe that the changes in attitudes appeared just after several years of a raging diphtheria epidemic. Children became severely ill, and a considerable number of the sick were torn away in a painful death. The cruel face of the contagious diseases, as experienced from 1885 onward, has probably never appeared in the same way in Norway in modern times. What did this experience mean to the public? Was there any connection between the child mortality and the birth rates? If so, what was the casuality? Did conceptions go down as a psychological effect of the mending of suffering children? Or the other way around, did conception numbers fall when the needs and wishes for replacement and securing succession posed by the epidemics diminished in strength?

5.5 *Health and Culture*

The last decades of the nineteenth century brought a turmoil of development in almost all segments of the Norwegian society. Politically, the ties with Sweden were strained, leading to the final dissolution of the union and establishment of national independence in 1905. The introduction of parliamentarism in 1884 was another sign of erupting forces beneath the surface.

In Norway, a national identity in the fields of visual arts, literature, and music also emerged at the same time. Heroic polar expeditions made Norwegians proud and made Norway known abroad.

It is interesting to contemplate the extent to which this cultural growth was a result of the processes of the demographic transition and the social changes: Gifted persons could now have opportunities to develop their talents. Artists described and made interpretations of what they saw. They looked upon their time with open eyes.

On the other hand, to what extent did the arts, the paintings, or the novels and plays from the era of social realism exert an impact on social development? Is there a process at work the other way around, too?

Reverting to medicine, when topics dealing with health and sickness appear in the visual arts, emotions and attitudes come out into the open, passing on from the sphere to the public field of action. Dramatic paintings of sick children, especially the favored motive of the sick girl, are an example of how human problems were put on the agenda.

Reviewing the medical and social history reveals an abundance of evidence of how health, disease, and misery were ever present as motives for artists and as the content of a new culture.

The end of the nineteenth century was indeed a fin de siecle.

References

Larsen, Ø., O. Berg and F. Hodne. *Legene og samfunnet*. Oslo: Den norske lægeforening, 1986.

Larsen, Ø, H. Haugtomt and W. Platou. *Sykdomsoppfatning og epidemiologi 1860–1900.* Oslo: Seksjon for medisinsk historie, Universitetet i Oslo, 1980.

Larsen, Ø. "Vekst i byen og helse på landet – noen trekk ved folkehelse og befolkningsutvikling på slutten av 1800-tallet." *Jord og Gjerning,* 5(1991):66–78.

CHAPTER 6

The Professionalization of Physicians in Nineteenth-century Norway

BENT OLAV OLSEN

6.1 Towards a Definition

In history and sociology, articles and books that in various ways treat the concept of "profession" are abundant, and the discussion of the issue is a scientific field in its own right. But in medical history professionalization is also important, because it makes up part of the framework that medicine and health develops within. And the interest is increasing. A sign of this is that professionalization was the theme of the Fielding H. Garrison lecture at the annual meeting of the American Association for the History of Medicine in Pittsburgh, Pennsylvania in 1995, where John C. Burnham reviewed how the concept of profession has evolved in the field of the history of medicine (Burnham 1996).

The chapters of this book treat and explain the development of the Norwegian medical profession in different ways. Here, however, the profession is seen in a national perspective: What is our history of the medical profession like?

This chapter is meant as an introduction to a discussion of some processes and trends related to the development of the Norwegian medical profession, with emphasis on the nineteenth century.

Norwegian sociologists and historians have been interested in physicians as belonging to the group of occupations which usually are termed professions. One of the most influential scientists in Norwegian studies of professions, Ulf Torgersen, stated in 1972 that important attributes of a profession are a long, formal education, aquired by persons who are oriented towards pursuing certain occupations, occupations where such education, as dictated by social norms, is obligatory for entrance. The profession has in fact an occupational monopoly.

He also held the view that medicine was the most typical profession, because in medicine, education, motivation, and occupational monopoly were closely tied together.

In the 1990s, however, Torgersen writes that his original interest in the linkage of higher theoretical education and occupation, and the distinction between profession and non-profession, has been somewhat tuned down (Torgersen 1994).

But from the point of view which seems sensible in medical history, the elements mentioned by Torgersen in 1972 still serve as a useful and operational definition.

6.2 The Term Profession, Some Comments

6.2.1 Different Use of Words

The variations in the use of the term *profession* is somewhat confusing. Using the concepts profession and professional without an explicit definition is problematic, because some clues automatically adhere from everyday use of both the word *profession* and the word *professional*, from the use of the concepts by different theoretical traditions, and from the use of the concept by the professions themselves. And the attributes of the "original" professions, medicine, theology, and law differ in many respects from professions on the make, semi-professions, or what ever we choose to call them.

Is the distinction between professions and other occupational groups really a good tool for examining the social division of labor? Has it turned out that since the theoretical work on professions, including the definition or listing of attributes of professions, has been so closely connected to the "original" professions, there will be no room for other full-fledge members of this group of occupations? Is there then a basis for the idea of professions, the idea that some occupations are, and still will be, basically different from regular occupations? Does the common concept of profession include possibilities for change, for a development of the definitions? In other words, is the idea of professions, as commonly held, linked to a particular historical situation, so that at some future time perhaps professions in the present sense will not exist?

The title of this book, "The Shaping of a Profession," is meant to indicate that, in our view, "profession" is not a static concept. By reading other chapters, the reader will learn how the role of the physician in Norway has changed, and that the processes that shape the profession have been subject to continuous change. Although some aspects of the profession's view of being a professional, being a doctor, remain stable for long periods, so that the professional self-image probably is the most stable part of the concept, it has been influenced by developments in medicine, in science, and in society at large. Concepts such as these are dynamic; "profession" changes, and the complex process of professionalization contributes to it.

Most readers would probably easily agree with Greenwood in the following description of what the sociological approach to professions is: This approach views professions as an organized group, which is constantly interacting with the society that forms its matrix, which performs its social functions through a network of formal and informal relationships, and which creates its own subculture, requiring adjustments to it as a prerequisite for career success (Greenwood 1957, p. 45). The problem is that this approach would more or less fit sociological approaches to many other groups in society. Such a definition is hardly precise enough to fit the special traits of the group of physicians.

One can treat the concept of professions as a "folk concept." Professions exist in the way that the term is widely used; people have an idea of what a "profession" is. For example, most people would categorize physicians as members of a professional group. And the physicians themselves certainly do; the idea of belonging to a profession has been internalized. Consequently, members of professions often defy attempts to locate them within the context of traditional social categories; they worry about signs of decay in their professional status, or they react against attempts by other occupational groups, or by the state, to limit their power. The fact that the concept is widely used is one of the main reasons for still using it.

Most views of what a profession is have one important trait in common: They describe a unified group, which the members are socialized into. To be a member of the profession therefore also includes maintaining this socialization. This explains the occasional defensiveness that members of professions sometimes display.

6.2.2 Attributes of a Profession

The task of defining *profession* often leads to setting up a list of attributes. Greenwood and other scientists in what we might call the "attribute school" of the sociology of professions, typically set up lists like this: "all professions seem to possess: (1) systematic theory, (2) authority, (3) community sanction, (4) ethical codes, and (5) a culture" (Greenwood 1957, p.45).

Writers within this school could be criticized because they do not study the process of professionalizing, but they participate in it, and have borrowed the professions self-conception as a basis for their analyses and that they have become dupes of the established professions, helping them to justify their dominant position (Roth 1974).

But such lists may have valuable information, so let us take a closer look on some of the attributes that are meant to be typical of the professions.

6.2.3 Skill and Theory

Professional skill in itself is not the main difference between members of the professions and members of non-professional occupations. The important matter is the fact that professionals have obtained an almost monopolistic possession of their specific skills; they hold the knowledge of how something is done, which most other people do not. And the way this control is obtained and guarded is an important matter. In medicine, this monopolistic possession of skill and knowledge is a reflection of the Hippocratic oath, where the oath-swearer swears to teach only those who are also oath-swearers.

The profession's skills are supported by a fund of knowledge that has been "organized into an internally consistent system, called a *body of theory*" (Greenwood 1957, p.46). The understanding of theory is one of the reasons why intellectual as well as practical experience is important. The education of professionals is not merely the learning of skills. A partial effect of education is that students are being socialized; education is like being initiated into a lodge.

6.2.4 Research and Rationality?

In the professionalization of an occupation, research is important, and the function of research is diverse. One important function is the symbolic raising of an occupation to a more fully professional standing.

A science-based rationality is closely connected with the professions. This is a view that is also held by many professionals. And many would agree with Greenwood that "rationality is the antithesis of traditionalism" (Greenwood 1957, p.47). This might be true, but for many professionals, traditionalism and a reverential attitude towards their own theoretical system, their scientific "beliefs," is part of belonging to a profession.

6.2.5 Customers and Clients. Commercial Attitude Versus Professional Attitude.

Parsons states that the commercial attitudes are the antithesis to the professional attitudes (Parsons 1937). But Parsons makes explicit that both professional members and businessmen are motivated by a desire for success (Parsons 1939). And that encouragement of the professional attitude is one of the most effective ways of promoting disinterestedness in contemporary society, because valuing knowledge for its own sake is an integral part of the professional spirit.

What comes close to this idea of the professional attitude in contrast to the commercial attitude is the idea of the professional as having some sort of a calling. No longer do law or medicine make a strong claim to be motivated by some sort of calling. Commitment to a set of values is no longer in itself a dominant or general motivation for entering and working in these professions. Of the original professions, priests are the ones who, understandably, claim a calling as their central motivation. But, in the nineteenth century, the idea of calling probably was a more central element in the physicians self-image, although this assumption is difficult to document.

To Greenwood, the knowledge held by the professional contrasts with the layman's comparative ignorance, and this is the basis for the professional's authority (Greenwood 1957, p.47). In line with other researchers, Greenwood makes a distinction based on the fact that non-professionals have customers and professionals have clients. Greenwood states that whereas the customer is always right, the client is dictated to by the professional. The client has little choice but to accept a professional judgment; however, this is an authority limited to the professional sphere.

Greenwood probably overestimates the power of the customer, as he turns slogans into theory. Making a living in medicine may sometimes mean giving the patients what they want. It may also be that since the time of Greenwood's article in 1957, a new breed of patient has emerged; patients are now more involved in their own general health care than before. And the lack of dictatorial professional power is shown even more clearly when "potential clients are frequently in a position to decide whether or not they will use a professional service and the extent to which they will follow the advice given" (Roth 1974, p.8).

By limiting the professional power to the professional sphere, the power of the professional in real life probably is underestimated. There seems to be no doubt that in other fields of life professionals "borrow" authority from their professional status, and that "key professionals are becoming generalized wise men" (McKinlay 1973, p.74).

6.2.6 Some Other Characteristics

Knowledge monopolies the ability to control how their work is to be accomplished, to master the theoretical base for it, and to control the development are among the major sources of professional power.

Another characteristic of professional power is gatekeeping, that is, institutionalized control over desired resources or entitlements. Professional judgment becomes a tool and a professional marker. As may be seen from other chapters in this book, the authority inherent in the role as a public health officer, a representative of the state, reinforced the gatekeeping role of the district physician, and probably contributed to the general reputation and status of Norwegian physicians in the second half of the nineteenth century.

Greenwood, among many others, in his list of characteristics of professions stresses the importance of a professional culture. And while it is not certain that the culture of the professions differs basically from that of other occupations, some aspects of this culture obviously have contributed to the shaping of the professions. In Norway, this culture among the physicians was strong from the earliest years of a national medicine, with the history of the Norwegian Medical Association and its predecessor being an important element (Larsen, Berg, Hodne, 1986).

Attributes of professions might be interesting, but mainly as outcomes of professionalization.

6.2.7 Professions and Closure

Closure as a concept was first outlined by Max Weber (1864-1920), and social closure is closely linked to the study of professions. Professions seek to achieve market control and collective social mobility by this means. In a Weberian sense, closure refers to the monopolization of advantages by one group, by closing of opportunities to other groups. Parkin, a neo-Weberianist, identifies two reciprocal modes of closure:(1) exclusion, that is, power directed downward; and (2) usurpation, power directed upwards.

There is basically one thing that makes professions different from other occupations: the process whereby a group of people, by different methods, gains nearly monopolistic control over some tasks in the social division of labor. Professions, for Freidson," are those occupations exercising the capacity to create exclusive shelters in the labor market for accepted practitioners through the monopolization of educational training and credentials required for the attainment of economic opportunities in the market" (Brint 1993, p 262).

But the power of the professions goes beyond that. They also set the terms for how central aspects of life are thought about. This is probably a main element in the modern attacks on the medical profession; surrounded by highly educated fellow citizens, and existing in a society with strong democratic traditions, the profession no longer is in the position to set the stage for thinking about medical matters.

6.2.8 Time and Place Make a Difference

Professions in different countries follow different paths. The different professions change with time and place. The literature on professions is dominated by the Anglo-American tradition. Some of the differences in time and place shall be highlighted: "The nineteenth century professional ideology of public service developed in a society in which the professions were typified by the independent practitioner in the twentieth century most professionals work for large scale organizations" (Duman 1979, p.131).

In this quote from Duman, the profession is a dynamic concept, but the generalization is not sensitive to place and not sensitive to the differences between professions. In a discussion of de-professionalization and proletarization, Freidson (1983) said that salaried employment has been the rule for professionals, not the exception. He also noted that only the legal and medical professions were typically self-employed in the past. But in Norway there has been a long tradition of salaried employment for the medical profession, and the district physician, who as a rule has been at least partly paid as a civil servant, constituted an important image of the physician in the eyes of both the public and the professionals themselves. In comparison to other countries, source of payment is not a typical profession marker in Norway, and in the course of time it has become even less important, because a major part of the physicians are salaried in one way or another. It is not likely that a possible shift in a liberal direction would be able to change this.

6.3. Norwegian Physicians and the Struggle for Professional Control

6.3.1 Norwegian Physicians, Both Liberal Professionals and Civil Servants

At the beginning of the nineteenth century, the Norwegian society was dominated by the state, and the state by its civil servants. In the ideology of civil servants, this dominance was not oriented toward group interests; they felt a national responsibility, and saw themselves as the class that was carrying the burden of promoting national development and modernization (Larsen et al. 1986). In such a society, there was a limited need for academics to organize. The civil servants were already part of the strongest institution in society, the state. Professionalization would only loosen this association.

There is reason to question whether or

not the physicians in the early nineteenth century could be termed a profession. Previously the surgeons had been organized in guilds, that had a strong control over their part of the work market. Surgeons guilds were comparable to the guilds of other craftsmen, but to call them a profession would be to push the similarities in organization too much. When a national medicine was established in Norway, medical work was no longer a craft calling for a guild-like organization. In the minutes of the Medical Society in Christiania from 1848 onwards, there is some material that supports the idea that physicians as a group were aspiring for more power. In 1849 Professor Christen Heiberg (1799–1872) started a discussion about whether the Society should take an initiative to improve the position of physicians in relation to the state. Later in the same year there is a reference to a feeling among physicians that they were not being heard in matters that concerned them and where they were the experts. As a result of both these discussions, a committee was being set up, but the important thing to notice is the emergence of the thought that physicians as a group had interests that conflicted with those of society at large.

The newspaper *Morgenbladet*, aimed several attacks at the physicians. In 1850, Frans Christian Faye (1806–1890) referred to an article in this newspaper in which it had been proposed that physicians should be obliged to perform official duties for a fixed price. This was strongly objected to, because physicians were said to have a moral obligation to do these tasks. Even so, this moral obligation should not be used to degrade the calling of the physician, or to turn him into a slave. Physicians were used to doing salaried work, but they reacted whenever new regulations were placed on their work.

Beginning in 1854, as a reaction to what the physicians regarded as low wages and few possibilities for advancement in the army and navy, all candidates refrained from applying for military posts. The physicians boycott of the military from 1854 on was the first strong professional opposition to the state. The boycott was not terminated until the parliament voted an increase of wages in 1861. One hundred fifty-eight physicians participated in this group in 1859, nearly half of all Norwegian physicians. This can be seen as the first example of a reaction by the physicians as a professional body.

The "civil servant state" gradually eroded during the nineteenth century, but the physicians still sought association with it.

6.3.2. Monopoly or Liberalism?

The controversy between folk medicine and physicians in Norway also involves the problem of effectively creating and maintaining a professional monopoly. During the first half of the nineteenth century, traditionally important groups of health personnel, the surgeons, army-surgeons and barber-surgeons, were no longer allowed to practice. Midwifes and dentists had their education increasingly controlled by physicians. In the nineteenth century, both the closure process directed toward, and also the control over, other professions was successful, but the problem of quacks remained throughout the nineteenth century, partialy due to politics.

Quacks represent a peculiarity when it comes to defining the bounderies of a profession. For example, in Norway in the eighteenth century, there were women who had been married to a physician, a surgeon, or a barber, and who had inherited their husband's right to a medical practice, but were not allowed to perform any of the tasks of the profession. A few of these women are named in the first edition of Norges Leger (The Physicians of Norway). They were included in the profession by the editor, because with this right to a medical practice, they could employ a qualified professional who could practice under their name. It is not known whether these women practiced themselves.

6.3.3 The Politics in Legalizing Folk Medicine

In the nineteenth century, little risk was involved in the practice of folk medicine, in spite of the decree of 5 September 1794. This decree proclaimed that treatment of sick people by non-physicians was subject to punishment.

In Norway, especially in the first half of the nineteenth century, access to physicians was limited and difficult. Throughout the nineteenth century, it was possible for some practitioners of folk medicine and mere quacks to have a rather profitable practice. Although physicians reported quacks who were practicing in their area, lawsuits against them were often stopped before they even came to court. Without any serious consequences for the unauthorized practitioner, even an undisguised practice could be kept up for a long time.

Folk medicine was not something that was solely or even predominantly a phenomenon in the peripheral regions. The most famous Norwegian female practitioner of folk medicine was Anna Sæther (1793–1851), who practiced in Christiania. Her qualifications were uncertain; some articles mention that she had learned anatomy by assisting students in the anatomy room (Nordhagen 1984 and Haugholt 1958). One of her descendants alleged that she had studied medicine under Doctor Jens Essendrop Knoph (1792–1829) (Haugholt 1958). The lawsuit against her revealed that Anna Sæther was consulted by all strata of society (Bø 1972).

In principle, the physicians had a monopoly on medical practice. The farmers and their parliamentary representatives, especially Søren Jaabæk (1814–1894), attacked the doctors' monopoly and also district physicians during the second half of the nineteenth century. On principle, the farmers were opposed to monopolies. The wish to limit government expenditures and a quest for an absolute liberalism were at the core of the farmers' opposition to professional monopolies (Seip 1994). This development was feared by the physicians, and several of them pointed to the comparable, but even more drastic development in America. In 1871 some changes were made in the laws on quackery, in principle opening up the practice of medicine to anyone who got a license from the king. As far as we know, no one ever got such license, but the signal given by this law was rather clear, and certainly understood by both physicians and quacks alike.

And it is clear that if we find certain forms of exclusion necessary or legitimate, we only say that they are accepted as necessary and legitimate in a particular context. There is no reason to believe that the role of the physician and the nature of professional power will remain unchanged, or that we have seen the end-point of a development.

6.4. *Challenge and Dynamics*

It is crucial to maintain the dynamic aspect when looking at the history of a professional group such as the physicians. The intention of this book is hopefully in line with the strategy outlined by Freidson: "studying occupations as individual empirical cases, rather than as specimens of some more general fixed concept" (Freidson 1983).

During the last decades there have been evident changes in the role and power of the professions. From the perspective of the profession these threats may be of different types, which will be further discussed in the other chapters of this book.

Deprofessionalization (see Haug 1973 and 1975) is the decline in the distinctiveness of the professions as a special kind of occupation. It means loss of the special position of public esteem and trust. However, as Friedson observes, "There is no evidence that professions have been singled out for special opprobrium" (Freidson 1983, p.285). A declining "competence gap" is felt, with the consequence that there is less willingness to accept the authority of professional expertise. But it is certainly a fact that "The professions have not stood still while the public has advanced in sophistication" (ibid.). Traditional professional services have become so simplified and routinized that lay people may do it themselves, or nonprofessionals or computers may take over the tasks. And yet "there has been a concomitant development of new, more complex areas of work that require highly professional skills" (ibid.). Finally, more and more professionals are employed by large organizations, becoming vulnerable to the control of their work by bureaucratization. But the important question is whether the bureaucratization is in the hands of the profession in question? "The consequence of credentialing for large organizations, is that who may perform what tasks, is in part determined from *outside* the organization. This means that the work professionals do, the way they do it, and the technical criteria by which that work is organized and evaluated, remain the domain of the professions" (ibid., p.286).

The other interpretation of the trend, proletarization, is "the process by which an occupational category is divested of control over certain prerogatives relating to the location, content, and essentially of its task activities and is thereby subordinated to the broader requirements of production under advanced capitalism" (McKinlay & Arches 1985, p.161). Or put more simply: "professions joining other occupations in the process of proletarianization drift down into the ranks of the working class, exploited by and in opposition to the interests of capital" (Freidson 1983, p.282)

In Norway, as well as in many other parts of the world, for a long time the professions enjoyed relatively uncritical public esteem, important influence on legislation, and economic rewards far less dependent on the normal marketplace than other occupations" (ibid., p.279). The uncritical public esteem, if it ever existed, has more or less disappeared, but the protected market, the monopoly, is still there.

The readers of this attempt to look at the development of a national medical professional group, a profession in the theoretical sense described here, should have the dynamics in mind, look at how it is continuously challenged, and certainly make their own judgment of the outcome.

References

Brint, S. "Eliot Freidson's Contribution to the Sociology of Professions," *Work Occupation*, 20(1993):259–278.

Burnham, J.C. "How the Concept of Profession Evolved in the Work of Historians of Medicine," *Bulletin of the History of Medicine*, 70(1996):1–24.

Bø, O. *Folkemedisin og lærd medisin: nordisk medisinsk kvardag på 1800-tallet*. Oslo: Samlaget, 1972.

Duman, D. "The creation and diffusion of a professional ideology in nineteenth century England," *Sociological Review* 27 (1979):113–138.

Freidson, E. "The Reorganization of the Professions by Regulation," *Law and Human Behavior*, 7(1983):279–290.

Greenwood, E. "Attributes of a Profession," *Social Work*, 2(1957):45–55.

Haug, M.R. "Deprofessionalization: An alternative hypothesis for the future," *Sociological Review Monograph*, 20(1973): 195–211.

Haug, M.R. "The Deprofessionalization of Everyone?" *Sociological Focus*, 8(1975):

197–213.

Haugholt, K. "Mor Sæther," *St. Hallvard*, (1958):270–287.

Larsen, Ø. O. Berg and F. Hodne. *Legene og samfunnet*, Oslo: Den Norske Lægeforening (1986):151–330.

McKinlay, J.B. "On the professional regulation of change," *Sociological Review Monograph*, 20(1973):61–84.

McKinlay, J.B. and J. Arches. "Towards the Proletarization of Physicians," *International Journal of Health Services*, 15(1985): 161–195.

Nordhagen, R. "Fra legekvinne til lege, og litt om det som har hendt siden Livius Smitt talte det Medisinske fakultet midt imot og skaffet kvinnen adgang." *In: Kvinner på Universitet 100 år.* Oslo: Likestillingsutvalget Universitetet i Oslo, 1984, p. 69–97.

Parsons, T. "The professions and social structure," *Social Forces*, 17(1939): 457–467.

Parsons, T. "Remarks on Education and the Profession," *The International Journal of Ethics*, 47(1937):365–381.

Roth, J.A. "Professionalism: The sociologists decoy," *Sociology of Work and Occupations*, 1(1974):6–23.

Seip, A.L. *Sosialhjelpstaten blir til. Norsk sosialpolitikk 1740–1920.*Oslo: Gyldendal, 1984.

Seip, A.L. *Veien til velferdsstaten. Norsk sosialpolitikk 1920–1975*. Oslo: Gyldendal, 1994.

Torgersen, U. *Profesjoner og offentlig sektor*, Oslo: Tano, 1994.

C H A P T E R 7

Medical Practice and Medical Enterprise

ØIVIND LARSEN

When the development of a medical profession and a health care system in Norway started from scratch at the beginning of the nineteenth century, one of the reasons why the introduction of medical services was hampered, was that physicians had to be paid by a population whose liquid assets were scarce. To set up a private practice and make a living from it was difficult for a long time during the early years of a national medicine, and salaried posts for physicians were few.

The building of a national health care system in Norway would take different directions. In many ways, the field lay open. When looking back on what happened, it is noteworthy to find that private-run health services eventually only got a diminutive share of the medical activity in Norway, in spite of initiatives and projects. No law of nature made it so. Why did the Norwegian society and most of the Norwegian physicians choose a development that was directed more towards a comprehensive health care system based on public budgets?

The explanation as to how the Norwegian health care system developed has multiple facets. Among the factors that ought to be discussed are the national economy, the social structure, the political processes, and the mentality of the population, including the attitudes of the physicians and the policy of the strong Norwegian Medical Association after its establishment in 1886.

Many of the social reforms that made the Norwegian medical care system into a mainly public one were prompted by economic backlashes that inevitably occurred during the social remodeling of the country in the nineteenth century. Another force, however, was the dominant social democratic ideology of the twentieth century, in which social equality in health matters as well as other areas has been a general, albeit disputed issue. This point has been so strongly argued over the years that by the 1990s almost part of the moral framework of the mind of every Norwegian. Therefore, it might be said that the necessary economic and ideologic base for a completly privatized medical service and the emergence of a large-scale private health care system, never was at hand.

Professional ethics, perhaps especially the unwritten codes, in a way may curb the creativity and initiative of physicians. There are limits to what you can do and what you cannot.

An example: in extending the commitment to the health of patients, there are some invisible borders that come into play, for example, when the patients' problems are a matter of wanting to feel good or to satisfy their vanity. Cosmetic surgeons will be familiar with this kind of thinking on the part of patients.

Another restriction: an ordinary citizen would hardly be met by objections if he gave some well-meant, but undocumented commonplace medical advice to a fellow human being. But a physician is expected to stick to his science. And to profit from working with the sick and suffering, at least above a certain level, has got an dubious quality.

Today, medicine may seem as though it has been prostituted if the physician violates a complicated pattern of norms. In the nineteenth century, however, the situation was not necessarily the same. The profession was searching for its profile. Options were still open.

Enterprises of all kinds were set up in Norway in the nineteenth century. Why not also exploit the medical market? Before the reader is presented with the further development of the profile of the Norwegian medical profession in the following chapters of this book, a closer look at some of those physicians who contributed to medicine and business would probably be useful. Our examples are taken from the spa branch of the medical enterprise, which also attracted interest in Norway.

The nineteenth century is the period when lots of spas were established in central Europe. Many of them were hybrids, their objectives lying somewhere between medicine and tourism, a balance sometimes so delicate that the role of physicians was at stake.

The social profile of the spas often aimed at the upper, more affluent classes. Balneology had a tradition that went back to ancient times. An old culture was revived. Institutions were established, where procedures of taking allegedly strenghtening baths, water drinking cures, fresh air exercise, special diets, and so on could be pursued together with such leisure activities as conversation and attending concerts. Doctors were engaged to supervise the activity. Some thought it might be a good idea to introduce spas in Norway, too.

The activity by the Norwegian physician Heinrich Arnold Thaulow (1808-1894) should be considered when looking at the Norwegian spa projects. Thaulow had in his background a high-ranking Danish family. He had started his medical studies in Kiel and passed the final medical examinations in Christiania in 1833. He opened a practice in the capital in 1834, and there he married the daughter of a high official.

Thaulow knew the German spas from having taken study tours, and he also knew conditions in Sweden. He found the shores of Sandefjord suitable for establishing a spa, and the institution was opened in 1837. Almost by accident a nearby source of mud was discovered that could be used in therapy. A well containing water with the taste and smell of sulphur was also found. Historically, the timetable should be noted. The spa was first; the mud and sulphur, important medical attractions, came later. A local specialty of Sandefjord was also introduced, namely the therapeutic use of stinging jellyfish for treating aching joints.

Although Thaulow moved to the inland municipality of Modum in 1838, he still became instrumental in the development of the spa in Sandefjord as a medical expert and as a major or sole shareholder. In Sandefjord, buildings for the bath were erected by famous architects; the spa had a nice park, and it arranged concerts, excursions, and theater performances for its guests during their stay, which usually lasted for six weeks. High-level guests and patients came to Sandefjord, and following a stay by the crown princess Louise in 1855, people from the uppermost layers of the population followed suit. The height of its fame was reached in 1917, when the spa, despite being open only in the summer, accomodated 1,300 guests.

Dr. Thaulow took over the job of industrial medical officer at the Modum cobalt mines in 1838, a position that was combined with that of the district physician. In Modum, Thaulow founded another spa. In many places in Norway traditional stories say that King Olav (995-1030), on his travels around the country in order to introduce Christianity, used or released wells, where the water later on proved to have healing properties. In Modum, Dr. Thaulow found a well named after Saint Olav, where the water contained iron, and established the bath of St. Olav on the site in 1857.

The process that was followed at Sandefjord repeated itself here. An establishment was founded where culture was very important, and the most elevated strata of society were attracted. Concerts, parties, and famous guests gave the spot its reputation. Dr. Thaulow had a special sense for arts and culture, and traveled widely in continental Europe. He had earned a substantial amount of money on investments in the mining industry in the neighboring district of Ringerike, and he reinvested his profit in the flourishing spa.

Although the baths may be ascribed a certain place in the treatment of such ailments as rheumatic diseases, the medical side of the activity was second to the cultural aspects. In a way, Dr. Thaulow, like other spa owners, used medical argumentation as a proxy for propagating a vivid tourist enterprise, one that was a profitable business for himself and for the local society as well.

A similar story could be told about a somewhat younger physician, Ingebright Lund Holm (1844-1918), and details about him are abundant in the literature. Dr. Holm was an entrepreneur of the same brand as Dr. Thaulow. He opened a spa in Larvik in 1880, a city on the southwestern shores of the Kristianiafiord, not far from Sandefjord. Again a well was sought as the core attraction, and again we hear of an institution that steadily gained in reputation; even a family from the Russian nobility spent time there in 1894. The fragance of high society was present.

From 1878 on, Dr. Holm lived in Christiania. From there he pursued his manifold business activities, among which were sanatoriums that he established in the Holmenkollen hills outside the capital. He also founded hotels, of which one the Dr. Holms Hotel in the mountains at Geilo in central Norway, now a winter resort, still bears his name.

Success in the spa movement was dependent on a leader who found the right attractions. The baths at Grefsen, on the eastern slopes overlooking the capital, opened in 1858. It was closed down in 1899, but had experienced a hard time. Even heroic attempts to run a steam-powered omnibus to take people from the city up to the bath had failed. The main asset, a well that gave water having a constant temperature of four degrees centigrade, never gained popularity.

After the turn of the century, and especially in the years following World War I, almost all the Norwegian spas declined in popularity and were converted for other uses or simply closed down.

There are several reasons for this. Of course the appearance of new leisure activities for the affluent classes was an obvious reason. Neither the climate nor the culture in Norway was favorable for spas, even if guests could be recruited from the more ordinary layers of the population. As a consequence, the clientele that still came to the spas was gradually made up more of patients than of guests, which in turn made the stay less attractive for those who were purely vacationists.

But medical reasons have to be discussed, too. The old forms of balneology never achieved a good reputation as a medical discipline. From the scientific perspective, the methods were seldom properly documented, and on the social side the scent of luxury threw certain shadows across its credibility. Local social status could not compensate for that. This could be detected as a problem when bath therapy was developed more specifically as something that could be offered to rheumatic patients. Andreas Martinius Tanberg (1873-1968), who was later to become president of The Norwegian Medical Association, has been called the founder of modern Norwegian rheumatology. He was physician at the Sandfjord bath, and found it a difficult task to convert the medical work at the spa into modern medicine.

The growing economic equality among the Norwegian population, as well as the health economy, where refunds through public or insurance money for medical treatment became the rule, changed the market for the old type baths.

At the turn of the century, tuberculosis took over much of the public interest. A new law on the handling of the disease had been passed, and sanatoriums and nursing homes for the sick were built all over the country. This drew on local initiative and resources. Patients with tuberculosis came from all layers of the population; in fact, the social character of the disease was visible and caused concern. Medical institutions built in the countryside, in pleasant surroundings, with parks and fresh air, were not spas for the rich people but resorts for the really sick.

It might perhaps be concluded that the development within medicine after the turn of the century not only focused very strongly on important public health problems, and made them the prime obligation for the medical profession, but also turned the moral codes somewhat away from the economic exploitation of a medical training, and toward what we have called serve the patient, serve the science, and serve the society attitudes.

References

Falkum, E. and Ø. Larsen. *Helseomsorgens vilkår*, Oslo: Universitetsforlaget, 1981.

Munthe, E. and Ø. Larsen. *Revmatisme - gamle plager - ny viten*. Oslo: Tano, 1987.

CHAPTER 8

The Establishment of a Public Health System

HANS P. SCHJØNSBY

8.1. Political Background

The basis and need for organizing a public health system was rooted in changes in Norwegian society which started early in the nineteenth century, a period that politically was characterized by the transition from a centralized autocracy to economic and political liberalism.

8.2. Socio-demographic Changes in Norway

The excess of births in the years after the Napoleonic wars had a great impact on both public health and society as a whole. The Norwegian populations increased by two-thirds from 1815 to 1855, while production methods remained largely unaltered. This, in combination with an already weak economy, led to a growth in the unpropertied class, limiting a large part of the population's possibilities to obtain work and make a living. With the new poor-laws of 1845, responsibility for the poor was passed on to the local authorities, thus strenghtening the local autonomy, but at the same time weakening the legal protection of the poor, and exposing them to the fact that the municipalities did not have the necessary funds to implement the measures mentioned in the law (Seip 1974).

It was obvious that this development would adversely affect public health; key words are overpopulation, poverty, poor nutrition, poor quality of drinking water and sanitation, and poor housing conditions. Resistance to disease was low, and, as in most of Europe, cholera swept through Norway several times early in the nineteenth century. The epidemics in 1832–33 and 1853 were the most important. The Health Act of 1860 was in many ways a reaction to the experience with the cholera. With this act the government turned away from the passive role, characteristic of a liberalist state, which it so far had taken, to a more active role. The government took on responsibility for public health. Thus the Health Act can be seen as the precursor of the social legislation later in the century.

8.3. The Sanitary Movement

Environmental factors' influence on morbidity and mortality was documented in France and England from the 1820s onwards (Porter 1993). Thus the prevailing moralistic attitudes and the tendency to place responsibility on the individual, which were characteristic of the time, and thus of most of the doctors, were gradually counteracted (van der Korst 1988).

In England, Edwin Chadwick (1800–1890), a lawyer and humanist, used modern public health methods to demonstrate different environmental factors' effect on public health (Chadwick 1842), and proposed political solutions to health problems. He played a central part in the development of the Sanitary Movement, in which socially conscious doctors in Europe, including Norway, were involved. In addition, Chadwick carried out cost-benefit analyses that documented potential economic gains from public investments in drinking water, renovation, housing conditions, and so on, because of the health benefits of such measures.

8.4. Epidemics, Social Unrest, and Legal Reforms

It is obvious from the preparatory drafts to the Health Act (Ministry of the Interior 1860), that the Norwegians were familiar with the European sanitary movement which, assisted by interested doctors, began to obtain a footing in Norway. The British Nuisances Removal Act (1845), the Public Health Act (1848), and the "Local Government Act" (1858) are all mentioned in the proposals for the Norwegian Health Act. Porter points out that there were several reasons for the reforms in Great Britain. She mentions, among other things, philanthropy and political expediency, but above all utilitarian economic motives based on Chadwick's cost calculations (Porter 1993). These factors probably influenced the decision-making process in Norway as well.

Another factor which probably contributed to the development of the public health service from 1850 onwards was the uneasiness and fear among the people caused by the serious cholera epidemics. Andreas Christian Conradi (1809-1868) analyzed the cholera epidemic in Christiania in 1853, when 65 per cent of those who became sick died (Conradi 1854). The analysis showed that even though the upper social classes were not affected as often as the working class, the death rate among them was just as high. Morbidity and mortality had thus become common property. The Norwegian historian Jens Arup Seip (1905–1992) describes the situation by stating that, in the course of the 1850s, the people who were well off discovered that diseases prevalent among the poor threatened themselves as well. There is good reason to assume that these epidemics led to public pressure on the authorities to take action, and that the pressure came from the upper classes (Seip 1974).

It is also possible that the government feared social unrest as a consequence of the epidemics; that had happened in England in 1832 (Porter 1993). Besides, Europe was still experiencing the aftermath of the revolutionary year of 1848. The Norwegian authorities could act quickly when social unrest threatened, – an example is their expeditious treatment of the Thrane movement. (Marcus Møller Thrane, 1817–1890, was a left-wing activist and leader of the first Norwegian "workers" union.) Later in the nineteenth century, the authorities changed their tactics; Midré, among others, has pointed out that rendering the masses "socially passive" by improving the living conditions of the working class was part of the rationale for the social reforms, as seen in the Bismarckian social legislation of the 1880s (Midre 1990).

8.5. Economic Growth and Professional Development

Another characteristic of these times was the growth in importance of professions, and especially of those with a scientific basis, such as the medical profession. The professionalization of physicians, of which scientific development was an important part, provided a basis for their demand for influence on the emerging public health service. The committee of six which drafted the Health Act was greatly influenced by its three physician members. These physicians, who were respected and regarded as knowledgeable and well-informed, thus contributed to the development of a health service largely based on the terms of the medical profession (Mellbye 1960). Later in the century, as their prestige increased, doctors played a more significant role both in developing health legislation and other preventive health measures.

From the 1840s onwards, the country experienced a period of economic growth. This was an essential condition for a public policy which was expansive and demanded high expenditures. Around 1860, a modern health service began to develop in Norway as a result of political, economic, cultural, and professional factors. The social responsibilities of the State grew, making health not only an individual, but also a social issue. Driven by the need for collective measures to combat diseases, a public health system was formed that was based on three cornerstones: health personnel, health institutions, and administration (Seip 1984).

8.6. Central Administration

In 1809, Norway got its first bureaucracy, or "Health Collegium," specifically devoted to health care. This was dissolved in 1814, and the health service became controlled through a medical office, placed in changing Ministries. Up until the end of the 1840s, this office had no medical expertise. However, the medical faculty had a duty to act as a medical and professional advisor, though they did not have the right to give advice unless they were asked for it. In other words, advice was given on the Ministries terms, when the Ministries' asked for it.

8.7. Professional Interest

New professions emerged, characterized by the new scientific way of thinking. They wished to influence the decision-making processes and the bureaucracy. The government administration, which mostly consisted of lawyers, was characterized by passivity and traditional routines, as opposed to the new ideas of specialization and efficiency. This applied especially to medical services, the educational system, and the church (Benum 1979).

It was the medical profession that first put forward a well-founded proposal for a new medical administration. In 1833, Professor Fredrik Holst (1791–1871), a pioneer in the field of socially related health problems, voiced the need for a Health Collegium in Norway with medical expertise. The collegium should be comprised of professionals, that is, physicians and pharmacists – and should deal with two types of cases: those which were to be presented to higher authorities, and those which the collegium could deal with themselves. With regard to the former, the influence of the profession would be seen through the Ministry participation in the negotiations of the Collegium. When the matter was to be dealt with by the Government, the head of the Collegium should participate in the governmental meetings (Benum 1979).

8.8. The Balance Between Medical Influence and Political Control

The doctors attempted to promote and secure professional considerations within the bureaucracy, and to create a new balance between the parts in the decision-making process. The historian Trond Nordby describes a clash of interest between three poles: professional leadership, democratic leadership, and the constitutional state (Nordby 1987). This obviously was, and still is, a difficult tightrope to walk, and a number of later conflicts up to the present time have their background in this balance of, or struggle for, power.

In 1834 a Medical Law Commission was appointed, which submitted its report as late as 1847. The Commission recommended the establishment of a Medical Collegium, outside of the concerned Ministry, under which the management of the medical services should be placed. The Collegium should consist of three members who were medical experts. The recommendation was rejected by the Storting (the Norwegian Parliament), partially for financial reasons (Report of the Royal Commission for Doctors of 1898). Other reasons were that the Storting looked upon a professional management as undemocratic, and they thought that the collegial strucure was inefficient. The Ministry of the Interior did not pursue the matter, because in 1846 a doctor was appointed as Executive Officer in the Ministry. As a compromise, a temporary medical advisory committee with professional members was appointed by the Ministry in 1850. The committee was made up of three prominent phycisians under the leadership of Professor Conradi. The final decision was made in 1857, when medical expertise gained a place in the Ministry of the Interior with the appointment of the physician C.T Kierulf (1834–1874) as Director General. He was the leader of the medical office in the department, and medical expertise therefore gained a more prominent position in the central decision-making process. After Kierulf's death, this arrangement came to an end.

8.9. Medicine and Central Administration

There were several reasons why the Storting in 1875 recommended separating the medical section from the Ministry of the Interior and turning it into an independent unit. Politically, this was undoubtedly part of the program of decentralization and reduction of Government influence. One must keep in mind that this period, which preceded the introduction of parliamentarism in Norway, was politically unstable and characterized by the antagonism between the Storting, with its majority consisting of liberal members that were pro decentralization, and a conservative Government, consisting mostly of former senior civil servants, appointed by the King. Thus, the Parliament wanted a Director of Medicine independent of the Ministry. The result, however, was that the Directorate of Medicine from 1875 to 1891 as a temporary arrangement remained within the Ministry. It had the authority to make decisions in professional matters, and the Director of Medicine functioned as Director General in matters which were to be decided on by the department. After the death of the Director of Medicine, Ludvig Vilhelm Dahl (1826-1890), the Directorate of Medicine was placed outside the Ministry. The reasons for this were, among other things, the Parliament's original terms of 1875, but also the fact that it had become apparent that the double role of Director General and head of an independent administrative body was indefensible (Svalestuen 1988).

The Director of Medicine now gained a more independent position in relation to the department and its Medical Office, even though, according to §1 of the mandate, he was directly subordinate to the department. According to the mandate, the Director of Medicine had five tasks: surveillance of the nation's health conditions and health services, recommending measures to improve these, advice and guidance to the Health

Boards, supervision of health personnel, and consulting with the department on those medical matters for which the department had responsibility.

This arrangement, which lasted from 1891 to the Second World War, meant that the political role of the Director of Medicine both formally and in reality was reduced (Nordby 1987). The system gave doctors little influence with regard to health policy. Thus it is not surprising, in light of their increasing influence generally, that the arrangement was constantly criticized until it was finally changed. A system in which physicians had a strong influence existed from 1945 on in the Directorate of Health, and it lasted until 1983. This represented a fusion of the section for health matters in the ministry and of the Directorate of Medicine in the Ministry of Health and Social Affairs.

8.10. *Local Administration*

The idea of mandatory local health bodies was voiced by the Medical Committee in 1853. Previously, regulations for health commissions existed. These commissions could be set up at specific times and in specific places for special diseases, particularly cholera. According to the Act of 1857, certain districts were to establish commissions for leprosy. This act must be regarded as a precursor of the Health Act.

8.11. *Aims of the Health Commission*

The establishment of permanent municipal committees with a strong professional input was then debated. The committees were to have general prevention as their area of concern. Professionally and administratively, they were to be linked to the emerging central medical administration. This concept was taken up and developed by the Law Commission that prepared the Health Act (1858). It was assumed by those who prepared the legislation that there were two important factors that could threaten general health, namely, on the one hand "barbarism and ignorance" and on the other hand "civilization and industry." Because of this, the health commissions (from c. 1905, the health boards) in rural and urban areas were given different tasks and composition. In rural areas the "barbarism and ignorance" had to be counteracted with health related information; in the urban areas the unwanted health effects of population growth, "civilization and industry," had to be fought. In the proposal for the Act, the importance of sanitation, light and air, prevention of overcrowding, and improved personal hygiene are specifically mentioned. The composition of the commissions reflects these concerns. The municipal councils or the municipal executive board functioned as health boards in the countryside, with the public medical officer as chairman. It was determined that health information – "a continuous influence and awakening in every district"- was to be disseminated throughout the villages by the board members (Ministry of the Interior, 1860). In the towns, the boards were to be composed of three laymen chosen by the municipal council, – an engineer ("technician"), a lawyer, and the public medical officer; in other words, a suitable composition of different professions, in relation to the tasks to be undertaken.

The new form of health legislation was characterized by democratization, decentralization, and a clear division of responsibility (Evang 1955). Democratization was achieved by allocating responsibility for health matters that were of public interest to a democratically elected body. Decentralization was accomplished by transferring the decision-making process from the Ministry and the County Governor to the municipalities. Division of responsibility was introduced by transferring primary responsibility for developing health care from the central authorities to the municipalities.

8.12. *Tasks, Problems, and Working Methods*

In the first decades following 1860, the importance of the health commissions was probably the greatest in the urban areas. The problems in the towns were more concrete than in the countryside. For example, typhoid fever was endemic in Hamar from 1853 to 1882; out of a population of 2,334 (in 1875), 2,712 people were infected, especially during the 1870s; and 291 of those who were infected died. The Health Commission and, in particular, the city medical officer were deeply involved in this matter. As early as the beginning of the 1870s, they pointed out the importance of a new water supply for the town. When the town eventually got a new water supply, the disease disappeared (The Director of Medicine 1885).

The city medical district (Stadsfysikatet) and the Health Commission in Christiania were active as early as the 1860s, and took the initiative in confronting different environmental problems – drinking-water, inadequate control of food, and so on – which were brought to light through the frequent epidemics and high morbidity in the capital. Early on, the city had passed adequate health regulations, and the commission's political support was satisfactory. These conditions were, and still are, very important for a body with the task of preventing disease. Looking back, the measures that they recommended were forward-thinking and relevant, but at the time they caused much debate (Grøn 1933), a debate that shows that both society and the medical profession's understanding of disease was changing.

However, the rural health administrations seemingly worked somewhat slower. The minutes from the commission meetings, which on average were held between one and three times a year, give the impression of widespread political passivity. During the meetings, the commission's chairman usually gave a report on the health situation in the municipality, and if there was an epidemic, necessary precautions were dealt with. Most of the chairmen of the commissions tried to follow the intention of the Act: to disseminate information. In the medical report of 1867 from Solør and Odalen health districts, we find: "In most of the Health Commissions in the district, Eilert Sundt's report on the cultural condition of the general public was read, and the members were encouraged to make ordinary people understand the importance of cleanliness and order." (Eilert Lund Sundt, 1817-1875, was as Norwegian theologian and social researcher.)

It is difficult to evaluate the health information work of the commissions. However, a local health administration was now established, became known, and could later be used both by doctors and by the public authorities (Seip 1984).

8.13. *The Role of the Health Commissions*

It was not always easy to carry out preventive health measures in country districts. Municipal health regulations were not mandatory in rural districts at that time. In addition, there was a certain concern in the municipal councils that the new system would interfere with ownership rights, municipal economy, and personal autonomy. The majority of farmers supported a policy of savings and cut-backs in public expenditure. Quite a few municipal politicians undoubtedly regarded the health commission more as a state body than as a municipal body, particularly when considering that the chairman was a senior government official.

State intervention, particularly if it involved expenses for the municipality, was not automatically accepted. It was preferable to find compromises, as the Ringsaker Municipal Executive Board did in 1882: Instead of approving new and binding regulations of health, the council requested the Health Commission to print a sufficient number of copies of the proposed rules, and to recommend that the public abide by them (Ringsaker Municipality, 1860–1942:42–43).

8.14. The Growing Importance of the Local Health Bodies

Seen in a broader perspective, the local health administration, through the public medical officer and the Health Commission, probably exerted most influence on local health policy and on measures to prevent disease during the decades around the turn of the century.

This development was also taking place in other European countries. The main reason for this was the new scientific knowledge that documented the importance of preventive measures for ensuring public health. Thus, the local health administration's workload and importance grew from the middle of the 1880s. Here we can briefly mention the new legislation on meat control (1893), which occupied the commissions in the towns; school legislation around 1890, which delegated control and supervision to the health commissions; and the Factory Inspection Act of 1892, which delegated obligatory supervisory tasks to public medical officers. Moreover, the public medical officer was a member of the urban municipal building board. In addition, the Tuberculosis Act of 1900 delegated an important role to the health commissions.

8.15. Draw-backs of the Legislation

During this period, the short-comings of the Health Act became apparent. The act provided a framework only. Because adequate financial support for municipal health work was not laid down in the act, and because the act in addition provided no possibilities for relevant sanctions, it did not have sufficient controlling powers over many of the problems that had to be solved. This was one of the reasons why practice under the Health Act varied from place to place and depended too much on the contribution, knowledge, and personality of the individual district medical officer. This was well known at the time (Benneche 1909). An analysis of the health commissions shows that when the local health administration functioned well, the district medical officer exercised an initiating and active role. However, he could not play this role in improving the health of the local population without the backing of the health commission (Schjønsby 1985).

The conditions for local health administration were altered by the introduction of the new national insurance legislation (1909), the Public Medical Services Act (1912), and a shift from collective to more individual and socio-medical preventive measures.

8.16. Institutions

Medicine as it was practiced during the time of the French Revolution, introduced completely new principles regarding the organization and role of hospitals. The earlier function of "social storage" was reduced, clinical work was to have a central place and was to be connected with teaching, and the doctors were to be employed full-time as clinicians and teachers (Johannisson, 1990:78–92). Seen from a professional perspective, this coincided with doctors now perceiving the importance of connecting disease and symptoms with pathological changes that were found during the post-mortem. In this way, the hospitals became essential for the education of doctors and the advancement of medicine (Granshaw 1993).

8.17. The Growth of Hospitals

The hospital's new role led to the establishment of large hospitals and particularly of university hospitals. In Norway, Rikshospitalet (the National Hospital) opened in 1826. It gradually expanded, grew out of its premises, and a new hospital on a new site was completed in 1883. The National Hospital dominated the institutional health services in Norway during the nineteenth century, though modern hospitals such as Kroghstøtten and Ullevaal were built in 1859 and 1887, respectively. The National Hospital was not the first Norwegian hospital. Because of, among other factors, "radesyken" (probably a Norwegian non-venereal variety of syphilis), a range of county hospitals were established from the middle of the eighteenth century up to 1815, with about 500 beds altogether (Reichborn-Kjennerud 1936). They were often small, with varying quality, and often without real treatment possibilities. Some of these hospitals were closed down; others continued as county hospitals after radesyken disappeared in the early nineteenth century.

Some data about hospitals from the middle of the nineteenth century and up to the turn of the century are shown in Table 8.1 (Department of the Interior 1856 & 1863, the Director of Medicine, 1902). The data are from somatic hospitals, in other words, county hospitals and urban municipal hospitals. Military hospitals, asylums and hospitals for lepers, and so on are not included. The figures show that great changes occurred in the institutional health services during this period. Throughout fifty years, the number of admissions more than tripled and the number of hospitals doubled. Efficiency improved, as indicated by the fact that the mean duration of stay per patient was halved.

However, the quality of hospital service varied dramatically. Around 1850, Rikshospitalet was by large the most important hospital in Norway, with 212 constantly occupied beds and eleven permanently employed doctors (Elster 1990). We do not have exact data, but no other hospital, with the exception of military hospitals, seems to have had doctors employed full time. Usually, the local public medical officer provided medical supervision, and the quality of the hospital services was variable (Reichborn-Kjennerud 1936, Wyller 1990).

With industrialization, urbanization, and improved economic conditions, most towns now saw the need for and had the possibility of establishing their own hospitals. This process started in the 1850s, probably aided by the period of prosperity that came after the Crimean War (1854–1856). As shown

TABLE 8.1
Norwegian Hospital Statistics 1853–1900

Year	Number of hospitals			Number of admissions	Mean duration of stay (days)
	County	Town	Total		
1853	13	5	18	4,523	81
1860	17	10	27	5,202	67
1900	17	19	36	14,898	45

in Table 8.1, the number of municipal urban hospitals doubled in 40 years.

By the turn of the century, the National Hospital was no longer the largest hospital in the country. All the large towns now had well-equipped institutions, which were of a standard equal to that found in other countries. Many of the county hospitals had now developed into modern local hospitals with a professional staff, usually consisting of surgeons.

The development was also spurred by a range of other social and professional changes. Earlier hospitals had, as already mentioned, a social function and were often used by the community to intern poor people and others in need of help. This practice continued well into the nineteenth century, and hospital patients were mostly from the lower classes of society. The middle-class was usually treated at home (Conradi 1860), something that among other things can be attributed to the fact that hospitals of the periods that followed did not have much to offer in the way of treatment. In the middle of the nineteenth century, there was a widespread mistrust of hospitals in Norway, as in the rest of Europe. The dissatisfaction was caused by "hospitalism," that is, the high frequency of hospital infections, and by the high mortality, especially in the surgical and the obstetric wards (Granshaw 1993).

Hospital conditions improved during the following ten to twenty years. This was not only due to advances in medical science, but also to the new recruitment of highly skilled and well trained caregivers, particularly nurses. This led to an acceptance of hospitals by the middle class, with the result that the patient population eventually came to be representive of the population as a whole. The population's increasing trust in hospitals during the second half of the nineteenth century was a basic requirement for the expansion of health care institutions that continued throughout the next century.

8.18. Doctors

The framework for medical education as we know it today is based on the medical ideology of the last decades of the eighteenth century. During the Napoleonic rule, a centralized and uniform system of medical education, with a state examination and licensing, was established. Other European countries followed suit. In England, which was traditionally more liberal, unregulated medical practice was much more widely accepted, a practice that lasted until the 1880s, when medical education became uniform (Gelfand 1993).

8.19. Social and Professional Characteristics

In Norway, this development began early on. The old distinction between surgeons and university-educated doctors quickly disappeared when the medical faculty was established. Thus, the foundation for a homogeneous medical profession was laid down early on. Practically all doctors had studied at the nation's only university, their professional qualities and attitudes were basically the same, and they belonged to the same social class. In the small country of Norway, doctors were part of the social-elite, though some time was yet to pass before they achieved a position equal to that of the clergy, lawyers, and officers. In other words, their position was promising, though a few difficulties lay along the way. For a long time the number of physicians was too low. The therapeutic possibilities that could be offered to the population were few, even at the end of the nineteenth century, when the scientific understanding of many diseases had attained a high level. In addition, doctors faced competition from people who practiced folk medicine and quackery, though the doctors had some professional protection through a decree of 1794. Many of the alternative practitioners probably did a good job (Bø 1980). Considering this, as well as the shortage of physicians and the deregulatory policies of the time, it is not surprising that the new Act on Quackery of 1871 in principle gave everyone the right to practice medicine.

8.20. Political Responsibility and Growth of the Health Service

Early on, Parliament perceived that it was important for the nation to be adequately supplied with public medical officers. In 1816, out of a total of about one hundred authorized doctors, only twenty-three worked in rural districts (Reichborn-Kjennerud 1936). That year, Parliament agreed to subsidize public medical posts in the north by granting the public medical officers a minimum salary substantially higher than for those in southern Norway (Hodne 1981), a decision of importance to northern Norway. With this decision, Parliament acknowledged a public responsibility for health services.

It was the need for curative services which, naturally enough, was the primary motivating factor for politicians. This was the case when, in 1603, Christian IV (1577–1648) nominated Norway's first public medical officer, the chief city medical officer in Bergen. The same argument was used in Parliament when the District Physician Act was discussed in 1911. It must be pointed out here that state involvement in health services during the first half of the nineteenth century was primarily concerned with regional medical services. Hospital services were mainly represented by the National Hospital and the Maternity Hospital. Even in 1900, when the process of establishing modern hospitals had started, hospital doctors accounted for only ten per cent of the total number of doctors (Evang 1955). The fact that, up until the 1840s, between 70 and 80 percent of the national health expeditures were allocated to regional medical services illustrates the importance of the district physicians (Royal Commission for Doctors, 1898).

The number of new public medical officer posts in Norway from 1815 to 1900 is shown in Table 8.2 (Royal Commission for Doctors, 1898). One reason why this increase in posts was possible was the increased availability of educated doctors. The number of inhabitants per doctor in 1824 was 8.127, while in 1854 this number had decreased to 4.495 inhabitants per doctor, and in 1904 to 2.025 inhabitants per doctor (Reichborn-Kjennerud 1936).

There was a genuine desire in Parliament to cover the increasing need for doctors within the population, and particularly to achieve as even a distribution as possible. Thus the majority of new posts from 1870 onward were allocated to northern Norway. At the same time, public economy allowed for expansions of the public medical service from 1850 to 1870. Hodne has shown that allocations of resources by Parliament were almost proportional to income from import tariffs (Hodne 1986).

8.21. Private Medical Practice or Public Doctors

However, Parliament did not always agree on which policies to pursue, and these dis-

TABLE 8.2
Number of new public medical officer posts in Norway from 1815 to 1900

Year(s)	New posts
1815	38
1824–1847	30
1848–1869	64
1870–1900	21
Total	153

sagreements grew stronger from the middle of the nineteenth century. In 1848, the question of state subsidies to private doctors' salaries was brought up in Parliament for the first time. It was discussed whether state subsidies should be given to parishes whose members wanted to establish their own medical service (Esmarch and Utheim 1901). In 1868, the Parliamentary Salary and Pension Committee stated, in a true spirit of liberalism, that if one goes too far in appointing public medical officers, it is feared that private enterprise and development of private medical practices may be inhibited, since when comparing doctors working in the same place or in the same district, public medical doctors will have more advantageous conditions than the others.

Dissatisfaction with the coverage of doctors probably lay behind this, and opposition to the public medical service came mainly from the rural districts. The Act on Quackery, mentioned above, is an example of this. In 1886, Søren Pedersen Jaabæk (1814–1894), a controversial politician who is mostly remembered for his consistent policy of saving and making cut-backs, moved that the whole system be abolished, justifying this by the plentiful number of doctors and the development of communications. Jaabæk wanted to turn the medical profession into a private business (Seip 1984). The final result, after a long and tortuous process, was the Public Medical Services Act of 1912.

With this act, Parliament affirmed and strengthened the policy of a public medical service, in accordance with the framework laid down in the nineteenth century. This attitude has characterized the development of the health service in Norway throughout the whole of the twentieth century.

8.22. Midwives

In 1814 there were 54 midwives in Norway. They had been educated at the Maternity Hospital in Copenhagen ever since its foundation in 1761. The events of 1814, when the Norwegian constitution was passed by the National Assembly at Eidsvoll on 17 May and a union with Sweden was formed on 4 November after a break with Denmark, made it necessary to establish a school for midwives in Norway. In 1818 this was done, with the opening of the new Maternity Hospital in Christiania. This school was transferred to the National Hospital in 1837 (Bjøro et al. 1993).

In 1810, the midwives were the first profession in Norway to get legal protection. In the Rules for the Arrangement and Management of Midwife Services, midwives obtained the exclusive right to practice midwifery, assuming that they had received an authorized education. The nation was now divided into midwife districts. Remuneration was meant to be based on a basic salary paid by the county, later by the municipality, supplemented with a fee per birth, based on ability to pay. In 1839, Parliament withdrew the monopoly of the qualified midwives, in line with the political philosophy of the farmers who were in the majority. However, in practice, the monopoly was reintroduced in 1898, with the new Midwives Act. The new act came as a response to the increasing dissatisfaction of midwives with the unfavorable economic conditions and competition from unskilled persons. The act introduced a public grant in addition to the municipal basic salary and effected a substantial improvement in the working conditions of midwives.

In the nineteenth century, births took place at home, and the nation was in need of qualified midwives. The number of midwives that were being educated increased significantly. In 1857 there were 435 practicing midwives, of whom 360 were public employees. By the turn of the century, there were 1,144, of whom 735 were public employees (Ministry of the Interior 1856 &

63 & The Director of Medicine 1902). The number of births per midwife was reduced from 115 in 1857 to 57 in 1900.

8.23. Nurses

There are no statistics on nurses among the statistics on health personnel in the yearly health reports in the nineteenth century. However, the picture was dominated by doctors, with midwives in second place, then dentists, veterinary surgeons, and vaccination assistants for smallpox.

Nursing as a medical discipline is young, and it's professionalization did not start until the establishment of the Norwegian Nurses' Association in 1912. Thus a separate act for the nursing profession, with uniform criteria for education, licensing, legal protection, and so on, is a phenomenon that belongs to the twentieth century; but the foundation was laid in the second half of the last century.

The need for a qualified nursing staff was partly the result of the expansion of the hospital service and the advances in medical science. The earlier use of untrained women who attended to the basic needs of patients in hospitals did not sufficiently satisfy the patients, increasing demands for humane treatment. Moreover, the untrained women could not carry out medical tasks according to instructions from the doctors.

In Norway, modern nursing was primarily the result of a religious movement. The Johnson Revival (Gisle Christian Johnson, 1822–1894, Norwegian theologian), which swept over the nation during the 1850s, led, among other things, to a reawakening of the Christian virtues of charity and the calling to serve (Molland 1968).

The education of deaconesses is associated with the name of Cathinka Guldberg (1814–1919). She had studied nursing in Kaiserswerth in Germany, where Florence Nightingale earlier had received inspiration for her pioneering work. The deaconess ideology and the more administrative and profession-oriented Nightingale school were later to be reunited in the important transition from calling to profession.

The Deaconess Institution began to operate in 1868, and in 1871 the first two deaconesses were appointed at the National Hospital. By 1874, as many as 53 deaconesses had been trained. Usually, they went directly into leading positions in the hospitals (Wyller 1990).

During these years, the issue of nurses was brought up many times, both in doctor assemblies and in medical journals. Doctors were very interested in helping to get the educated nurses into rural districts (Kaurin 1905). From the mid-1880s doctors – together with leading people in the villages, religious and humanitarian orgainizations, and so on – were instrumental in establishing several local organizations that helped suitable people from the villages get nursing training at the Deaconess Institution, paid for by the organizations. By 1900, 70 such parish deaconesses had been educated at the Institution. The deaconesses were the forerunners of the present home-nursing system.

During the 1890s, many other schools were established: Diakonhjemmet (the Deaconess House), the Red Cross, Betanien and Sanitetsforeningen (the Norwegian Association of Women Voluntary Workers). All of them were private and established as the result of private or humanitarian initiatives. It was not until 1900 that the two first publicly funded nursing schools, the Public Schools of Nursing in Kristiania and Bergen, were established. These schools ran three-year courses, compared with the one – to two – year courses at the other schools, something that set a new standard in the education of nurses and contributing to the beginning professionalization of the group.

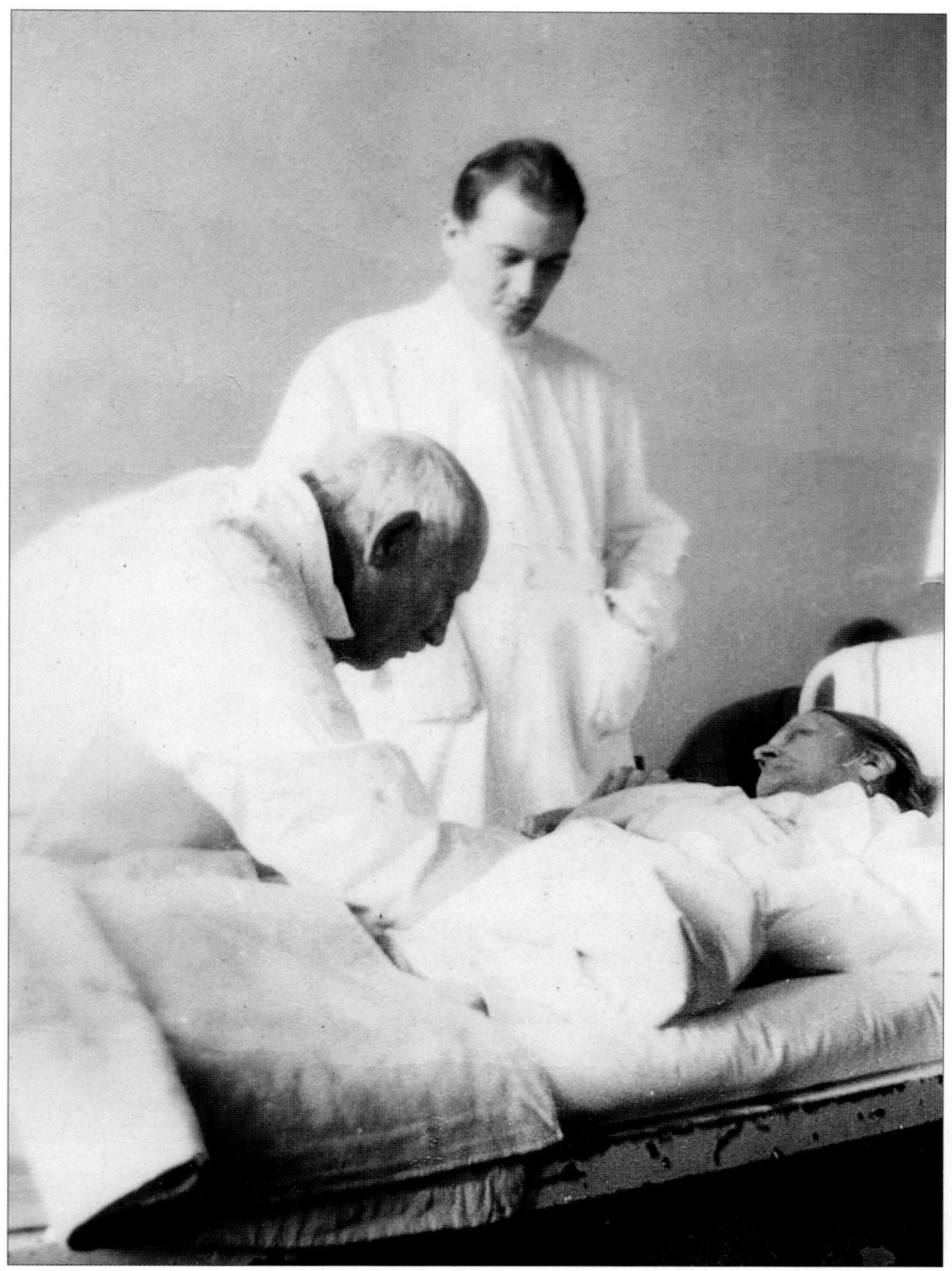

Figure 9: The image of a doctor: Hjalmar Schilling (1867-1946) was head of one of the surgical departments of Ullevål Hospital in Oslo 1917-1934. He was highly respected, and his clinical skills are clearly indicated in this old snapshot, taken by one of his students, Johs. Hagtvet (1904-1989).

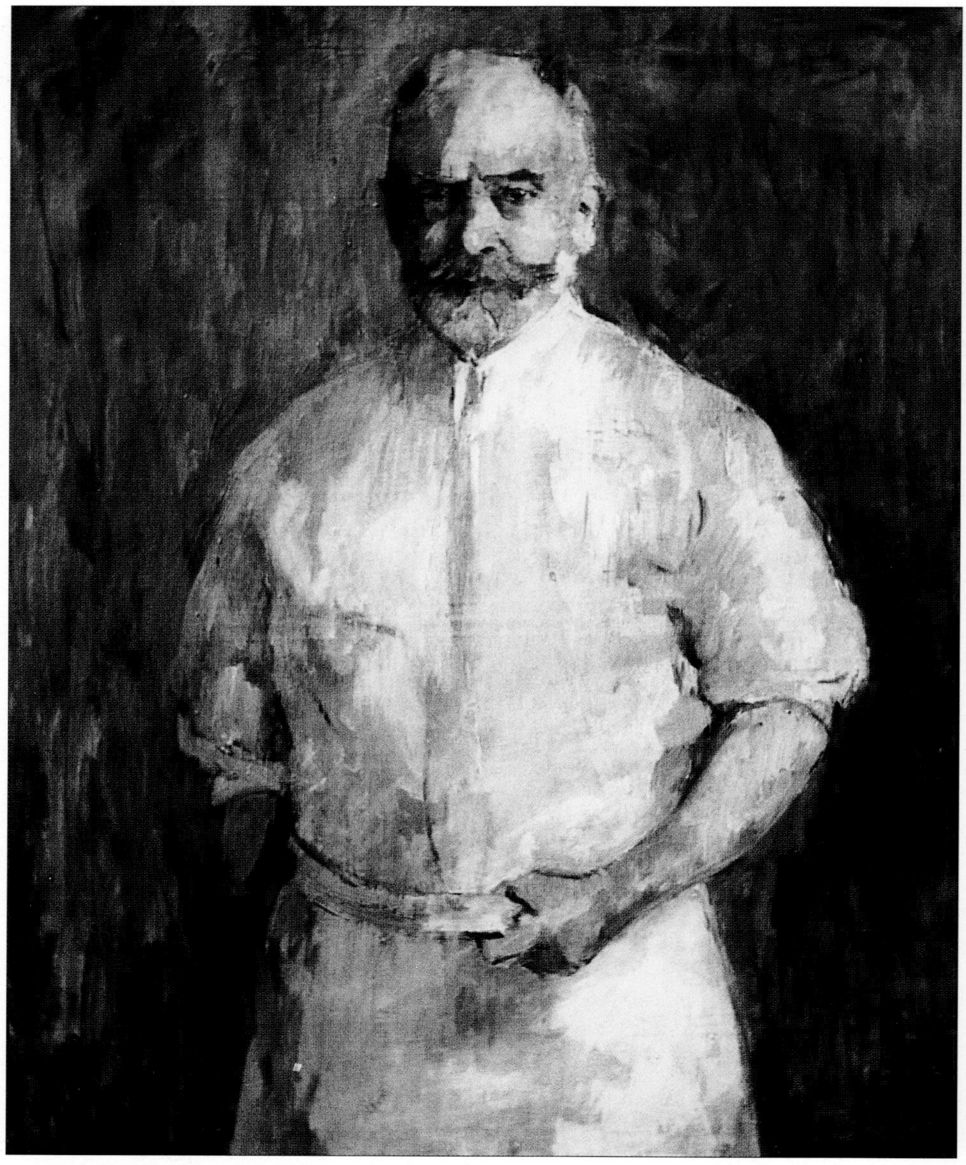

Figure 10: An artist's perception of a surgeon: Dr. Alexander Malthe (1845-1928), portrayed in 1910 by the well-known painter Henrik Lund (1879-1935). A dramatic composition and vivid colors emit strength and decisiveness (Private collection, photo: Øivind Larsen 1996).

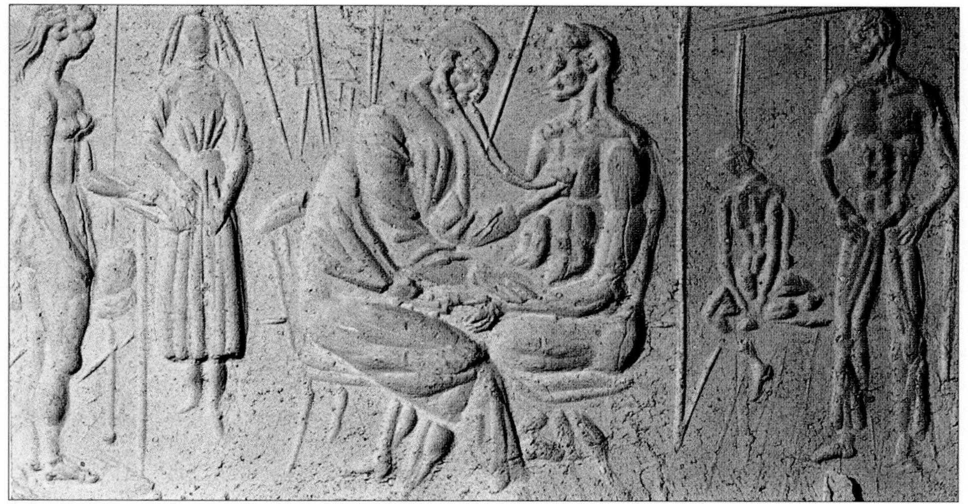

Figure 11: Health screening and preventive medicine: A clay cast for a bronze relief with motive from the occupational health services between the two World Wars, sculpted by Ørnulf Bast (1907-1974). The final version is exhibited in the Freia sculpture park in Oslo (Private collection, photo: Øivind Larsen 1996).

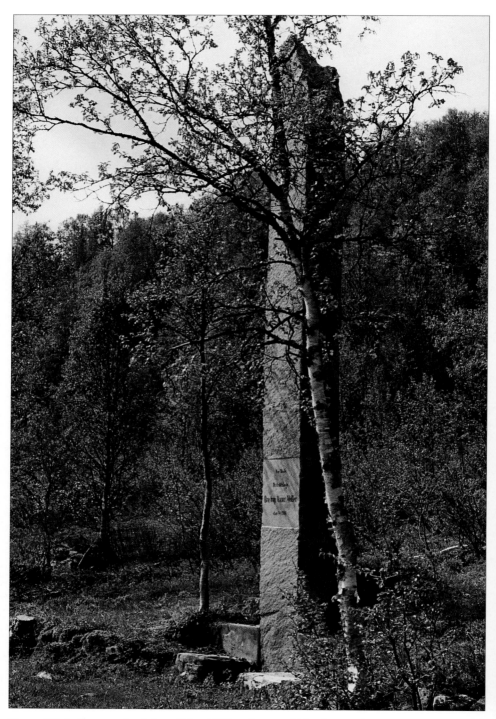

Figure 12: Is there a physician of the 1990s who would be honored with a monument like this? Dr. Brostrup Marius Müller (1841-1908) at Røros, a beloved person who took an active part in almost everything in the society, suddenly died when out on a house call, and the stone was erected on the spot (Photo: Øivind Larsen 1989).

8.24. *Technical Staff*

The Medical Act Committee (Ministry of the Interior 1860) recommended that an engineer ("a technician") should be one of the members of the urban health commissions. The reason given by the committee was that it was considered to be of great importance that a man of technical knowledge, when available, should assist the Commission in questions of a technical nature, about which there would often be discussion, when the Commission had to make regulations concerning sewage disposals, unhealthy dwellings, ventilation, and so on.

Usually it was the city engineer who was given this seat in the urban health commission, and this was undoubtedly beneficial with regard to the competence and credibility of the commissions. Apart from the larger cities (Christiania, Trondhjem, and Bergen), we know little about how the commissions functioned. For example, we do not know whether engineers took part in the work of the commissions in all places. It is, however, reasonable to suppose that the multi-professional composition of the towns' health commissions gained a special importance after the benefit of hygienic measures had been documented by bacteriology. This breakthrough also led to increased efforts in the prevention of food and water-borne diseases from the end of the 1890s onward. The Meat Control Act of 1892 is an example of this. The large municipalities invested in preventive measures, and around the turn of the century systems for controlling meat and other foodstuffs were being developed in many cities and densely populated areas. This was one stage in preventive health work, and other groups, like chemists, and particularly veterinary surgeons, became involved in the public health service. More professionals were to become involved, but this is a development that primarily belongs to the twentieth century.

8.25. *Conclusions*

Norway emerged from the political turmoil at the time of the Napoleonic wars as a free and relatively independent nation. However, the country had to start a fresh development of the government and the infrastructure, including a democratic governing system and an adequate bureaucracy. The existing system was built on absolutist principles from the previous four centuries of union with Denmark. The first Norwegian university was established as late as 1811, and the public health service was very weakly developed. In 1814, there were about twenty public medical officers in Norway, serving a population estimated to be 880,000.

Considering this, most other European states had a flying start in developing a modern health system in the nineteenth century. Nevertheless, this process went surprisingly fast in Norway, and in the later part of the century, Norway was in step with the rest of Europe.

There were probably several reasons for this development. As early as the 1820s, Parliament accepted that public health was a public responsibility. This was exemplified by the approval of the Health Act in 1860. Improvement in the economic situation of the nation from the 1840s onward made public investment in the health services possible. The medical profession also played an important part: as early as the 1820s prominent members of the medical society were aware of the relationship between health and society and were able to influence attitudes and legislature.

The homogeneous class of medical professionals was important as well, socially and professionally. Nearly all of them were also educated and trained at the same university.

The coverage of public medical officers in Norway increased from three to seven per 100,000 inhabitants in the period between 1825 and 1900, an increase significantly higher than in the neighboring countries

(Hodne 1981).

There is good reason to say that at the turn of the century the coverage, structure, and quality of the medical services in Norway did not lag behind those of the other European countries.

References

Benneche, O. "Det civile lægevæsens omordning," *Tidsskrift for Den norske lægeforening*, (1909).

Benum, E. *Statsadministrasjonens historie. Vol 2 ch 1*. Oslo: Universitetsforlaget, 1979.

Bjøro, K., B. Berg, K. Kjærheim, B. Hem, and T. Negaard. *Jordmorutdanning gjennom 175 år.* Oslo: Jordmorhøgskolen, 1993.

Bø, O. "Folkemedisinen – signekjerringer og bygdedoktorer." In *Norsk Kulturhistorie, Vol 5.* Oslo: Aschehoug, 1980.

Chadwick, E. *Report of an Inquiry into the Sanitary Conditions of the Labouring Population of Great Britain.* Edinburgh 1842. Quoted in Rethinking Community Medicine. London: Department of Community Medicine, Guy's Hospital Medical School, 1979.

Conradi, A. C. "Cholera i Christiania og Omegn 1853." *Norsk Magazin for Lægevidenskaben, 1854:433–460.* Quoted in Falkum, E. *Sykdomsoppfatning, helseomsorg og samfunn.* Oslo: Universitetsforlaget, 1978.

Conradi, A. C. "Om Sygelighedsforholdene og Sygdomsconstitutionerne i Christiania." *Norsk Magazin for Lægevidenskaben,1860.* In: Falkum E. *Sykdomsoppfatning, helseomsorg og samfunn.* Oslo: Universitetsforlaget, 1978.

Elster, T. *Rikets Hospital.* Oslo: Aschehoug, 1990

Esmarch, L., and J. Utheim. *Oversigt over Det norske civile Lægevæsens historiske Udvikling og nuværende Ordning.* Supplements to Ot. prop. 39, 1911. Ministry of Justice 1901

Evang, K. "Helsestellets utvikling i Norge i 75 år," *Tidsskrift for Den norske lægeforening*, 2(1955).

Gelfand, T. "The History of the Medical Profession." In *Companion Encyclopaedia of the History of Medicine, Vol 2*. eds. W. F. Bynum and R. Porter, London: Routledge, 1993.

Granshaw, L." The Hospital". *In Companion Encyclopaedia of the History of Medicine Vol 2.* eds. W. F. Bynum and R. Porter, London: Routledge, 1993.

Grøn, F. *Det Norske Medicinske Selskab 1833-1933. Festskrift til selskapets 100-års jubileum.* Oslo: 1933.

Hodne, F. *Norges økonomiske historie 1815–1970. Ch 8.* Oslo: Cappelen, 1981.

Hodne, F. "Medisin og miljø – nye synspunkter". *In Legene og samfunnet,* eds. Ø. Larsen, O. Berg, and F. Hodne. Oslo: Seksjon for medisinsk historie, Universitetet i Oslo og Den norske lægeforening, 1986.

Johannisson, K. *Medicinens öga, Ch 3.* Stockholm: Norstedts, 1990.

Kaurin, E. "Sygepleiesagen," *Tidsskrift for Den norske lægeforening*, (1905):291–293.

Mellbye, F. "Sunnhetsloven av 1860 og de menn som skapte den," *Liv og Helse*, 5(1960).

Midre, G. *Bot, bedring eller brød.* Oslo: Universitetsforlaget, 1990.

Molland, E. F*ra Hans Nielsen Hauge til Eivind Berggrav. Hovedlinjer i Norges kirkehistorie i det 19. og 20. århundre.* Oslo: Gyldendal, 1968.

Nordby, T. "Profesjokratiets periode innen norsk helsevesen – institusjoner, politikk og konfliktemner," *Historisk Tidsskrift*, 3(1987):301–323.

Porter, D. "Public Health", in T*he Companion Encyclopaedia of the History of Medicine Vol 2,* eds W. F. Bynum and R. Porter. London: Routledge, 1993.

Reichborn-Kjennerud, I., F. Grøn, and I. Kobro. *Medisinens historie i Norge*. Oslo: Grøndahl & Søns forlag, 1936.

Schjønsby, H. P. Helserådet. *MPH thesis.*

Göteborg: Nordiska Hälsovårdshögskolan, 1985.

Seip, A-L. "Helse som samfunnssak", in *Sosialhjelpstaten blir til 1740–1920.* Oslo: Gyldendal, 1984.

Seip, J. A. *Utsikt over Norges Historie Vol 1 ch 4.* Oslo: Gyldendal, 1974.

Svalestuen, A. "Medisinalvesenets sentraladministrasjon 1809-1940", in *Norsk Arkivforum. Administrasjonshistoriske oversikter.* Oslo: Arkivarforeningen, 1988.

van der Korst, J. K. *Om lijf en leven. Gezondheotszorg en geneeskunst in Nederland 1200-1960.* Utrecht: Boon, Scheltema & Holkema, 1988.

Wyller, I. "Det 19. århundre", in *Sykepleiens historie i Norge.* Oslo: Gyldendal, 1990.

Official documents:

Director of Medicine. 1885. Medicinal report of the county of Hedemarken 1882.

Ministry of the Interior, 1860. Ot.prop. no.34, 1859–60.

Minute Book of the Health Commission of the Municipality of Ringsaker 1860–1942.

Reports on the Public Health in Norway 1853, 1860 & 1900. Ministry of the Interior 1856 & 63 & The Director of Medicine 1902.

CHAPTER 9

Health Challenges in a Changing Society – Regional Patterns of Epidemic Diseases, and the Attitudes Towards Them, 1868–1900

CHAPTER 9.0

Diseases, Geography, and Attitudes

ØIVIND LARSEN

Health as a public concern was a growing issue in the nineteenth century. As a medical profession emerged, one might assume that three factors, viz. the health conditions, the perception of the health problems, and the new scientific achievements and practical possibilities, including economy, social infrastructure, and so on, would excert a heavy influence on the development.

However, trends in attitudes, perceptions, and conceptions are not readily studied, at least not if one wants to get beyond generalizations from individual impressions, and especially if one wants to apply some quantitative measures to what was going on. Trends in morbidity on a local level, that is, on a level rather close to the situation which was perceived, and which was the basis for the generation of attitudes, are not so easily detected, even from existing statistics and narrative sources.

One approach might be to study the annual reports (Medicinalberetningene) submitted by the district physicians. Here, figures were presented for a series of diseases occurring in the district, together with accounts on the general situation, the health services, and so on. These reports are first-hand sources about health and living conditions on the grassroot level, about conditions as they were experienced by the population.

A way of assessing the conditions described is to compare the verbal judgment and considerations in the text to the numerical information on the same situation in a systematic way. The infectious diseases were a dominant group of diseases, and it is therefore sensible to use this group as a proxy to the health conditions.

Reports by the district physicians from the nineteenth century are at hand in abundance in the Norwegian State Archives because the physicians had a professional duty to send them in. Quantitative studies, however, based on individual reports for the whole country, or even for such a large part of it that geographical comparisons are meaningful, are almost prohibitive to undertake, because of the immense amount of local data that has to be included, especially if one also wants to cover a span of time with such width that trends are allowed to appear. The local reports, as a rule recorded in the old, gothic handwriting, are best suited for local studies, and they are often used for this purpose.

The reports that were sent in were also compiled on the county level by the health authorities, and were supplied with a general review for the whole country before they were published by the central authorities. Occasionally, some of the local reports by individual district physicians occur as appendices in the published statistics.

Although the first-hand impressions by the individual physicians therefore mostly appear in a condensed, edited and collective form in the printed version, and on the county level, the editing work has been performed by contemporary health officials. Further, the grouping of information from single districts into a larger region, a county, smoothes occasional differences and particularities, and makes the material more suitable for study on an accumulative level. The source value of the printed reports is regarded as quite good in relation to the questions asked in our investigations. Of course, a gradually more complete registration over time and certain geographical variations may be present, a fact that may influence the results of the compilations, but anyhow, the figures available show some interesting trends. For looking at the situation on an agglomerate level, a possible minor failure of this type in parts of the source material should not be of any great importance.

The period from around 1860, the crucial year when the law regulating the district physician system was passed, and up to the turn of the century, is of special interest for reasons already described. Annual reports had been submitted by the district physicians for a long time prior to that, but from now on the reports gain a new source value: they tell the story about the effects of the new reform in the local public health system introduced in 1860.

The reporting was also upgraded: beginning in 1868 the reports were requested in a more systematic format than before, and they are therefore especially suitable for studying from this year onwards.

In a previous study (Larsen et al. 1980), data were compiled for important infectious diseases from the printed statistics on county and nationwide levels for the period 1868-1900 in a set of tables. Then the data from the tables were compared to an assessment of the verbal impressions given on the corresponding health conditions.

By means of a content analysis method, verbal evaluations of the health conditions, given in the reports, were ranked and given a numerical score, which in turn was combined with the rates for morbidity, mortality, and lethality to calculate health concern indexes, where a high value of the index pointed at, indicated a higher degree of concern about the situation than a lower one, given the same morbidity, mortality, and lethality.

Of course, this method has its faults and weaknesses, and registration procedures and other factors have to be taken into consideration, but the approach nevertheless ought to give some indications.

In the following, some of the general conclusions are referred to, and in the subsequent chapters the conditions lying behind the figures in the different counties are described in more detail.

A general impression, apparent to everyone who goes even superficially into Norwegian nineteenth-century history, is that the health conditions in the various parts of the country include an abundance of diseases

Diagram 9.1
Epidemic diseases in Norway 1868–1900. Incidence, mortality, and lethality

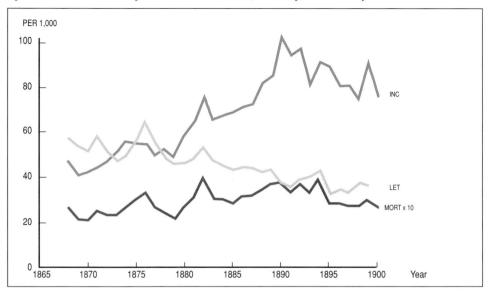

Diagram 9.2
Acute diarrheas in Norway 1868–1900. Incidence, mortality, and lethality

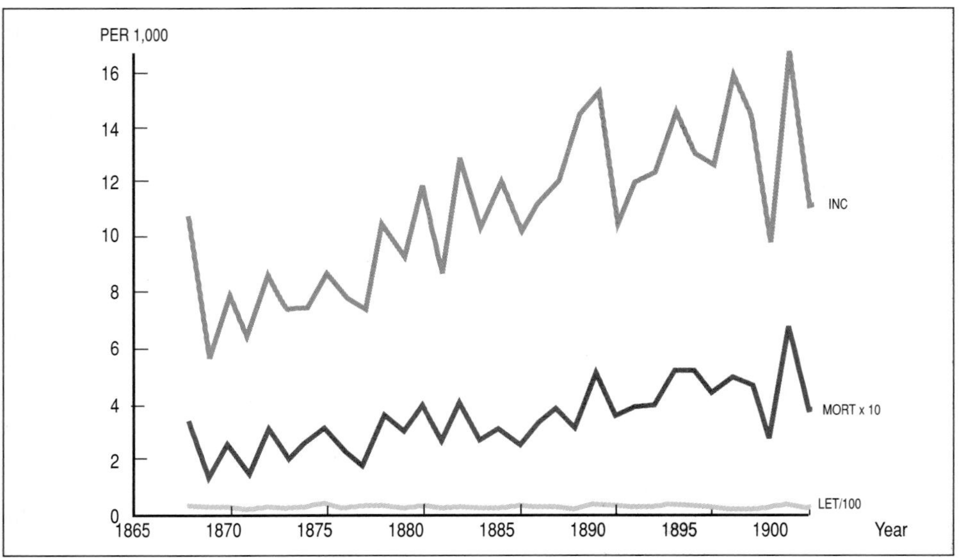

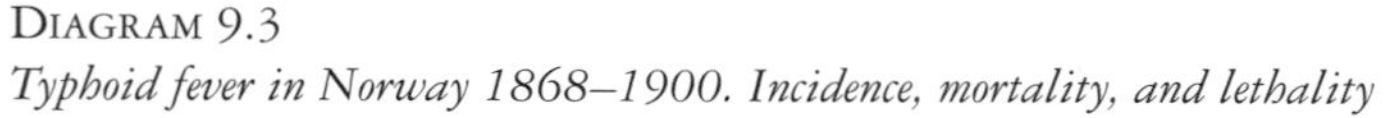

DIAGRAM 9.3
Typhoid fever in Norway 1868–1900. Incidence, mortality, and lethality

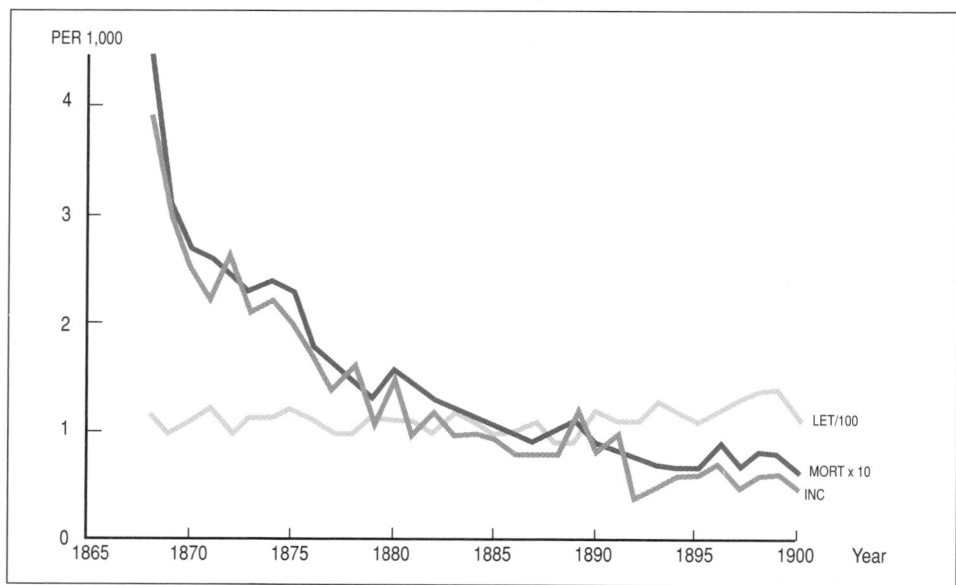

and misery, measured by any standards. Probably what happened was that the population gradually became more aware of this fact, mainly because of the activity of the district physicians.

According to the reports by the district physicians, the incidence of contagious diseases increased steadily in the period up to 1890, when a culmination took place (Diagram 9.1). The mortality from these diseases was more unaffected through the period, and the lethality declined.

Acute diarrheas were prevalent throughout the period, and statistics show an increasing incidence (Diagram 9.2), but a more serious gastro-intestinal disease, typhoid fever, showed a diminishing importance in the course of time (Diagram 9.3)

Diphtheria (Diagram 9.4) was a true scourge from the early 1880s until the mid-1890s. Incidence and lethality reached frightening levels; it frequently occurred that one out of four of the afflicted died.

The geographical differences follow the degree of urbanization, and the degree of migration and social unrest. So the figures are generally larger in the urbanized areas than in the countryside, with the capital of Kristiania as the most typical among the densely built-up areas (Diagram 9.5). There are more similarities between the county of Smaalenene in the south and Finnmark in the north than between Smaalenene and the nearby capital of Kristiania. The urban-rural effect is clearly demostrated here. This effect is most clearly visible for the incidence statistics, but also appears for mortality (Diagram 9.6), while lethality, the number of deaths among the affected, does not differ as much (Diagram 9.7).

Due caution is necessary as to the pitfalls inherent in evaluating the attitudes occurring in the reports when calculating a health concern index. However, it seems appropriate to conclude from the pattern of the indexes that for the country as a whole, the

DIAGRAM 9.4
Diphtheria in Norway 1868–1900. Incidence, mortality, and lethality

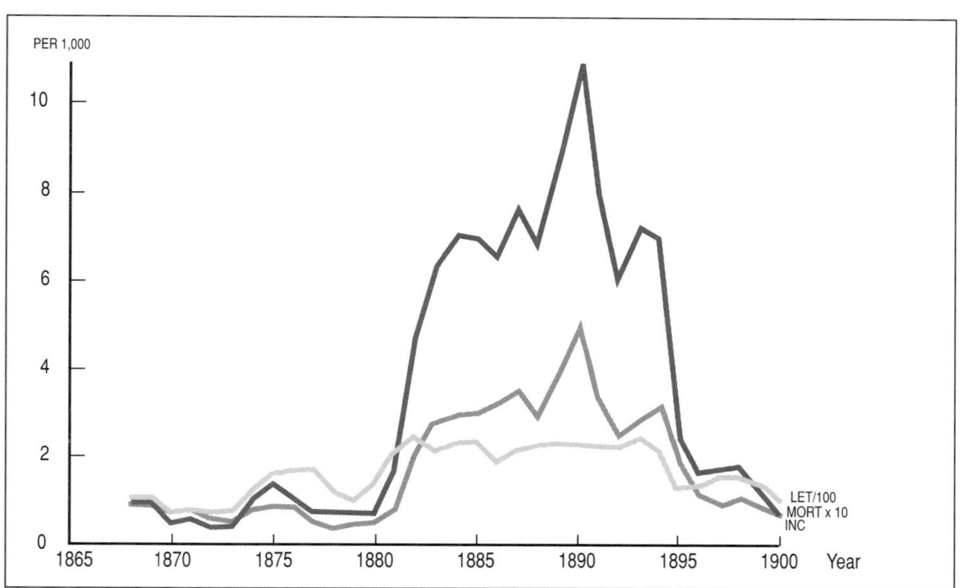

DIAGRAM 9.5
Incidence of epidemic diseases in Norway 1868–1900. Regional differences

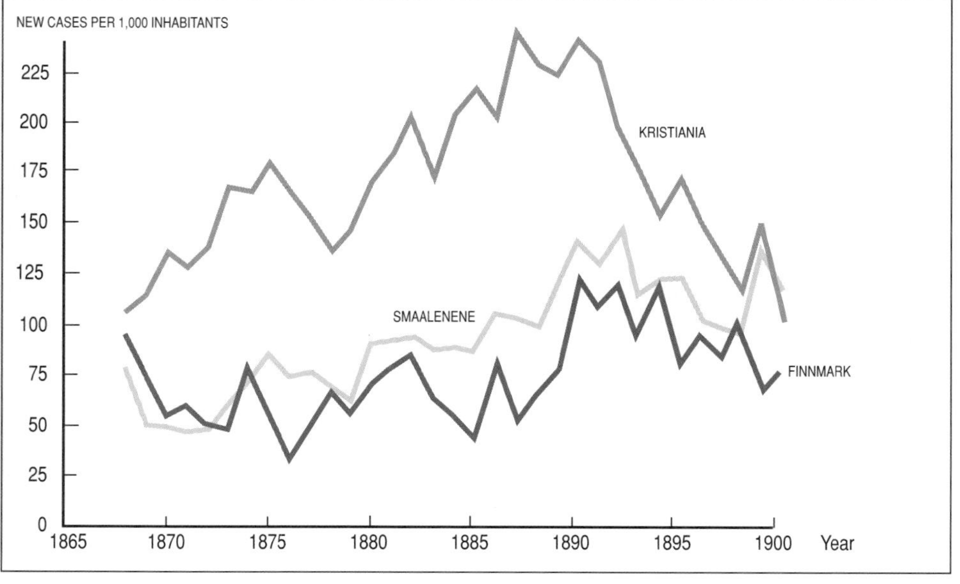

DIAGRAM 9.6
Mortality of epidemic diseases in Norway 1868–1900. Regional differences

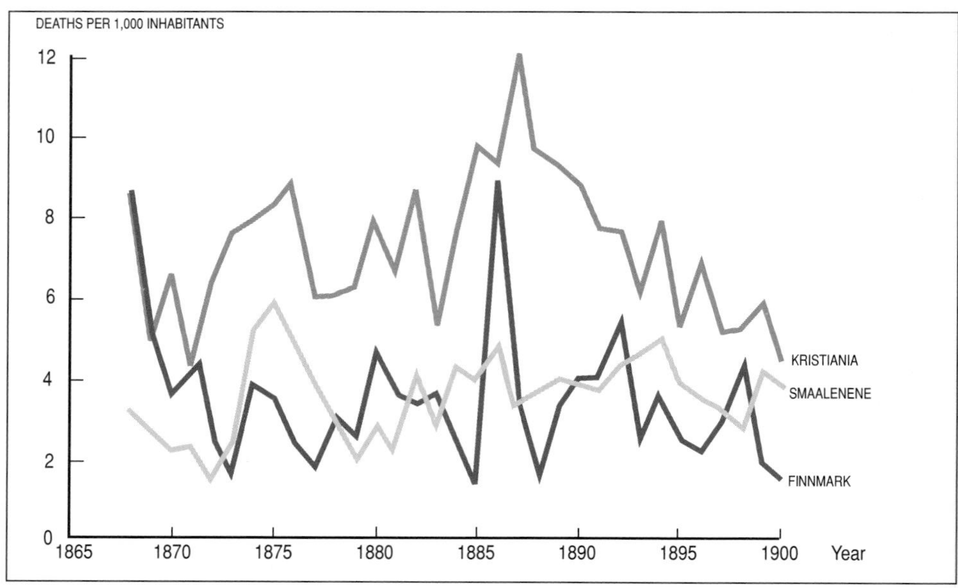

DIAGRAM 9.7
Lethality of epidemic diseases in Norway 1868–1900. Regional differences

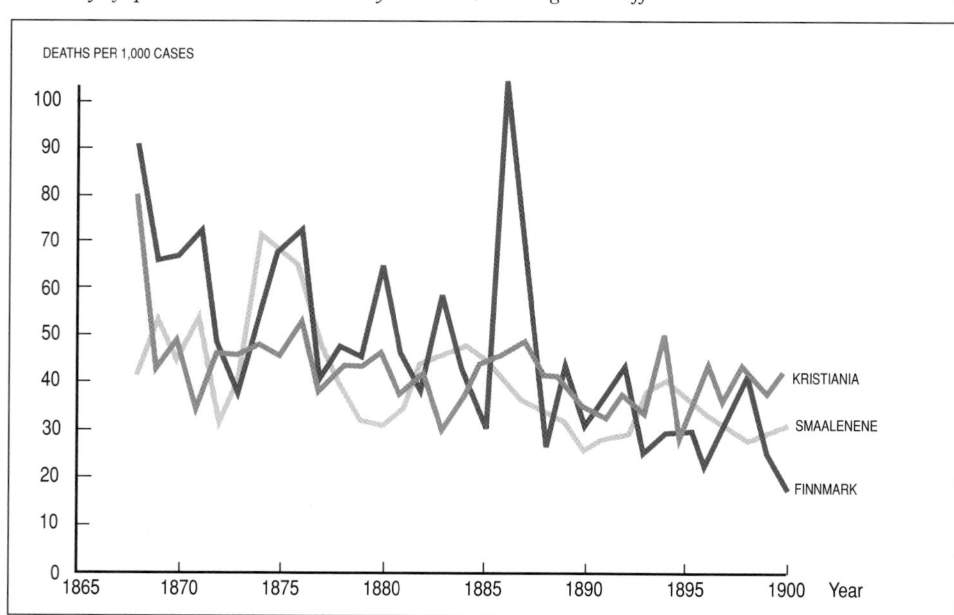

DIAGRAM 9.8

Health concern index for epidemic diseases in Norway 1868–1900. Calculation based on incidence (v/inc), mortality (v/mrt), and lethality (v/let). (For calculation of index see Larsen et al. 1980)

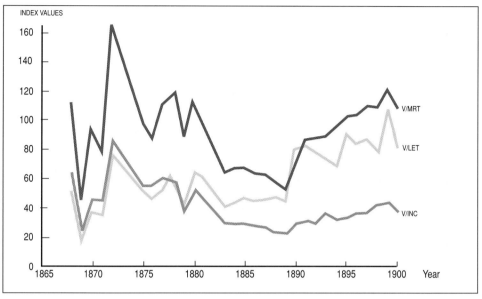

DIAGRAM 9.9

Health concern index for acute diarrheas in Norway 1868–1900. Calculation based on incidence (v/inc), mortality (v/mrt), and lethality (v/let). (For calculation of index see Larsen et al. 1980)

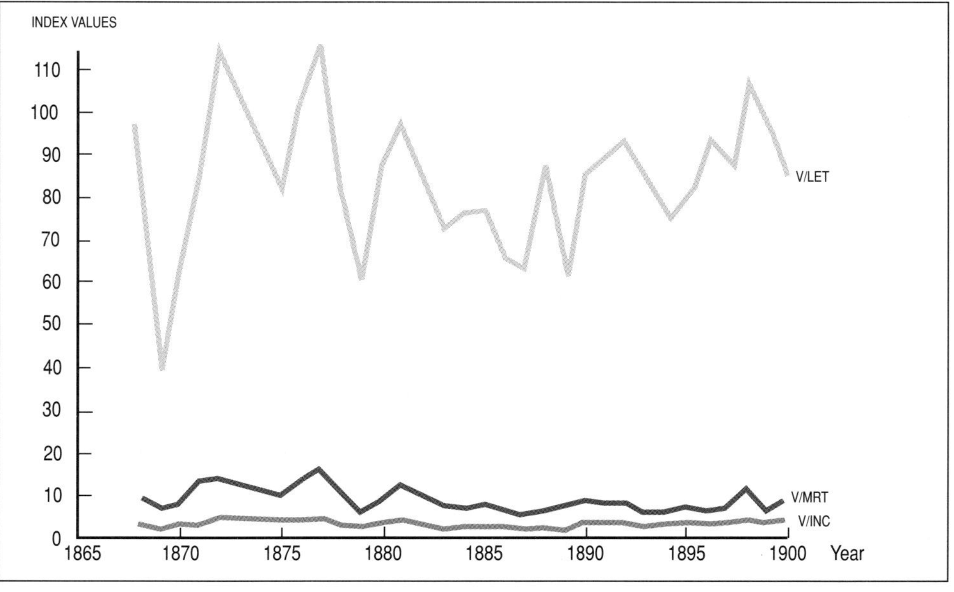

DIAGRAM 9.10
Health concern index for typhoid fever in Norway 1868–1900. Calculation based on incidence (v/inc), mortality (v/mrt), and lethality (v/let). (For calculation of index see Larsen et al. 1980)

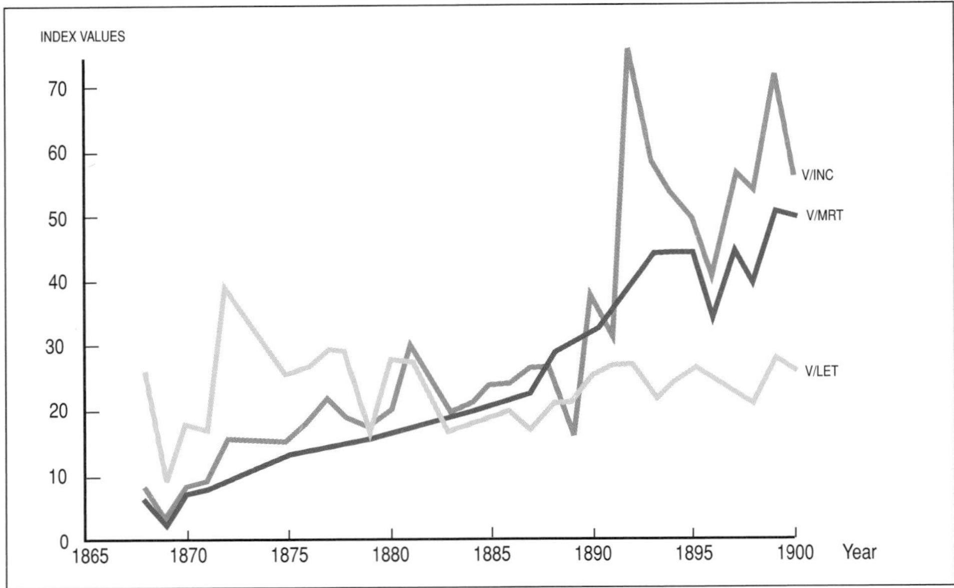

DIAGRAM 9.11
Health concern index for diphtheria in Norway 1868–1900. Calculation based on incidence (v/inc), mortality (v/mrt), and lethality (v/let). (For calculation of index see Larsen et al. 1980)

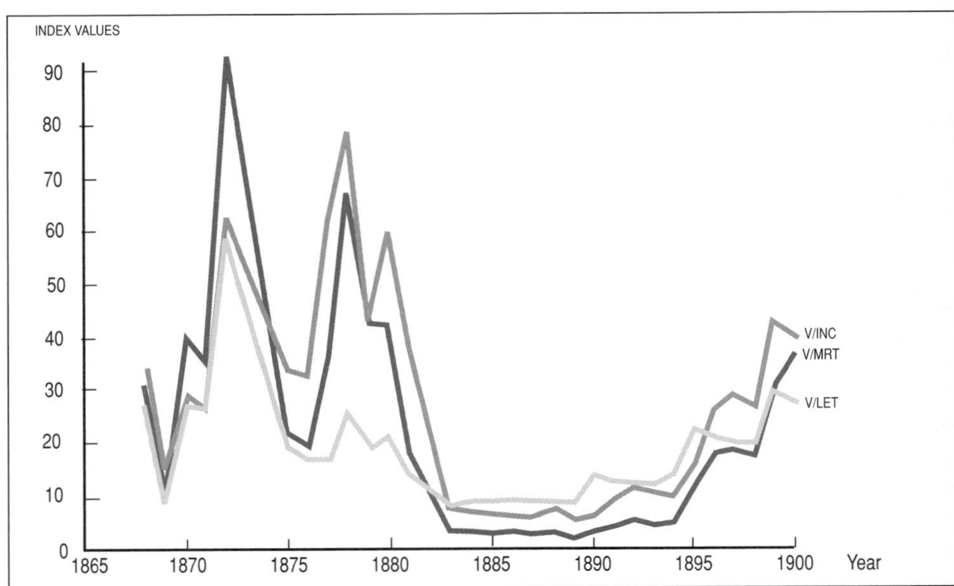

DIAGRAM 9.12

Health concern index for epidemic diseases in Norway 1868–1900. Calculation based on incidence (v/inc), mortality (v/mrt), and lethality (v/let). (For calculation of index see Larsen et al. 1980)

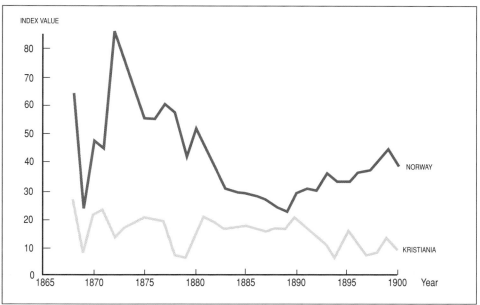

concern about the diseases seems to diminish gradually up to around 1890, when the tide turns (Diagram 9.8). In the case of the capital, the concern was on a lower level throughout the entire period.

Mortality as a basis for the calculation of the index seems to give a special visualization of the effect. A health concern index calculated on the basis of the statistics on acute diarrheas does not show any differences over time (Diagram 9.9); however, the more serious typhoid fever (Diagram 9.10), and diptheria (Diagram 9.11), indicates the perceived importance of the more dangerous infections.

Two questions arise: were diseases regarded as a more or less inevitable cost in the process of modernization and economic growth experienced by the Norwegian society? Diagram 9.12 indicates this. And why did a change occur around 1890?

As to the first question, a lot of factors may be discussed, among them that in the contemporary epidemiological situation, an increase in contagious disease was almost unavoidable when a society was intermigled. This was common knowledge at the time, based on experience through the centuries: a fact that the population had accepted and adjusted to.

The answer to the second question is that around 1890 several cultural changes took place in the Norwegian society. One of them was that by then society had obtained such a degree of maturity that the final phase of the demographic transition started the fall of the birth rate. A possible shift in the perception of the importance of diseases may also be an element in this maturation, but it is only one of the threads in a complicated lace.

References

Larsen, Ø., H. Haugtomt, W. Platou. *Sykdomsoppfatning og epidemiologi 1860–1900*. Oslo: Seksjon for medisinsk historie, Universitetet i Oslo, 1980

Medicinalberetningene. *Avlevering fra medisinaldirektoratet 1932*. Medicinalberetningen og innberetninger om epidemiske sykdommer, kolera etc. 1835–1921. Riksarkivet i Oslo.

CHAPTER 9.1

Modum: Health in an Industrialized Country Municipality

INGVILD STOKKE ABRAHAMSEN AND VICTORIA HØEG

9.1.1. An Interesting Mixed Economy

The municipality of Modum is situated in the eastern part of the county of Buskerud in eastern Norway. It has an area of 517 square kilometers, mostly consisting of farmland and forests. Two major rivers, one coming from the great lake of Krøderen, the other from the lakes of Tyrifjorden, Sperillen and Randsfjorden, unite here in a river that continues some forty kilometers downstream to the outlet in the City of Drammen. Thus, Modum is a rather central municipality situated in Norway.

Farming conditions in Modum are, and have been good, and farming, together with forestry, had a dominant position in the local economy in earlier centuries. In the 1770s "Modum Blaafarveverk" (The Modum Blue Dye Factory) was established, bringing industry to Modum. The company produced a much- sought-after blue dye processed from cobalt ore. Ore was mined from the nearby hills, but the factory and the main dwelling area for the workers were located at the nearby river, close to the waterfall of Haugfoss. For years "Blaafarveverket" was a cornerstone of the local economy, with its production peaking in the period 1822–1848. Later, production was closed down, mainly because of international competition from other and cheaper substitutes.

Modum's early mixture of industrial and more traditional rural occupations makes the municipality special and therefore an interesting object of study. The sources give us the possibility, within a small geographical area, to study the medical problems following the urbanization and industrialization of a rural community, and to compare the health problems of an urbanized group with those of a rural population. To start with, there were six medical districts in Buskerud: Buskerud Landsfysikat (later Drammen Lægedistrikt [medical district]), Ringerike Lægedistrikt, Modum Lægedistrikt, Hallingdal Lægedistrikt, Sandsvær Lægedistrikt, and Rollag Lægedistrikt. Modum medical district consisted of the administrative counties of Eker, Sigdal, and Modum. Hence, the numbers for Modum include these counties as well. Eker had the most inhabitants (11,783 in 1865), followed by Modum (7,556) and Sigdal (6,582). Differences that separate Modum medical district from the other two are not necessarily due to conditions in Modum county, but might arise from conditions in Eker or Sigdal. Up to 1879, Hallingdal medical district consisted of Næs, Aal, and Gol. In 1879, it was divided into Næs medical district, which included Gol, and Aal medical district, which included Hol.

From 1842 to 1867 Heinrich Arnoldus Thaulow (1808–1894) was a physician at "Blaafarveverket" and at the same time the district physician in Modum. His handwritten medical reports for the years between 1842 and 1868 are valuable sources on the health conditions. These reports consist of only limited statistical material, something that makes it difficult to give precise figures describing the state of health during this period.

From 1868 onwards a more systematic reporting of epidemic diseases is available. The studies of the period from 1868 to 1899 are based on the county reports.

But for the district of Modum there exists a quite special source: In the years between 1829 and 1855 a French scientist by the name of Frédéric Le Play (1806–1882) conducted a comparative study of the living conditions of 57 working-class families from different European countries. These studies were published in 1855. Among the communities studied was Modum in Norway. The field work here was carried out in 1845 by A. de Saint-Léger, a co-worker of Le Play. The objective of the studies was to study what influence factors such as geography, occupation and family life had on the people, both physically and socially. This was done by studying the working conditions, wages, household economy, family life, customs and morality and so on of what was considered to be a representative family over an extended span of time (de Saint-Léger and Le Play 1877).

Le Play's studies give us an interesting account of the life in Modum. It could be stated that, even though the work at the Blaafarveverket brought the workers in contact with poisonous arsenic, the work in itself obviously was not unhealthy. Actually, the health conditions were considered to be good, something that probably could be attributed to social measures at the work place, which also were described. Le Play's studies have often been used as support for the view that hygienic conditions were particularly good at Blaafarveverket. This may of course not be true if we compare them with modern hygienic standards, but it seems beyond doubt that the conditions were better than those in most factories and workshops elsewhere in the country.

Modum may be compared to the nearby parts of the county of Buskerud. For the years 1870–1873, we have the numbers of illnesses in the town of Drammen, but we lack such information for the periods of 1868-1870 and 1874–1878. From 1879 the numbers from Drammen Lægedistrikt (medical district) have been used, because there are no figures for the town alone. The numbers therefore contain information from some districts around the town as well. Until 1879 we have related the number of diseased in Drammen to the population in Buskerud Landsfysikat (medical district). When we compare numbers of diseased in Buskerud Landsfysikat with numbers from Drammen, we see minor differences; this source of error is therefore unsignificant.

9.1.2. Health and Disease

9.1.2.1. Health in Modum 1842–1868

In general it seems that health conditions in Modum from 1842 to 1868 were good. The dominant epidemic diseases were pneumonia, diphtheria, scarlet fever, and diarrhea. Pneumonia and pleurisy were particularly common during the winter. In the spring, common colds were prevalent, while in the summer and autumn, diarrhea and cholera were the dominant diseases. There were individual cases of chicken-pox, measles and mumps during the whole year.

9.1.2.2. 1842-1852

In 1842, 1,313 cases of illness were reported

in the district, while there had been 2,200 cases the previous year. At that time, 7,500 people lived in Modum. The number of cases of illness during the other years of this period is not given. The state of health in 1847 was described as "less than good." Cases of respiratory diseases, diphtheria, measles, and croup appeared all year. In 1851, there was a major epidemic of dysenthery from the beginning of September to the end of the year. This disease particularly affected children and was often fatal.

9.1.2.3. 1853

From 1853, county reports with information on the whole of the county of Buskerud are readily available. In 1853, health was described as generally good throughout the whole county. Typhus was the dominating disease, particularly in Drammen. Cases of typhus were also mentioned in Modum, Ringerike, and Sandsvær. We do not know whether the incidence in the country districts was lower or higher than in Drammen. Otherwise, it seems as though throat infections and bronchitis were more common in Drammen than in other municipalities. Overall, the level of illness was low.

9.1.2.4. 1854

1854 was an interesting year. The state of health in Modum was particularly good, better than in previous years. No epidemics occurred, and there was no increase in chronic illness. Thaulow ascribed this to the fact that agriculture prospered well. The bankruptcy of Blaafarveverket led to an increase in the number of people who moved away from the district. This led to less crowded living conditions among the workers, and the farmers gained access to larger areas of agricultural land. The farmers and crofters produced more than before. According to Thaulow, most people lived better than they did before. The health status for the rest of Buskerud is also described as good for this year.

9.1.2.5. 1855

In the county report for 1855, there is a report of an epidemic of scarlet fever at Modum, which spread to the nearby valleys of Sigdal and Eggedal. There were few who sought help, and there were many who died. There were no similar epidemics in other districts. Unfortunately, Thaulow's report for this year is missing, so we do not know what the general health status in Modum was considered to be. There was a typhus epidemic in Kongsberg, the mining town west of Modum. The epidemic could also be detected in Drammen and in other places in Sandsvær. The health status in Drammen was otherwise dominated by pneumonia and diarrhea. The latter two diseases had a consistently higher incidence in Drammen than in the other health districts. This applies to all the years of this period.

9.1.2.6. 1857

In 1857, there was reported an outbreak of Asiatic cholera in Drammen. The epidemic was confined to a single neighborhood in the town. There was not a single case of this disease in Modum in 1870. The reason could be that few people moved into the district, since there were few employment possibilities there.

9.1.2.7. 1859

In 1859, there was an epidemic of plague in Drammen, which probably was malaria. It affected 121 persons. Twenty-five years had passed since the last time the disease had been widespread in the town. The epidemic was considered to be associated with a swamp in a tributary of the river Lier. However, in Modum only a few cases of illness were reported this year.

9.1.2.8. 1860

For 1860, a table (Table 9.1) is available giving the number of deaths from different dis-

Table 9.1
Causes of death in Modum in 1860

Causes of death	Age Males	Age Females	Numbers Males	Numbers Females	Total
Phthisis	28–68	32–58	2	3	5
Angina Membranosa	1.5	1.5	2	1	3
Typhus	68	19–36	1	2	3
Pneumonia	26–58	–	2	0	2
Apoplexia	–	58–82	0	2	2
Bronchitis	2	3	1	1	2
Hydrops	–	65–68	0	2	2

eases in Modum. This is included to give a picture of which diseases were the most serious.

Health status was regarded as extremely good in 1860, despite the fact that it was a poor year for agriculture. There was a long and rainy autumn, and the crops were small and poor. Pneumonia was less common than in the previous year, both in Modum and in several other districts. Thaulow mentions that there were minor epidemics of typhus and whooping cough in Modum. The county medical reports show that the state of health was also good for the rest of Buskerud. Whooping cough was common in Drammen during the first half of the year. The incidence is not known, because poor people rarely sought help from the doctor for this disease. The epidemics during this year were reported as small, contained, and mild.

9.1.2.9. 1861–1863

Thaulow's reports for 1861-1863 are missing. Comments for these years are therefore based on the county medical reports. 1861 was, like the previous year, a good year for most of Buskerud. Sandsvær and Hallingdal were exceptions, since there was more sickness there than in the previous year. Whooping cough was the only epidemic disease with an increase in incidence. It occurred in all the health districts. There was a minor epidemic of scarlet fever in Ringerike and Modum. This ravaged the farms of the crofters, and took many lives.

In 1862 and 1863, the status of health was poor in the whole of Buskerud. There were several epidemics, mainly diphtheria and scarlet fever. In 1862, there was also an epidemic of measles, which occurred in more scattered cases in the following year. These epidemics were to be found in all the municipalities.

9.1.2.10. 1864–1867

From 1864, there is little information on sickness in Modum in Thaulow's reports. He refers more and more to the building of the spa at Modum, and writes less about illness in the district. Therefore, for the last years up to 1868 we have obtained information mainly from the county medical reports.

In 1866, a few cases of Asiatic cholera appeared again in Buskerud, mainly in the town of Drammen. There was only one case in Modum, and three in Sandsvær.

In 1867, there was a large typhus epidemic in Modum and Buskerud. It started in 1866, and the number of cases increased during 1867. There is reason to believe that the epidemic started in Drammen, and that it spread from there to Modum.

In the summer of 1866, there was a large fire in the town of Drammen. Many workers from Modum traveled to Drammen, because of the opportunity to obtain work in rebuilding the town. They obviously brought infection back with them to the rural districts. There was also a scarlet fever epidemic in 1867. Perhaps this disease was brought to Modum and further on to Sigdal in the same way as the typhus epidemic.

9.1.3. Illness Among the Workers at Blaafarveverket, as Compared to the Farmers

According to Thaulow, there was no more illness among the workers at Blaafarveverket than among the farmers. It seems that working conditions at Blaafarveverket were not especially damaging to the workers health, apart from the people who got skin disease as a result of cleaning the ovens. The miners were subjected to eye infections, because of the dust created when crushing the ore. They delayed contacting the doctor, which led to the development of an ophthalmitis. There was little that could be done for this condition.

In the medical report for 1842, Thaulow states that there was no evidence that arsenic fumes were dangerous. Neither was there any reason to believe that the new oxidation process, which had been introduced into the factory around 1847, had any negative effects on the workers' health. However, many workers were bothered by "chronic frailties," such as arthritis, rheumatism, cardialgia (heartburn) and "hysteri"(hysteria). Thaulow found that these diseases were more common among the workers than among the rest of the population.

In the medical reports, little is told about accidents in the mines. The historian Eli Moen has looked at the frequency of accidents at Blaafarveverket. She found very few fatal accidents. From 1830 to 1845, there were 12 deaths due to rock falls, explosions and falls. 1854 was the worst year for accidents, when six people died and two were injured in a rock fall (Moen 1984). The figures for fatalities was much lower at Blaafarveverket than at the nearby Kongsberg Silver Mine, for example.

9.1.4. The Importance of the Social Measures at Blaafarveverket

Industry obviously did not have the same negative influence in Modum as in the large towns. It is tempting to associate this with favorable social measures at Blaafarveverket. As mentioned earlier, all workers and their families were given free medical help and medicine. Treatment could be given at an earlier stage in the disease, which meant that the workers could recover more quickly. In addition, this could have limited the spread of epidemic diseases. Such diseases could be detected earlier, giving the doctor the chance to initiate necessary measures. Thus, to a large extent, serious epidemics could be avoided. However, it has been shown (Imhof and Larsen 1975) that even though the doctor was available free of charge, the tendency of people to consult the doctor for ordinary diseases was low. This fact tells something about the general attitudes toward disease and toward the services offered by the medical profession.

Many workers were provided with housing. The standard of such housing was relatively good. Compared to the crofters' homes, the workers had better houses (Sæter 1976). They lived in much less crowded conditions than the workers in Drammen, for example. In addition, they were able to use wood that could not be used for anything else then firewood. These factors could also have helped to prevent diseases from flourishing and spreading.

The management in Blaafarveverket recognized the importance of good hygiene. As an example, they provided free soap to the workers. Perhaps the cleanliness in Modum was better than in Drammen? Thaulow reports that there were few workers who had scabies. Hygiene was probably a significant factor in explaining the differences in the level of illness between the two districts.

The management at Blaafarveverket was built on paternalistic principles. The managers took responsibility for the workers; their concern extended beyond the payment of a salary and providing a working environment. They also cared for the workers when they were sick or elderly, and ensured that they had a healthy lifestyle. In addition, they made the workers feel a sense of solidarity with the factory, both while they were at work and during their spare time. The lives of the workers were followed up and arranged in order to keep them healthy and enable them to do a good job. Many of the social rights were laid down in the Mining Acts, but there was much variation in how well the management in the different works followed up these rights. In this respect the workers at Blaafarveverket obviously were fortunate in having good management.

9.1.5. Blaafarveverket's Influence on the Farmers' Living Conditions

The favorable state of health in Modum was not caused by the relative prosperity of the workers alone. The farmers also had good living conditions during the boom years. The farmers could sell their produce at the factory's market, every fourth week, when it was payday. Many of them also worked as seasonal workers, for example, transporting ore. A general trend at this time was that farms had been divided up into smaller units. This meant that many farmers no longer could earn a living from farming alone. During the summer and the winter there was less to do on the farms, which meant that the excess labor force was available to the industry. Farmers in Modum began to use cash money as a more integrated part of their economy somewhat earlier than farmers in other parts of the country. The combination of farming production and wage labor stabilized the social and economic situation of the farmers. The whole community clearly benefited from the company's progress.

9.1.6. The Impact of the Bankruptcy in 1848

The level of illness in Modum remained low, even after the factory went bankrupt in 1848. One would have expected the level of illness to increase when unemployment soared and people suffered. But this was not the case. Unemployment led to people moving away from Modum, so that those who remained had more spacious living conditions. Since few people moved into the district, few diseases were brought into the area. Perhaps this is why there was not a single case of Asiatic cholera in Modum during the major epidemic in 1853. Even when cholera occurred in Drammen in 1857, no-one in Modum was infected. In 1866 and 1867, more people moved in, and then the epidemic diseases, typhus and scarlet fever, flared up. This does not necessarily mean that there were few sick people in Buskerud during these years, even though the state of health was generally good. It is important to realize that "good health" was different then it is today. Disease was something that people had to live with, and people visited the doctor only when the situation was serious.

9.1.7. Industry with Positive Health Effects?

As we have seen, the state of health in Modum and the rest of Buskerud was generally good in the years from 1842 to 1868. There was no more illness in Modum than in the other municipalities, but the level of illness was on the other hand not markedly lower. Modum was mentioned less frequently than neighboring Sandsvær in the reviews of diseases. Generally, the incidence of disease was slightly lower in Modum, but this varied from year to year, so the trend is not clear.

However, it is obvious that there was much more illness in the city of Drammen than in the other municipalities. This particularly applies to pneumonia, bronchitis, and diarrhea. This was probably due to the overcrowded housing conditions in Drammen. Industry provided work for many people, so many moved into the town. Overcrowding was conducive to the spread of epidemic diseases, which therefore became more widespread. Towns are often characterized by much through-traffic, so that many diseases are brought into the town, and this applied to Drammen as well.

When looking at how the growth of industry influenced illness, there are several factors that must be taken into account: the type and level of industry, the working environment, and social measures at the work place. Our findings indicate that the growth of industry did not necessarily have a negative influence on the state of health of the population. Industry which causes little pollution, both for the workers and the surrounding area, and which has good safety routines and a responsible management could actually improve health conditions in the population. By living conditions, we here mean how people live, their access to social services, for example a doctor, poor relief, sickness benefits, and schools and the possibilities for a good nutrition. It seems that Modum Blaafarveverk was a company that obviously had a positive influence on the economy and the living conditions in the district.

9.1.8. Illness in Modum 1868–1899

From this period, the information given in the county medical reports is more detailed. The number of cases of different diseases is given for each health district. We have here selected the most common diseases, because these provide most information and probably also contain the least errors in diagnostics.

It is of interest to compare Modum with the districts of Sandsvær, where the town of Kongsberg is, and Ringerike. The silver mine in Kongsberg, not far away from Modum, was closed down in 1805. It started up again in 1816, but was never as big as it previously had been. Flour mills, saw mills, and brick works had a minor influence on the employment situation in the district. In 1873, two wood pulp mills were established, which helped the employment situation a little. Agriculture expanded, particularly from 1850 onward. Kongsberg and the surrounding rural area had an industrial history resembling that of Modum. (The health conditions in the mining period in Kongsberg are discussed by Larsen [1994] and will not be covered here.) People in the nearby district of Ringerike earned their living mainly from agriculture. Saw mills made up the most important industry. Ringerike also had mines. Dr. Thaulow was the medical officer for Ringerike's nickel mine.

The most common disease was bronchitis, probably acute bronchitis. The incidence of bronchitis generally increased during this period. This could be due to the increasing industrialization that occurred over the whole of Norway and that led to increased instability in the society. People moved more, and diseases therefore became more widespread. Perhaps people also visited the doctor for less serious diseases, or contacted the doctor earlier. An important question, however, is to what extent the diagnosis of bronchitis was confused with cases of tuberculosis. If this was the case, this could explain some of the epidemic pattern.

The incidence was highest in Drammen and Sandsvær (Diagram 9.13). The level in Modum was lower, at about the same level as Ringerike. The Drammen health district included the town, with much through-traffic and overcrowding, factors which contributed to the spread of major epidemics. There was high unemployment in Sandsvær, and alcohol consumption was high there, which could have led to decreased resistance to disease among the population.

For diarrhea and what in the reports was called cholera (but not in the sense of Asiatic cholera), the trends were the same as for bronchitis: a low level of disease in Modum and Ringerike, a constantly high level in Drammen (Diagram 9.14). For many years, the poor sewerage system in the town was discussed in the county medical reports. In 1887 it was pointed out that poor sewerage conditions led to ill health. Little was done in Drammen to prevent epidemics. In 1891, the lack of a place for isolating cases of epidemic diseases was highlighted. They had to use an unsuitable hospital in Strømsø. The worst year in all districts was 1889. According to the medical reports, this was due to the warm summer. The warmth and the drought led to a water shortage, and the epidemic spread quickly. At the end of the summer, when the rain came, the epidemic quickly subsided. The same thing happened in 1899, with a warm, dry summer and poor drinking water. Warm summers also provided ideal conditions for bacteria and caused food to spoil.

The graph for scarlet fever (Diagram 9.15) shows clear waves of epidemics. The

DIAGRAM 9.13

Incidence of bronchitis in the county of Buskerud 1868–1899

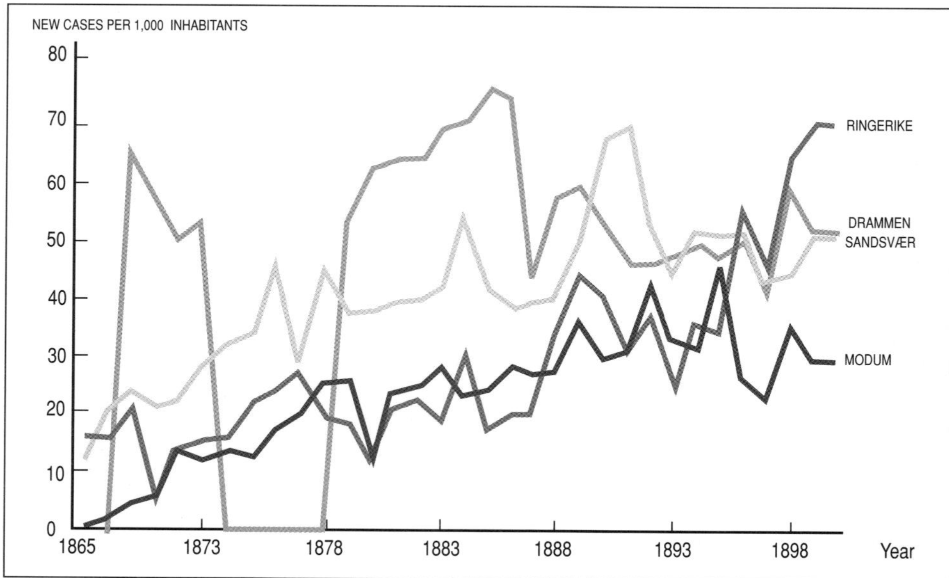

Diagram 9.14
Incidence of diarrhea in the county of Buskerud 1868–1899

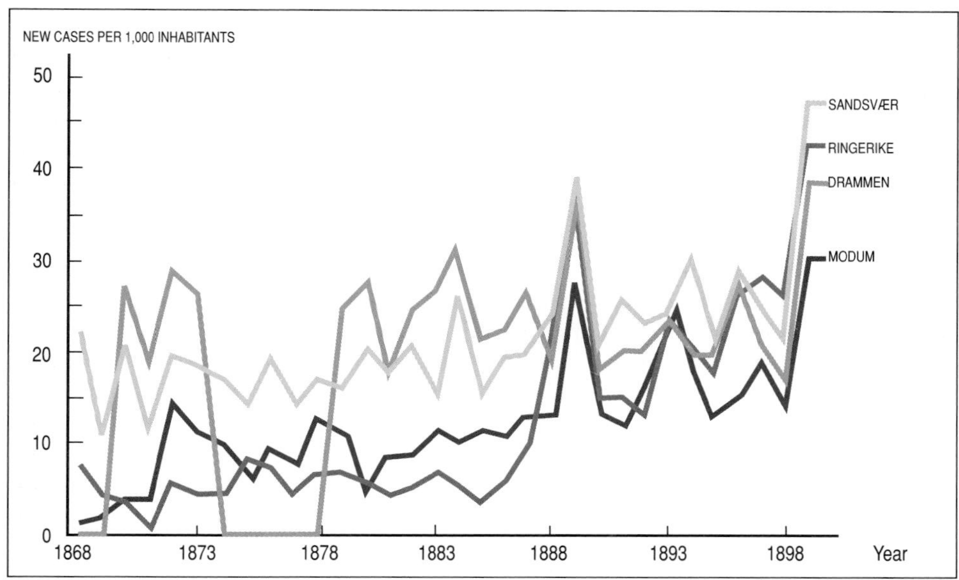

Diagram 9.15
Incidence of scarlet fever in the county of Buskerud 1868–1899

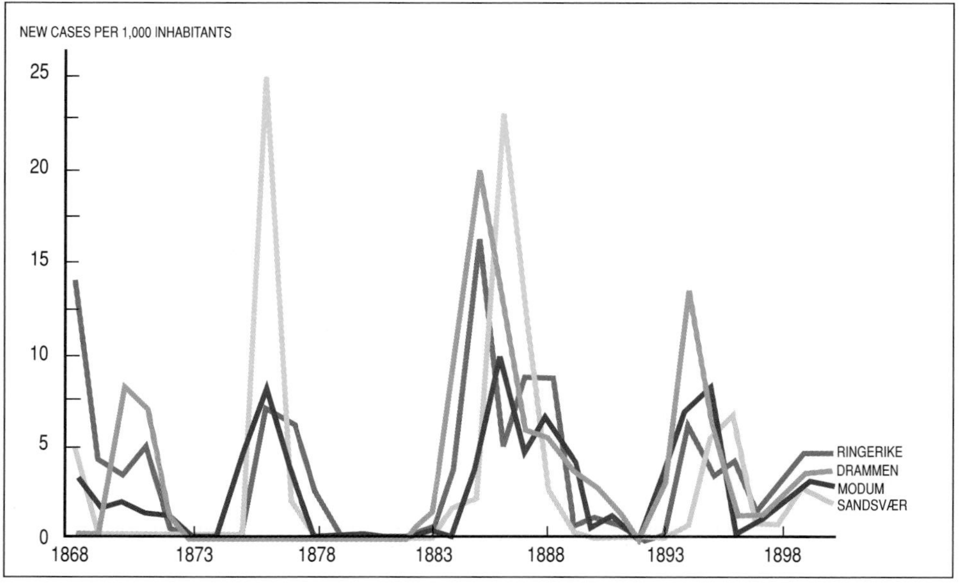

epidemics reached all districts, but were milder in some districts than others. The trends in Ringerike and Modum were similar, and at a lower level than Drammen and Sandsvær. In both Modum and Ringerike, people were appointed to supervise disinfection and isolation of places where there were cases of infectious diseases. This arrangement was very important during the diphtheria epidemic in 1891. When infection occurred, the house was disinfected and strict isolation had to be observed.

A major epidemic of scarlet fever broke out in 1876. The epidemic was mild in Modum the first half of the year, but became more serious during the autumn. Dr. Hans Gabriel Sundt Dedichen (1836–1899) points out that the risk of transmission was great in the small, crowded crofters' cottages. The disease was widespread and often very virulent in Sandsvær, often leading to complications. Overcrowding was also indicated as the reason why the disease was so widespread there. Better housing conditions in Modum was probably the reason why the epidemic was less serious there, in addition to the generally good nutritional standard.

There was an epidemic in Drammen and Ringerike in 1885, and in 1886 there was a mild epidemic in Sandsvær and Modum. The epidemic in Ringerike was the largest one since 1868, with a large number of fatalities. There was a scarlet fever epidemic in Drammen and Modum in 1893, but it was mild. It was spread from Drammen to Modum by a family with a sick child, who went to a party in Vikersund, from where the disease spread further on. The epidemic lasted throughout 1894 in Modum, it waned in the autumn, but blew up again at the end of the year, probably again because of spread from Drammen. The graph shows that the waves of epidemics in Modum followed those in the other districts, but they were milder than in Drammen and Sandsvær.

From 1873 to 1898, the level of typhoid

Diagram 9.16
Incidence of typhoid fever in the county of Buskerud 1868–1899

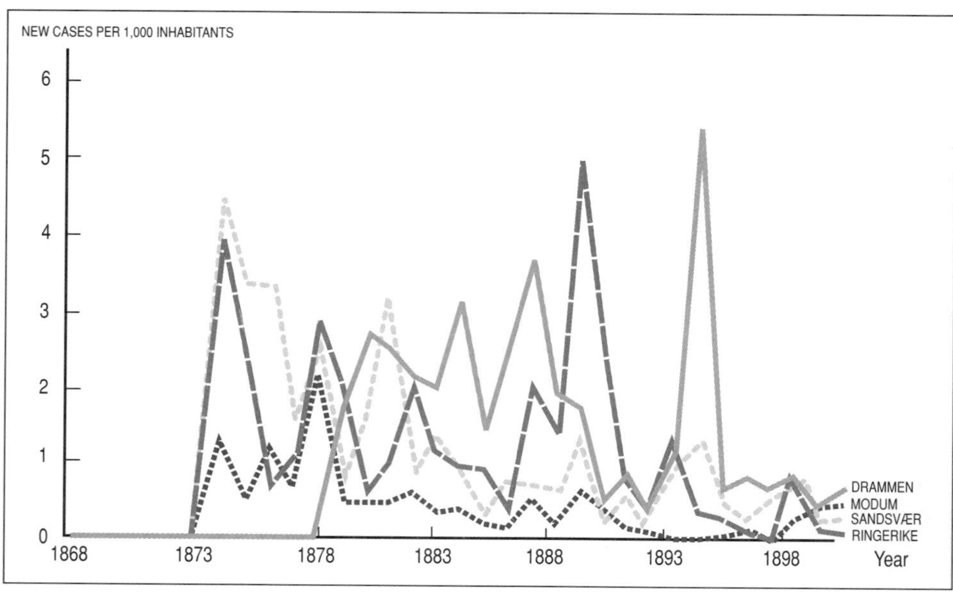

DIAGRAM 9.17
Incidence of scurvy in the county of Buskerud 1868–1899

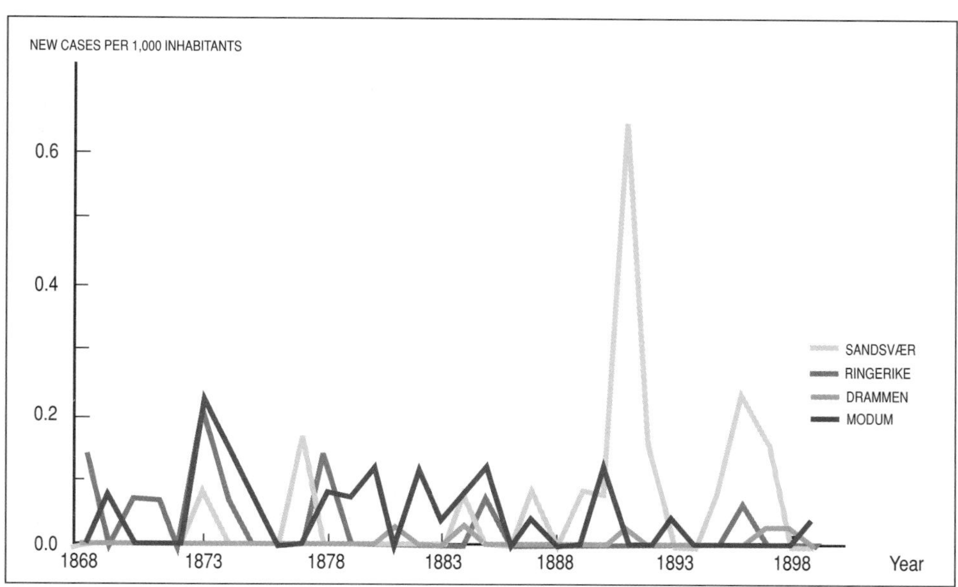

fever was generally low in Modum and higher in Drammen, where the disease usually started (Diagram 9.16).

Scurvy was the only disease which was more prevalent in Modum than in the other districts (Diagram 9.17). From Le Play's studies, we know that potatoes and vegetables, important sources of vitamin C, only made up 6 percent of the diet of families in Modum in 1845. Perhaps vitamin C intake was lower in Modum than in the other districts?

References:

Christophersen, H.O. *Eilert Sundt, en dikter i kjensgjerninger.* Oslo: Gyldendal Norsk forlag, 1962.

Hodne, F. *Norges økonomiske historie 1815–1970.* Oslo: Cappelens forlag, 1981.

Imhof, A.E. and Ø. Larsen *Sozialgeschichte und Medizin. Probleme der Quantifizierenden Quellenbearbeitung in der Sozial- und Medizingeschichte.* Oslo: Universitetsforlaget, 1975 and Stuttgart: Gustav Fischer Verlag, 1975

Kosthold og helse. Oslo: Landsforeningen for kosthold og helse, 1956.

Larsen, Ø., O. Berg, and F. Hodne, *Legene og samfunnet.* Oslo: Seksjon for medisinsk historie og Den Norske Lægeforening, 1986.

Larsen, Ø., H. Haugtomt and W. Platou. *Sykdomsoppfatning og epidemiologi 1860-1900. Epidemiologiske sykdommer i Norge og helsemyndighetenes vurdering av folkehelse – presentasjon av data.* Oslo: Seksjon for medisinsk historie, Universitetet i Oslo, 1980.

Larsen, Ø. *Berglege Henrik Rosted og levekårene på Kongsberg på slutten av 1700-tallet* Kongsberg: Sølvverkets Venner, 1994.

Lunde, Aa. *Sandsværs historie, bind 1.* Sandsvær bygdebokkomite, 1973.

Moen, E. *Rift om brødet? Thesis in history,* University of Oslo, 1984.

Moen, E. *Modum – ei bygd, tre elver.* Caspersens trykkeri, 1993.

Natvig, H. "Blaafarveverket på Modum. Kosthold og leveforhold i en arbeiderfamilie på Modum i 1845." *Liv og Helse, 1963.*

Natvik, H. "Kosthold, levevilkår og arbeidsforhold blant arbeidere ved Modum Blaafarveverk i 1845." *Norsk bedriftshelsetjeneste*, 1985, 6, 292–302.

Natvig, H. and E. Thiis-Evensen sen. "Arbeidsmiljø og helse." *Norsk bedriftshelsetjeneste,* 4(1983):1–333.

Nerbøvik, J. *Norsk historie 1870 – 1905.* Oslo: Det Norske Samlaget, 1986.

Norge vårt land. Den vide bygd – der fjerne åser blåner. Oslo: Gyldendal Norsk Forlag, 1984.

Saint-Léger, A. de and F. Le Play, "Fondeur des usines à cobalt du Buskerud.", in *Ouvriers Européens. Etudes sur les Travaux. La vie domestique, et la Condition Morale de Populations Ouvriers de l'Europe*, 2em édition. Tome 13, Les Ouvriers du Nord. Paris, Marne. 1877, Chapter II.

Sæther, P. *Modum Blaafarveverk, et verkssamfunn i 1830 – 40 årene.* Oslo: Thesis in ethnology, University of Oslo, 1976.

Tveiten, G. *Hole Herred Ringerike.* Kristiania: Centraltrykkeriet i Kristiania, 1914.

CHAPTER 9.2

The Remote Regions – Northern Norway

ANDERS FORSDAHL

9.2.1. Geography and Climate

Northern Norway, which in 1866 was divided into the three counties of Nordland, Troms, and Finnmark, is a huge geographical area of about 120,000 square kilometers, comprising about 37 percent of Norway's land mass. In comparison, the whole kingdom of Denmark covers about 43,000 square kilometers. Northern Norway is long, the distance between Bindalen in the south and Vardø in the north-east is, in a straight line, about 1,000 kilometers. Because the coast line winds round numerous small fjords and islands, it is actually 24,000 kilometers long. In comparison, the equator is about 40,000 kilometers long.

The climate is severe, becoming more severe the further north one travels. Even though the Gulf Stream brings reasonable temperatures to the coastal regions, winter temperatures become very cold in the interior. In the inner areas of Finnmark, temperatures down to minus 51°C have been measured. Summers can be warm and friendly, with mild temperatures and midnight sun in most of Northern Norway; but in winter, weather conditions can be tough and stormy, with polar nights lasting more than three months in the northernmost regions.

9.2.2. Population, Trade, and Industry

Even though Northern Norway comprises about 37 percent of Norway's total area, there were only 160,000 people living there in 1865, 10 percent of the country's population at that time. In 1900, the percentage had risen to 12.2 percent, with a registered population of 257,000.

The population of Northern Norway is made up of several different ethnic groups. Sami people live in the whole area, but the proportion increases towards the north. In 1865, about 8,100 Norwegians lived in Finnmark, as well as 7,500 Sami people (of whom about 1,000 were nomadic), 1,300 people of mixed background, and 3,400 people of Finnish origin. Thus a considerable proportion of the population had an insufficient or lacking command of Norwegian.

With very few exceptions, none of the doctors learned to speak Sami or Finnish, so interpreters had to be used during consultations. Bearing this in mind, it is surprising how seldom language problems are mentioned in the medical reports. In the published medical reports, this issue is covered only once, in a report from Vadsø in 1891, where more than half the population were of non-Norwegian background. The medical report states that help from doctors seemed to be rather unsatisfactory; the doctor did not even understand the patients' language sufficiently well to check the often inadequate interpreter.

The most frequent way to make a living during the whole of the second half of the nineteenth century was fishing, which was very often combined with agriculture. To a large extent, the men were involved in fishing and the women in agriculture. Agriculture gradually became more important, so that by the turn of the century it had become economically more important than fishing in Nordland and Troms. But fishing continued to be the primary industry in Finnmark.

Small, open boats, propelled by sails and oars, were used for fishing. The distances to the fishing grounds were generally short, and small fishing villages lay spread out all along the coast. In places where fishing and agriculture were combined, farms were also widely scattered. Often, only a narrow coastal strip could be cultivated.

Inland, in Nordland and Troms, commercially viable forests were to be found, with the area of Saltfjellet at the Polar Circle forming the border between spruce and pine. Attempts were made to grow grain as far north as Troms, but with unreliable results.

Most Sami people also combined fishing and agriculture, though many had reindeer as their primary or secondary industry. With the exception of the building of small boats, there seems to have been few crafts. In the second half of the nineteenth century, mines were established in many places in northern Norway. This provided many people with the opportunity of earning money outside the fishing season, but there were also social costs: in the course of a short time, there were many people living in poor housing and facing tough and risky working conditions.

9.2.3. Availability of Doctors

In the 1860s, there was a total of about 25 doctors in Northern Norway, that is, one doctor for every 6,600 inhabitants. The number of doctors gradually increased up to the turn of the century, when there were a total of 79 posts. This was partly due to the establishment of hospitals, and partly because the largest health districts were subdivided. At the same time, the population increased by 60 percent. The number of inhabitants per doctor was by then 3,250, which was no worse than in many other parts of the country. But the distances were longer, and most visits to the sick were undertaken by sea in small, open boats. There were few roads, and those that existed were poor, but visits to the sick could be done by means of horse-carts in the summer, and, in some districts, reindeer sledges could be used in winter.

Being a doctor in Northern Norway was a hard and toilsome life. Even though the district physicians as a rule lived in the central area of the district, visits to the sick, even under normal weather conditions, could take a couple of days or more. The distances in some districts could be over 150 kilometers each way, and in poor or stormy weather, the district medical officer and his helpers could be weather-bound for over a week. Several doctors perished during such journeys.

It is impressive to see how well the district physicians kept themselves updated on advances in medicine. This updating was done both through reading medical literature and taking study tours to places where medicine was taught in Europe. Behring's serum-treatment for diptheria started in Germany in 1891, and within three years the serum was in use in Northern Norway.

9.2.4. Social and Hygienic Conditions

The population in northern Norway was generally poor. This is clear from all reports from the districts, including the medical reports. Poverty seems to have been more extreme the further north one went. Because

TABLE 9.2
Live births and infant mortality (deaths under 1 year of age per 1,000 live births) in the health districts in Finnmark in 1890 and 1900

District	1890	1890	1900	1900
	Live births	Infant mortality	Live births	Infant mortality
Alta	204	88.2	198	101.1
Loppa	59	397.9	71	169.0
Hammerfest	153	189.5	149	147.7
Måsøy	89	269.7	109	137.6
Kistrand	125	128.0	155	129.0
Tana	102	225.5	84	84.5
Vardø	140	250.0	168	113.1
Vadsø	138	130.4	153	104.6
Sør-Varanger	61	114.8	38	26.3
Finnmark	1,071	179.3	1,125	115.6

people were dependent on the primary industries, unsuccessful fishing expeditions or a cold, wet summer could quickly lead to dire poverty. Many people lived at the minimum subsistence level. In many northerly parts, there were periods of famine.

Houses were generally small, overcrowded, damp and poorly ventilated. Many people lived in mud huts, and in several places there were huts where people and domestic animals lived in the same room.

Often, privies did not exist, making the area surrounding the houses rather unpleasant. The residents often lacked understanding of the importance of pure drinking water. There was also a lack of knowledge about a varied and adequate diet. And, even if they had had the knowledge, they probably would not have been able to keep their diet varied and sufficient. Clothing was often inappropriate, and vermin flourished. Here, as in other places, poverty often led to resignation and apathy.

The infant mortality rate is regarded as a fairly reliable indicator of social conditions, a fact that is confirmed by looking at the conditions in Northern Norway. Compared to other places in the country, conditions in Nordland were not particularly bad, but the infant mortality rate indicated that conditions became worse the further north one went. Infant mortality in Nordland was at about the same level as the average for the whole country; that is to say, that 10-13 percent of the newborn babies died during their first year up until 1890. But infant mortality in Troms and Finnmark was higher. Only the largest towns in the country came anywhere near such a high infant mortality (Backer 1961). The large variation in infant mortality that occurred in the health districts (Table 9.2), resulted less from variations in social conditions than from different epidemics that ravaged the districts from time to time. It was not until the 1920s that Finnmark had an infant mortality rate under 10 percent (Backer 1961).

Fishing was a dangerous occupation, and many fishermen drowned. Between 1877 and 1900, 5,600 "unfortunate incidents" were registered in Northern Norway, which primarily were due to drowning while fishing or traveling by sea (Backer 1961). This gives an average of 233 cases per year. In 1893, 244 such cases were registered in Nordland alone, and that year over 120 fishermen died in a single storm that struck the Lofoten fisheries.

Moreover, the women also struggled. Their work was heavy and endless as they tended the land and looked after children. They were poorly and inadequately nourished, and if the fishing went bad, they received no money from their fishermen husbands. Many of them were widowed, often as a result of drowning accidents. A system for fostering children was developed in Northern Norway. We know little about how this system functioned, but it seems to have been a good and humane arrangement.

Some district physicians pointed out how deleterious it was that boys as young as twelve years old had to go out on the fishing expeditions. The children often suffered badly on these trips. In the period when the fish were hung up on the drying racks or spread out to make clipfish (dried cod), children as young as ten years took part in the work.

However, it is important to have in mind that poverty was widespread in the whole of Norway, as was poor housing and inadequate nutrition. Slovenliness and poor clothing is described in reports from districts all over the country (Holst 1955).

9.2.5. Medical Reports

In 1803, the health authorities in Copenhagen decided that public medical officers should submit a yearly report on the "health situation and medical conditions." This included dangerous epidemics, mortality, serious accidents, the number of doctors and midwives and their conditions, quacks and pharmaceutical services. Before the regulations came into effect, this function was assigned to the ministers. They had not only to report to the county governor on infectious diseases, mortality, and so on, but they also were required to take measures against epidemics by giving out information and distributing medicines.

In 1830, a new directive was published, which now included all doctors. They had to report on a much wider range of conditions than before: the influence of the weather on health conditions; meteorological observations; nursing care of the poor; sanitary facilities in the district; legal autopsies; and medical, natural historical, chemical and physical observations of interest to medical science. Later, additional factors were added to the list of conditions that had to be reported on, such as general hygienic conditions, housing, mode of living, trade and industry, nutritional status, moral standards, alcohol abuse, and presence of vermin. Many district medical officers used the opportunity to give a more comprehensive account of medical, hygienic or social problems in the district, and some of them also gave a more general report of people's way of life. From 1860, the chairman of the board of health, which in practice meant the district physician, was given the duty of submitting the health report.

It is reasonable to suppose that these numerous additions to systematic reporting had a positive influence on the doctors' practice. Doctors were forced to become familiar with the local environment and the living conditions of the population from a broad perspective, which gave them increased understanding of the relationship between social conditions and the occurrence and development of disease.

From the middle of the nineteenth century and up until 1930, extracts of the medical reports were published by what was called the Ministry of the Interior, in the annual publication on medical conditions and the health situation in Norway. Of course, not all the extracts are equally good. Some seem to be rather superficial and others give perhaps a better impression of the doctors' social background than of the population's life and struggle to survive. But most doctors seem to have taken their duties seriously. The wealth of information gathered in these reports gives a comprehensive picture of the population's standard of living throughout the country, and the reports represent the only source of information in several areas. District physician Anders Bredal Wessel in Sør-Varanger published extracts of the reports from Finnmark in the magazine *Sydvaranger* up until 1912. In his introduction, Wessel stressed how valuable the reports were for everyone who wished to study development not just medical and hygienic development, but cultural and social as well.

9.2.6. Statistical Material

The ministers reported births and deaths, and most often the cause of death as well. With regard to their statements of cause of death, there were certainly many mistakes. Very often, the deceased had not been seen by the district physician during their fatal illness, so a reasonable diagnosis could not be set. But it seems as though the ministers did their best to obtain information from the district medical officer on the cause of death.

During epidemics, the district physician did not manage to see everyone who was sick. In addition, there were many people, particularly the poor, who did not contact the doctor. It is reasonable to assume that this led to prevalence and incidence figures that were too low, and hence lethality figures were too high.

In 1883, the district medical officer in Sør-Varanger reported that only five out of 38 people who died had been visited by the doctor during their last illness. According to the Central Bureau of Statistics, district medical officers at around 1860 had received notification of only 40 percent of all deaths in the country. This situation gradually improved, and by the turn of the century, doctors' mortality statistics included about 81 percent of all deaths (Backer 1961).

9.2.7. Infectious Diseases

Poverty, inadequate nutrition, and general poor health made the population susceptible to infectious diseases. One could perhaps be misled into believing that, because the population was so widely scattered, infectious diseases which came to a district could easily be contained. But this was not the case. The fishing industry involved a lively traffic during the whole year. During the great fishing expeditions, large numbers of fishermen congregated, primarily from Northern Norway, but also from the Trøndelag coast and further south. In 1860, 22,000 fishermen were registered in Lofoten, and at the height of the fishing expeditions in 1893, 32,000 were registered. The district medical officer in Vardø reported that while the town normally had about 1,200 inhabitants, 4,000–5,000 fishermen from other places would gather there in the season. They lived under wretched hygienic conditions. When infectious diseases broke out, the fishermen took the diseases home with them to all parts of Northern Norway. The district physician in Alta reported in 1871 that it was rare to have consecutive months without some kind of infectious disease breaking out within the district.

Another special feature of Northern Norway, particularly for the two northernmost counties, was the close contact with Russian traders and fishermen from the coast around Murmansk and the Barents Sea, the so-called Pomor people. This trade was very beneficial to the region. The Pomores could supply the population with cheaper rye and building materials than the local tradesmen, and they bought fish at a good price from the Norwegians during periods when it was difficult to sell the fish elsewhere. During particularly difficult years, this trade in fact helped large sections of the population of

Finnmark to survive. A special language developed, "Russian-Norwegian."

But, the Russian traders and fishermen could also bring infectious diseases with them, leading to both major and minor epidemics in Northern Norway. We know less about which diseases the Russians took home with them from Norway.

During the years of typhus and famine in Finland in the 1860s, many Finnish people emigrated to Finnmark, and this also probably led to some epidemics. In the medical reports from Finnmark, there are some reports about cases of diphyllobothrium latum, fish tapeworms, and these seem always to have been associated with people of Finnish origin. The immigrants have otherwise always been mentioned as a positive addition to the population. The Finnish immigrants were regarded as skillful, energetic, and more hygienic than Norwegians. They brought with them the sauna, better agriculture, and better animal husbandry.

9.2.8. Leprosy

Leprosy was very sporadic in Northern Norway. The disease was not uncommon in the south of Nordland in the second half of the nineteenth century. In 1865, 148 cases were reported in Nordland, 42 in Troms, and 12 in Finnmark, the latter all in the western part of the county. Even taking the size of the population into account, the disease was less common the further north one went. No cases have ever been reported in eastern Finnmark. Otherwise, the social and hygienic conditions in coastal districts in Northern Norway were conducive to this disease. As in the rest of the country, the incidence of leprosy rapidly declined towards the end of the century (Irgens 1980).

9.2.9. Tuberculosis

In the first half of the nineteenth century, tuberculosis was most prevalent in southern Norway, but it gradually spread northward. Pulmonary tuberculosis and scrophulosis seem to have spread at first in Nordland. Tuberculosis was seldom reported in Finnmark until about 1870-80, but from then on it was registered more and more often, until by the end of the century it was the most common cause of death. Conditions were conducive to tuberculosis.

9.2.10. Diphtheria

There were frequent outbreaks of diphtheria and croup throughout the whole area, in one district or another. It seems often to have been very virulent, with up to 30 percent lethality. But as mentioned previously, figures for incidence and lethality are unreliable. In the 1890s, treatment using serum was introduced, which led to a great reduction in lethality. In the medical report from Hadsel in 1894, it was reported that Eastern Lofoten (149 cases, 34 deaths) and Hadsel had been ravaged to a tragic extent. In the latter district, the disease was relatively benign in the beginning, but then became fairly lethal. On the farms Kvitnes and Brotøen in the district of Hadsel, everyone who caught the disease died, and in the district of Bø 52 of the 72 who were infected. After diphtheria serum was obtained, no further deaths were reported in Bø. In the district of Loppen in Finnmark, 7 out of the 39 people infected in 1897 died. Notwithstanding that the epidemic was very virulent, only one person died out of the 32 who were treated, since serum was widely used. In all places where there were children who had not been infected, prophylactic injections were given with undoubted success. In the same year, 16 cases in Hammerfest were treated, without any deaths. These favorable results were also ascribed to widespread use of serum.

The official statistics in particular show a sudden fall in mortality from the disease during the 1890s (Backer 1961), which presumably was the result of serum treatment.

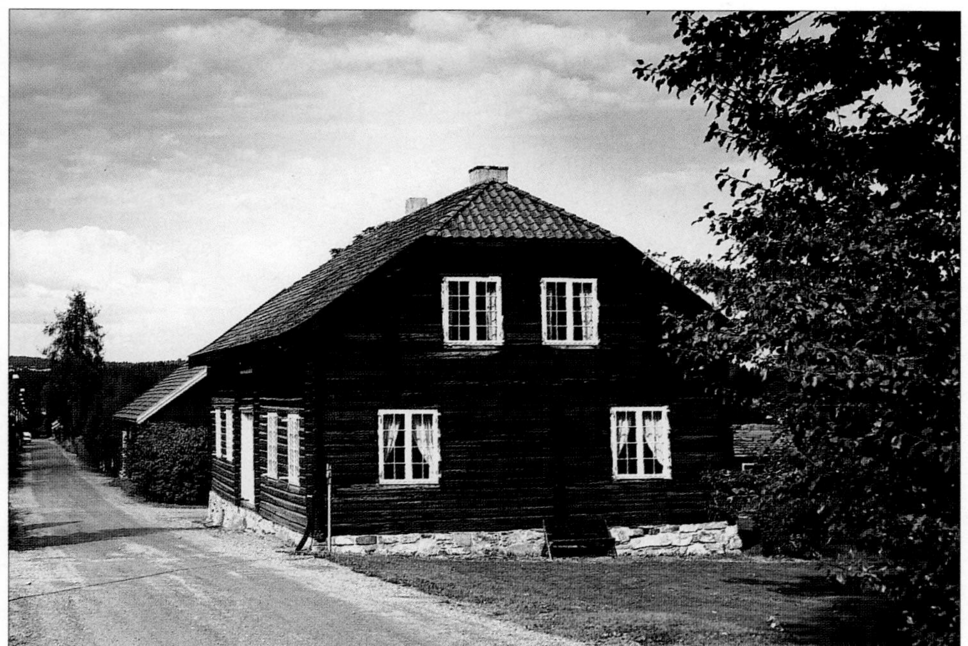

Figure 13: The old mining municipalities of Norway often had set up an organized health system at an early stage. The buildings shown here are from the Modum cobalt miners' village in Southern Norway (Photo: Øivind Larsen 1996).

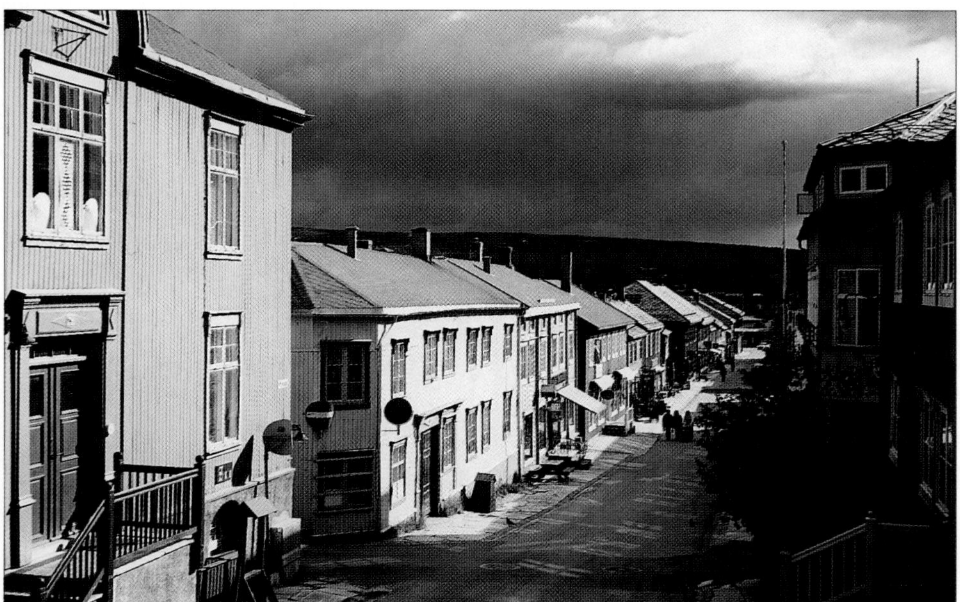

Figure 14: The health system of the silver mine city of Kongsberg is often mentioned in medical history (Larsen 1994), but the copper mine city of Røros also has long traditions in this respect. The picture shows one of the main streets of Røros in 1996 (Photo: Øivind Larsen).

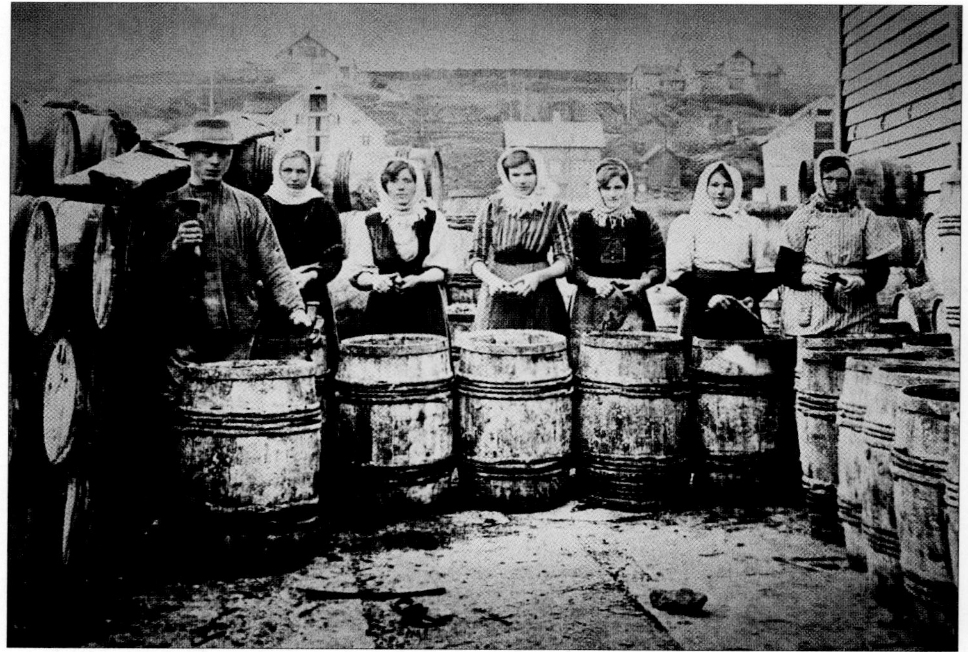

Figure 15: The fisheries off the coasts of Norway have a special part in the development of the morbidity in the nineteenth century. The amounts of catch were sometimes enormous, and the fisheries attracted fishermen from far away during the season. On the one hand the fisheries gave prosperity and better living standards for the population; on the other hand the vivid seasonal migration and clustering of people led to an efficient spread of infectious diseases. On the island of Karmøy at the Western coast, there are two small museums that feature the fishery, and the three pictures printed here were reproduced there.

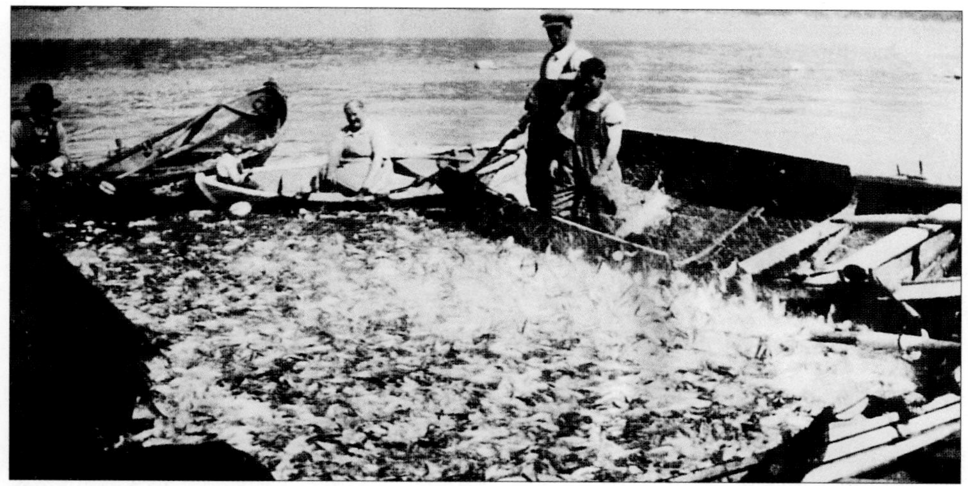

Figure 16: Dangerous work.

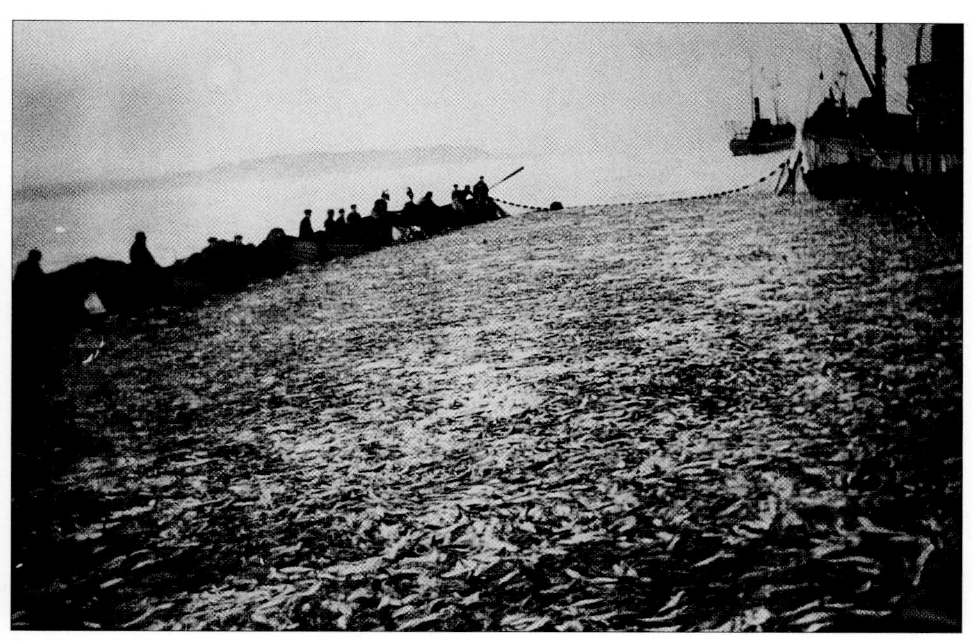

Figure 17: Immense amounts of fish.

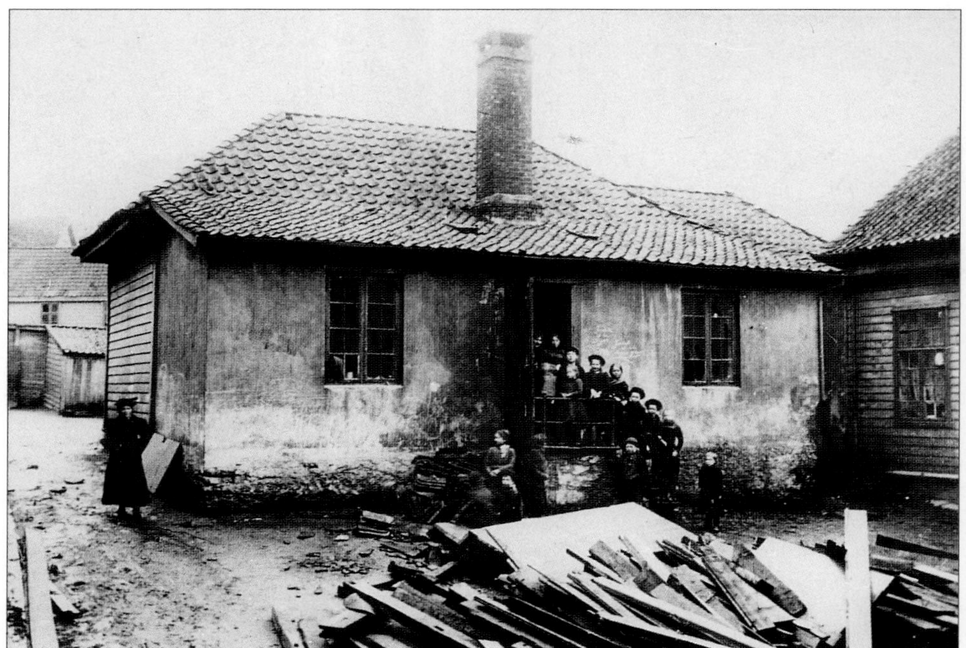

Figure 18: The so-called "Combined Institution" in Stavanger at the end of the nineteenth century. These rather simple buildings served both as a hospital and as a disciplinary institution (Courtesy City Archive, Stavanger).

9.2.11. Typhoid Fever (Nervefeber, Tyfoidfeber)

Typhoid fever was common in the last half of the nineteenth century, and major and minor epidemics broke out throughout the area, with many cases and high lethality. It was often stated that the disease began in a district when a sick person returned home from one of the large fishing expeditions. In addition, the district physicians throughout the whole area regularly complained about the sanitary conditions and poor drinking water in all the fishing villages.

9.2.12 Exanthemic Typhus, Spotted Fever

This serious disease was first registered in the 1870s and seems to have spread rapidly throughout the whole area, often in major epidemics with high mortality. Conditions were conducive to the spread of infection. There were lice everywhere. Doctors also caught this disease and died from it.

9.2.13 Febris Recurrens, Relapsing Fever

This was a serious disease, with high lethality. After district physician James Calder Danchertsen (1825–1904) had read about an epidemic of relapsing fever in Saint Petersburg (Irgens 1980), he realized that an epidemic in Vadsø in 1858–61, which he had registered as typhoid fever, had undoubtedly been febris recurrens.

There were several subsequent outbreaks in eastern Finnmark. In his medical report in 1871, district physician Lauritz Bernhard Thams (1839–1876) in Sør-Varanger described an epidemic in this district.

District surgeon Niels Cristopher Suhr (1768–1816) wrote in his medical report for 1804 about major epidemics in Finnmark of a very serious disease, with a large number of people infected and many deaths. We do not know for certain which disease this was, but it could also have been febris recurrens (Holck 1987, Wessel 1928). The disease was not mentioned in medical reports after 1876.

9.2.14 Smallpox

Despite a very active vaccination effort, several minor smallpox epidemics occurred throughout all of Northern Norway in the 1860s. The most serious epidemic was in Troms in 1866–67, with 395 reported cases and 60 deaths. There is said to have been a major epidemic, with 50–100 deaths in the spring of 1867 in Sør-Varanger, but the information on this is uncertain. At that time there was no district physician in the district. But the incidence dwindled, and after 1873, no new cases were reported in Nordland or Troms. The last cases were recorded in Finnmark, where minor epidemics broke out right up to 1892. Infection was almost exclusively spread by Russian fishermen and traders from the coast around Murmansk and the Barents Sea. District physician Lars Olsen Follum (1822–1905) in Alta gave a thorough report of smallpox and use of smallpox vaccine in his medical report in 1871. He pointed out that when the human lymph was used from one person to another it could lose its effect, and that there was a danger of transmitting other diseases.

9.2.15. Scarlet Fever

Almost throughout the whole period there were constant outbreaks of major epidemics of scarlet fever, with high mortality and dangerous complications (ettersykdommer). During the 1880s, the lethality of the disease seems to have become markedly reduced (Backer 1961). No special treatment was introduced at that time, so either the previously high incidence had resulted in a generally high level of immunity among the population, or else the bacteria must have become less virulent.

9.2.16. Other Infectious Diseases

Epidemics of other infectious diseases, such

as influenza, whooping cough, measles, and German measles, seem to have prevailed, as in the rest of the country.

9.2.17. Scurvy

Scurvy was not uncommon, especially in Finnmark. In 1865–67, 663 cases were reported, with 14 deaths. This was associated with crop failure, with poor harvests of potatoes and cloud berries, and with general suffering and misery. There were isolated cases of scurvy among the Norwegian fishermen, and particularly among the Russian fishermen along the coast of Finnmark. The district physician Johan Theodor Salomon Østberg (1841–1907) in Sør-Varanger reported in 1869 that scurvy was not found among the Sami people in the district, who almost exclusively had a diet consisting of fresh food. But the district physician in Loppa in the years around 1870 reported that he himself had had scurvy several times.

9.2.18. Summary and Conclusions

The district medical physicians' reports are, without doubt, the most important source we have with regard to descriptions of the life and activities of Norwegian people in the second half of the nineteenth century. Even though the district physicians belonged to the class of senior government officials, they had a close relationship with the people. When visiting the sick, they met people in their own homes and obtained insight into traditions and living conditions through personal observation. They often made dangerous journeys, many times accompanied by their coachmen. No other group was in a position to provide information for posterity about the daily lives of ordinary men and women.

However, one must be aware of the fact that the instructions concerning what the medical reports should contain meant that the reports mainly dealt with serious diseases, poor hygiene, and other adverse health-related conditions that the district medical officers wished to correct. This meant that negative aspects might have been highlighted. Positive developments more clearly appear in the statistical material, and developments were indeed positive during this time. People gradually became less dependent on fishing alone; agriculture developed and mining and other industries blossomed. Nevertheless, there is no doubt that people in Northern Norway were poor and had a hard time in the last part of the nineteenth century, and conditions were harder the further north one went.

The life of a district medical officer was difficult, and one becomes filled with respect for those who somehow managed year after year. Few of them stayed in Northern Norway for their whole lives, but they dedicated the best years of their working life to this area.

References

Backer, J.E. *Dødeligheten og dens årsaker i Norge 1856-1895.* Oslo: Statistisk Sentralbyrå, Samfunnøkonomiske studier nr.10, 1961.

Danchertsen, J.C. "Febris recurrens i Vadsø Lægedistrikt i 1858–1861," *Norsk Magazin for Lægevidenskaben (1865):746–751.*

Holck, P. "En Finnmarks-lege," *Tidsskrift for Den norske lægeforening*, (1987):107; 3006–3012.

Holst, P.M. "Helseforholdene i Norge omkring 1880," T*idsskrift for Den norske lægeforening*, Jubileumsnummer, 1955

Irgens, L.M. "Leprosy in Norway. An epidemological study based on national patient registry," *Leprosy Review*, 51(1980), Suppl 1.

Wessel, A.B. "Epidemier og Lægeforhold i Finnmark i slutten av det 18de og begynelsen av det 19. aarhundre," *Tidsskrift for Den norske lægeforening*, 48(1928):118–133.

CHAPTER 9.3

The Trøndelag Counties and the County of Romsdalen

HÅKON LASSE LEIRA

9.3.1 Epidemics, Population and Doctors

King Carl XV (1826–1872, king of Norway and Sweden 1859–1872) was crowned in Trondheim Cathedral on August 5, 1860. One of the reports covering this great event appeared in the medical records, where it is said that just after the coronation, an unusually high number of cases of syphilis occurred in Trondheim, where people from different parts of the country had congregated. Thirty-seven cases of primary, 44 cases of secondary and 63 cases of tertiary syphilis were admitted to the hospital. And the hospital mentioned was Trondheim's municipal hospital.

The town also had in the later half of the nineteenth century a cottage hospital for epidemics (lazaret), a Catholic hospital, a municipal asylum, the State asylum for criminals (1895), and a private surgical clinic, in addition to Trondheim's isolation hospitals for people suffering from leprosy. Just outside the town was Reitgjerdet Pleiestiftelse (1861) (the Reitgjerdet Foundation for Lepers), and some years later the Rotvold Sindsykeasyl (Rotvold Asylum for the Insane) was opened in 1872.

Around 30,000 people lived within the area which today makes up the city of Trondheim. There were 96,300 inhabitants in the whole county (Sør Trøndelag), slightly more than in Møre og Romsdal (the county of Romsdalen) which had 90,300 inhabitants, while in Nord Trøndelag (the county of Nordre Trondhjem) there were 73,500 inhabitants, according to calculations made in 1855. There was one hospital in Møre og Romsdal, Reknes Hospital in Molde, where leprosy patients were treated. Nordre Trondhjem had one hospital in the Namdalen valley and one in Innherred, as today, and there was also an ordinary hospital in the small town of Molde. Otherwise, the hospital structure remained largely unchanged until the turn of the century.

In Møre og Romsdal, the number of doctors increased from 12 to 38 during the period 1860–1900, in Sør Trøndelag from 21 to 57, and in Nord Trøndelag from 11 to 28. At the same time, the populations increased to 134,800 (Møre og Romsdal), 133,800 (Sør Trøndelag), and 82,200 (Nord Trøndelag).

9.3.2. Fishing, Agriculture, and Industry

The 1860s were introduced with an event in which many people gathered in one place, something that was quite uncommon at that time, except for the gathering of fishermen during the fishing seasons. In those days, travel by land was both time-consuming and expensive so making sea voyages was the main way of traveling. The sea was also an important source of income. In this area, fishing and agriculture were the most important sources of income for most people throughout the period; in fact, they were slightly more important than for the rest of the country. In 1891, 76 percent of the people were occupied in the primary industries, whereas in the country as a whole 60 percent were.

As in other coastal counties, the annual fishing expeditions were of great economic importance. But the fishing expeditions for cod and herring were also of great importance for the spreading of epidemic diseases. It was also mentioned that traveling lay preachers spread more than just the gospel. The spring fishing expeditions for herring were often uncertain. No one knew where the herring would appear, but fishermen equipped their boats and sailed to where there had been the most fish the previous year. The fishermen lived on-board their vessels or in accommodation ships, which could have come from far away. The standards of hygiene were poor, and infectious diseases were effectively spread.

The spring herring disappeared from Western Norway toward the end of the 1860s, but remained in Sunnmøre until 1872. Thirty to forty thousand men took part in this fishing, and even though prices varied, they earned money from their work. Deposits in the bank in the town of Kristiansund increased fourfold between 1860 and 1868 and doubled during the 1870s.

When the herring disappeared, fishing for cod became increasingly important. In Lofoten, 20,000–25,000 men took part in cod fishing, while in 1870, along the coast of Møre, 13,000 men took part, 12,000 of them from the county. It was estimated that 50 percent of all employed men in Møre and Romsdal took part either in fishing or in processing the fish to make clipfish (dried cod).

Agriculture was the dominant occupation in Trøndelag. The rural districts around the Trondheim Fjord were known for their reliable harvests, and prosperity increased, if we are to believe the descriptions given by the medical officers. Commercial forestry started around 1840, followed by a period of heavy investments in the period between 1845 and 1865. In the area of Namdalen, investments amounted to 200,000 speciedaler, a substantial amount at that time. However, investors demanded a quick return on their investment, causing a rapid exploitation of the available resources. By around 1885, the timber resources had been used up and commercial forestry came to an end.

As in the rest of the country, there was little industry in this middle part of Norway, and most of it was located in Trondheim. The dominating industry there was a mechanical workshop, which began to operate in 1844. It had about two hundred employees at the beginning of the 1860s (Sandvik 1993). As late as in 1895, there were only nine factories in Nord Trøndelag, seven of them in Stjørdal, with a total workforce of 122 men (Vanebo 1982). But a change was under way. A medical report from Romsdalen in 1896 tells us that more and more butter dairies were being established, many of them powered by small water turbines that were usually connected to a combined separator and butter churn. There was a superfluity of small, water-powered flour mills and sawmills, and a couple of larger steam-powered sawmills. The manufacture of clothes and shoes for the fisheries in Nordland and Finnmark was a significant activity that took place in Indre Romsdal, in tailoring and shoemaking workshops.

9.3.3. Living Conditions

The medical reports leave an impression of steady progress, a process that probably started in the 1860s, since the medical reports from the 1850s could be dramatic, especially the reports from Vestre Søndmøre. One report from 1858 states that the living conditions of ordinary people were still regarded as quite poor. The diet was not varied enough, and the food was often poorly prepared. In most places the diet mostly consisted mainly of herring and salted fish, often so poorly processed, that it went bad. This, combined with food made from flour that was often served with bad milk and a lack of fresh meat does not impress one as being a healthy diet. The rare meat meals consisted mostly of salted or dried meat.

In addition to this, hygienic conditions were also described mentioned as poor. Houses were usually cleaned only on Christmas Eve, and even the slaughtering of animals was done inside the cottages. A general filthiness seems to have been widespread. Diseases are described, and in connection with menstruation and uterine disorders it is mentioned as a sign of progress that woollen underwear had come into more general use.

But things were not only described as being bad. In 1859 it was reported that the use of spirits had been significantly reduced, and the previously widespread nightly activities, with dancing and disorderly conduct, were said to be less common than before. And just two years later there are accounts of improvements in Vestre Søndmøre. Larger and more comfortable houses were being built in more suitable places, and with better foundations. We also learn that privies were built on several farms in the parish of Vanelven. People were moving out of the large farms, where the houses lay huddled in an untidy cluster between puddles and heaps of manure.

In the better parts of Herø, the Health Commission passed a resolution demanding that floors be washed every Saturday. The incidence of scabies also was reduced. The level of education was reported as quite good, most people could read, and all adults could write and do arithmetic. However, the information most people received, was considered to be narrow minded and solely religious. The Christianity of the residents was considered fanatical, and all education about nature and the forces of nature was regarded with suspicion.

In the counties of Nord and Sør Trøndelag, there was a steady progress in the agricultural rural districts, but progress was more uneven along the coast. At times there was great poverty on the islands of Hitra and Frøya and in several places in Fosen. In the valley of Namdalen there were two major ways of making a living: The people who lived along the coast usually were occupied with both fishing and agriculture. Here and there, agriculture was of greater importance, but almost all of the farmers took part in the cod and herring fisheries. It is reported that they suffered badly while working in the fisheries and acquired a whole range of skin diseases, especially leprosy, to a pitiful degree. The inhabitants of the inner valleys were not occupied at sea anymore, but worked in agriculture or forestry. Work in the forests was especially difficult because of the cold nights spent in the primitive forest huts. Even so, these people were better off than those who lived by the sea.

In the valley of Stjørdalen, living standards and hygiene were described as unfavorable. The economy was bad, and the agitation for emigration to America found a fertile soil. We hear that in 1880 the workers did not earn much, since work on the railways had been cut back more and more. Forestry was at a stand still. When the hard winter came it resulted in an unusually large number of beggars along the roads. Emigration to America increased yearly.

The proportion of the population that went to America was greatest from Nord Trøndelag in the 1860s and 1870s, just as

TABLE 9.3
Annual number of poor receiving medical treatment

	1865	1870	1875	1880	1885	1890	1895
Romsdalen	377	884	1,211	1,193	1,402	2,523	2,418
Sør-Trøndelag	1,642	2,471	1,537	2,111	2,129	3,069	3,251
Nord-Trøndelag	683	995	859	793	1,168	1,604	1,799

great in Sør Trøndelag from 1875 on, while emigration started later in Møre og Romsdal, and reached the level of Nord and Sør Trøndelag after the turn of the century.

9.3.4. Poverty

In 1845 parliament passed a law on poverty, a law that followed the prevailing ideology of decentralization and local autonomy. First and foremost people had to rely on themselves and their closest relatives. If that failed, the municipalities were responsible for the poor. The central government only had marginal responsibilities. Thus, poor relief was variable and dependent on local economy and policy.

In Steinkjær there were only a few poor people who were actually supported by the municipality. According to the report, they were well housed in a house for the poor under irreproachable hygienic conditions. This, however, may have been a special case, as confinement to poor houses often was reported to be looked upon with resentment.

DIAGRAM 9.18
Mortality in the counties of Møre og Romsdal, Sør-Trøndelag, and Nord-Trøndelag 1860–1900

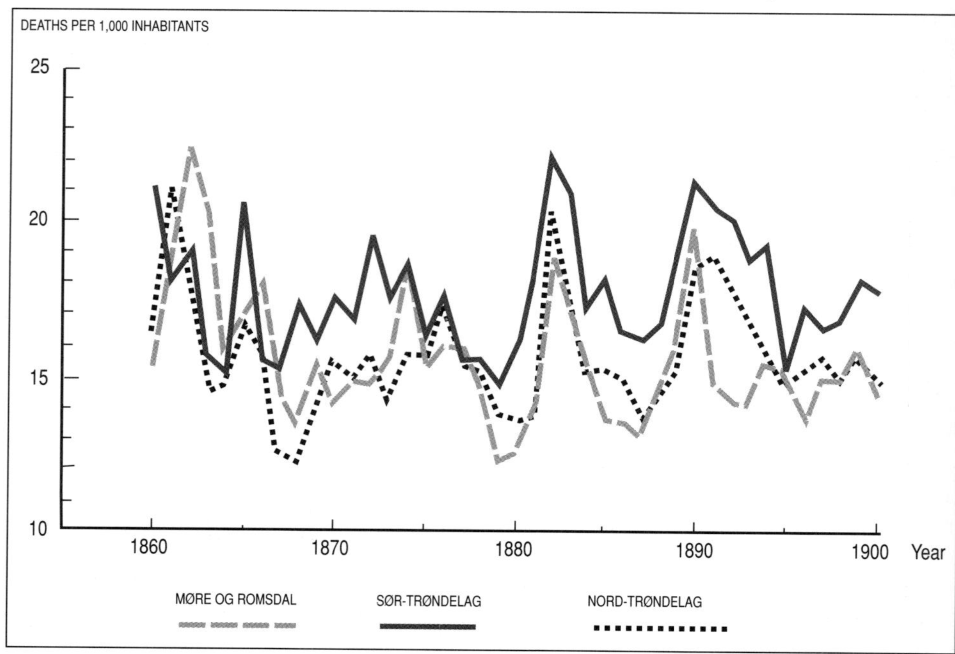

DIAGRAM 9.19

Incidence of typhoid fever in the counties of Møre og Romsdal, Sør-Trøndelag, and Nord-Trøndelag 1860–1900

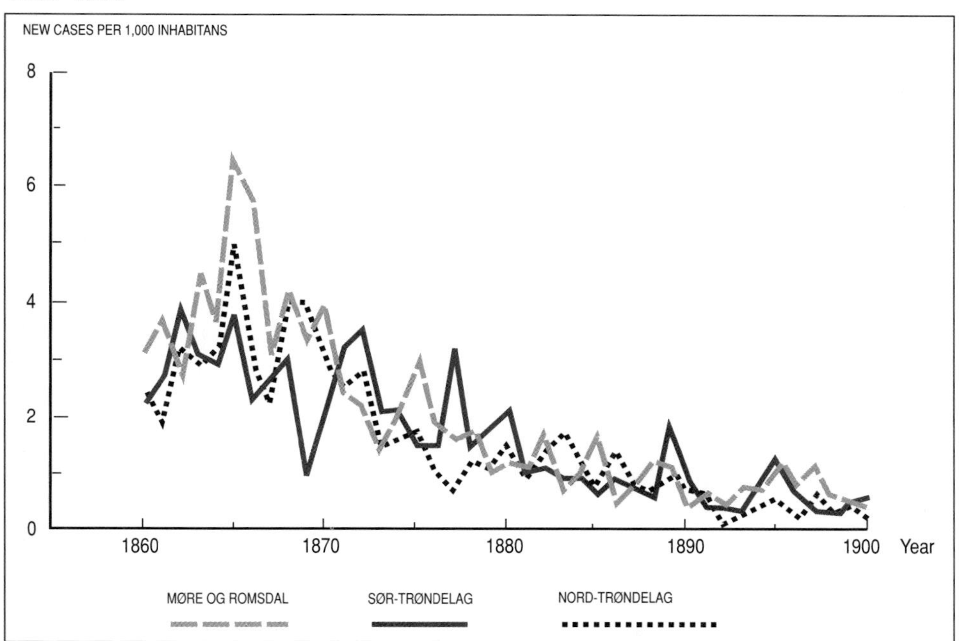

DIAGRAM 9.20

Incidence of scarlet fever in the counties of Møre og Romsdal, Sør-Trøndelag, and Nord-Trøndelag 1860–1900

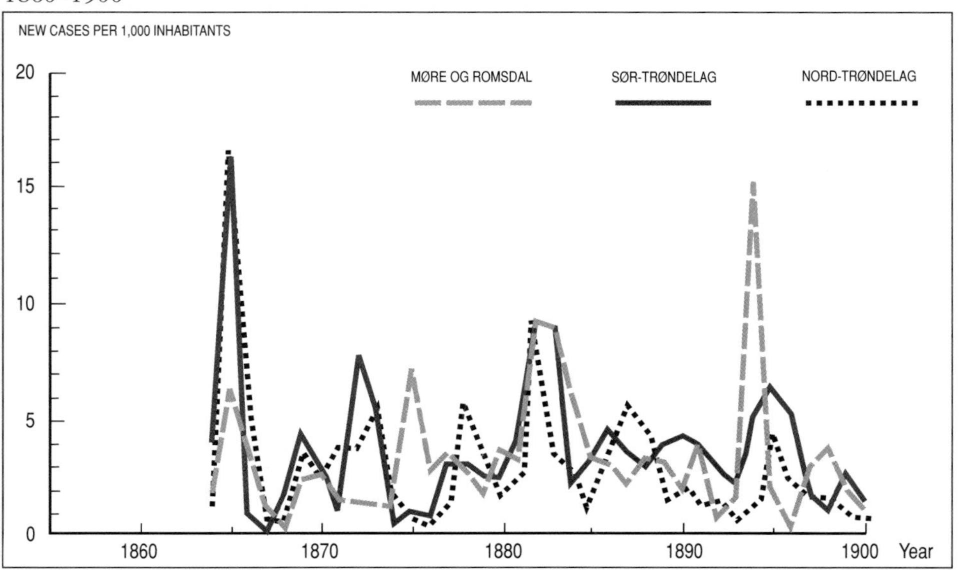

DIAGRAM 9.21

Incidence of diphtheria in the counties of Møre og Romsdal, Sør-Trøndelag, and Nord-Trøndelag 1860–1900

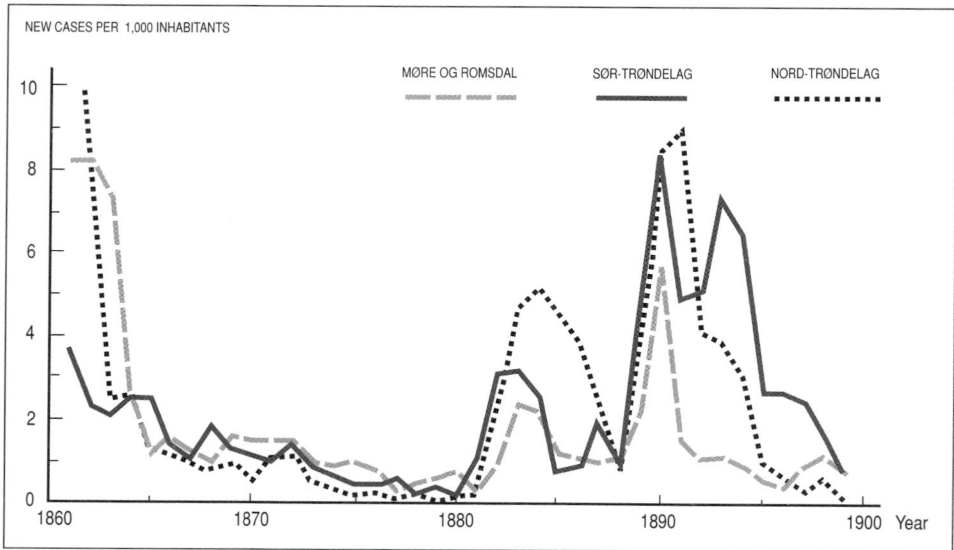

DIAGRAM 9.22

Incidence of pneumonia in the counties of Møre og Romsdal, Sør-Trøndelag, and Nord-Trøndelag 1860–1900

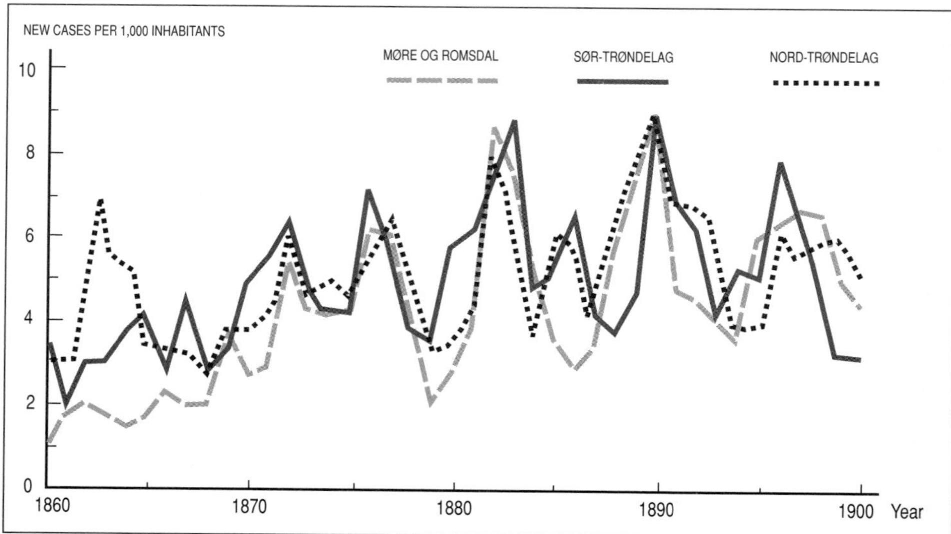

DIAGRAM 9.23
Incidence of tuberculosis (svindsot) in the counties of Møre og Romsdal, Sør-Trøndelag, and Nord-Trøndelag 1860–1900

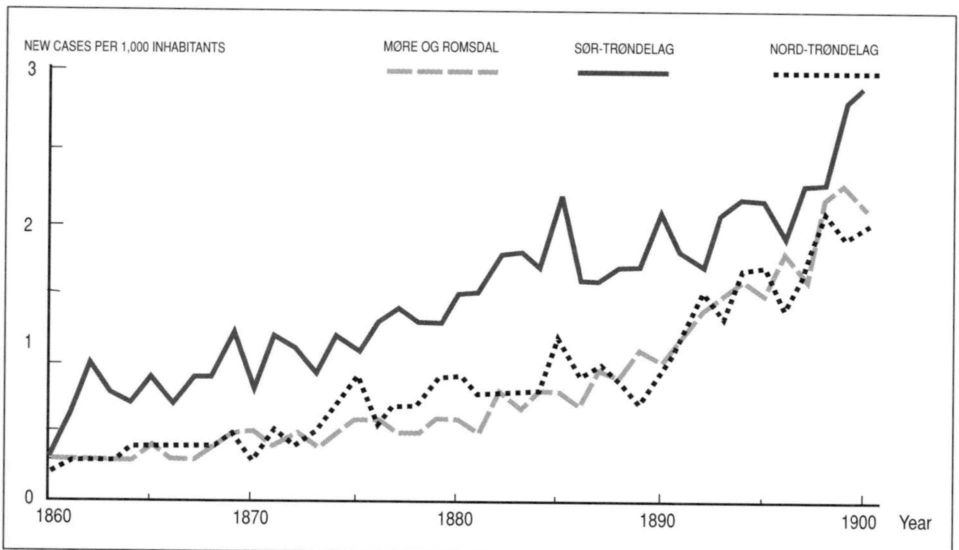

After 1895, the number of poor people who were sick is no longer in the reports. As can be seen from Table 9.3, treatment of the poor was a significant part of the work for the physician.

9.3.5. Epidemics

The mortality in the three counties is shown in Diagram 9.18, while Diagram 9.19 to 9.23 show the incidence of typhoid fever, scarlet fever, diphtheria, pneumonia, and tuberculosis. The spread of epidemic diseases was frequently discussed in the medical reports. Although medicine still was at the beginning of the bacteriological era, interesting observations were made by the local doctors as to the contagiousness of the diseases. The impact of geographical conditions on the occurrence of diseases was also discussed.

Implementation of new evidence or new theories could be difficult. In a report from 1867, Dr. Sophus Høegh (1827–1880) complained that the propagation of a more hygienic behavior in order to halt an epidemic of scarlet fever met with heavy resistance among the population, which would not accept the fact that disease was contagious. Dr. Høegh also remarked that he had observed that some people seemed to be resistant to the disease – an early observation of immunity.

References

Sandvik, P.T. *Fabrikken ved Nidelven*, Thesis in History, University of Trondheim, 1993

Vanebo, J.O. "Trøndersk industri i går, i dag og i morgen," in *Trøndelag – 82*, Trønderlaget, Trondheim, 1982.

CHAPTER 9.4

Western Norway

HOGNE SANDVIK

9.4.1 General Introduction

Western Norway consists of the counties of Rogaland (previously Stavanger Amt) in the south, Sogn & Fjordane (Nordre Bergenshus Amt) in the north, and Hordaland (Søndre Bergenshus Amt), with Bergen, the main city of Western Norway, in the middle. In 1869 the pioneer sociologist Eilert Sundt (1817–1875) noted that while Christiania had a lively exchange with the surrounding relatively developed rural districts, Bergen was isolated in the center of a district of populous villages. A person needed only to go a short distance outside the city gates to find a way of life so old-fashioned and rough that he would believe himself to be many miles from a civilized town (Sundt 1869).

Sundt's impressions of Western Norway and its people were shared by most Norwegians. Many disparaging remarks were made about farmers from Western Norway and their lack of order and cleanliness, and doctors were among their harshest critics.

Conditions were particularly bad in the fishing districts. When the men were away fishing, the women were responsibile for the farm and the home, and therefore the doctors' criticism of household and hygiene was directed mainly at them.

In 1879 district physician Karl Ephraim Nilssen (1838–1906) in the district of Sand noted that it was the women who carried a large part of the blame for the poverty and wretchedness of the people who lived along the coast. According to him, the women were ignorant, lazy, careless, and gossiping and had an ingrained propensity to roam about.

Unbalanced, offensive criticism of this type was fairly prominent in the physicians' descriptions of the farming population of Western Norway. The physicians were deeply and sincerely shocked by the widespread lack of cleanliness, and they impatiently applied pressure for improvements in hygiene. Words like "old-fashioned" and "conservative" crop up many times in their reports. With the exception of the farmers in Jæren (southern part of Rogaland), farmers from Western Norway were also slow to adopt new technology (Pryser 1993).

South-western Norway became a hot bed of oppositional, pietistic laymen's organizations and temperance movements. A huge, deeply-moving religious revival spread over the whole of Western Norway during the 1870s and 1880s (Furre 1990). This mixture of lay Christians, teetotalers, and adherents of the linguistic movement propagating and developing a national language based on rural, mostly Western dialects, gradually entered the political arena.

The building practices of Western Norway, which were considered special, also occupied the district physicians. Johan Vilhelm Midelfart (1835–1898), a physician in Middle Sogn (Midtre Sogn), wrote in 1865 that the houses usually consisted of only one room, and that they were clustered in wild disarray. On a single farm there could be up to 19 dwellinghouses in addition to all the barns and other farmhouses. There were only narrow passages separating the different houses, and these were often used as lavatories, as privies were unheard of.

The district physicians advocated the replacement of these old clustered country courtyards. Not only was this reform of great significance to the hygienic standards in this part of the country, but it also had a positive effect on farming productivity and thus on the prosperity of the region. Once again, the farmers in Jæren were the first to adopt the new ideas (Pryser 1993).

Fishing was an important factor in the economy of Western Norway. As elsewhere along the Norwegian coast, people flocked to the big fisheries, sometimes as many as 40,000. The hygienic conditions during these annual gatherings were extremely bad, making them not only an important source of income, but also an important source of disease.

In order to avoid the spread of disease, temporary hospitals were set up during the big fisheries, for exampel, in Espevær, Haugesund and Florø. Finding a proper place to sleep was difficult, and those lucky enough to get a roof over their head often had to rest in an upright position in drenched clothes, supporting each other in overcrowded fishermen's shacks. Those who were not so lucky had to spend the night under an overturned boat or without any cover at all (Hannestad, Nordhordland 1843). The men who fished for spring-herring usually returned home in the late spring, many of them carrying contagious diseases. In this way epidemics were efficiently distributed throughout Western Norway.

In the beginning of the 1870s, the herring suddenly disappeared from the West Coast of Norway. This had dramatic consequences for the fishing population, since many people, especially the coast farmers and villagers, were totally dependent on this annual income. In 1881 district physician Nilssen described poor villagers who approached him in the hope of receiving some help. The villagers, many of whom suffered from dyspepsia and anemia, complained that food was scarce and health conditions were poor.

Apart from the fisheries, there was an active traffic to and from Bergen, where the population increased considerably during the last part of the nineteenth century (Ertresvaag 1982). The sanitary conditions in the town were poor and the relatively young population, with many children, often became victims of severe epidemics. The great amount of traffic between the rural districts and the towns led to a continuous exchange of infections. The district physicians over and over again described how local epidemics broke out after somebody had "collected" the diseases in town. The mortality in Bergen was among the highest in the whole country, and considerably higher than in Hordaland and Sogn & Fjordane (Diagram 9.24). The somewhat more urbanized Rogaland gradually took up an intermediate position.

A description of some important diseases is given in the following sections. However, one must bear in mind that while this chapter concentrates on the serious epidemics, there were also large groups with "ordinary" illnesses. The district physicians often heard complaints about rheumatism, dyspepsia, and scabies, yet only a few of the afflicted went to see the doctor. "Modern" causes of death, such as cardiovascular diseases and cancer, are hardly mentioned in the medical reports from this period.

9.4.2. Smallpox

Vaccination against smallpox was made compulsory in 1810, but many years passed before the vaccination coverage was sufficent to prevent new epidemics. There are several reasons for this. One reason is that the vaccination probably did not produce sufficient protection against the disease. Children who had been infected earlier (and this included most of them) had better protection against the disease than the ones who were only vaccinated. The vaccine was reported to fail if the vaccination assistants did not do their job properly. This was the case in Fjell, where in 1859 one could observe an astonishingly high mortality from smallpox among people between the ages of 22 and 26. On closer investigation one could ascertain that the vaccination assistant practicing 20–25 years earlier had been both old and a compulsive drinker (Holmsen, Midthordland 1859). Perhaps his vaccination practice was to blame?

Many villagers put little faith in vaccination and attendance at vaccinations was low. Another reason for the low attendance was the religous beliefs held by many of the villagers. Vaccination was considered an unreasonable meddling in the Lord's affairs; God had a reason for sending disease (Sandvik 1993c).

Unexpectedly, there were also some farmers who vaccinated their family and neighbors themselves. They did this by using pus from the vaccine pustules of those who had been vaccinated by the vaccination assistants (Thesen, Northern Ryfylke 1864). Some doctors were afraid that unskilled vaccinating could contribute to the spread of tuberculosis and leprosy. Two of the doctors in

DIAGRAM 9.24

Mortality in the four counties of Western Norway 1860–1900

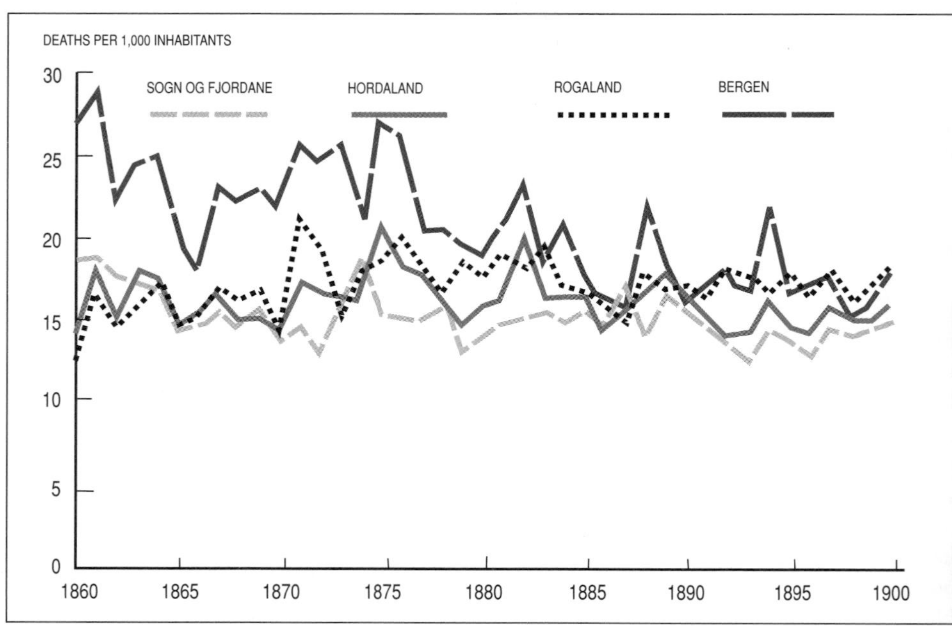

Stavanger practiced homeopathic medicine and advised against smallpox vaccination. They claimed to have found both preventive and remedial means against the disease in homeopathy (Dr. Kaurin, Stavanger 1853).

Generally, however, the vaccination coverage was sufficient to prevent large outbreaks of smallpox after 1860. The most severe epidemic was registered in Rogaland in 1864. Infection through homecoming fishermen contributed to the extensive spreading of this epidemic. It was also in Rogaland, where many of the cases could be attributed to the ship traffic from abroad, that later outbreaks were most frequent (Diagram 9.25). This was also reported from Bergen. There was practically no smallpox in Hordaland and Sogn & Fjordane after 1864.

9.4.3. Leprosy

In the last century, leprosy was a considerable health problem in Norway, especially in the rural regions of Western Norway. A law was implemented in 1856 which required that districts with leprosy establish local health commissions to fight the disease. The health commissions, in cooperation with the district physicians, were made responsible for registering all leprosy patients in a nationwide leprosy register.

Thanks to this register, we have detailed knowledge of the epidemiology of leprosy in Norway (Irgens 1980). However, in the beginning the district physicians had considerable problems with the registration of infected people. The patients feared that the information in the register could be misused to implement coercive measures, and that they would be stigmatized and expelled from society. There were actually good reasons for such fears, and the patients therefore reasoned that they would be better off keeping their disease a secret (Dr. Krohn, outer Nordhordland 1858). But gradually most of the

DIAGRAM 9.25
Incidence of smallpox in the four counties of Western Norway 1860–1900

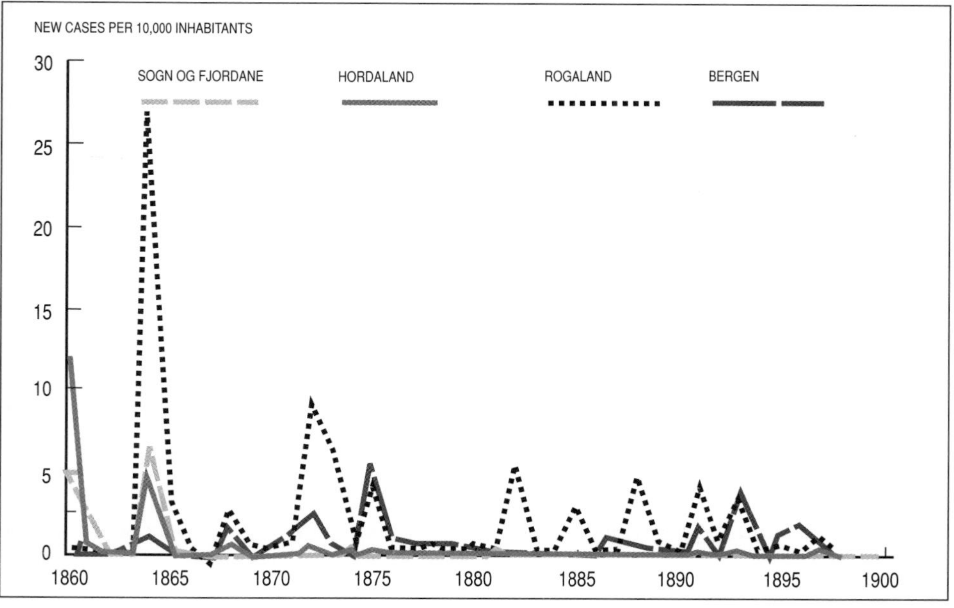

patients were registered, numbering 8,000 during the period from 1856 to 1945.

The disease was not evenly distributed. Leprosy was most frequent in Sogn & Fjordane. The highest incidence ever appeared in Naustdal, but further south the disease was less frequent.

In some families, the disease was conspicuously frequent. However, only a few spouses of lepers became sick. The personnel in the leprosy hospitals also showed little tendency towards contracting the disease. Because of this it took some time before all physicians acknowledged that leprosy was an infectious disease. Even after Gerhard Henrik Armauer Hansen (1841–1888) in Bergen discovered the leprosy bacillus in 1873, some doctors claimed that heredity was of considerable importance (Sandvik 1992a), a fact that admittedly has been confirmed by modern genetic research. This could be one of the explanations for the uneven geographical distribution of the disease, but various environmental factors may also have contributed.

The understanding of leprosy as an infectious disease led to the use of more restrictive and effective measures against it. According to new laws, more patients could be permanently isolated in leper hospitals, and this probably contributed to the swift decline of the disease (Irgens 1980)

9.4.4. Typhoid Fever

Typhoid fever was probably the disease that demanded the most effort from the regional doctors of Western Norway. The disease was called the "nervous fever", and it had a dominating position in the statistics, especially up to the 1870s.

The statistics for typhoid fever are probably more reliable than those for most of the other diseases. This was a serious and protracted disease, and people were afraid of catching it. In addition, since the government paid for the doctor and the medicine, one had less objections to calling a doctor, wrote district physician Nils Torgersen (1844–1889) in inner Nordfjord in 1879.

District physician Michael Krohn (1822–1888) described the course of the disease during a serious epidemic. He noted severe intestinal bleeding, bronchitis, pneumonia, terrible bed sores, and complete deafness. The convalescence was protracted, with dropsy, ascites, and fluid accumulation in the thoracic cavity. It took a long time for the patient to recover mentally. Memory loss was common, which led to patients wandering around lethargic and indifferent (Dr. Krohn, outer Nordhordland 1859).

There seems to have been a heated discussion about whether typhoid fever was caused by miasma or infection. The district doctors around Bergen obviously were strong supporters of the infection theory.

The big fisheries were also an important factor in the spreading of typhoid fever in Western Norway. The spring herring fisheries usually ended in April. Subsequently the doctors could register an increase in cases of typhoid fever in their districts. This was particularly striking in outer Nordhordaland (Diagram 9.26). After a powerful increase in infections in April, the epidemic would continue with further secondary cases through spring and summer. After 1870, the pattern changed. From then on, most cases were noted in the winter, as was usual for the rest of the country (Larsen 1879). The annual incidence of typhoid fever decreased considerably in the early 1870s (Diagram 9.27), probably due to the fact that the spring herring fisheries stopped around 1870, when the herring disappeared (Sandvik 1993b).

It was not only the fisheries that caused the spreading of typhoid fever. The infection could often be traced back to Bergen, this "hole of plague," as the town was called by the peasants (Vidsteen, outer Sønhordland 1878). A source of infection that was not so easy to detect was the countless "Bergen bar-

DIAGRAM 9.26

Typhoid fever in Ytre (Outer) Nordhordland. Annual distribution of cases in the health district

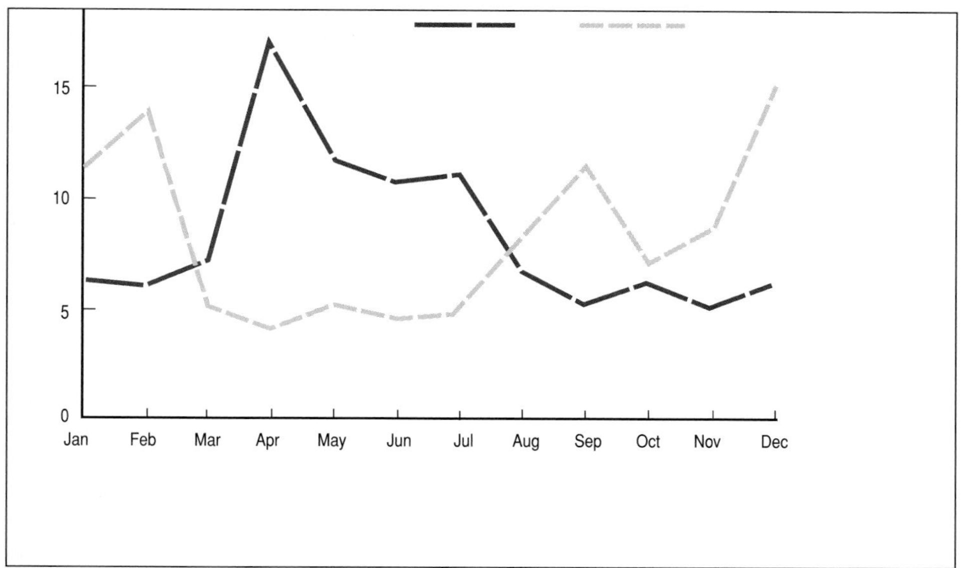

DIAGRAM 9.27

Incidence of typhoid fever in the four counties of Western Norway 1860–1900

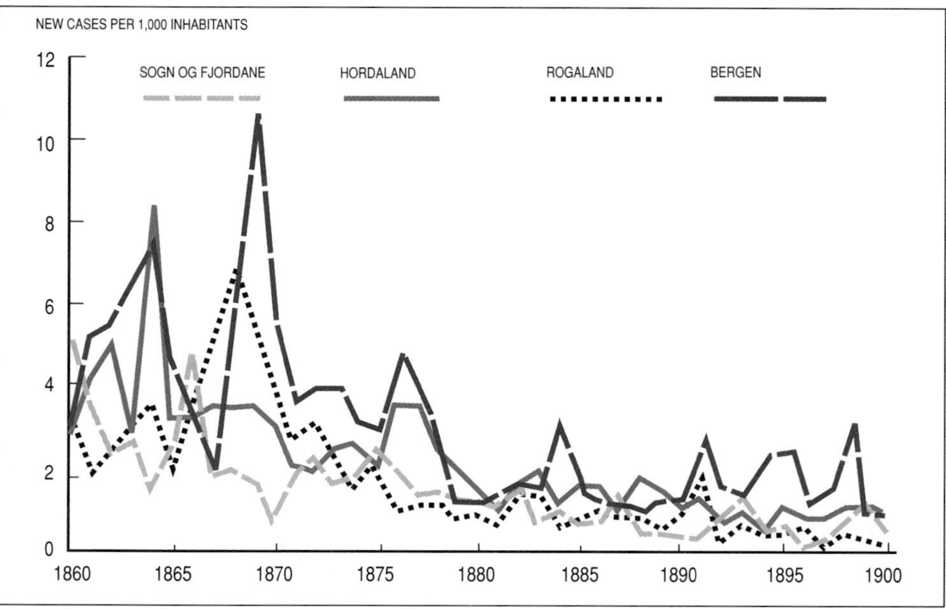

rels" of privy contents that were distributed as a fertilizer to farmers all over Western Norway (Geirsvold 1914).

The spreading of typhoid fever can be considered an index of cleanliness. Contaminated food, milk, and drinking water are the most common vehicles for transmitting the infection, and district physicians all over Western Norway complained about the population's lack of cleanliness. District physician Johan Ludvig Møinichen (1838–1915) reported that only a small minority of the farms had a privy. It was quite common to see, even by the roadside, people sitting side by side without being embarrassed by passersby (Dr. Møinichen, Lærdal 1876).

9.4.5. Tuberculosis

Towards the end of the nineteenth century, tuberculosis was a main cause of death in Western Norway. Apparently more people died from tuberculosis in Bergen than in the rest of the area, but this is probably due to a more complete registration of death causes in Bergen than elsewere. If we make corrections for the uneven percentage of reporting, the picture is somewhat different (Diagram 9.28). From about 1875 it was Rogaland that had the most deaths from tuberculosis, whereas Sogn & Fjordane differed in the opposite direction. It seems like there was an inverted relation between the frequency of tuberculosis and leprosy.

Once again, the doctors at first emphasized the hereditary aspect of the disease, but gradually they realized that infection was the cause. And again the doctors traced the disease to the towns (Brandt-Rantzau, outer Sogn 1883).

Poor housing often was connected with tuberculosis. Some of the houses in Jæren were described as terrible. District physician

DIAGRAM 9.28

Mortality of tuberculosis in Western Norway 1860–1900. The figures have been adjusted in accordance to the fact that there was larger percentage of physicians that filled in reports in Bergen than in the counties. A reporting ratio was calculated for this purpose.

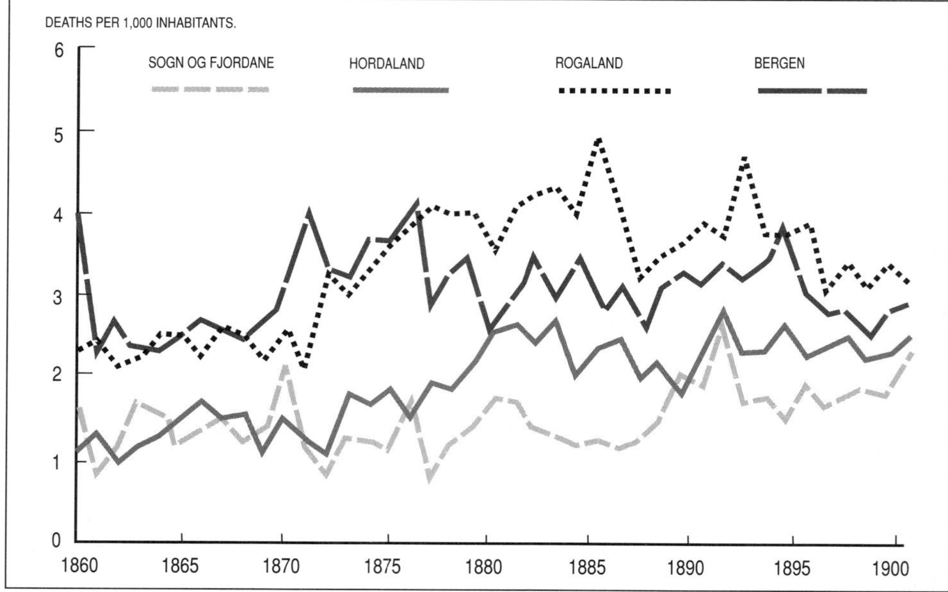

Bentzen in Sandnes wrote of houses where "anyone who moved in, died." Working conditions were also important in this respect. The frequency of tuberculosis was especially high among the factory workers at the Arne and Dale factories, and at the potteries in Egersund (Borge, inner Nordhordland 1884), (Heiberg, Egersund 1874).

The school was an important arena for the struggle against tuberculosis. Children were taught good hygienic habits, but they also had to be protected against infection within the schoolroom. One district physician described a case in which pulmonary tuberculosis appeared in a ten-year-old girl from an otherwise completely healthy family. The infection was probably contracted in the school. She had been forced to wash and brush away the half-dried sputum that the teacher, in spite of warnings and knowing better, quite inconsiderately had spread around her place in the classroom. There were also complaints that the teachers were bad examples for the children when it came to personal hygiene (Dr. Østvold, Sand 1899).

District physician Johan Fredrik Larsen Nielsen (1855–1941) noted that most cases of pleurisy did not subsequently develop into lung tuberculosis. According to Nielsen's experience, almost all the pleurisy patients recovered completely and remained healthy and strong. After nine years he could only remember one patient who later showed signs of tuberculosis. When hospitals abroad and, as far as he could remember, also our own National Hospital indicate that more than half of pleurisy patients are suffering from tuberculosis, one has to take into account that usually the grave cases of the disease are hospitalized, whereas most are treated and cured at home (Dr. Nielsen, Gulen 1896).

9.4.6. Scabies

"There are few people of whom one can say that they are free from this skin disease. It is called 'the itch' and it is with a certain well-being that they satisfy the urge which the name implies" (Dr. Collett, outer Norhordland 1863).

A large part of the population of Western Norway was infected with scabies in the latter part of the nineteenth century, but we do not know exactly to what extent the population was infected. The sick-list does not give a realistic picture of the situation, because only a few of the people infected went to see the doctor. On the other hand, the medical reports often leave the subjective impression that most of the population was infected. Eilert Sundt organized extensive investigations of soldiers in order to clarify this question, and he found that only 6 to 7 percent of the soldiers from Western Norway suffered from scabies. Most who were infested by 'the itch' were recruits from Sogn, at a rate of 57 percent (Sundt 1869). In 1865 more than 400 soldiers with scabies were admitted to the hospital in Bergen. However, it was reported that some people from Sogn returned home immediately, when they discovered that a bath was mandatory at admission (Thorsen, Outer Sogn 1867).

Physicians tried to fight the disease by giving people free ointment or recipes for such ointments (Sandvik 1993 a). The physicians also wanted the local teachers to help fight the disease, since children often were infected at school. Unfortunately, the teachers showed little interest in this work. One measure that could be taken was to deny the already infected children admission to the school, but this was considered useless. Having children at school was a burden to many parents, and they would be only too happy if the children had to stay at home (Engh, Inner Sogn 1862).

In some cases, scabies could lead to disablity. A woman in Håland had been considered leprous and unfit for employment for 20 years. At a meeting of the local health commission she was presented to the district physician in order to be included in the leprosy register. The physician then discovered that her disease definitely was not leprosy but was "scabies crustosa." After 42 days of treatment at the county hospital, she was discharged as healthy and fit for work (Stang, Stavanger 1859).

9.4.7. Venereal Diseases

Veneral diseases were mainly an urban phenomenon (Diagram 9.29), and the prostitutes of Bergen and Stavanger were blamed for the explosive increase of these diseases. In spite of this, district physician Johan Nicolay Cappelen (1818–1887) in Outer Nordfjord registered many cases of gonorrhea in the years around 1860. However, these cases could probably also be traced to the town prostitutes, since most of the patients as Cappelen exercised great care to emphasize were fishermen and sailors passing through. They had as a rule been infected in Bergen, Ålesund, or Trondheim.

The absence of organized brothels made satisfactory control of the prostitutes difficult. In Stavanger an attempt was made to organize prostitution, in order to force the women to live on the outskirts of the town and to subject them to regular inspections. This attempt had to be abandoned because the town's clergy felt that such inspections actually legitimized prostitution (Stang, Stavanger 1881). Bergen introduced weekly inspections of prostitutes, but attendance was low. It was particularly difficult to catch the dangerous novices, the girls 16 to 19 years of age. They managed to instigate a long line of infection before they were caught by the control. There was a heated discussion in Bergen as well about the moral aspect of the inspections. Chief Medical Officer Joakim Nikolai Krej Lindholm (1832–1907) wanted to institute raids

DIAGRAM 9.29

Incidence of gonorrhea and syphilis, treated outside the hospitals in Western Norway 1860–1900

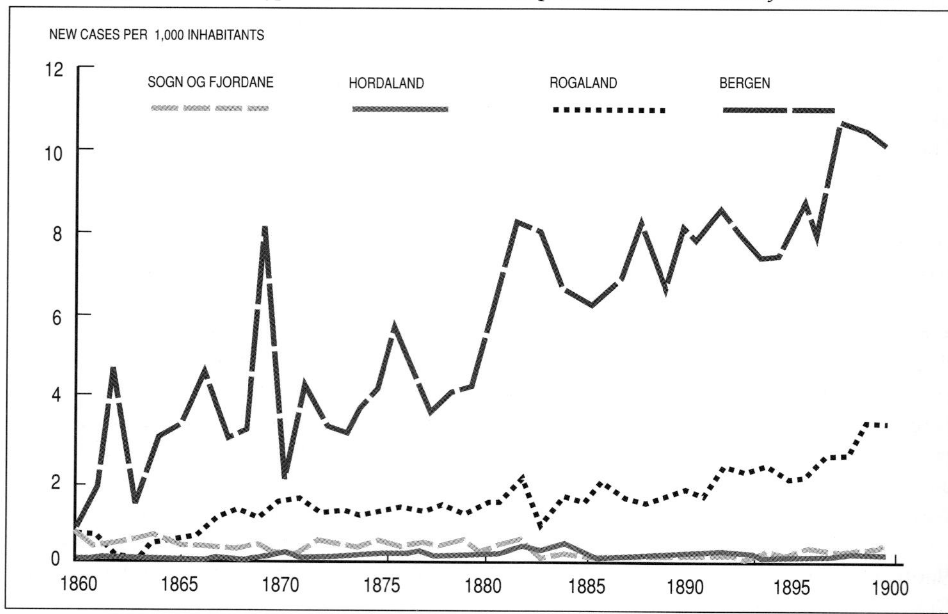

against the prostitutes, but was met with opposition. Obviously frustrated, he complained that society was not allowed to protect itself against "such women" (Lindholm, Bergen 1898).

Scattered cases of non-veneric syphilis radesyke, which earlier was so frequent, were reported until the end of the 1850s, but according to Chief Physician Daniel Cornelius Danielsen (1815–1887) in Bergen, it was not possible to differentiate between this sickness and secondary syphilis. He was of the opinion that syphilis and "radesyke" were the same disease (Danielsen, Bergen 1854).

9.4.8. Insanity

District physician Gerhard Christopher Broch (1813–1859) in inner Hardanger noted that there was a disproportionately large number of mentally deranged people in his district. According to a rumor, a number of them were kept on a leash. Broch also wrote that two chretins from Telemark roamed around in the district (Broch, Inner Hardanger 1854).

The treatment of psychiatric patients was considerably humanized as a consequence of the insanity law of 1848 (Ericsson 1974). Loony bins gave way to asylums, and patients who were cared for privately were entitled to medical supervision. Most of the patients were taken care of by their own families, but in some places private nurses also took care of people unrelated to them (Sandvik 1990).

District physician Collett in outer Nordhordland worked hard to transfer the incurable patients from the asylums into private care. His experience was that the patients functioned better and became calmer when they were taken out of the asylum (Collett, outer Nordhordaland 1875). District physician Johannes Mauritz Thorsen (1863–1892) in outer Sogn, who in 1885 changed his name to Brandt-Rantzau, had the same experience. Long treatment in an asylum had a negative effect on the patients and moreover was much more expensive for the county (Thorsen, Outer Sogn 1880). The county medical officer in Stavanger argued that it was easier to adjust private care to individual needs than hospital care (Hagemann, Stavanger 1899). Thus, in addition to being less expensive than hospital care, the buildup of private care also was grounded on medical considerations.

In the medical reports, mental disorders are mainly described in individual case reports, making it nearly impossible to construct any statistical material on the frequency of these diseases. However, many district physicians reported a sudden outbreak of mental disorders in connection with the religious revival in Western Norway. Two cases were reported after people had been exposed to a roaming lay preacher's description of the punishments in hell (Østvold, Sand 1888).

The counties' accounts clearly show that mental disorders were a considerable item in the health budgets. Since a single patient could require a lot of care and resources, it was considered most just to distribute the expenses on the basis of the whole county, instead of charging the patient's district. The accounts for Hordaland show that expenses for the care of the insane claimed 65–75 percent of the county's health budget (Sjurseth 1937).

9.4.9. Scarlet Fever

Scarlet fever was perhaps the most dramatic of the acute epidemics during this period. The highest number of deaths was registered in 1871 in Rogaland, with a total of 466 registered deaths (Diagram 9.30).

Once these epidemics broke out, there were many deaths. As usual, Bergen got the blame. New infections were regularly imported from Bergen, where the disease raged uncommonly severe, but it seemed as if the disease did not get a proper grip there. In 1882, however, it got more and more out

DIAGRAM 9.30
Incidence of scarlet fever in Western Norway 1860–1900

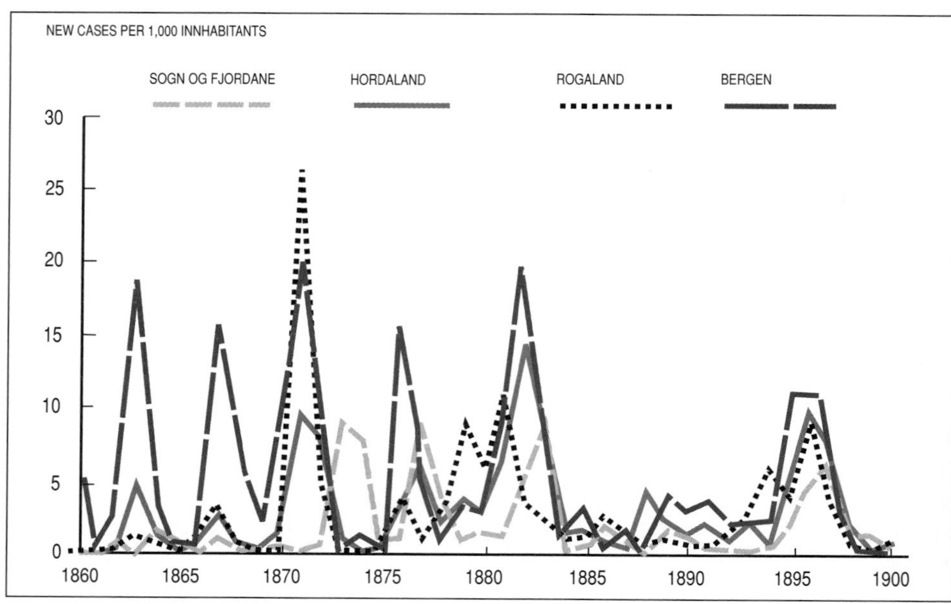

of control, and in the second half of the year it seemed as if most of the district was in flames. When an epidemic exerted such grip, the district physician, who worked alone among a population of 15,500, felt quite powerless (Collett, outer Nordhordland 1882). That year, 94 deaths from scarlet fever were registered in Outer Nordhordland (Sandvik 1992b).

The deaths were largely caused by kidney failure, but local purulent tissue necroses could also result in death. When the glands suppurated, there were frequent pus collections with subsequent gangrene of the skin. Dr. Collett reported one case where the sternum and the costal cartilage were totally exposed by the time the child died (Collett, outer Nordhordland 1871).

The physicians had very little therapy to offer, but they tried as best they could to restrict the epidemics through strict isolation of the sick. Isolation was often rejected by the population. It was in many cases considered unreasonable and difficult to implement. Tradition of people gathering at funeral parties was an especially deeply rooted custom. Epidemics could also be so severe and lengthy that people became exhausted and fatalistic, allowing the disease to take its toll (Krohn, inner Nordhordland 1871).

A better period followed once the severe epidemic in 1882 was over. Around 1895 a new outbreak occurred, but this time in a much milder variety. Lethality, which earlier was around 15–20 percent, was only 3–4 percent in the 1890s.

9.4.10 Measles and Whooping Cough

Of the many dangers small children faced, measles and whooping cough were the worst ones. As late as 1894, 117 children died of measles and 71 of whooping cough in Bergen. Epidemics broke out with only a few years between intervals during the whole period (Diagram 9.31). The infection proceeded rapidly, so that the epidemics

Diagram 9.31
Incidence of measles in Western Norway 1860–1900

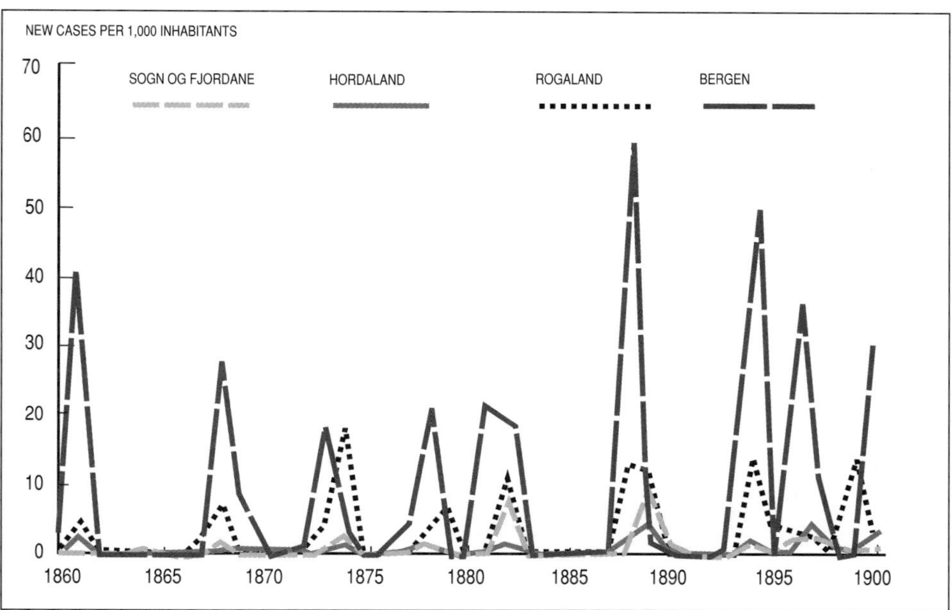

raged almost at the same time in the whole of Western Norway. As so often before, it was the towns, especially Bergen, that were the hotbeds.

From the physicians' statistical reports, measles seems to have been considerably more widespread in the towns than in the countryside. However, these statistics may be deceptive, they may mostly reflect the density of physicians. Children's diseases were a part of life, and as a rule they ran their course unhindered. The doctors could give very little help, and in the countryside there were not many who would call a physician for a sick or dying child. It was easier to call a physician in the towns, and a lot of different treatments were tried. Chief Physician Danielsen in Bergen tried, among other things, to treat whooping cough by letting the children breathe in the air from the gas works (Danielsen, Bergen 1864).

District physician Cristopher Alfred Louis Reinsch Habel (1847–1898) in the rural community of Lindås did an epidemiologic investigation in his district. The members of the local board of health were set to work registering all cases of measles in their part of the district. Altogether 1,204 sick were registered, out of which 90 percent were children. During the same period, only 59 (that is, 5 percent) contacted the district physician (Habel, Lindås 1889).

9.4.11 Diphtheria

Western Norway was not among the areas that were hardest hit by diphtheria, even though a lot of children died from the disease. This disease appeared especially during two periods, in the 1860s and the 1880s (Diagram 9.32). During the first period, it seems to have been confined to Bergen, but in the 1880s diphtheria was as frequent in the countryside. The districts of Kinn and Outer Nordfjord were hit particularly hard,

DIAGRAM 9.32
Incidence of diphtheria in Western Norway 1860–1900

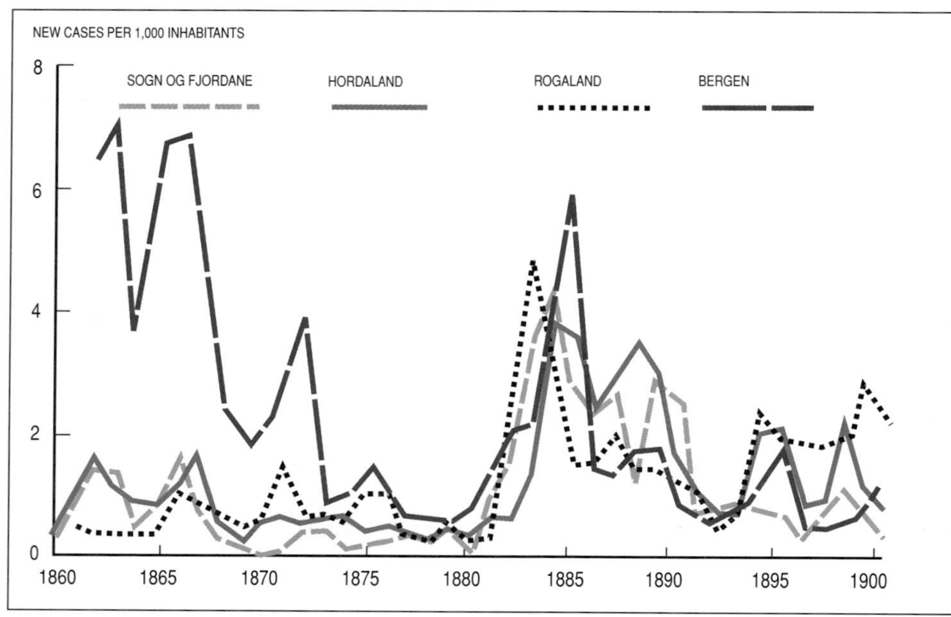

possibly because of the influx of fishermen in the 1880s (Lorentzen, Kinn 1887).

Diphtheria is a disease that can develop very fast, and this may explain why the doctors in the countryside registered relatively few cases in the earlier period. Again, there were fatalistic attitudes among the people, and measures for restricting the epidemics could be met with opposition (Dr. Paasche, Lyster 1889). Distance was also a problem: it simply took too long to call a physician.

Remedies were few. Tracheostomy saved some patients from choking to death, and many believed that there was a positive effect from swabbing the throat with lapsis. But treatment had to start early in the course of the disease. Medicine was therefore stored with trustworthy men around the district. They were instructed to start treatment as soon as they suspected the beginning of a diphtheria outbreak (Krohn, Inner Nordhordland 1864).

Diphtheria serum came into use in the 1890s, something that revolutionized the treatment. For the first time a specific therapeutic remedy was at hand for this disease. Enthusiastic descriptions of patients being miraculously cured are reported by the physicians (Falkenberg, Alversund 1895).

9.4.12 Epilogue

It is difficult to attribute the health trends during this period directly to the build-up of a local public health service. Vaccination can probably take the credit for the combat of smallpox, but the reduced lethality from scarlet fever was probably due to less virulent bacteria. Better transport, changes in economic life, urbanization, and education were probably the most important factors. Replacement of the clustered courtyards limited the spreading of infectious diseases in the countryside, as did the disappearance of the herring. Finally, school and education made the rural population more receptive to information about health and preventive measures.

References

Ericsson, K. *Den tvetydige omsorgen. Sinnsykevesenets utvvikling – et sosialpolitisk eksempel.* Oslo: Universitetsforlaget, 1974.

Ertresvaag, E. *Bergen bys historie, bind III.* Bergen: Universitetsforlaget, 1982.

Furre, B. *Soga om Lars Oftedal.* Oslo: Det Norske Samlaget, 1990.

Geirsvold, M. "Bergens sundhetsvæsen" in *Bergen 1814-1914*, eds. Geelmuyden, C. and H. Shetelig. Bergen: John Griegs Forlag, 1914.

Irgens, LM. "Leprosy in Norway. An epidemiological study based on a national patient registry," *Leprosy Review* 51 (Suppl 1) (1980):1–130.

Larsen, CF. "Om forekomst av Tyfoidfeber i Norge indtil 1876," *Norsk Magazin for Lægevidenskaben* 9 (Suppl)(1879): 1–123.

Pryser, T. *Norsk historie 1800-1870. Frå standssamfunn mot klassesamfunn.* Oslo: Det Norske Samlaget, 1993.

Sandvik, H. "Psykiatriske pasienter i privat pleie. Historisk analyse fra en Vestlands kommune," *Tidsskrift for Den norske lægeforening*, 110(1990):1666–1668.

Sandvik, H. "Spedalskhet og arv. En distriktsleges betraktninger fra 1884," *Tids skrift for Den norske lægeforening*, 112 (1992a):3799–3801.

Sandvik, H. "Ingen sammenheng mellom skarlagensfeber og giktfeber. Historisk analyse fra Ytre Norhordland 1862-84," *Tidsskrift for Den norske lægeforening* 112(1992b):3803–3805.

Sandvik, H. "Bekjempelse av skabb i Ytre Nordhordland legedistrikt. Et samfunnsmedisinsk eksperiment i 1860-årene," *Tidsskrift for Den norske lægeforening,* 113(1993a):40–43.

Sandvik, H. "Tyfoidfeber i Ytre Nordhordland legedistrikt. Smitteveier, insidens og letalitet i perioden 1854-83," *Tidsskrift for Den norske lægeforening*, 113-(1993b):1990–1993.

Sandvik, H. "De siste dødsfall av kopper i Ytre Nordhordland. En distriktleges erfaringer," *Tidsskrift for Den norske lægeforening,* 113(1993c):2096–2098.

Sjurseth, K. *Hordaland fylke 1837-1937.* Bergen: Hordaland fylke, 1937.

Sundt, Eilert. *Om Renligheds-Stellet i Norge.* Christiania: Chr. Abelsted, 1869.

CHAPTER 9.5

The Southern Coast – Aust-Agder and Vest-Agder

BÅRD AUSTNES

9.5.1. Geography, Trade, and Industry

Aust-Agder and Vest-Agder were previously called the county of Nedenes and the county of Lister and Mandal, respectively. These counties stretch all along the southern coast of Norway, with its rich coastal culture, and almost up to the deserted plains of Hardangervidda in the north, to the then fairly isolated communities in the Setesdal valley. Between these areas there are extensive moors and forests, intersected by many rivers, with some small villages and farms in places where it seemed possible to make a living. The two counties have a mild climate, with warm summers, mild winters and little rain. The numerous skerries along the coast have provided a place for sheltered settlements in close contact with the sea (Kristiansen 1977).

Most of the people who lived along the coast were farmers with small holdings, with fishing or seafaring as secondary occupations. The men could be at sea for long periods, so that the wives and children were responsible for running the farms. Many men also went to America for a period to earn money. When the farm had been expanded and paid for, the husband would come home and settle down as a fisherman and farmer (Medical report for the county of Lister and Mandal 1890).

Inland, the population did not have the same opportunities for secondary occupations as those the sea provided. Subsistence economy was more predominant there. Cash money was earned from seasonal work, such as stone breaking, land clearance, and road building. Emigration to America was common from these areas. Child labor was widespread, and many children from mountain districts worked as shepherds during the summer.

Another secondary occupation, particularly in the inner regions of the county of Lister and Mandal, was seasonal production of planks for making barrels. These were made of pine. The wood used to make the planks could not be floated down the rivers, as was usual for timber, because this would have washed the resin out of the logs. It was therefore necessary to produce the planks locally and then transport them by land to the coast. Production of such planks was an attractive way of earning extra income, although price fluctuations strongly influenced the people's purchasing power (Kristiansen 1977).

Timber was also exported. Norwegian timber had been exported for more than 300 years, and oak from Aust-Agder and Vest-Agder was sought after on the international market because of its use in shipbuilding.

Timber export gradually became profitable in the nineteenth century. The timber trade therefore experienced its last boom before the market for timber almost disappeared when wooden ships were no longer built. Timber export resulted in economic growth from 1860 to 1880, which benefited both the forest districts in the central parts of the counties and the coastal districts (Hodne 1981).

9.5.2. Shipping

Shipping was an important industry in the towns along the southern coast, and changes in the shipping industry influenced people's way of life and the development pattern in the southern coastal communities. Shipping also had an influence on people's health, either directly through transmission of infections or indirectly through changes in economy, and through cultural exchange.

Throughout different periods, shipping has been important for the Norwegian economy, and the growth in international trade that began in the middle of the nineteenth century gave the Norwegians the opportunity to utilize their seafaring experience in commercial shipping. The abolishment of international protectionist measures increased international trade, and thus led to increased demand for Norwegian shipping services.

The first regular production of steamships began in England in 1839. However, in 1907 half the Norwegian tonnage was still made up of sailing ships. Thus, Norwegian shipping concentrated to a large extent on second-best technology. Norwegian ships were mainly small wooden ships, often run by shipping companies in which both the skipper and the crew were joint owners. These ships had low running costs and the cost of labor was also low. The low costs made Norwegian ships competitive for freight that was not dependent on speedy transport. The ships often sailed in the tramp trade, that is to say, not on regular routes.

However, conditions for running sailing ships gradually deteriorated towards the end of the nineteenth century. Freight rates for both sail and steam fell. The steamships were built of steel instead of iron, which meant significant reductions in fuel costs. And steamers were faster, bigger, required fewer crew members, and had greater storage capacity per gross ton than sailing ships. Many factors contributed to sailing ships gradually losing their share of the market in competition with steamships. However, in spite of this, for a long time Norway was reluctant to adopt the new technology.

Steamships were more capital intensive than the older sailing ships. This can to some extent explain why the transition from sail to steam took so long in Norway. In the Norwegian jointly owned shipping, there was usually one company for each ship. Profits and losses were divided according to the number of shares in the vessel, and often all the profits from one expedition were paid out in dividends. This kind of organization made it possible for many people to contribute toward the capital needed for one ship or shipping expedition. It can also be looked upon as an attempt to spread risk. However, another result of this ownership structure was that little or no joint capital was built up, something that was needed to run a modern steamship company.

Falling freight rates and the problems associated with the transition from sail to steam led to stagnation in the shipping industry in the 1880s. Shipping companies began to lose money, and there was no longer an increase in the number of people employed. For many people, the sea was no longer a possible source of income, and they had to look elsewhere to earn a living. Many looked to America, where there was said to be work, a prospect that led to a great increase in the number of emigrants.

As a result of the shipping companies' ownership structure, income had been distributed rather evenly. Profits had been divided among many people, so that everyone had prospered to a relatively similar degree. The new, more capital-intensive steamship companies that eventually came into being, had few owners and income was divided among fewer people. This led to greater divisions by class. A few people earned a lot of money from steamships, while the majority received only a very small share of this income (Hodne 1981).

Shipping also had an influence on health. A strengthened economy gave people the possibility of investing in proper housing and to have better clothes and food. Thus, the good times for shipping in the 1860s and 1870s led to a better standard of health. Shipping also provided money for the municipalities, something that made possible investment in health promoting measures, such as improved sewerage and an adequate water supply.

In foreign ports, sailors easily came in contact with infectious diseases, and in many cases they brought these infections back to Norway with them. In this way, shipping became a source for importing epidemic diseases. Many examples on this are given in the medical reports.

Shipping also led to cultural exchanges and the importation of influences from the rest of the world, making the people of Southern Norway often fairly well-informed and knowledgeable. Thus, new ideas about hygiene and nutrition were often better received and accepted along the southern coast than in other parts of the country.

9.5.3. Hygiene and the Spread of Infection

People lived in crowded conditions in the nineteenth century, and the worst overcrowding was in the cities. According to the census in 1891, the mean number of persons per dwelling in the county of Nedenes was 5.78 in the rural districts and 7.77 in the towns. The corresponding figures for the county of Lister and Mandal were 5.16 and 8.07. Dwellings with two or three rooms were common, but the sitting room was hardly ever used, except on special occasions and when there were visitors. Thus, the whole family often lived in one room, where they ate, slept, and carried out their daily tasks. Such crowded living conditions were conductive to the spread of infection. Particularly, diseases such as diphtheria and cholera affected most of those who lived in the same house (Helland 1903; Medical report for the county of Lister and Mandal 1894).

Physicians expressed strong criticism of the hygienic conditions several times in the medical reports. They meant that people did not clean the house often enough, that they too seldom took a bath, and that they were not good enough at using kitchen utensils. They also expressed some personal opinions, in which they described the population as uncivilized, dirty, and with little hygienic knowledge or motivation. The physicians' criticism can seem harsh at times, though it was probably justified in some cases (Medical report for the county of Lister and Mandal 1894).

Eilert Sundt (1817–1875) carried out thorough studies of living conditions in Norway in the 1850s. In his book about hygienic conditions in Norway (1869), he expressed an understanding attitude towards hygienic conditions. He thought that the physicians were too pessimistic about hygienic conditions, and that they demanded too much of the population. On a small farm, everyone was dependent on everyone else doing his or her share of the work on the farm, leaving little time for the cleaning of the house. Sundt was therefore of the opinion that in many cases it was not lack of knowledge or laziness that led to poor hygiene, but lack of resources.

In 1868 he wrote an article in the newspaper *Morgenbladet*, entitled, "On the occasion of the planned home management school in Romsdal", in which he opposed the physicians' views on the hygienic conditions. In his article, he maintained that the view that women were hardly able to prepare food and had little understanding of cleanliness, which was expressed in the physicians' reports, was wrong. This was probably the result of physicians' writing only about their negative impressions, and was not based on accurate observations and considerations. Eilert Sundt wrote that he personally had observed how women scrubbed and tidied up. He ascertained, by staying for a few days, then leaving the village and returning later to see if the situation was the same, that this was not an isolated incident.

Sundt also claimed that the physicians had an unrealistic view on proper hygiene. He tells about a district near Kristiansand where the Health Commission had adopted a paragraph that everyone should take a daily bath, either in warm water, or in a lake or a river. Only the English upper class observed such a habit, and he believed that it was too ambitious to try to implement this behavior in a mountain district in Norway. If doctors used such customs as their standard of reference, it was not surprising that they often were disappointed and wrote in a negative way (Sundt 1869).

It appears that people became more conscious about hygienic conditions towards the end of the nineteenth century. After the great fire in Kristiansand in 1892, the district physician was eager to build a complete underground sewerage network. This plan was carried out. Hygienic conditions were also improved in other ways. Many towns got new water works that obtained water from sources far away from the towns. In 1894, meat inspection was introduced in Kristiansand (Medical report for the county of Lister and Mandal 1893).

Physicians were often the strongest proponents for improved hygienic conditions, perhaps because they were the ones who most clearly could see how important hygiene was for health. It is therefore also understandable why they were sometimes rather resigned when people received advice over and over again, and then obviously did not follow the advice that was given.

The district physicians had a rather extensive authorization to implement measures for preventing the spread of infection. Intervention could involve isolation of infected people, closing schools, disinfection of houses and personal property, and in the most serious cases, burning furniture. If necessary, these measures could be implemented with force, with the permission of the county (Medical report for the county of Nedenes 1880; Medical report for the county of Lister and Mandal 1894).

9.5.4. Tuberculosis

Tuberculosis was the most common cause of death during the second half of the nineteenth century. One death out of every four or five was caused by this disease. As early as 1866, tuberculosis was registered in a separate table in the medical reports, indicating awareness of tuberculosis as an important fatal disease. However, in the beginning, there were few thoughts about what caused the disease in the medical reports. Such thoughts first appeared around the middle of the 1870s.

A prevailing theory was that tuberculosis had a hereditary element. In addition, the connection between poor hygiene, overcrowding, and tuberculosis was pointed out. The tubercle bacillus was discovered by the German doctor Robert Koch (1843–1910) in 1882, and the confirmation that tuberculosis was an infectious disease quickly became known. As early as in 1882, it is stated in the medical reports that the infectious nature of the disease was well known in the population. However, this knowledge did not lead to any fall in the number of deaths from the disease. It is one thing to know that a disease is infectious, quite another to do anything about it, especially when months can pass between being infected and the manifestation of the first symptoms. It can also be difficult to limit the spread of the disease when people live in overcrowded conditions, especially since tuberculosis is infectious over a long period (Medical report for the county of Nedenes 1882).

Towards the end of the nineteenth century, the pattern of tuberculosis in urban and rural areas changed. Earlier, mortality from tuberculosis had been higher in the coastal towns than in the country districts, but from about 1890, mortality fell in the towns and increased in the country districts (Diagram 9.33). A similar trend can also be seen for the epidemic diseases, though not so pronounced.

One explanation for this could be improved registration of mortality from tuberculosis in the country. But this assumes that registration was previously poor. The low rate of doctor coverage in the districts supports such an assumption, while the stable and easily surveyed conditions dispute this. It is thus difficult to say whether registration was previously poor and whether there was potential for improvement which could be reflected in an apparent worsening of the situation.

Another possible explanation for the increase in mortality in the country districts is the economic recession in Southern Nor-

DIAGRAM 9.33

Mortality of tuberculosis in the county of Lister and Mandal during the period 1865 to 1900. The diagram shows an increase in mortality in the countryside, and a decline in mortality in the towns throughout the period. (Date are collected from the tables on deaths by tuberculosis and the information on population number in the medical reports for the county of Lister and Mandal 1865 to 1900.)

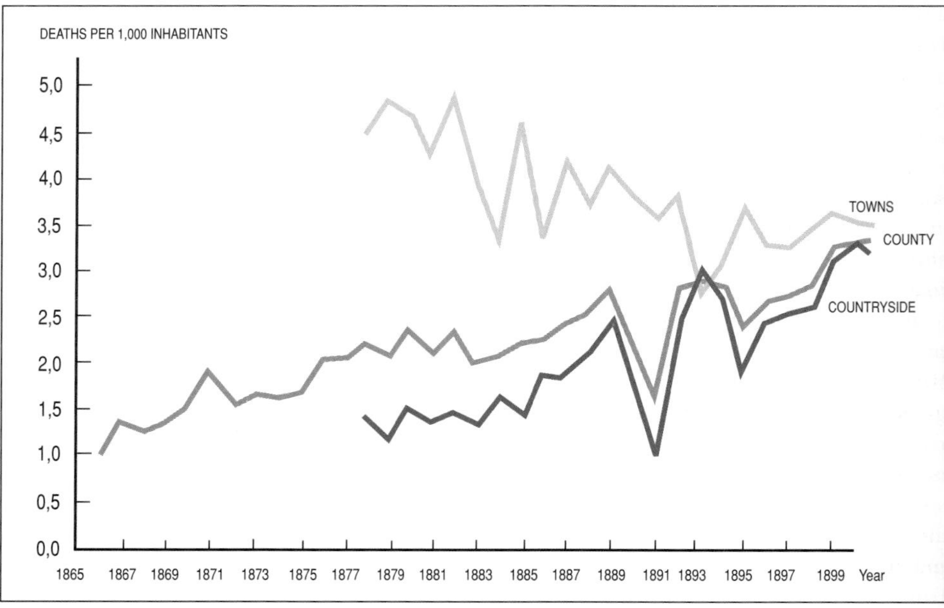

DIAGRAM 9.34

Incidence of typhoid fever in the county of Lister and Mandal and the county of Nedenes during the period 1865 to 1900. The diagram shows a steady decline in incidence through the whole period. It begins as a disease with high incidence and eventually becomes insignificant. (Larsen 1980.)

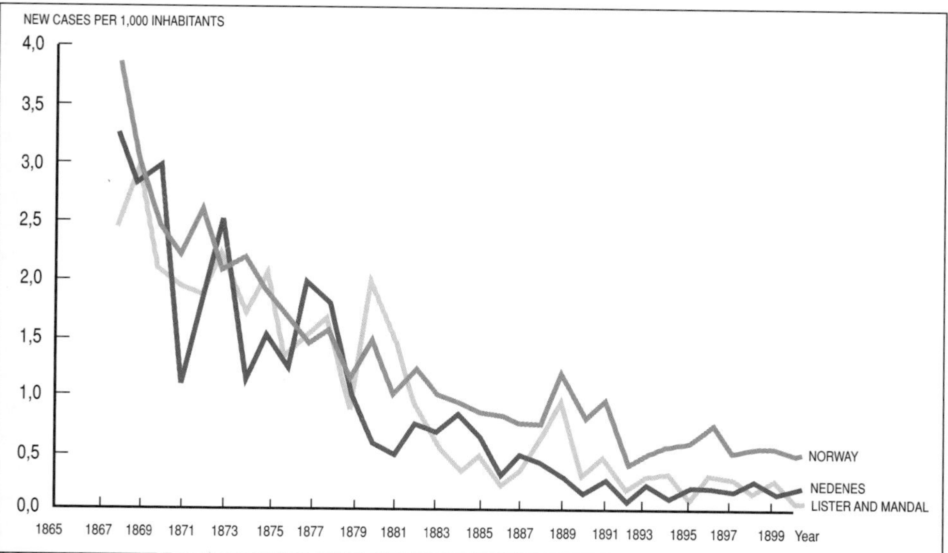

way during the 1880s and 1890s. The shipping industry had stagnated, and many shipping companies went bankrupt. Many sailors lost their jobs. The economic recession also affected the timber trade. People's economy worsened, this affected their health status, and this in turn led to increased morbidity from tuberculosis.

A partial explanation of the fall in mortality from tuberculosis in the towns can be improved hygienic conditions and improved nutritional status. Sanitary conditions and water supply improved. Better nutrition led to improved general health, which influenced mortality from tuberculosis. The theories of McKeown seem to apply here. Measures against the spread of infection were also strengthened. An effective way of containing infection was to isolate the sick. The number of isolation wards increased and they were used more frequently towards the end of the nineteenth century.

9.5.5. Typhoid Fever

While the incidence of epidemic diseases showed a general increase between 1870 and 1890, and a small decrease up to 1900, the incidence of typhoid fever in the country was about 2.5 per 1,000 inhabitants, but this fell to 0.5 in 1900. The incidence in the county of Lister and Mandal and the county of Nedenes was slightly lower than for the country as a whole, and in 1900 it was down to about 0.025 per 1,000 inhabitants (Diagram 9.34). There were two outbreaks of typhoid fever in the county of Lister and Mandal in 1880 and 1889. These outbreaks occurred at the same time as epidemics occurred in Kristiania.

Typhoid fever is caused by the salmonella bacterium. This was demonstrated in 1884. Previously, it had been shown that typhoid fever was infectious, and that the main mode of transmission was through food, milk, or water that had been in contact with feces (Degré 1994).

The disease seems to have been a phenomenon of the towns, which is where the major epidemics were described. In the country districts, and especially in isolated areas far from the coast, only a few isolated cases are described. The cases which are mentioned can usually be traced back to infection from vagrants, transmission of infection from travelers who caught the infection in the coastal towns, or drinking water from known infected sources.

Much of the explanation for the steady decrease in the incidence of typhoid fever could be associated with its mode of transmission, and with the fact that the disease was a city phenomenon. In order for typhoid fever to be transmitted, feces from infected persons must come in contact with food or water. This was not so difficult to avoid in country districts, but was a greater problem in the towns, where there was overcrowding and open gutters. Measures such as improved personal hygiene, better sewerage, improved water supply, and isolation of sick people were implemented at the end of the nineteenth century. Such measures were probably particularly effective against diseases with a fecal-oral mode of transmission, such as typhoid fever (Medical report for the county of Lister and Mandal 1900).

The risk of infection was also great in the overcrowded conditions on board the sailing ships. If one person on board was infected, it was not uncommon for the whole crew to become sick. These sick people were, in turn, a potential source of infection if they were not isolated when the vessel landed (Medical report for the county of Lister and Mandal 1873).

9.5.6. Malaria

Malaria was different from the other epidemic diseases, in that it appeared exclusively after being imported from abroad. Each year, there were about 20–30 cases in towns along the southern coast. In the early medical reports, a few local epidemics are described, but the later reports refer exclusively to imported cases. Sailors were infected in foreign ports, particularly in South America and Africa. They became sick on the way home and were admitted to hospital when they arrived in Norway. However, they did not catch malaria only in South America and Africa: the disease was also to be found in European cities in the nineteenth century. In the medical report from 1882, there are reports of six sailors who caught malaria in America, Holland, or Sweden (Medical report for the county of Lister and Mandal 1882).

9.5.7. Scarlet Fever

Scarlet fever was first described in Norway in 1787. The disease primarily affects children, and in much of the nineteenth century it was one of the most common causes of death among children. Around 1890, the character of the disease changed and became milder and less lethal. Epidemics of scarlet fever occurred during the whole of the second half of the nineteenth century (Diagram 9.35). In some years there were only a few cases, while in other years large groups were afflicted. Particularly in urban areas along the southern coast, there were large fluctuations in incidence. In rural districts, conditions were more stable, and it was easier to limit the spread of infection, so that there was a lower and more even number of cases (Holst 1954).

Statistics on scarlet fever in the medical reports are relatively incomplete, particularly with regard to the minor, less serious epidemics, during which few people sought medical help. During the winter of 1875–1876, a virulent epidemic of scarlet fever ravaged a large part of the southern coast. In Kristiansand, which at that time had a population of about 12,000, 421 cases were reported, of which 48 died. Oddernæs and Undal also were badly hit by the epidemic, but there was a significant under-registration of both morbidity and mortality from

DIAGRAM 9.35

Annual cases of scarlet fever in the county of Lister and Mandal and the county of Nedenes during the period 1865 to 1900. The graphs shows that scarlet fever was a disease with typically epidemic fluctuations. (Date are collected from the tables on epidemic diseases in the medical reports from the county of Nedenes and the county of Lister and Mandal.)

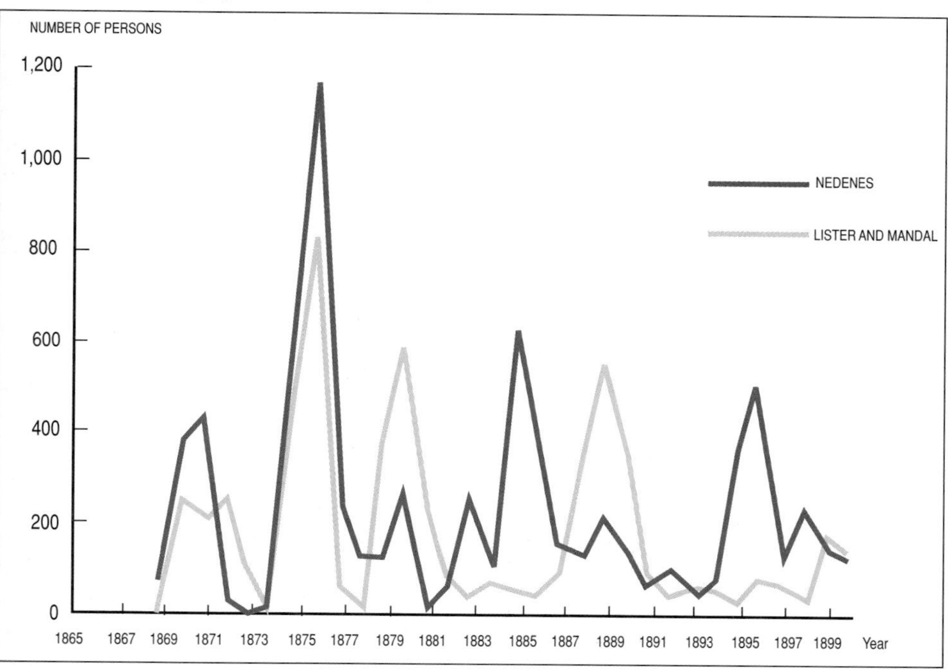

scarlet fever in these townships. Thus scarlet fever was possibly a greater burden to the population than is indicated in the medical reports (Medical report for the county of Lister and Mandal 1876. Medical report for the county of Nedenes 1880).

9.5.8. Scabies

Scabies was a disease that was well known among people during the nineteenth century, but was rarely treated by doctors. People had known for a long time that it was caused by a small animal. Eilert Sundt (1817–1875) related that people called this animal "klåemakken" (the itchy mite). Eilert Sundt was surprised at how well-informed people were about the cause of scabies. He tells about a visit to Sætesdalen in 1866, during which a woman plucked out a scabies mite and showed it to him. Later, he observed that people had this knowledge in many places.

Even though people knew about the scabies mite, this did not mean that they knew how it was transmitted, or how to protect oneself against it. Earlier, scabies was regarded as something that everyone had and as nothing to be ashamed of. Later, as the mite's mode of transmission became known, and people found out how to protect themselves against it, the disease became stigmatizing. Scabies came to be associated with dirtiness and poor hygiene. However, there were differences from district to district. In 1877, it is stated in the medical report that, in the district of Aamli, it was regarded as a disgrace to have scabies, while in the valley of Setesdal it was regarded as quite natural (Medical report for the county of Lister and Mandal 1877).

9.5.9. Summary

The health situation improved steadily in the last four decades of the nineteenth century, both in the county of Nedenes and in the county of Lister and Mandal. But infectious disease still affected the everyday life of people around the turn of the century, and mortality was still relatively high. The major epidemics that had previously ravaged the population had obviously disappeared. There were indeed great variations in the number of people who caught diseases such as scarlet fever, but there were no longer epidemics that affected large segments of the population, although such epidemics still remained as a threat even during the century to come.

The time of prosperity in the first half of this period had contributed to speeding up the improvement in health-related conditions, while stagnation in the economy from about 1880 on probably slowed down this development. However, a positive trend in improved hygiene is not easily halted by a few years of poor economy. Diseases such as typhoid fever demonstrate this. The incidence of this disease fell steadily throughout the whole period. By reducing crowding, emigration to America perhaps also contributed to the positive development for those who remained in Norway.

References

Degré, M. et al. eds. *Medisinsk mikrobiologi.* Oslo: Universitetsforlaget, 1994.

Helland, A. ed. *Norges land og folk*, bind 9 (del 1 og 2). Kristiania: Nedenes amt: H. Aschehoug & co (W. Nygaard), 1903.

Helland, A. ed. *Norges land og folk bind 10 (del 1 og 2)* Kristiania: Lister og Mandals amt: H. Aschehoug & co (W. Nygaard), 1904.

Hodne, F. *Norges Økonomiske historie 1815-1970*. Oslo: J.W. Cappelens forlag, 1981.

Holst, P.M. *Våre akutte folkesykdommers epidemiologi og klinikk.* Oslo: H. Aschehoug & co, 1954.

Kristiansen, A. ed. *Bygd og by i Norge – Agder.* Oslo: Gyldendal norsk forlag, 1977.

Larsen, Ø., H. Haugtomt, and W. Platou *Sykdomsoppfatning og Epidemiologi 1860-1900.* Oslo: Seksjon for medisinsk historie, Uiversitetet i Oslo, 1980.

Medisinalberetningene for Lister og Mandals amt for årene 1865 til 1900.

Medisinalberetningene for Nedenes amt for årene 1865 til 1900.

Sundt, E. *Om Renligheds-Stellet i Norge.* Oslo: Gyldendal norsk forlag, 1975 [1869].

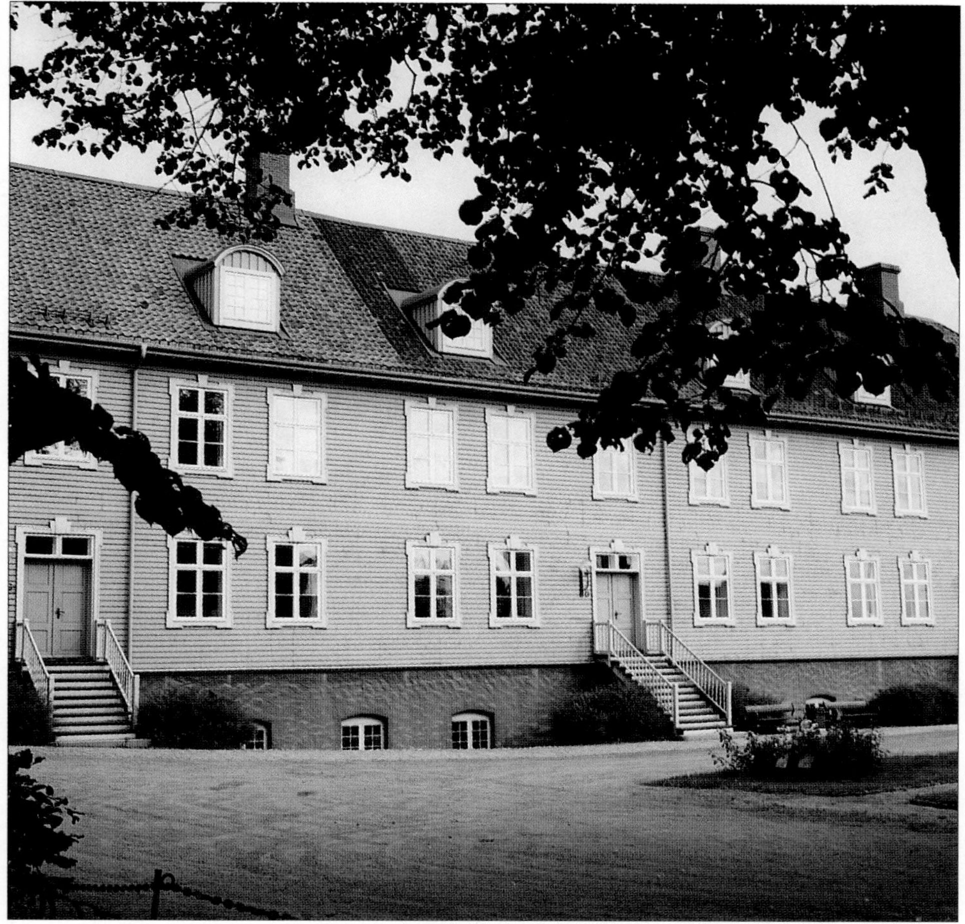

Figure 19: The military hospital in Christiania, built in 1807, was the first teaching hospital in Norway. The large empire-style wooden building was taken down 1954-1962, and was rebuilt on another site. It was finished in 1983, but no longer serves as a hospital (Photo: Øivind Larsen 1996).

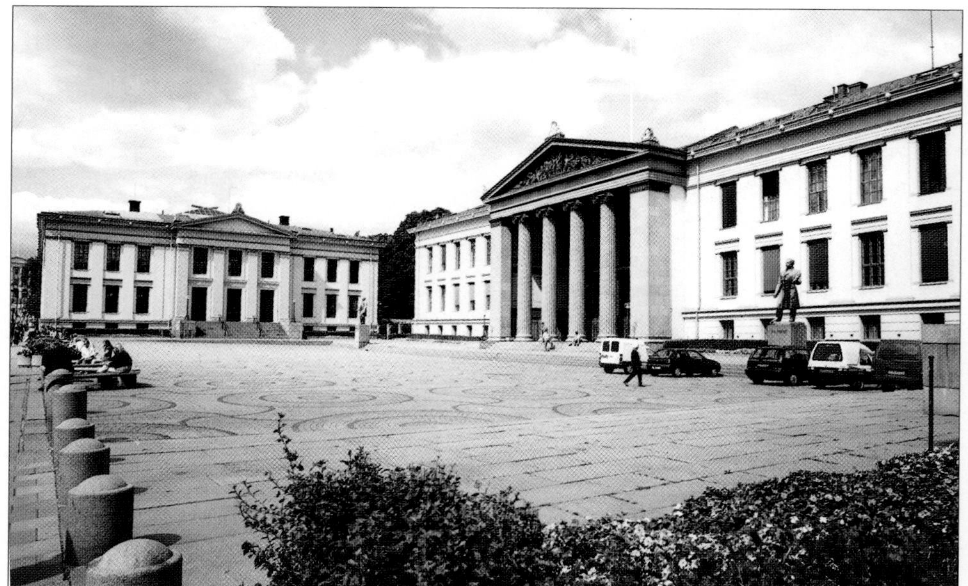

Figure 20: The University of Oslo, buildings from 1852 (Photo: Øivind Larsen 1996).

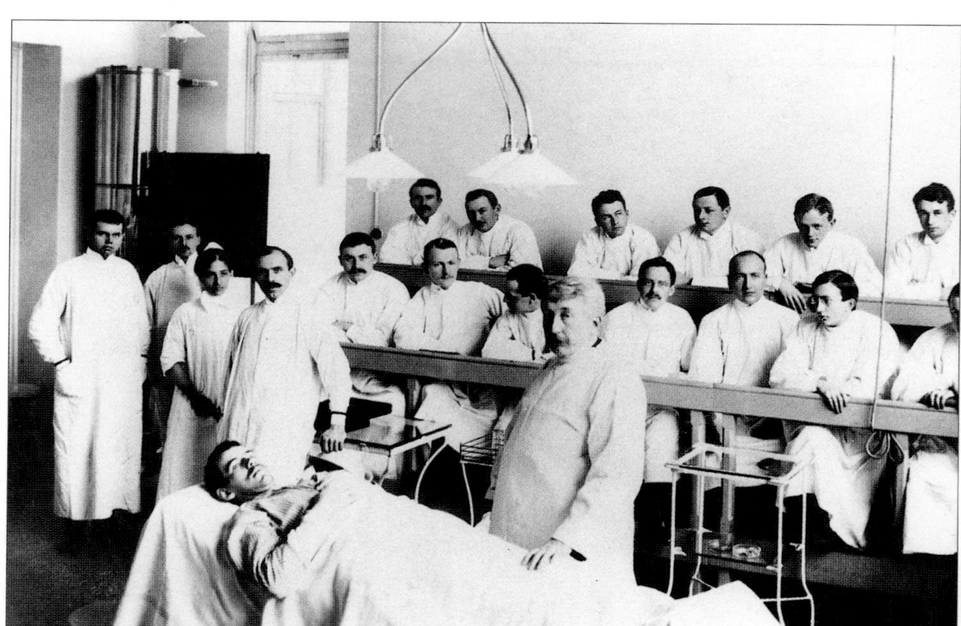

Figure 21: In the surgical theatre, Surgical department B, The National Hospital, Kristiania 1910. Professor Hagbarth Strøm (1854-1912) is teaching. First row from the left hand side: H. Haugseth, T. Schönfelder, Sister Hanna, Dr. Asbjørn Nilsen, E. Grønning, A. Jermstad, G. W. Keyser, S. Haug, J. Carlsen, H. Harmens, E. Aaser. Second row from the left: A. Rinde, A. Dahlø. F. A. Johannessen, C.A.B. Vemmestad, E. Julsrud, H. Kloumann. The patient and the photographer are the only unknown persons (Courtesy Dept. of Medical History, University of Oslo).

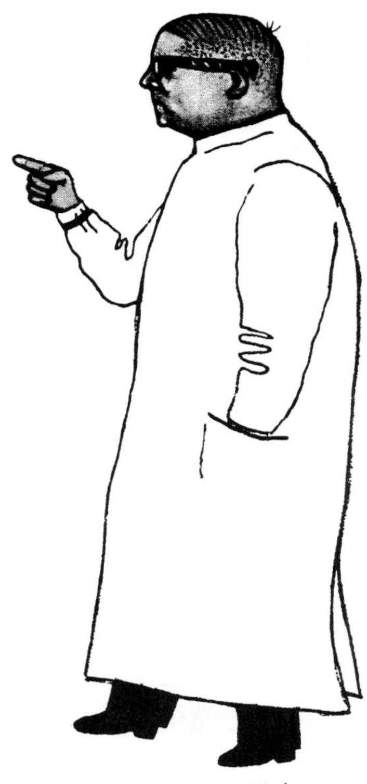

Figure 22: A teacher in dermatovenerology well-known by many Norwegian physicians, professor Niels Danbolt (1900-1984) of the University of Oslo, drawn by one of the medical students, Rolf Gärtner (1927-).

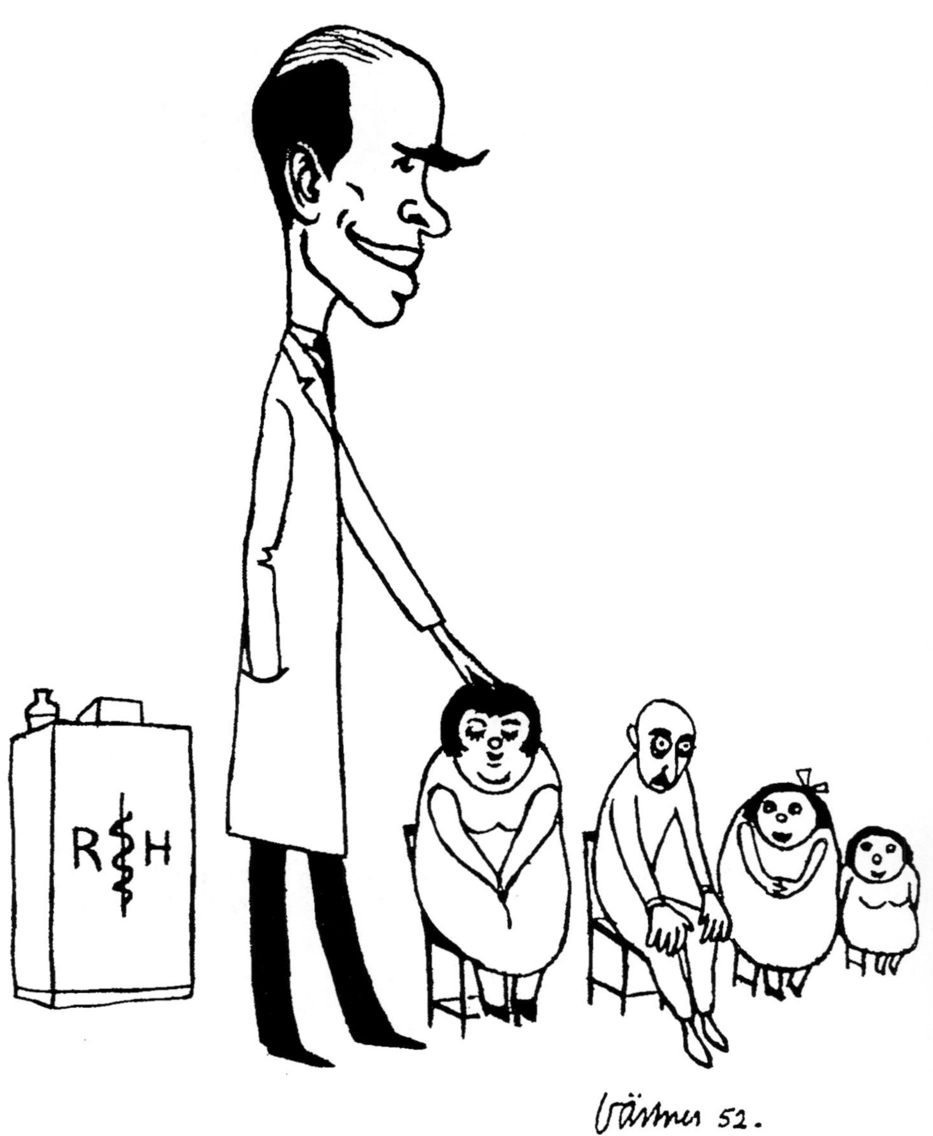

Figure 23: Professor Paul A. Owren (1905-1990), professor of internal medicine in Oslo and internationally highly esteemed blood coagulation researcher, drawn by the student Rolf Gärtner (1927-).

C H A P T E R 9 . 6

The County of Bratsberg. Epidemic Diseases in a District of Stability, Decline, and Progress

ASBJØRN STORESUND

9.6.1 Agriculture and Growing Industry

During the last thirty years of the nineteenth century, the County of Bratsberg, which is now called the county of Telemark, was divided into seven health districts. The boundaries were mainly based on the administrative boundaries, which remained unaltered during the period. Social development were very different in the seven districts, which provides the possibility for discussing differences in health development in relation to differences in demography, social conditions, economy, communication, and other factors. In this context, the health districts can be grouped into two outer districts (Skien and Kragerø), two central districts (Hollen and Kviteseid), and three inner districts (Laardal, Sauland, and Tinn) (Diagram 9.36 and Table 9.4).

Of the two outer districts, the population increased rapidly during the whole period in the Skien district, particularly when new industries were established after around 1880. This applied both to the towns and the large rural municipalities in the district. The population in Kragerø district stagnated after around 1890, as a result of the depression in the shipping industry after 1876, and the problems involved with transition from sail to steam (Diagram 9.37). The depression particularly affected the town of Kragerø and to some extent Bamble. The central and inner districts were farming communities, with either a decreasing or stable population. Exceptions to this were the industrial area of Ulefoss in Hollen, and to some extent Aamdal works in Laardal, which experienced population growth in the 1880s. The town of Notodden in Sauland district was also an early industrialized area. Apart from these, the other towns of the county were situated in the two outer districts.

The great changes in Norwegian society during these years are clearly reflected in Bratsberg, as new industry was established early here. The increase in activity and communication are also described in the medical reports. There is no typical central valley in Bratsberg, as is often found elsewhere in Norway. In the nineteenth century, the villages therefore lay scattered and relatively isolated. There is reason to believe that this dispersion created special conditions for the development of epidemic diseases and health status in the population. Another aspect is that the doctor's work often was hindered by impassable roads to isolated places, particularly during the spring, as was the case in 1876 in Tørdal, to the far north-west in Kragerø health district (BSM 76). This could

DIAGRAM 9.36
Health districts in the county of Bratsberg 1870–1900

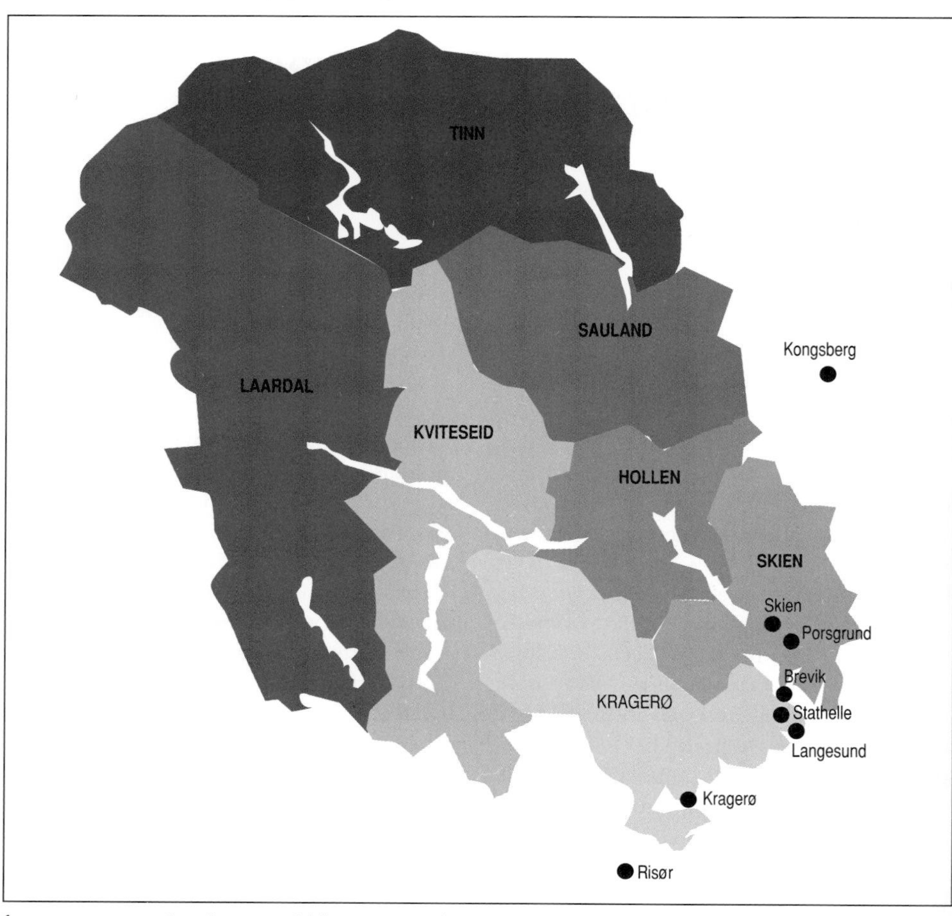

be one reason why there could be many sick people in such places, without them appearing in the doctor's statistical reports.

9.6.2. Mortality and Epidemic Diseases

According to the ministers' lists in Bratsberg, total mortality fell from just under 20 to about 15 deaths per 1,000 during the period 1870–1900. The reduction was greatest during the 1890s, in line with the development in the rest of the country (Backer 1961). This is particularly characteristic for the district of Skien, while in the Kragerø district, it seems that mortality began to fall in the middle of the 1880s. The reasons for this have not been investigated, but could be associated with the difference in population growth in the two districts.

In the central districts (Hollen and Kviteseid), the trends in mortality were similar to those in the outer districts. The inner districts were different. In Sauland and Laardal, mortality hardly fell, but remained at around 15, with the exception of Sauland, which had a period of high mortality during most of the 1880s. Mortality increased in theTinn district throughout the whole period from the lowest level in the county during the 1870s, to just

TABLE 9.4
The health districts in the county of Bratsberg, in area and population as per 01.01. 1891. (Source: A. Helland: A Topographic Statistical description of the county of Bratsberg amt I, Kristiania 1900.)

Health districts	Corresponding town communities and administrative communities	Area in km^2	Population
Skien	Skien kjøpstad Porsgrund kjøpstad Brevik kjøpstad Eidanger Solum Gjerpen Slemdal (Siljan)	1,066.24	30,429
Kragerø	Kragerø kjøpstad Langesund ladested Stathelle ladested Bamle Sannikedal Skaatø Drangedal	1,650.41	23,386
Hollen	Hollen Lunde Bø Saude	1,141.81	12,138
Sauland	Hitterdal Hjartdal Gransherred	1,716.04	6,759
Kviteseid	Seljord Kviteseid Nissedal	2,256.07	7,837
Laardal	Laardal Fyresdal (Moland) Mo Vinje Rauland (except the parish of Møsstranden)	4,214.11	7,952
Tinn	Tinn Hovin The parish of Møsstranden	3,144.42	3,533

Kjøpstad = provincial town Ladested = small coastal town

over the mean for the county in the years just before the turn of the century (Diagram 9.38). But, variation in mortality was great in Tinn, with peaks in 1877 and 1882. At the end of the 1860s, mortality reached a peak of 25–30 deaths per 1,000 in the populous outer and central districts. The inner districts, particularly Tinn, did not experience this.

Trends in mortality in the different health districts correspond well with mor-

DIAGRAM 9.37
Population in the county of Bratsberg 1866–1900

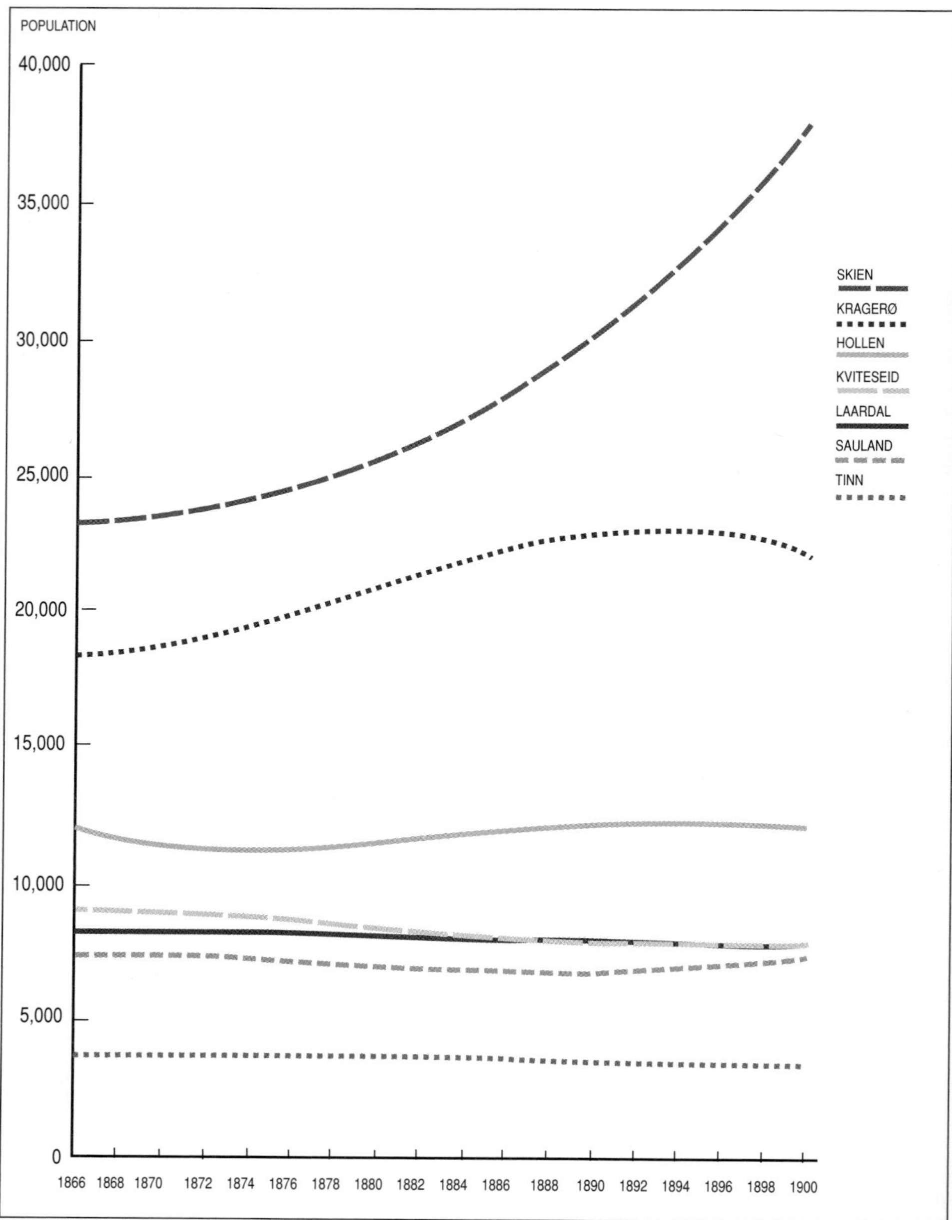

tality from epidemic diseases calculated from the reports of the district medical officers. The example of Tinn demonstrates this (Diagram 9.38 and 9.39). Since the reports of the doctors and ministers probably can be regarded as independent sources, this can be

DIAGRAM 9.38
Mortality in the district of Tinn, as compared to the county of Bratsberg except for Tinn, 1866–1900

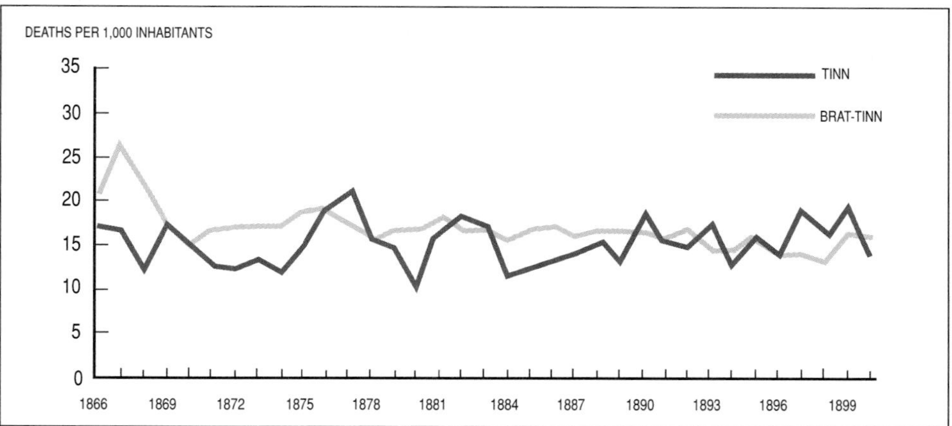

interpreted as indicating that mortality from epidemic diseases provides a reasonably correct picture of the main trends, even though the absolute figures for each district for individual years are low. This does, of course, not necessarily mean that the epidemic diseases totally explain the increased mortality from other causes, particularly among the weakest groups, children and elderly people. Apart from this, other factors, such as weather conditions with subsequent failing harvest, undoubtedly were important in accounting for variations in mortality in different years.

9.6.3. Differences in Morbidity According to District

In the most populous district of Skien, epidemic diseases reached a peak around 1890 and then diminished, as in the country as a

DIAGRAM 9.39
Mortality of epidemic diseases in the district of Tinn, and in the county of Bratsberg except for Tinn, 1868–1900

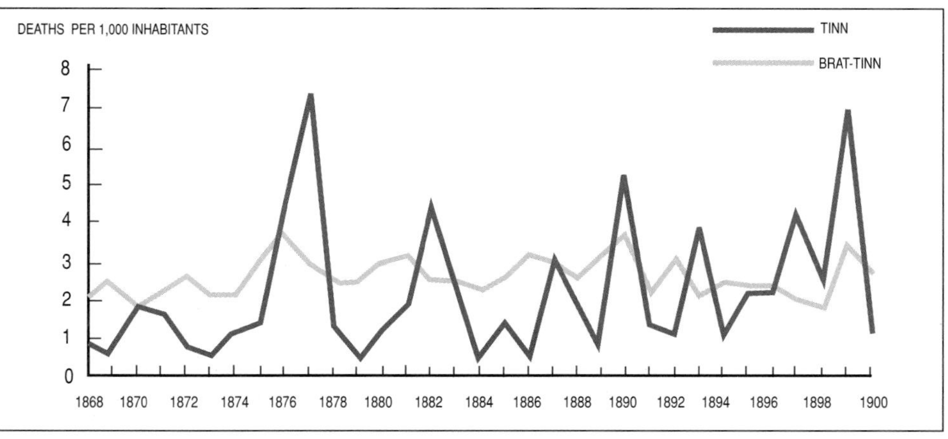

DIAGRAM 9.40A
Incidence of scarlet fever in Skien and Kragerø 1868–1900

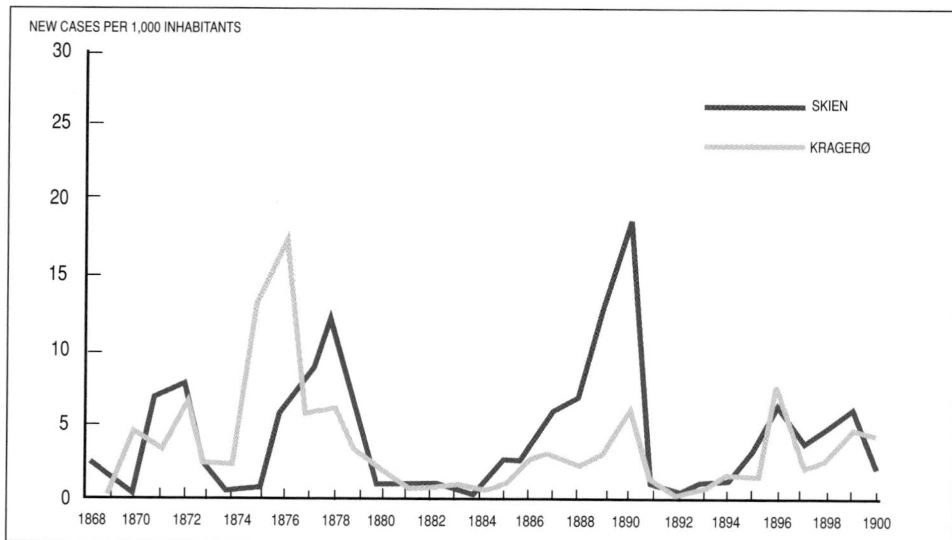

whole (Larsen et al. 1980). The incidence of epidemic diseases was less in the Kragerø district than in Skien during the whole period, with the exception of a few years in the middle of the 1880s. In the other districts, the incidence of these diseases was either constant or slightly increasing, but much lower than in the outer districts. It is, however, difficult to know to what extent the registration was incomplete here.

There is also a range of differences in the occurrence of different diseases throughout the period in the seven health districts in Bratsberg. Some of the most important diseases will be described here, with a certain emphasis on scarlet fever, since this disease is among the best documented and played an important role throughout the whole period.

9.6.4. Scarlet Fever

Scarlet fever broke out as a virulent epidemic in 1867–1868, with three subsequent major outbreaks during the period 1870-1900 (Diagram 9.40a-d). As in other parts of the country, the disease dominated the disease panorama in Bratsberg, causing significant mortality among children and young people due to complications. Cases were registered each year during the whole period in the two outer districts, so that the disease was more endemic than epidemic there. But in the other districts, particularly in the three inner districts, many years elapsed when the disease was not registered at all. This could, of course, be due to incomplete registration, as several doctors reported that there were many cases that were not registered during epidemics (BSM 76).

A minor outbreak of scarlet fever with low mortality peaked in 1872, affecting only the districts of Skien, Kragerø, and Hollen.

The major epidemic started in 1875 in Skien and Kragerø. The following year, the disease was present in all the districts in Bratsberg, with varying mortality. Kviteseid had the highest registered incidence from 1876 to 1879. It was assumed that the disease came into the district from three or four different places during the first half of 1876. In Seljord, the disease spread during the

DIAGRAM 9.40B
Incidence of scarlet fever in Hollen and Kviteseid 1868–1900

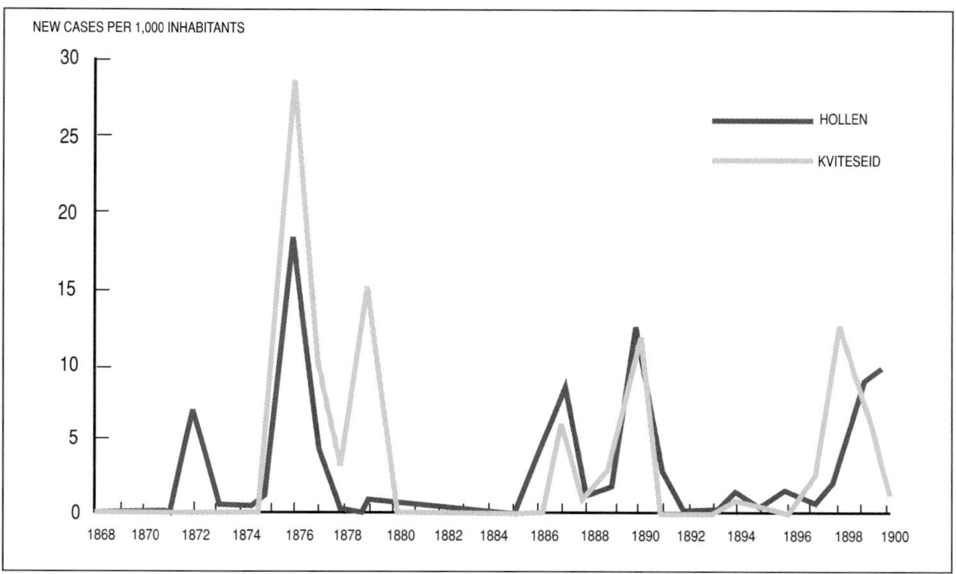

DIAGRAM 9.40C
Incidence of scarlet fever in Sauland and Laardal 1868–1900

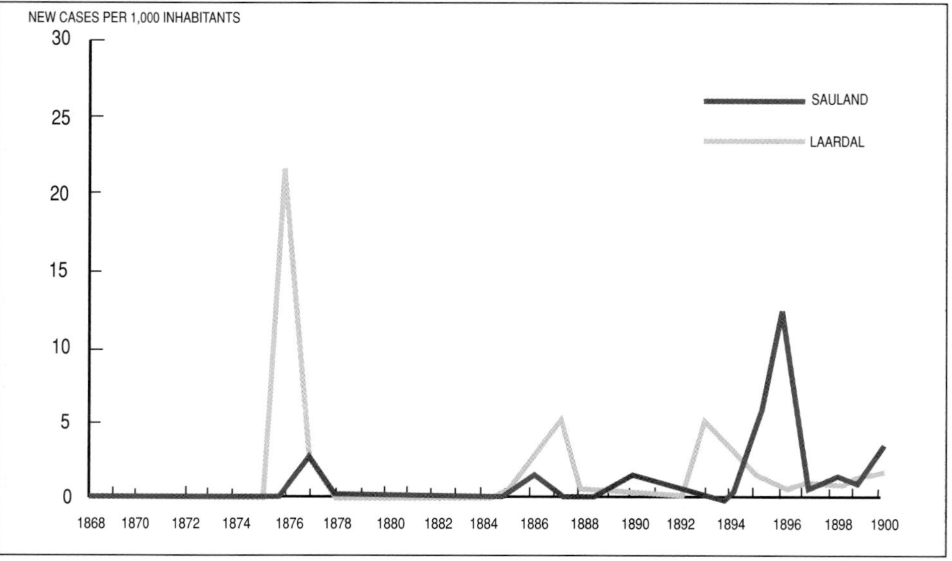

DIAGRAM 9.40D

Incidence of scarlet fever in the health district of Tinn, and the county of Bratsberg except for Tinn, 1868–1900

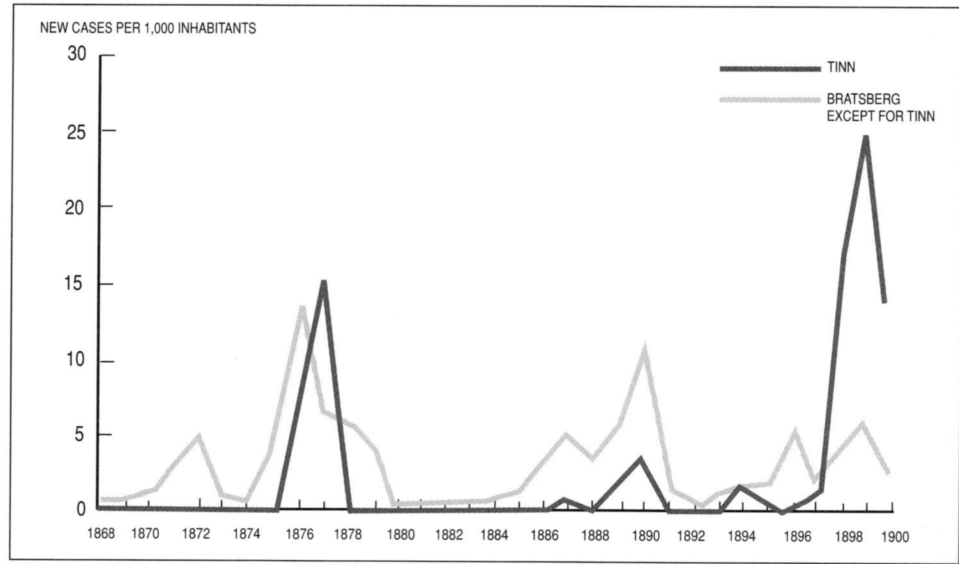

summer to remote villages, and was reported to be more virulent than in Vrådal or Kviteseid. After a remission in 1877, the disease flared up again in 1878 and 1879, with serious consequences. The infection was assumed to have spread from the southern part of the county. The inner districts were also affected by this epidemic, but not as severely as the district of Kviteseid. In Laardal, where the disease had not been present for many years, the disease was assumed to have been imported from the south, through Fyresdal in the spring of 1876, and at the same time to Høydalsmo from lower Telemark. The development in Tinn was the same as the one in Laardal, but the disease did not break out until the late autumn. In both these districts, the disease was mild to begin with, but became more virulent after a few months (BSM 76). The district of Sauland seems to have been the only district that remained relatively free from scarlet fever during the 1870s. A few cases were assumed to have been transmitted from Tinn (BSM 77).

The next outbreak of scarlet fever in Bratsberg started in 1885. It began in the south-western regions, in the districts of Kragerø and Laardal. It was assumed that the disease had originated in Arendal. During the year 1886, the disease spread to most of the surrounding districts, but it was locally limited and benign. A year later the disease reached a preliminary peak in the outer and central districts, as well as in Laardal. There were a great many local variations within each district. The counties in the north of the district of Laardal, Vinje and Rauland were reported to have avoided the epidemic, as they had done during the epidemic of the 1870s. There weren't any registered cases in the north-east (Sauland and Tinn). The disease culminated in 1889 and 1890, when especially the district of Skien, where the disease acquired a more serious nature, was affected. In the other districts, the epidemic was so mild that relatively few of the cases were registered. For instance, this was true of Tinn, where the settlement was widely spread out(BSM 90)

A third major outbreak of scarlet fever occurred in Bratsberg in the second half of the 1890s, but the disease was generally mild, as compared to the previous epidemics. It was reported that in several districts the actual number of sick was much higher than was registered, because the relatives of the sick did not think that it was necessary to report the disease. Except for in Skien, the disease was first registered in 1893 in the district of Laardal, when a laborer on the roads between Dalen and Vinje was infected, and the disease then spread to Vinje and Rauland, where scarlet fever had not been registered since 1870. Later the disease became confined to these two areas (BSM 93/95). In the two outer districts, it seems as though new cases continually appeared in different places, but generally the disease appeared as "house epidemics" (BSM 97). In some years, however, there was a relatively high incidence in the central and inner districts, such as in Sauland in 1896, Kviteseid in 1898, Hollen in 1899, and particularly in Tinn in the same year. Taking into account that many cases were not registered because the disease usually progressed without complications, it is possible that the disease had an endemic nature during the 1890s in the central and inner districts in Bratsberg. Even though scarlet fever was widespread at this time, mortality was reported to be low, as shown in the statistics (Diagram 9.41a-d). The development described here is in accordance with the general supposition that the scarlet fever virus became less virulent from around 1890 (Holst 1954).

9.6.5. Measles and Whooping Cough

Measles appeared regularly in the outer districts in the form of eight outbreaks at three- to four-year intervals from 1874 to 1899. There were fewer outbreaks in the other districts, with periods when no or very few cases were registered. There were four

Diagram 9.41a
Mortality of scarlet fever in Skien and Kragerø 1868–1900

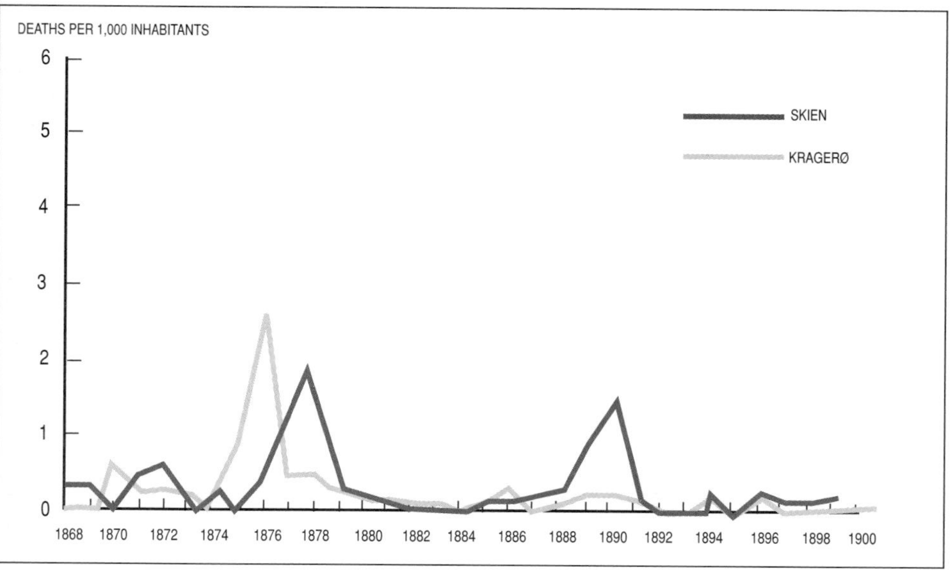

DIAGRAM 9.41B
Mortality of scarlet fever in Hollen and Kviteseid 1868–1900

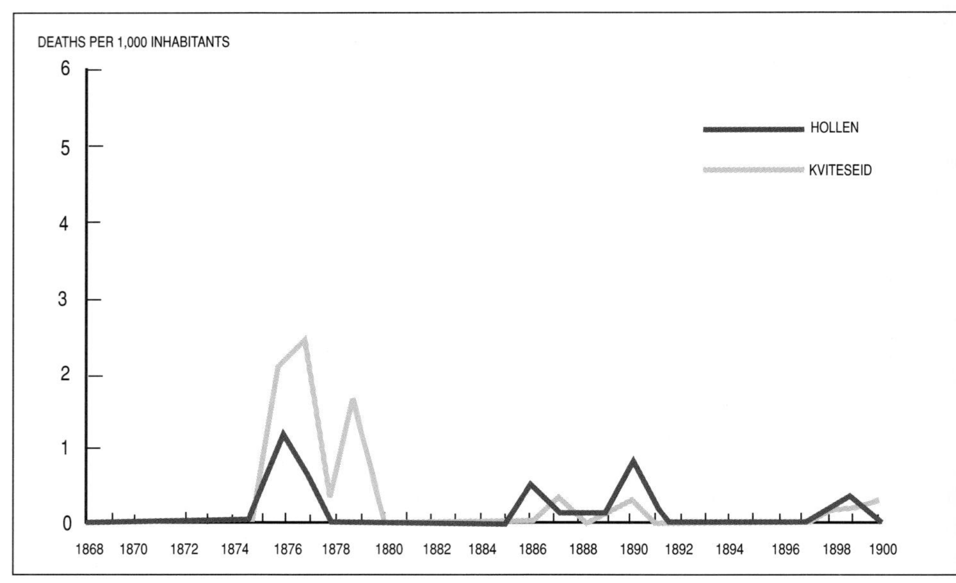

DIAGRAM 9.41C
Mortality of scarlet fever in Sauland and Laardal 1868–1900

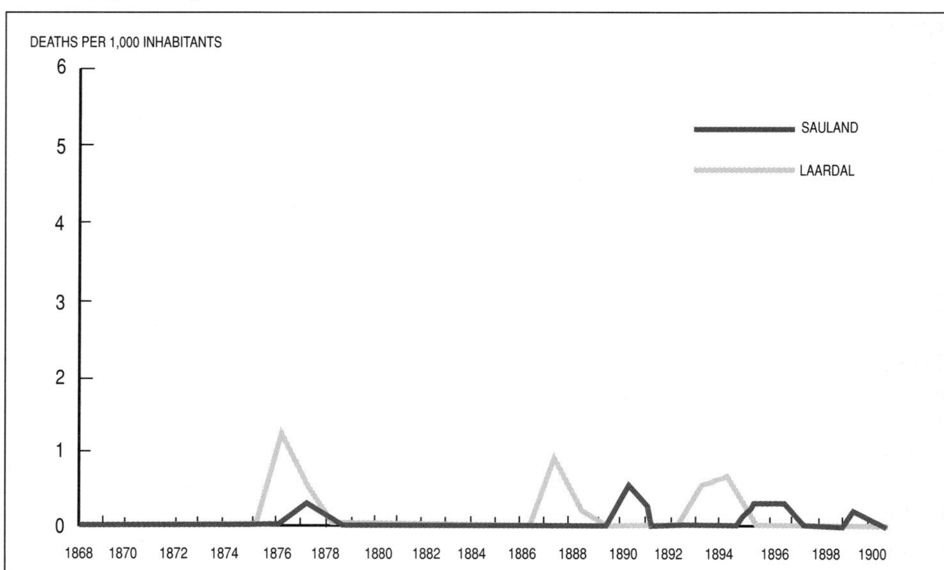

DIAGRAM 9.41D

Mortality of scarlet fever in the health district Tinn as well as the county of Bratsberg except for Tinn, 1868–1900

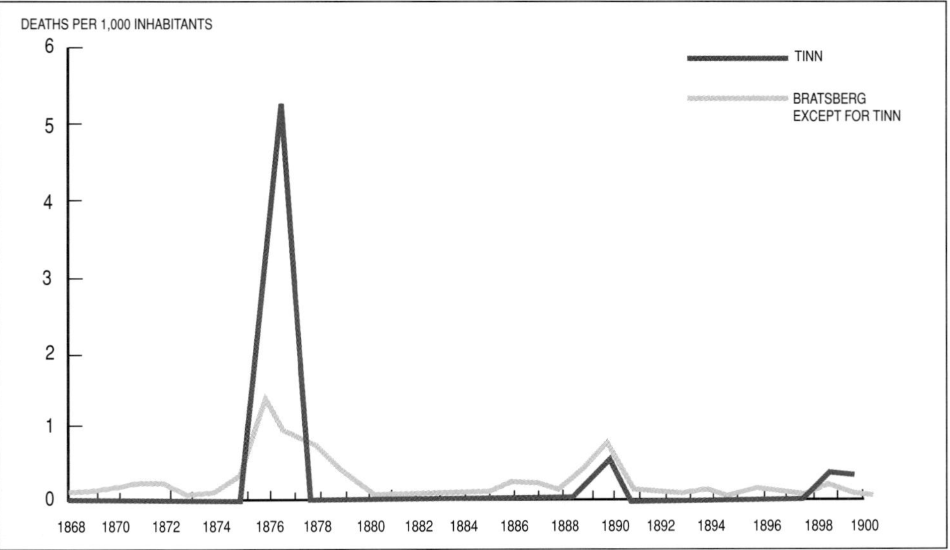

outbreaks in Laardal, three in Sauland, and only two in Tinn. The number of deaths due to measles was less than ten per year, and mortality from the diseases was low throughout the whole period. Cases were registered in Tinn only in 1877 and 1892. However, nearly all the children in the district were affected in these two years. In 1877, the infection was said to have been imported by a school child from Kristiania, and the disease was relatively virulent with significant complications (BSM 77). A similar event had occurred in Laardal two years earlier (BSM 75). Measles broke out again in Tinn in 1892, probably transmitted by a soldier from Gråtenmoen near Skien, but this time it was a mild form of the disease, and only a few children received treatment (BSM 92).

Whooping cough seems to have followed a pattern similar to that of measles, but the out breaks seem to have appeared somewhat more continuous.

9.6.6. Diphtheria

In the 1880s and the first half of the 1890s, diphtheria broke out in Bratsberg, as in other parts of the country. In the early 1880s, the disease appeared mainly as isolated outbreaks in the outer and central districts; later it also appeared in the other districts apart from Laardal. The cases gradually became more serious, with higher mortality. Infection spread to the other districts from the east, from the Numedal and Kongsberg areas (BSM 83), and it seems as though this pattern was repeated in the following years. From 1884 to 1887 higher incidence and mortality were registered in the northeastern districts of Sauland and Tinn than in any other district in Bratsberg. Subsequently, the disease rapidly disappeared there. A few years later, around 1890, the number of cases greatly increased in the districts in the south west – Kragerø and Kviteseid. The infection in Kviteseid was said to have come from the north, through Seljord (BSM 89). Not until 1891–1892 did the disease gain a foothold in

Laardal, and then only for a short period. The diphtheria period culminated in Bratsberg with a fairly major out-break in the area around Skien that lasted for a couple of years just before 1895.

9.6.7. Typhoid Fever

Of the food- and water-borne diseases, typhoid fever was known and feared throughout the nineteenth century (Holst 1954). From the medical reports, it is clear that the doctors in Bratsberg paid a lot of attention to this disease in the 1870s, in order to be able to isolate the sick quickly. People in the country districts were afraid of being infected and avoided contact with infected families (BSM 73). In Bratsberg, as in other parts of the country, the disease was very common in certain districts from the 1870s on, since there had been several years in a row with warm summers, followed by rainy months in the autumn. The number of sick then usually increased during the autumn (BSM 70 and 72). The incidence was generally higher in the towns than in the country districts, but high incidence was also registered in Sauland and Tinn. The disease reached a peak in Tinn in 1870–1872, but after that hardly any cases were registered in this district. In the outer districts, the disease gradually declined up to the turn of the century. At the end of the 1890s, a slight increase in typhoid fever occurred in Sauland and Tinn, the infection supposedly coming from Kristiania via the market in Kongsberg (BSM 99).

9.6.8. Diarrhea and Cholera Nostra

Gastro-intestinal diseases, registered as diarrhea and cholera nostra, were very common in Bratsberg as elsewhere in the country during the second half of the nineteenth century. These diseases are similar to typhoid fever in mode of transmission. Even though a significant number of cases were registered each year, the diseases were given little attention in the medical reports. The reason is probably that these diseases were so common that they were given attention only when they appeared as major outbreaks. As late as 1899 in Laardal it was reported that only a few cases were treated, because people were so accustomed to the disease, which appeared more or less epidemic almost every summer (BSM 99). The doctors' reports show the highest incidence in the populous outer districts, but of course an uneven registration may possibly be a source of error. The statistics show that incidence and mortality for this group of diseases fell in the district of Kragerø when the population began to decrease in the 1890s, but this did not occur in the district of Skien. This is to be expected, as population density is probably a contributory factor in the incidence of these diseases, which are spread via food and water, and also in more serious cases through direct contact (Holst 1954). In some years with warm, dry summers and dried-up water sources, individual, isolated epidemics with high incidence were also registered in the inner districts, especially in Kviteseid and Laardal (BSM 80/81). The same happened in Tinn in 1899. In Laardal, several such epidemics broke out among the workers at the Aamdal Copper Mine (BSM 88/95).

9.6.9. The Physicians' Work in Mapping out and Preventing the Spread of Infection

9.6.9.1. Detailed Mapping of the Spread of Infection

Detailed mapping of the spread of infectious diseases was essential for the district physicians, in order to be able to implement measures to contain these diseases. It seems that great care was taken to register infected people during the repeated outbreaks of typhoid fever in Bratsberg in the 1870s. Each year, sailors brought infection with them to the districts of Kragerø and Skien, and infection was spread to the inner districts by merchants and soldiers returning home from the outer districts or from towns in the neighboring counties (BSM 74/78).

From the major scarlet fever epidemic in the second half of the 1870s, we have an example of mapping the spread of infection in the district of Kviteseid. The disease spread over two of the three administrative areas in the district during the course of five months, and its progress was carefully followed from month to month. At the end of October 1878, the disease was brought to a place at the southern end of the lake Seljordsvannet by a woman from Porsgrunn. From there, the disease spread from one place to the next along both sides of the lake. In December 1878, a man brought the infection from there to a farm called Bjørge at the northern end of the lake. From Bjørge, the disease was spread by pupils from a nearby school to the farm of Nordgarden in the Seljord village, and from there to the pupils' homes in Brunkeberg. The infection could then be traced into the valley of Morgedal. From Seljord, the disease spread north-east to Flatdal, and in February 1879, it was spread from there to Ordal in Brunkeberg by a girl who went there seeking employment. On March 22, 1879, the disease was carried to the parish of Kviteseid by a woman from Morgedal, whose children had not been confined to the house when they had the disease. The woman brought milk to relatives in Solberg, near Opsund, one afternoon. The next day, on March 24, the children at Solberg were ill. From there, a farm laborer in Opsund caught the infection. After this, the spread of the disease was halted. It was reported that the district physician on a daily basis checked that isolation was strictly observed and that infected places were disinfected (BSM 78/79).

During the second major outbreak of scarlet fever at the end of the 1880s, the disease was milder than it had been before. The district physician in Hollen believed that this was the reason why the disease spread so rapidly, since people omitted to report it. Thus, during this epidemic, posters were hung up, ordering people to report the disease (BSM 87). During the epidemic in Skien in 1889–1890, the physicians' work was made difficult because the initial phase of the disease was mild. Consequently, children were not ordered to stay inside during the initial phase of the disease, and the doctor was not called before more serious complications occurred.

Throughout the whole period, the most commonly used preventive measures were isolation of infected persons, admittance of cases to a cottage hospital, bans on attending school and meetings, and finally disinfection of places where infected people were found.

9.6.9.2. Isolation

Isolation of sick people, or people who were suspected of having been in contact with infection, seems to have been widely practiced during serious epidemics of typhoid fever, scarlet fever, and diphtheria.

When the scarlet fever epidemic in 1876 and 1877 was at its worst, there was little that could be done in the way of prevention, as new cases constantly appeared in new places, often by spread of infection from neighboring counties. Nevertheless the district physician in Skien noted that, as was mentioned previously," the usefulness of isolation is confirmed; isolation both of individual patients within a family and of the houses where there was infection" (BSM 77).

Doctors worked actively to isolate patients, even when the outbreak was over, in order to prevent new outbreaks. There were complaints about lack of cooperation. In Skien, printed posters were hung up, giving information about the symptoms of the disease symptoms and about regulations for the population. The district physician in Skien reported that the working-class people in the towns and in the country made prevention difficult, because of their indifference and their fatalistic view, in addition to the persistence of inherited customs and established manners. The district physicians in Tinn had similar comments (BSM 76). As late as 1896, it was reported from Sauland that since the people had found out that isolation involved inconvenience, they tried to hide the disease for as long as possible (BSM 96). Isolation of patients must have been almost impossible in families with many children, because they often had only one room at their disposal. In Laardal district, the regulation about isolation was rarely observed (BSM 77).

During diphtheria epidemics, it was forbidden to sell milk that had been handled by people who were suspected of having been in contact with sick people, and posters warning about infection were pinned up on buildings where there were sick people (BSM 85). There were cases where people were fined because they left isolated houses before the isolation period was over. This happened in Nissedal, where diphtheria infection was brought from Åmli, south of the border with Aust-Agder, when some forestry workers went home for Christmas too early (BSM 89/90).

9.6.9.3 Isolation Wards

Special isolation wards do not seem to have been usual before the 1890s, and then they appeared first and foremost in the towns. Some patients with typhoid fever were isolated in the county hospital in Skien in the 1870s, but some patients developed typhoid fever after they were admitted to hospital, so that extensive procedures had to be adopted to eradicate infection (BSM 79).

In Skien, a couple of rooms in the poor house were reserved for people with scarlet fever, but only a few people seem to have been admitted to these rooms (BSM 76/78). However, separate isolation wards were used in Skien for patients who brought diphtheria from outside the district (BSM 92/99). People with diphtheria in the country districts outside Skien were isolated in a temporary cottage hospital and in a newly constructed empty barrack (BSM 91). In 1893, a cottage hospital for diphtheria patients was established in Porsgrunn, and in Bamble in Kragerø district; isolation wards were established the following year. In 1900, all patients with scarlet fever in Porsgrunn were admitted to isolation wards.

9.6.9.4. Closing of Schools

Schools seem to have been closed for short periods, often in connection with disinfection. The public shool in Porsgrunn was closed for a period, after a case of typhus was discovered. Sunday school and other church activities for children were forbidden in Skien during the scarlet fever epidemic in the 1870s, and children from infected houses were denied access to school and other acivities until disinfection had been carried out. Children from diphtheria-infected homes in the Skien district were denied access to school and, in the town of Skien, the school was closed to be disinfected against scarlet fever in 1890. The same happened in Tinn as late as in 1899.

9.6.9.5. Disinfection

Disinfection involved fumigating houses and furniture, and also clothes that could not be washed. Chlorine, or preferably sulfur, was used for fumigating, after which clothes and rooms were aired and washed. But it was often reported that disinfection had been inadequate, since the disease appeared again in the same house. Thus, in Porsgrunn, an inspector was appointed to carry out the disinfection and to be present to ensure that fumigation was done properly (BSM 78/79). In winter, it was difficult or impossible to disinfect poor people's flats or houses, since they often had only one room at their disposal (BSM 76).

During the diphtheria epidemic, sulfur

fumigation was shown to be inadequate, especially where there were uneven and cracked floors, so a strong solution of carbolic acid and hydrochloric acid was used instead, and this proved to be a more effective disinfectant (BSM 90). Another disinfectant that was used was warm linseed oil. Replacement of the floor, either at the owner's expense or paid for from the poor relief fund, could also be a solution. In order to prevent spread of infection by bedding, people in Laardal had the choice of either burning or disinfecting skin bed covers, with the amount of four kroner provided as compensation. Most people chose to burn bed covers, even though it cost between eight and sixteen kroner to replace them (BSM 92).

9.6.10 Concluding Remarks

Several of the most important epidemic diseases in the county of Bratsberg between 1870 and 1900 seem to have progressed rather differently in the seven health districts. Figures and accounts from the medical reports indicate that there were fewer epidemics of some diseases in the inner districts; the epidemics were often shorter, but in some cases the incidence was higher than in the outer districts.

It is necessary to consider the combined effects of biological, cultural, and other factors to explain differences in morbidity and mortality between the districts. There is reason to believe that an important role in the natural history of disease is played by biological factors, such as variations in virulence and reduced immunological defense in a sparse population with longer periods of time between each outbreak of diseases.

Differences in life style, in a broad sense, between the communities of farmers in the inner districts and communities of mainly workers, seamen, and others in the outer districts, have to be studied in greater detail to evaluate the significance of cultural factors. The annual reports give a general impression that the district physician officers in Skien and Kragerø were definitely more satisfied with the sanitary standards in their districts than were their colleagues in the inner districts.

As could be expected, infection was often imported from outside to the outer districts, but from time to time infection came from outside to the inner districts also, from Kongsberg and Numedal in the north-east, and from Arendal and the rest of the county of Nedenes (Aust-Agder) in the south-west. Geographical isolation seems to have given communities in the inner districts some protection against epidemics.

At a time when curative measures against infectious diseases had limited effect, it seems as though preventive measures were a central part of the strategy chosen by the health personnel. Even though these measures alone could not improve the health status of the population in the long run, there is reason to believe that experience gained during this period contributed to developments in society, such that the general health of the people gradually could improve in the years to come.

References

Backer, J. E. *Dødeligheten og dens årsaker i Norge 1856–1955*. Oslo: Samfunnsøkonomiske studier 10, Statistisk Sentralbyrå, 1961.

BSM: *Beretning om Sundhedstilstanden og Medisinalforholdene i Norge*. Kristiania: Norges officielle Statistik. (The two last digits in the references indicate the year.)

Holst, P. M. *Våre akutte folkesykdommers epidemiologi og klinikk*. Oslo: Aschehoug og Co, 1954.

Larsen, Ø., H. Haugtomt og W. Platou. *Sykdomsoppfatning og epidemiologi 1860–1900. Epidemiske sykdommer i Norge og helsemyndighetenes vurdering av folkehelsen – presentasjon av data*. Oslo: Seksjon for medisinsk historie, Universitetet i Oslo, 1980.

CHAPTER 9.7

The Counties of Hedemarken and Kristian. Health Conditions and Standard of Living 1860–1900

HANS P. SCHJØNSBY

> "For man is, to a great extent, what external circumstances make him."
>
> (Eilert Sundt 1855)

9.7.1. Registration of Diseases

Larsen and his colleagues (Larsen 1980) have shown an increase in epidemic diseases in the 1870s and especially the 1880s. Then follows a decline in frequency from about 1890, which may have something to do with the altered understanding of diseases by the health authorities. This applied first and foremost to the towns, and implied that these diseases were now taken more seriously, and that the increasing problems these diseases brought from the 1880s on was no longer to be accepted.

Based on the district physicians' reports, there are also other conditions that should be considered when investigating the course of acute contagious diseases during this period. The increase in the frequency of epidemics can be genuine, but may also be related to the fact that reporting from the 1860s onward was more systematic, comprehensive, and complete. Some time later the progress of the medical sciences led to a better quality of reporting, as the diagnoses became more rational and accurate. In addition, the number of doctors increased. There were 16 doctors in the county of Hedemarken in 1865, and 45 in 1900, whereas the population remained rather stable. This increased the precision of the information. It is also probable that more people sought the advice of doctors, something that can be substantiated by the fact that the number of deaths registered by doctors in the county of Hedemarken increased from 43 percent in 1876 to 88 percent in 1900 (Skappel 1914).

Skappel gives yet another indication, in his presumption that "this condition (the increase in deaths from tuberculosis) continues until the end of the 1870s, when deaths from (tuberculosis) increases both in absolute and relative numbers, although maybe only in the accounts, as a result of more extensive doctor consultations." During this period the legislation for the poor also resulted in a certain increase in consultations (Try 1979).

The reports on diseases earlier in the century are not very reliable sources of comparison with the years from around 1870 up till the turn of the century. However, the district physicians in the two counties reported that, on average, they considered health to be good or satisfactory during 13 of the years between

1853 and 1870, that is, 76 percent of the time. The corresponding percentage for the period between 1870 and 1900 is 53.

One should be careful with interpretations, but it seems that Skappel (Skappel 1914) could be right in saying that "during the (18)40s and (18)50s there were very few contagious diseases" and that this could strengthen the assumption that there was a considerable increase in epidemic diseases in the inland during the last 10 years of the 1800s. However, there were fewer doctors around 1850, diagnoses and the comprehension of sickness were more primitive, the statistics were incomplete, and the standard of living worse than 50 years later.

9.7.2. Ill-health in the Counties of Kristian and Hedemarken

The incidence and the mortality from acute epidemics in the inland counties, Hedemarken and Kristian, measured on average for 5-year periods from 1870 to 1900, are shown in Diagram 9.42.

From the numbers we can see that the incidence for Hedemarken and Kristian was lower than the average for the country as a whole. The difference also applies to mortality. An exception is the period between 1886–90, when mortality in Hedemarken is highest. This was due to a nationwide diphtheria epidemic, which was particularly severe in this part of the country.

Although interesting differences can be shown in mortality and also in lethality (lethality is somewhat higher in the county of Kristian), it is the consistent and systematic lower occurrence of acute contagious diseases in the county of Kristian, as opposed to the neighboring county, which is of interest.

Table 9.5 shows the average incidence (cases of new disease per 1,000 inhabitants) of the main acute epidemic diseases, and the total for the period 1870-1900 in the counties of Hedemarken and Kristian. The table shows that the total frequency of these diseases is 31.1 percent higher in Hedemarken. It is especially the higher occurrence of infections of the respiratory passage (bronchitis, pneumonia, influenza, etc.) that is decisive (43.9 percent).

A further analysis of the data revealed

DIAGRAM 9.42

Incidence and mortality of acute epidemic diseases in the whole country and in the counties of Hedemarken and Kristian 1870–1900

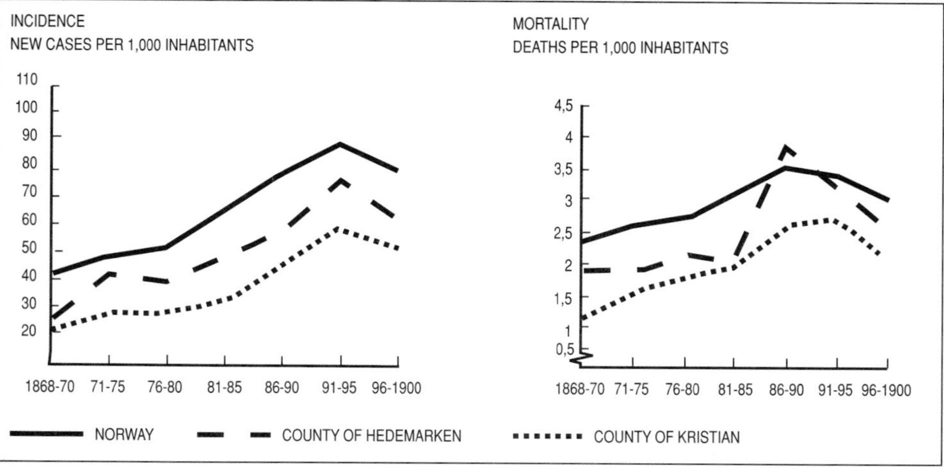

TABLE 9.5
Incidence of acute epidemic diseases in the period 1860 to 1900 in the counties of Hedemarken and Kristian

	Hedemarken County	Kristian County
Scarlet fever, Measles, Whooping cough, Diphtheria	9.0	6.7
Acute respiratory infections	43.7	24.5
Diarrhea	7.8	4.8
All acute epidemic diseases	55.3	38.1

that the incidence of epidemic diseases was highest in the district of Hedemarken. Today this district includes the municipalities of Ringsaker, Hamar, Stange, and Løten. Similarly, one observed low incidence in the valley of Gudbrandsdalen, especially in the districts of Ringeboe, Lom and Lesje, which are today the municipalities from Ringebu and northwards.

Diagram 9.43 gives information on sickness in the districts of Hedemarken and Gudbrandsdal in 1870–1900, and Diagram 9.44 for the remaining parts of the two counties. In Diagram 9.44 one observes that

DIAGRAM 9.43
Incidence and mortality of acute epidemic diseases in the districts of Northern Gudbrandsdal and the district of Hedemarken 1870–1900

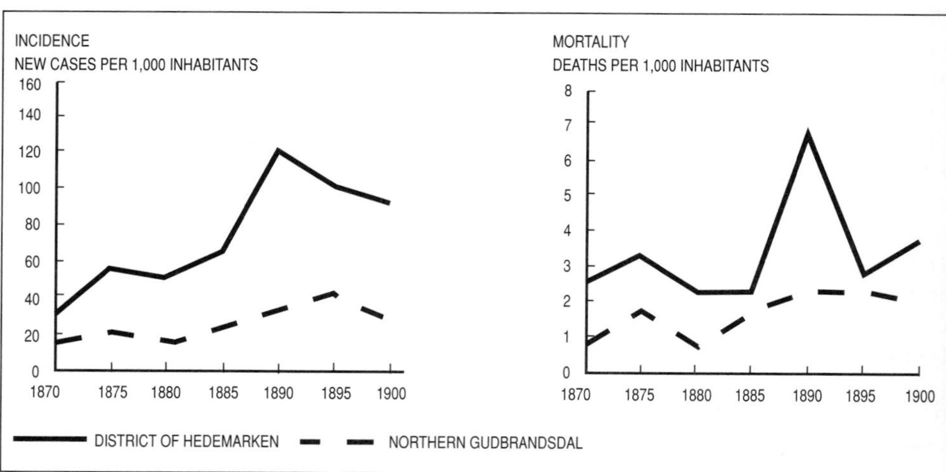

DIAGRAM 9.44

Incidence and mortality of acute epidemic diseases in the counties of Hedemarken and Kristian except the districts of Hedemarken and Northern Gudbrandsdal 1870–1900

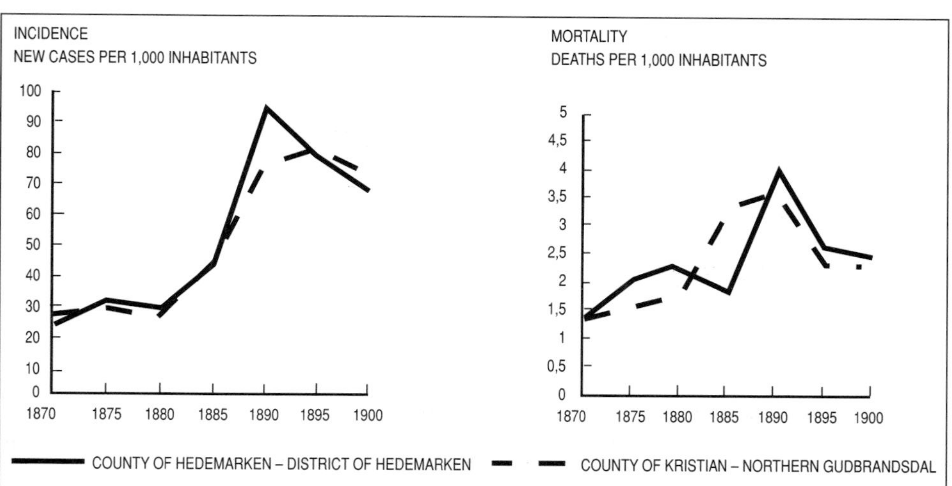

the graphs for both incidence and mortality are more or less merged. It seems therefore probable that the differences in sickness between the two counties can essentially be traced to the conditions regarding contagiousness in Hedemarken and Northern Gudbrandsdal, respectively.

This information corresponds to a series of other epidemiological observations from these areas. Jervell and his collaborators (Jervell 1965) pointed out in 1965 the low mortality of coronary heart disease in North-Gudbrandsdal in the county of Oppland (formerly the county of Kristian). More than 100 years earlier, Eilert Sundt (Sundt 1975) found a higher mortality in the deanery of Hedemarken than in the northern part of Gudbrandsdal during the period 1821-1850. He also calculated that the average life span of a newborn in 1848 in Gudbrandsdal was 53 years of age and in Hedemark 48 years of age.

9.7.3. Ill-health and Risk Factors

The reason for the outbreak of epidemic diseases could lie in the properties of the microorganism, in the individual, the individual's resistance, and in environmental conditions which can be conducive to the spreading of infection and disease; often, several factors are present at the same time. Some of the main factors are diet and nutrition, housing, and hygienic factors such as the quality and availability of drinking water and sanitation. The density of the population also plays a large part in the mechanism of spreading of contagious diseases. At the same time, circumstances such as economic basis, communications, the society's finances, health care services, working conditions, salaries, and other social conditions are taken into consideration. In other words, the living conditions are important factors.

By means of the medical reports and other sources of information, we may possibly find an explanation for the differences in sickliness between the two parts of the interior.

9.7.4. Diet and Nutrition

It is typical of the medical reports before the 1860s that information is given more frequently than in later years about crop failures and bad years, which disturb the delicate balance between availability of food and the population. There was often not enough food, and it is from this period that the district physicians give information about food substitutes. The last time this was reported was in 1870, from Tolga in the district of Tønset, where it is reported that the people mix "mask" (residues from the brewing of beer) and bark in the bread flour. Concern for the quality of the diet is often expressed in the 1870s and 1880s, and many are afraid that these unfortunate changes in diet contribute to the breakdown of people's health.

The district physicians were aware of the connection between diet and health conditions, and the medical reports also evidence the fact that they linked sickliness with people's nutritional basis. This is interesting, considering today's discussions and understanding of the relation between food and people's health (McKeown 1976). From Hedemarken it was reported in 1861 that the increased sickliness, to a large extent, was ascribed to the previous year's poor grain and potato harvest. And from Gudbrandsdal in 1877 it was reported from Lom, especially for Vaage, that living conditions for a large number of the crofters had been miserable, as they had been forced to use frozen flour due to the miserly grain harvest. The poor people's diet is described as bad from both these areas, and it was the composition of the food, rather than the quantity, that the district physicians were worried about. The district physician in Ringeboe wrote in 1885 that the main nourishment in the poor peoples' cabins was coffee, potatoes, and potato cakes. Coffee was regarded as indispensable, and, according to the district physician, the poor sold the flour they received from poor relief to buy coffee: "Coffee is the working man's alpha and omega; with coffee he feeds his children, and coffee he drinks at their funeral."

Complaints about the scarcity of milk are especially heard of from Hedemarken (1882): "still it becomes more and more difficult to get milk, especially for the poor, since milk is quite easy to sell at the dairies and condensation factory in Hamar." This situation, which illustrates that period's economic liberalism and the transition to a money economy, is commented on as follows from the valley of Gudbrandsdalen in 1893: "A direct result of our time's changing demands is, among others, the fact that our good old national thin wafer crispbread (flatbrød) is now replaced everywhere by the oven baked rye bread, which causes the peasants' previously strong and healthy teeth to be substituted with dentists' dentures."

It appears that the diet in Gudbrandsdal was generally somewhat more varied than in Hedemarken: "Meat, pork, cheese and butter are common the whole year round, often even for the poor classes" (1878), and "the way of life is simple and frugal. Wafer crispbread, butter, cheese, porridge, gruel, meat and pork constitute the daily diet. Though generally, one cannot afford to use meat" (1893). It is possible that this is related to the fact that Hedemarken was, at least until 1875–80, mostly a grain district, while the higher parts of Gudbrandsdal had a more varied nutritional foundation. Due to the marginal cultivation conditions the governor of the county of Kristian states in 1865 that, on an average, there was a crop failure every third year in the northern part of Gudbrandsdalen (Ministry of the Interior 1867–68) the inhabitants were mobile and both fish and game were a part of their diet, to a larger extent than for the people in the lowlands. Cattle breeding was fairly extensive among the inhabitants of Gudbrandsdal and temporary mountain farms were well-developed, which secured a better diet for the population. There were cattle breeding and mountain farms in Hedemarken as well, but to a smaller extent, and with poorer summer pastures (Tranberg 1993).

As for other differences in diet between Hedemarken and Northern Gudbrandsdal, it is important to mention the fact that there was an increasing number of hired laborers in Hedemarken. This was the case especially from the mid-1870s on, and this was due to changes in the running of the farms. In the same period the number of cottars with land declined (Gaustad 1935). This meant that agricultural laborers in Hedemarken, and to a smaller degree in Northern Gudbrandsdal, had to supply their own food, which was of a lower quality than previously, when food came either from their own land or from the landowner's farm. Skappel (Skappel 1914) describes it in this way: "The changes in diet have had a detrimental effect on the working classes, because the workers have gone over to supplying their own food, at the same time as their own farming has been reduced," and he moralistically adds, "any change in these conditions cannot be expected until the workers' wives are taught sensible cooking."

The medical reports and other relevant sources of information suggest that the quality of nutrition was better in Gudbrandsdalen in the last part of the nineteenth century, something that in turn could have contributed to the fact that the population there was less disposed to acute epidemics than the inhabitants of Hedemarken.

9.7.5. Housing

"the houses of the poor classes are one of the most important hotbeds of the epidemic diseases, which then threaten to spread to the rest of the population" (Holst 1892).

Even though Axel Holst's remark in this case is directed to the towns, it is beyond doubt that it also applied to the rest of the country. This is also a recurring theme in the medical reports.

There are plenty of accurate and mostly depressing descriptions of the sanitary conditions of houses from both Hedemarken and the districts in the valley of Gudbrandsdalen. It is, however, difficult to make qualitative distinctions between them, based on these descriptions. As early as in 1853, county physician Albert Blehr (1805–1872) from Hedemarken, writes that "the year was profitable but uncleanliness and stale air in overcrowded dwellings are still an important factor in the generation of infectious diseases (dyscrasic and zymotic diseases)" and in 1858 it is commented that "the narrow, small rooms are generally crammed with dwellers." The district physicians made a social distinction: "The landowners' houses are good and spacious, the cottars' small, without the necessary ventilation" (1867).

Descriptions such as "the mentioned classes (cottars and laborers) usually have one single room, which not only serves as a living room for the family day and night, but also as a working room, kitchen, and yes, much too often also as a hen coop and pigsty" and "the poor part (of the population) live under miserable conditions. Low ceilings, draughts all over, from walls, windows and doors, cold floors, in many places rotten due to the dampness of the foundations" are very common from both counties.

The district physicians are both descriptive and indignant about these humiliating conditions. They are, however, reluctant to make a closer analysis of the conditions, and very seldom offer any concrete suggestions for improvement. They were in no doubt that poor living conditions were the cause of sickness and misery, but the profession was generally conservative at least in their reports and they did not connect living conditions with political responsibility. Neither was this normal at the time. Attitudes were paternalistic with moralistic tendencies, and they imposed responsibility on the individual. One example of this was the district physician in Rendalen who in 1896 reported that the laborers' poverty is mostly due to a lack of any kind of economic sense, and to the women's incompetence in all domestic duties.

Conditions such as sanitation, drinking water and so on are seldom commented upon in the reports. That such sanitary conditions must have had disease-promoting qualities is evident in a report from Gudbrandsdalen, as late as 1891, where cleanliness was not in high favor. Privees could be found only porting stations and at the houses of the upper classes. Not even midwives and school teachers had acquired such for their homes. Many deemed it unhealthy not to perform such natural functions around the house walls, in the open. And pigs, sheep, and goats ate the excrements. Meanwhile, it seems that the hygienic standards, in both counties, gradually improved towards the turn of the century. Many district physicians attributed this to the economic growth and the improved level of knowledge: "The houses are as a rule healthy, and people become more and more aware of the necessity of washing floors and airing out rooms " (Lesja 1894). "Housing conditions are steadily improving, something that The House Loan Fund (Huslaanefondet) has contributed to." (Hedemarken 1900).

Sanitary and housing conditions were generally bad among the working classes in both counties during the period 1870-1900. However, based on the medical reports, it is difficult to find a relation between housing conditions and the differences in morbidity.

9.7.6. Population Density and the Structure of Settlements

Traditionally, population density is often used as a measure of the danger of infection in a population. The denser the population and the closer to each other people live and work, the greater the chance of catching an infectious disease. At the outset, one would think that one of the reasons for the higher incidence of contagious diseases in Hedemarken is because of the apparently higher population density. For example, in 1877 there were six times as many people per square kilometer in Hedemark than there were in Gudbrandsdalen. However, the situation evens out to a great extent when allowance is made for uncultivated areas. This is seen from the table 9.6.

The concentration of people at the work place and at home is of utmost importance to the spreading of infection. Infection has the best opportunity of swooping down on people in their local environment, and the higher the concentration of people, the more exposed one is to infection through water, food, and particularly droplet infection. The range of diseases (see Table 9.5) shows that droplet infection is the main way of infection in this connection. The structure of settlements and households is therefore an

TABLE 9.6
Population density in Gudbrandsdal and Hedemarken in 1877

	People per square kilometer	
	Gudbrandsdal	Hedemarken
Total area	2.5	15.2
Total area less uncultivated area	21.2	25.2

important factor in the degree to which infection is spread.

At this time, our two counties still had their traditional farming methods in common and intact. What we have in mind here is the farm as the center of a working and productive cooperative, consisting of the farmer, crofters and laborers. However, the structures were not completely identical, and the biggest difference was the size of the farms. Tranberg (1993) has calculated the farming communities' size in Ringsaker in 1801, and found that every fifth farm consisted of more than 20 people, and half of them had ten people or more. The average size was 13-14 people. The biggest farms had between 40 and 80 people, and were equal in size to whole settlements in other places.

The northern part of Gudbrandsdal was such a place. There, a greater number of smaller and equally sized farms were found that did not have as many cottars and servants as was usual in Hedemarken, and there were fewer people in the cooperative and in each household. Based upon data presented by Kjelland, it can be calculated that in Lesja in northern Gudbrandsdal in 1865, depending on social status, geographic position, and so on the size of the farmers' household averaged nine, and of the cottars' about five (Kjelland 1987 and 1992).

Another important structural difference lay in the economic basis. As mentioned earlier, Hedemarken was predominantly a grain district until well into the 1870s, whereas the districts of Gudbrandsdalen had more varied farming. Farming in Hedemarken required long periods of labor sharing (e.g., threshing teams) and specializing, with concentrated efforts and cooperation between the links in the productive cooperative.

Engelsen (1987) examined the possible differences in mortality according to social status in 1801 and 1802, and established that, from his material, he could not show that the poor had a higher death rate than the better-off classes. Engelsen claims that this must indicate the importance of the farm in the process of spreading infection, and points to the population density on the farms and its central position in the districts in terms of transport.

Together, these observations should be interpreted with care, but they do support the assumption that the higher occurrence of acute epidemics in Hedemarken can be related to larger and denser working and living conditions than in the districts of Gudbrandsdal.

9.7.7. Social Conditions

The present discussion of the influence of unemployment on public health has brought psychosocial factors into the picture, as risk factors for sickness (Ministry of Health and Soc. Affairs 1992). Life in the inland communities during the nineteenth century was often hard, and for the poorest it could be merciless. Fear, uncertainty and insecurity about their daily bread and the future, which often marked the weak groups, prepared the ground for sickness, together with other risk factors.

The county of Hedemarken and especially the county of Kristian were the two big cottars' counties. In 1855, which was the peak year, almost 9,000 cottars with land lived in the county of Kristian, and about 6,000 in the county of Hedemarken. At the turn of the century, there were less than 3,000 such cottars in both counties (Hovdhaugen 1976). There were many reasons for this decline both internal and international migration, re-organization and rationalization of farming, industrial development claiming workers, changes in salary conditions and so on, a series of processes that will not be dealt with here.

In connection with exposure to disease, it is important to pay attention to the fact that the farm laborers were not a homogeneous class. Cottars with land had a higher status. The really underprivileged and poor stratum where it was reasonable that disease and insecurity were at hand in abundance consisted of cottars without land, other landless navvies, day laborers, and other paupers. In 1885 there were almost 35,000 belonging to these categories, whereas there was a total of about 65,000 cottars with land (Hovdhaugen 1976).

It is also important to notice the fact that the overall standard of living was worst during the period between 1840 and 1860. The pressure from the population was then at its highest. Society had at this point little possibility of absorbing the excess population. Development, however, resulted in an increasing demand for labor, and an increase in salaries. From 1860 to 1900, salaries just about doubled in both counties, with relatively the most increases for the day workers and contract workers (Statistisk sentralbyrå 1969). In general, the cottars were financially better off during this period (Beitrusten 1976), and there was an improvement in the standard of living among the weakest groups. However, the number of people on poor relief did not decrease (Try 1979). Even though both counties were cottars' counties, and consequently had relatively more poor people than the rest of the country, there were differences between Hedemarken and the districts of Gundbrandsdal. Expenses for the poor were highest in Hedemarken. The county's parish statistics for 1885 reveal that of 659 parishioners, 500 came from the district of Hedemarken, a part of the county with the same name (Skappel 1914), whereas from the county of Kristian it is reported that Valdres and the northern Gudbrandsdal have relatively few poor on relief (Ødegaard 1918). This, however, does not mean that there was neither poverty nor beggars in Gudbransdal.

We shall take a closer look at the social conditions among these groups, and if possible establish differences which may have significance on the differences in the overall view of diseases.

In the case of the distribution of the working classes in the two counties, the number of landless cottars was highest in the county of Hedemark. Only Nordland had more in 1855 (Hovdhaugen 1976). The county of Kristian came further down the list, and considering that there was a larger total number of cottars in this county, the county of Hedemarken had decidedly more laborers of a lower social status and standard of living than the neighboring county. The conditions of employment, that is by the farmer, differed in the districts of Hedemarken and in the valley of Gudbrandsdalen. Arbitrariness was more widespread in the lowland districts. In Ringsaker the largest municipality in the district of Hedemarken- the most common type of employment conditions at the beginning of the 1800s was that the cottars had unrestricted work (Tranberg 1993). As the population increased, this created dissatisfaction and social unrest, and it is understandable that the Thrane movement had most supporters in the lowlands of the Eastern part of the country. These circumstances related to the increasing class distinctions in Hedemarken, led to conditions described in the following way (Helland 1902): "Generally, cottars, servants and ordinary day laborers receive little respect from their master and mistress," and "The relations between master and mistress and their workers are often strained." This description forms a contrast to the conditions in the district of Northern Gudbrandsdal.

Lifelong engagement of a cottars' farm was more common in the mountain districts (Ødegaard 1918). In Hedemarken the cottar's farms were rented out by the year. Even during the last part of the century, working obligations often lasted the whole year round, and the cottar could be summoned to work (Thorleifsen 1991). The relationship between farmer and worker in the valley of Gudbrandsdalen was characterized to a large extent by an old-fashioned paternalism and more equality, so there was less unrest: "Otherwise, one notices that class distinctions and dissatisfaction are, on the whole, less than in many other communities in the country. This is apparent from the fact that, among other things, the Thrane movement did not get much power here (Lesja)" (Einbu 1949).

9.7.8. Communications

The role of communications in the spreading of infections was also obvious one hundred years ago, and it was remarked about tuberculosis: "the steady development of transportation must necessarily generate a higher instance of the spreading of diseases" (Larsen 1889). This applies also to acute infectious diseases. The medical reports bear testimony of this. District Physician Morten Andreas Leigh Aabel (1830-87) wrote the following about the scarlet fever epidemic in the county of Kristian during the middle of the 1870s: "In the district of Southern Valdres, it started in December at the parish of Southern Aurdal, probably through infection from the town of Drammen."

Similarly, it is reported that same year from the districts of Hadeland and Land that the infection came from the town of Hønefoss. In 1876 from Lom in Gudbrandsdal, it is stated that "The disease came to the district of Lom with a travelling salesman."

Regarding the severe diphtheria epidemic in the county of Hedemarken around 1890, District Physician Hans Lemmich Juell (1839–99) reported from Kongsvinger (Solør og Odalen district): "that the epidemic was brought here from Kristiania by various carriers throughout the whole year," and in 1890: "The disease came also this year from the neighboring Swedish parishes, where it has been stationary for years."

We notice in these instances that the infection comes to the interior from outside, and most often from the districts' natural trading and town centers.

The development of the transportation network must of course be significant for the spreading of diseases.

The extent of driveable roads increased by 50 percent from 1850 to 1880, mostly in the Eastern part of the country (Try 1979).

The railway system in the inlands was also developed during this period. The main railway to Eidsvoll was opened in 1854, to Lillestrøm-Kongsvinger in 1862, and to Hamar-Elverum in 1863, while the railway from the South to Hamar came in 1880. Lillehammer got a railway as late as 1894, and Gudbrandsdalen some time later.

The improved communications network in the southern part of the counties probably to some extent accounts for the higher occurrence of diseases in Hedemarken. One should bear in mind, however, that, up until our century, contact between people took place first and foremost from hamlet to hamlet by the old roads that had been used for many centuries.

Both Hedemarken and the northern part of Gudbrandsdal have always been in the center of the public traffic system. The districts lie along the main road joining north and south, but also at the east-west crossing. Northern Gudbrandsdal has always been dependent on the supply of commodities and the sales of their own products, and the traffic did not only go north-south but they are also to a large extent to the coast, first and foremost to Bergen, but also to Romsdal (Steen 1942). For business reasons, the inhabitants of Gudbrandsdal were more mobile which is of importance to the spread of infection than the inhabitants of Hedemarken, who had a more secure economic basis, both as tradesmen and as laborers searching for work.

In general, increased mobility and

improved communications during the last part of the 1800s has undoubtedly had an influence on that period's increased epidemics. These circumstances, however, do not document the differences in morbidity between Hedemarken and the northern part of Gudbrandsdal.

9.7.9. Conclusion

There were obvious social differences between the working classes in Hedemarken and in Northern Gudbrandsdal. Class distinctions were more prevalent in Hedemarken, the society was less egalitarian, and there were more people in the lowest social ranks. The cottars in Hedemarken had less freedom and were at the same time bound by contracts over longer periods.

These conditions constituted a psychosocial risk factor, and could have contributed to the higher frequency of epidemics in Hedemarken.

We have also reason to believe that the more varied nutritional basis and diet in Gudbrandsdal, as well as the denser working conditions and structure of settlements in Hedemarken could have been additional factors.

The improved transport conditions during that period have probably had some significance on the increase in frequency of infectious diseases, but it is uncertain whether this has played any particular role in the differences in incidence between Hedemarken and the northern part of Gudbrandsdal.

So, it is probably not wrong to come to the same conclusion drawn by Eilert Sundt, who said that the differences were partly to be found in the way "in which the cottars' and all other working people's lives, are organized."

9.7.10 Epilogue

This attempt by a physician in social medicine to make a comparative analysis of these two districts, based on a disparity in the incidence of diseases, has resulted in the demonstration of a problem. A more thorough investigation of the frequency, mortality, and lethality requires better statistical material. Among other things, it is necessary to have information pertaining to age, sex, and social status.

The analysis also raises the question of cultural and constitutional differences between the two populations. Another complex problem could be the effect of the environment on adolescence and on the subsequent disposition to disease.

It is therefore recommended that further interdisciplinary research be carried out, a cooperative effort between, among others, researchers from the fields of ethnology, anthropology, history, sociology, and medicine. This would give a better basis for a closer look into this fascinating interaction between environment and disease, so clearly described by the old district physicians in their medical reports.

References

Beitrusten, G. *Husmannsvesenet under avvikling.* Hovedoppgave i historie. Oslo: Universitetet i Oslo, 1976.

Beretning om Rigets økonomiske Tilstand 1861–65. Christiania: Departementet for det Indre, 1867–68. (*Report on the Economic State of the Country*. Christiania: Departement of the Interior, 1867–68.

Einbu, S. and O. Skotte *Lesja. Litt frå den kommunale soga 1838-1938*. Lesja: Lesja kommune, 1949.

Engelsen, R. "Mortalitetsdebatten og sosiale skilnader i mortalitet", *Historisk Tidsskrift*. (1987), 161–202.

Gaustad, I. *Arbeiderklassen på Hedemarken 1850–1900.* Hovedfagsoppgave i historie. Oslo: Universitetet i Oslo, 1935.

Helland, A. *Topografisk-Statistisk Beskrivelse af Hedemarkens Amt. Bind 1*. Kristiania: Aschehoug, 1902.

Holst, A. "Om arbeiderhygienen i England", *Tidsskrift Den norske lægeforening*. 6(1892):225–240.

Hovdhaugen, E. *Husmannstida*. Oslo: Det Norske Samlaget, 1976.

Jervell, A., K. Meyer and K. Westlund. "Coronary heart disease and serum cholesterol in males in different parts of Norway", *Acta Med Scand* 177(1965):177: 13–23.

Kjelland, A. *Bygdebok for Lesja. Bind 1&2*. Lesja: Lesja kommune, 1987 and 1992.

Larsen, C.F. "Hvorfor tiltager Utbredningen af Lungetuberkulose i Norge?", *Norsk Magazin for Lægevitenskaben* (1889):4 :229–263.

Larsen, Ø., N. Haugtomt and W. Platou. *Sykdomsoppfatning og epidemiologi 1860–1900. Epidemiske sykdommer i Norge og helsemyndighetenes vurdering av folkehelsen – presentasjon av data*. Oslo: Seksjon for medisinsk historie. Universitetet i Oslo, 1980.

McKeown, T. *The role of medicine: Dean, Mirage or Nemesis*. London: The Nuffield Provincial Hospitals Trust, 1976.

Skappel, S. *Hedemarkens Amt 1814–1914*. Kristiania: Grøndahl & Søn, 1914.

SSB. *Historisk statistikk 1968/Historical Statistics 1968*. Oslo: Central Bureau of Statistics, 1969.

Steen, S. *Ferd og fest*. Oslo: Aschehoug, 1942.

Stortingsmelding nr. 37(1992–1993). Utfordringer i helsefremmende og forebyggende arbeide. (Parliamentary Report no. 37 (1992–1993) on Challenges in Health Promotion and Preventive Medicine.) Oslo: Ministry of Health & Social Affairs, 1992.

Sundt, E. *Om dødeligheten i Norge*. Oslo: Gyldendal, 1975.

Thorleifsen, M. *Husmannskår i Gålåskroken og Vang ca. 1780–1903. Magistergradsavhandling i etnologi*. Oslo: Universitetet i Oslo, 1991.

Tranberg, A. "Korn og klasseskille", in: *Bind 3. Bygdebok for Brøttum,Ringsaker & Veldre.* Moelv: Brøttum, Ringsaker & Veldre historielag, 1993.

Try, H. "Yrkesstruktur og sosial struktur", *Norges historie Bind 11*. Oslo: Cappelen, 1979.

Vinje, Aa. *Ferdaminne frå sumaren 1860*. Oslo: Gyldendal, 1967.

Ødegaard, N. *Kristians Amt 1814–1914*. Kristiania: Grøndahl & Søn, 1918.

C H A P T E R 9 . 8

The City of Kristiania and the Counties of Akershus and Smaalenene, 1868–1900

ARILD HAGESVEEN

9.8.1. Kristiania

As the old city of Oslo burned down in 1624, king Christian IV (1577–1648, king of Denmark and Norway 1588–1648) ordered it rebuilt a few miles further west, in the protective shadow of Akershus fortress, and gave orders securing a modern outline of the streets and regulations for the planning of new houses. He gave his name to the new city; thus Oslo was renamed Christiania in 1624. The spelling of this name was altered to Kristiania in 1877. However, in 1924, the original name of Oslo was taken up again.

According to the medical reports, 63,504 people, 3.7 percent of the total population of Norway, lived in Christiania in 1868. However, the population increased markedly in subsequent years, so that by 1900 it had risen to 227,735, which represented 10.2 percent of the total population (Diagram 9.45). Excess of births that is, live births minus deaths per 1,000 inhabitants increased from 14.6 in the period 1868–1872 to 18.9 in the period 1896–1900.

Apart from an increased birth rate and a reduced mortality, the population of Kristiania increased during the second half of the nineteenth century because of the large number of people who moved from the countryside into the town. For people in the countryside, times were hard. As described elsewhere in this book, population pressure led to a migration into the cities which was caused by a series of push and pull factors. Moving to towns, particularly Kristiania, seemed often to be the best solution when problems mounted. The city attracted people because of its workplaces within the metal, machine and timber industries, and in the rapidly expanding textile industry. New service professions also provided employment possibilities.

But what kind of life awaited people in Kristiania? The shortage of housing was acute. New housing areas had to be found, because the inner city was already overcrowded, and the traditional middle-class areas were too expensive. New housing areas for workers were established outside the city border. In 1860, it was reported that the houses in these areas were separated by streets of mud. Drinking water had to be fetched from a long way off, and sewage ran in the streets. Whole families lived in one or two rooms and many houses had fewer beds than inhabitants (Bull 1976). The construction of blocks of flats built of brick increased from the 1870s on. Although this was a step in the right direction, conditions were still overcrowded. Up to five people might live in one room, a situation which was conducive to the spread of air-borne infections. Many of these blocks had poor sanitary arrangements and gastro-enteritis flourished. High rents were also a problem; the consequence was that people did not have enough money for food and heating.

9.8.2. Akershus

According to the population census 31/12–1865, the county of Akershus at that time had a population of 107,422, which represented 6.3 percent of the total population of Norway. The population increased only slightly in subsequent years, so that by 1900 there were 111,300 people in the county, 5.0 percent of the total population (Diagram 9.45). The excess of birth was 13.8 in the period 1896–1900.

Akershus was divided into four health districts, which covered most of the population of the county: Aker district (34.7 percent of the population), Ullensaker district (34.1 percent), Høland district (14.4 percent) and Follo district (17.8 percent).

The county consisted of typical rural districts, but also had some small cities: Drøbak, Son, and Hølen. In 1865, 97.4 percent of the inhabitants lived in the countryside. Sixty-seven percent of the population earned their living from farming, about 21 percent from industry, and 6 percent from sea-faring and trade (Kjær 1921). However, 37 percent of the population in the towns earned a living from sea-faring and fishing.

One explanation for the low population growth in Akershus was that a large number of people moved to Kristiania. However, the competition for work was vigorous, and people who had neither professional training nor contacts in the city fared badly (Myhre 1990). In addition, a large number of people emigrated to America. Between 1866 and 1915, 29,645 persons emigrated from the county of Akershus.

DIAGRAM 9.45
Population 1868–1900

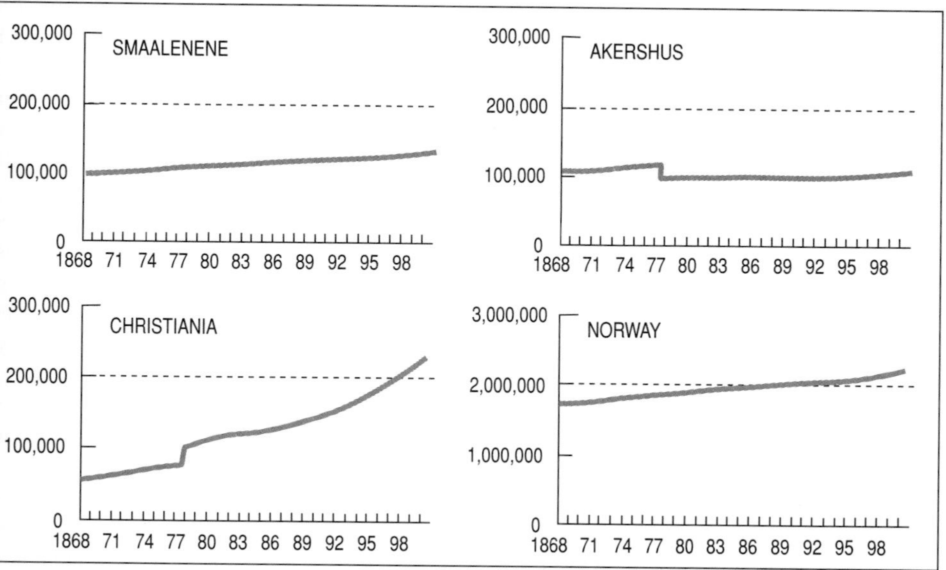

9.8.3. Smaalenene

According to the medical report for 1868, 101,569 people lived in the county of Smaalenene that year, that is, 5.9 percent of the total population of Norway. The population increased to 133,100 by the year 1900, representing 6.0 percent of the total population (Diagram 9.45). The birth rate increased from 12.8 in the period 1868-1872 to 16.7 in the period 1896-1900.

Smaalenene was divided into five health districts: Eidsberg district (25.6 percent of the population), Moss district (19.3 percent), Sarpsborg district (32.2 percent), Hvaløerne district (13.6 percent), and Fredrikshald town district (9.3 percent).

The county of Smaalenene was an agricultural county with a growing element of working-class people from the factories in the towns of Sarpsborg, Fredrikstad, Fredrikshald (Halden from 1927 on) and Moss. The factories were mainly sawmills along the rivers Glomma and Halden. The county gradually became more and more industrialized during the second half of the nineteenth century. As more and more factories sprang up along the rivers, the towns expanded and new towns and rural districts became industrialized (Medical report 1899).

Expansion was particularly marked when the industries began to produce for export. Certain waterpowered timber mills had cut timber for sale abroad for a long time, but when the timber mill privileges were repealed in 1860, the process of industrialization speeded up. Having timber mill privileges meant that one had exclusive rights to cut timber for export. Timber mills that did not have these privileges were allowed to cut timber only for the needs of the local rural district. Production of wood pulp and cellulose, which was also based on export, developed rapidly at about the same time as the timber mills, in the 1860s and 1870s. These

Diagram 9.46

Incidence of epidemic diseases in the city of Christiania and the counties of Akershus and Smaalenene 1868–1900

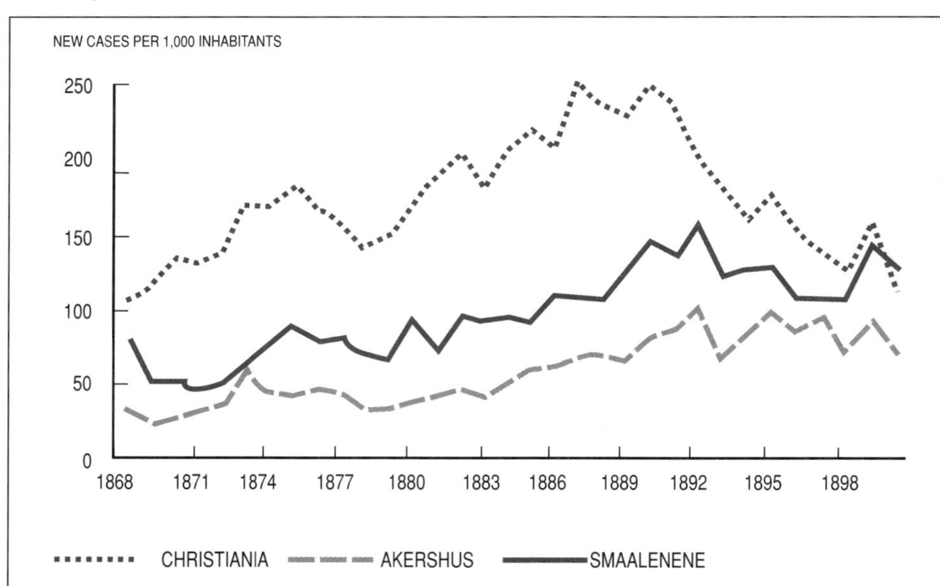

DIAGRAM 9.47
Lethality of epidemic diseases in the city of Christiania and the counties of Akershus and Smaalenene 1868–1900

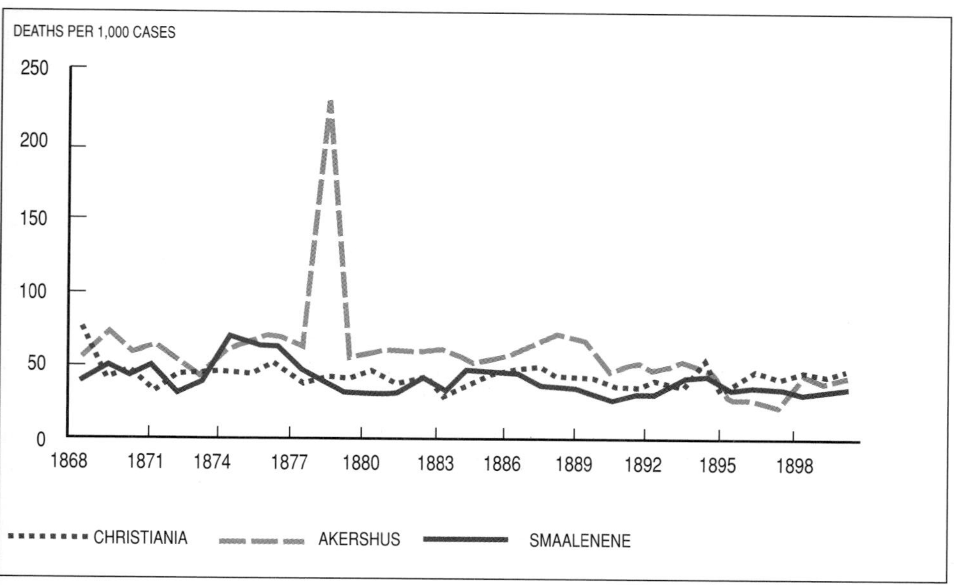

DIAGRAM 9.48
Incidence of typhoid fever in the city of Christiania and the counties of Akershus and Smaalenene 1868–1900

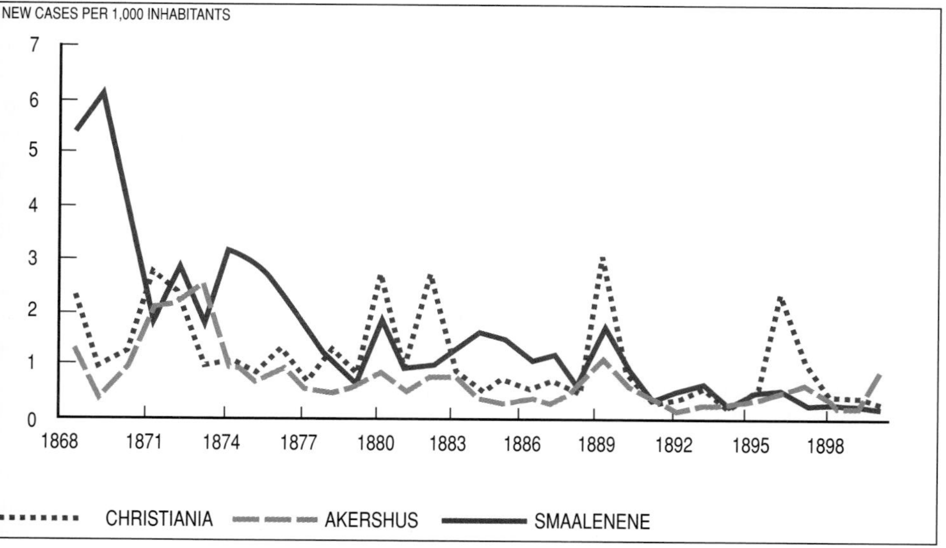

TABLE 9.7
The most common epidemic diseases in the city of Kristiania and the counties of Akershus and Smaalenene in the period 1886–1890

	Percent
Kristiania:	
Acute respiratory catarrh and bronchitis	37
Diarrhea and cholera	21
Catarrhal and follicular angina	14
Epidemics of diphtheria, measles, scarlet fever and whooping cough were also common.	
Akershus:	
Acute respiratory catarrh and bronchitis	26
Diarrhea and cholera	17
Catarrhal and follicular angina	11
Scarlet fever	9
Smaalenene:	
Acute respiratory catarrh and bronchitis	32
Diarrhea and cholera	15
Catarrhal and follicular angina	12
Measles	9
Diphtheria	5
Scarlet fever	5

new industries grew up at the mouths of the rivers, where it was easiest to obtain timber. At the mouth of the Glomma, in Fredrikstad and the neighboring districts, the population doubled from 1860 to 1870 as a result of this industrialization (Bull 1976). A significant number of workers came from Sweden, in addition to farm laborers from the farming districts in Smaalenene (Myhre 1990).

9.8.4. Epidemic Diseases

Diagram 9.46 shows that the incidence of epidemic diseases in Kristiania increased up to around 1890, and then showed a fairly rapid decline up until 1900. The incidence of epidemic diseases in the counties of Akershus and Smaalenene was lower than in Kristiania, and increased only slowly during the whole period. The death rate from these diseases (Diagram 9.47) was relatively stable and varied little between the three areas. However, figures must also here be interpreted with caution, since improved registration of epidemic diseases and an increasing number of people who sought help from a doctor towards the end of the century could have caused an apparent increase in incidence, which in turn would produce an apparent fall in cause-specific mortality.

From the medical reports for the five-year period 1886-1890, the epidemic diseases shown in Table 9.7 were the most common causes of illness.

9.8.5. Typhoid Fever

Diagram 9.48 shows that the incidence of typhoid fever shows a clear epidemic pattern. However, the incidence fell somewhat

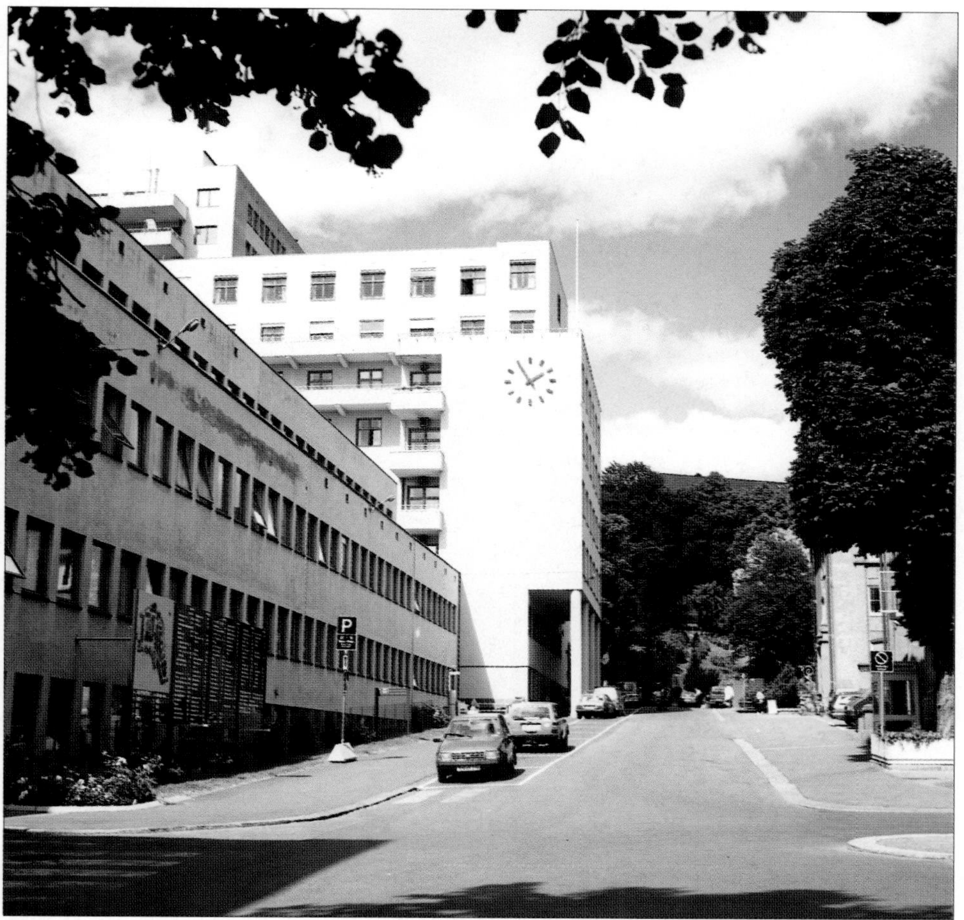

Figure 24: The National Hospital (Rikshospitalet) has been located in the city center of Oslo since 1883, and has in many ways been the central point of Norwegian medicine up to now (Photo: Øivind Larsen 1996).

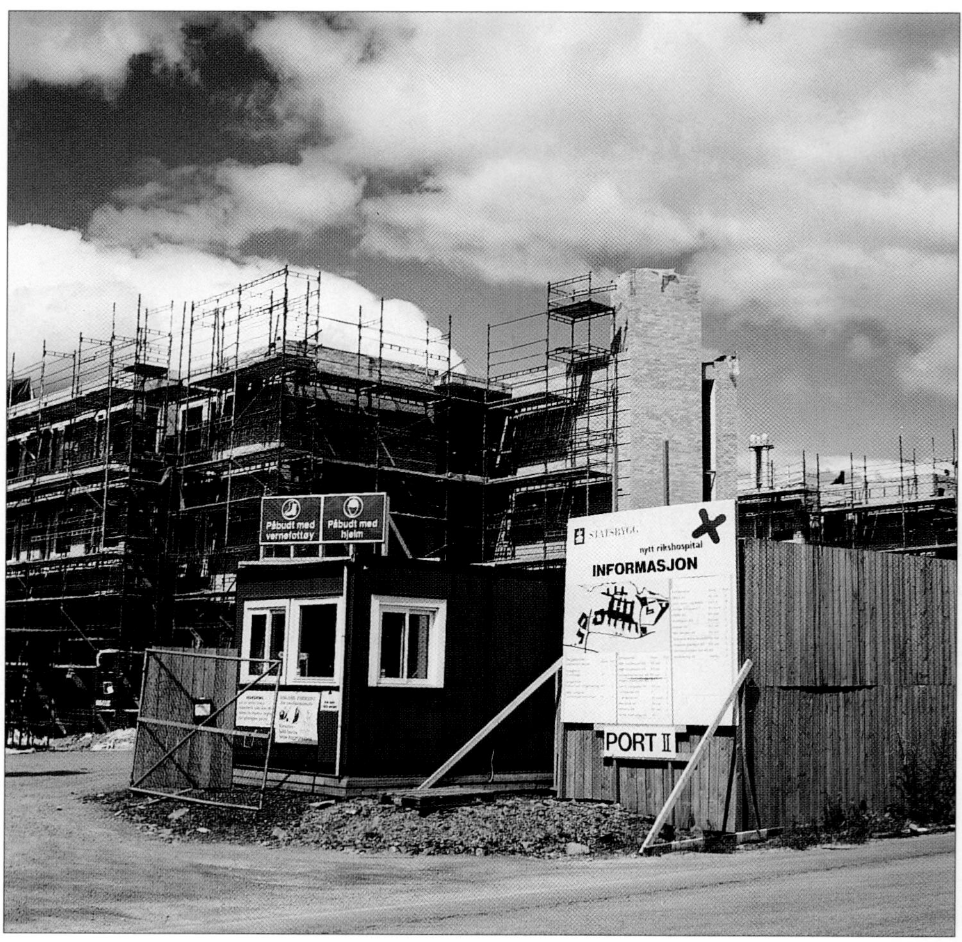

Figure 25: As of 1996, a new National Hospital is under construction just opposite the Gaustad psychiatric hospital in Oslo, and as can be seen through the scaffolding and from the information poster, the wings of the new buildings will match the old ones. When completed, the Gaustad area will become a new center in Norwegian medicine, as several University institutes already are on the site (Photo: Øivind Larsen 1996).

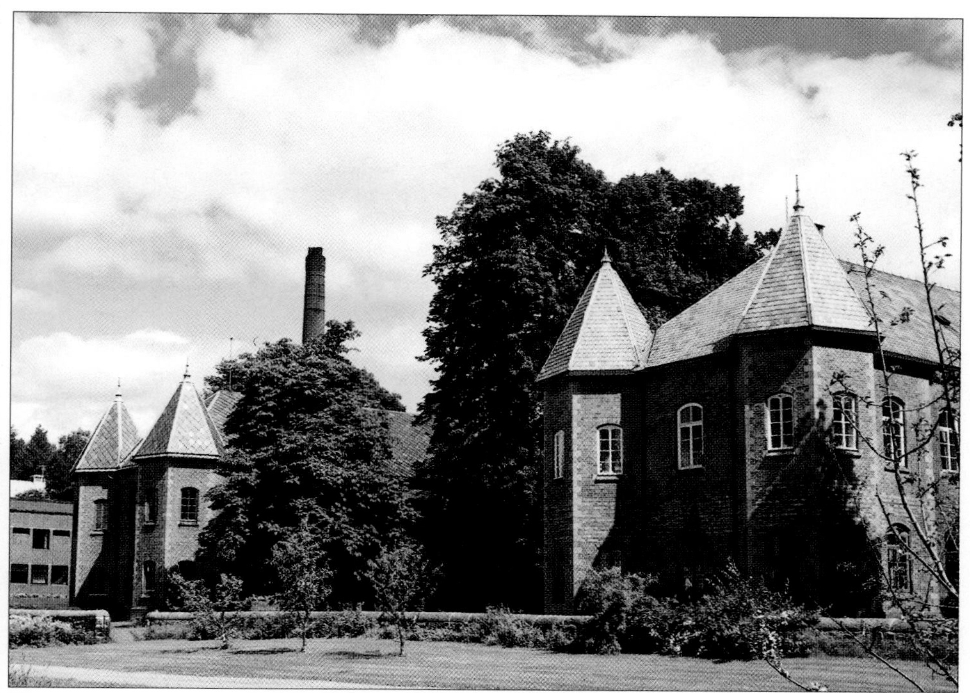

Figure 26: Gaustad, the psychiatric hospital on the outskirts of Oslo, had an advanced architecture when it was opened as the first state asylum in Norway in 1855 (Photo: Øivind Larsen 1996).

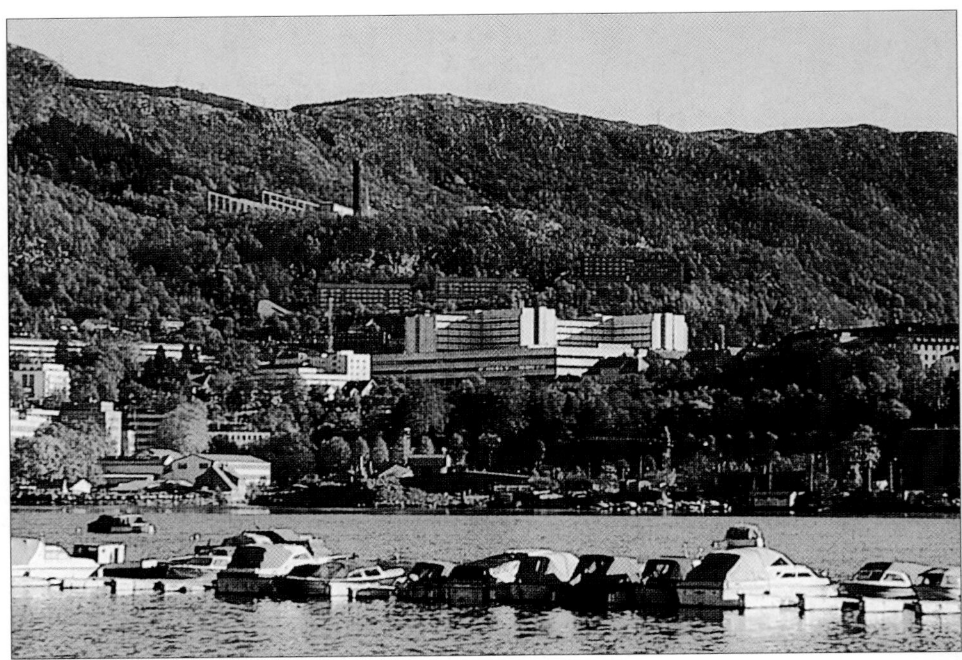

Figure 27: Most of the clinical and scientific medical activity in the city of Bergen on the Norwegian West Coast takes place in the Haukeland region. Around the old hospital that dates from 1912 a large, modern building complex with wards, laboratories, and institutes has been built over the years. This picture shows the situation as it was in the 1980s (Photo: Øivind Larsen).

DIAGRAM 9.49
Incidence of diphtheria in the city of Christiania and the counties of Akershus and Smaalenene 1868–1900

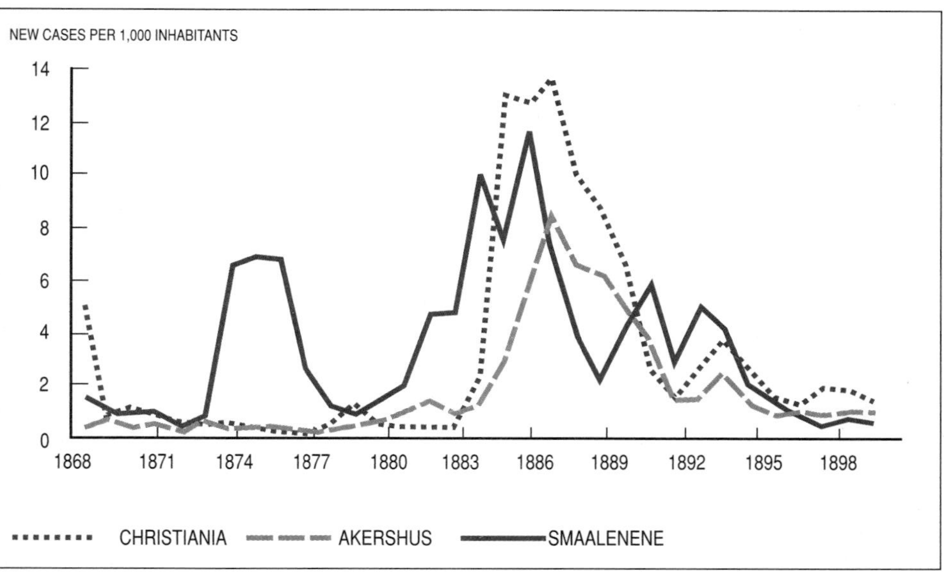

towards the turn of the century, and the epidemics became less frequent. Generally, the epidemics were more serious in Kristiania, an overcrowded city with poor sewerage, than in the counties of Akershus and Smaalenene.

9.8.6. Diphtheria

Diagram 9.49 shows that the incidence of diphtheria reached a peak around 1868 and 1886–1890, the last peak reaching as many as 13 cases per 1,000 in Kristiania. The most important epidemics in Smaalenene occurred in 1874–76 and 1884–86. During the major epidemic in Akershus from 1885–92, there were accounts in the medical reports of whole farms that were affected and had to be isolated. In most cases, the infection could be traced back to Kristiania and Drammen. Before the great epidemic at the end of the 1880s, the incidence of diphtheria in Kristiania was actually lower than in the county of Smaalenene. The death rate from diphtheria was high, particularly in the last great epidemic, when about one in four among those affected died. In the medical report for Smaalenene, it is reported that most deaths occurred among children under six years of age. Both the incidence and the health rate fell markedly in all three areas after the great epidemic and up to the end of the century. It is stated in the medical reports that there were no seasonal variations in incidence.

9.8.7. Cholera Nostras, Acute Diarrhea

This group of diseases includes a range of diseases that cause diarrhea. True Asiatic cholera was probably observed for the last time in Kristiania in 1853 (Knarberg Hansen 1985), when the incidence was 50 per 1,000 and the lethality was 651 per 1,000 cases (Holst 1954). "Cholera nostras" was the name given to mild cholera-type diseases, but as doctors could not always distinguish between various gastro-intestinal

DIAGRAM 9.50
Incidence of cholera and acute diarrhea in the city of Christiania and the counties of Akershus and Smaalenene 1868–1900

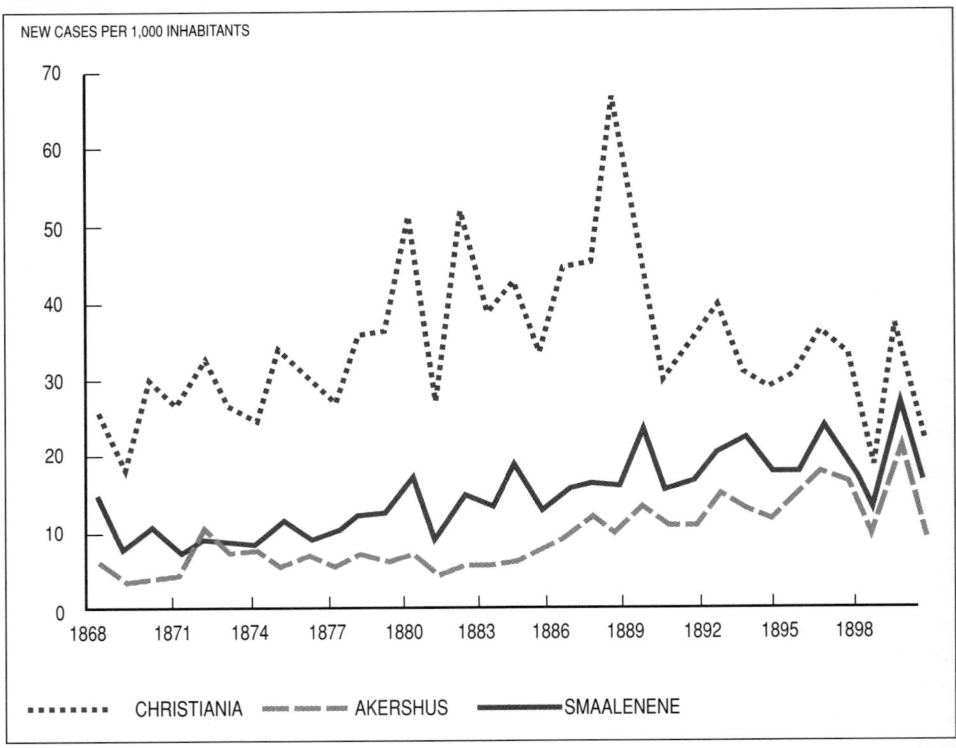

diseases, the different types are grouped together.

Diagram 9.50 shows large fluctuations in incidence, though the incidence was relatively high throughout the whole period, with a peak in Kristiania of 67 per 1,000 inhabitants in 1888. The incidence was much higher in Kristiania than in the counties of Akershus and Smaalenene, perhaps because this group of diseases, more than many others, was associated with overcrowding and poor hygiene. The epidemics in Kristiania were more widespread, because many people used the same source of drinking water. Control of these sources was often very poor. In some cases, sewage and dirty water could come in direct contact with drinking water (Holst 1954). The incidence of cholera nostras, the acute diarrhea, increased in Akershus and Smaalenene during the whole period, whereas the incidence in Kristiania increased up to 1888 and then fell until the end of the century. However, we must also assume that many cases were never reported, since diarrhea was so common at that time.

The lethality rate for this group of diseases was high for the reported cases, and showed an increase up to the turn of the century, when as many as 65 people per 1,000 cases died in Kristiania, which was a higher rate than for Akershus and Smaalenene. It is stated in the medical reports that the incidence was higher in the summer months and that all age groups were affected. However, it was particularly children who died of these diseases, since children are particularly vulnerable to dehydration.

9.8.8. Venereal Diseases in Kristiania

There were few deaths from venereal diseases, and people who did die from this cause were mainly children who had congenital syphilis. However, much time and money were spent on fighting the diseases in this group. For example, many prostitutes were frequently compelled to visit the police doctor. If they were infected with venereal disease, they were admitted for compulsory treatment. If they were healthy, they received a written certificate that they could show their customers (Emblem et al., 1983).

In 1878, 4,696 such compulsory visits were made by 53 prostitutes from brothels, and 2,149 compulsory visits by 27 independent prostitutes. In addition, 2,805 visits were made by women who did not have prostitution as their only occupation. Altogether, these visits revealed 508 new cases of diseases, one case for every 19 visits (Medical report 1878).

The authorities believed that this was the way to deal with venereal diseases, rather than to enforce the ban on prostitution in the Criminal Act of 1842. They were afraid to interfere with men's sexual needs. The Director of Medicine stated that measures to prevent prostitution could be compared to blocking a sewage pipe. The stinking contents would find other ways of escape through a series of unavoidable leaks, and thus infect the surroundings (Emblem et al., 1983).

In 1878, 1,546 cases of venereal diseases were detected (Medical Report 1878), giving an incidence of 14.7 per 1,000 inhabitants per year. The number of cases had risen to 3,297 in 1900, an incidence of 14.6 (Medical Report 1900). Most cases were reported among men (65–80 percent). In 1888, the responsibility for control of venereal diseases was transferred from the authorities through the police to the Board of Health (Medical Report 1888). The discontinuation of public control may be one explanation for the increase in the incidence of venereal diseases up to the turn of the century. Perhaps the frequent, humiliating visits to the police doctor, often with subsequent compulsory admission to the hospital, had had an effect. But the apparent increase may also be partly explained by better registration and diagnosis after control was transferred to doctors under the Health Commission.

9.8.9. Alcohol

Alcohol is mentioned specifically in the Medical Report for Akershus in 1877. It is stated that use of beer and spirits had not decreased during the previous years, despite the fact that the municipal administrators had done everything they could to prevent the situation from deteriorating. We can read about the result of their work in the Medical Report for 1886. It was reported that people who had become fat, and had huge bellies from drinking alcohol, had again become thin around the waist. The reason for this was that there was no longer any alcohol to drink. The authorities had limited the availability of alcohol by closing most of the places where alcohol was sold.

9.8.10. Other Factors that Affected Health

Many other factors that affected the health of the population were mentioned in the Medical Reports.

Nutrition was an important factor. In the Medical Report for Akershus for 1890, we can read that people used bread from the towns and the village bakeries. They drank too much coffee, particularly the adults, who drank large quantities. This pattern was evident among the poor families, who couldn't afford the change to a more nourishing food combination. The children became pale, were anaemic, and complained of cardialgia and other digestive problems.

The weather is also given special attention in the Medical Reports for Akershus and Kristiania. The average temperature for each month and the amount of rain were important factors that affected the quality and quantity of the harvest, which in turn affected food production and nutrition, which had a great deal of bearing on health.

People were aware that the environment could be damaging to health. In the Medical Report for 1879 for Akershus, the conditions around the Iron Works in Bærum are described as very dangerous to health, due to the sooty and dusty smoke from the factory, and the bad odor from the cow sheds and the out-houses. In addition, it is mentioned that the high hills around the factory cut out much of the sunshine and light.

The moral standards of the time, or lack of moral standards, are described as detrimental. In the Medical Report for Akershus for 1879, we can read that night wandering flourishes; it was common that girls left their windows open so that the boys could pay them a visit during the night. Many children were born outside permanent relationships, and in many cases it was difficult to determine who the father of the child was. As another explanation for this uncertain parentage, it was said to be that servants of both sexes slept in the same bedroom, so that sexual relationships could take place freely and uncontrolled. The youth from the neighborhood also often gathered in those bedrooms on Saturday and Sunday evenings.

Other factors that are mentioned in the Medical Reports are hygienic standards, water supply, sewerage, housing conditions, and economic conditions. However, these generally improved towards the turn of the century.

9.8.11. Causes of Death

Diagram 9.51 demonstrates that the death

Diagram 9.51

Mortality in the city of Christiania and the counties of Akershus and Smaalenene 1868–1900

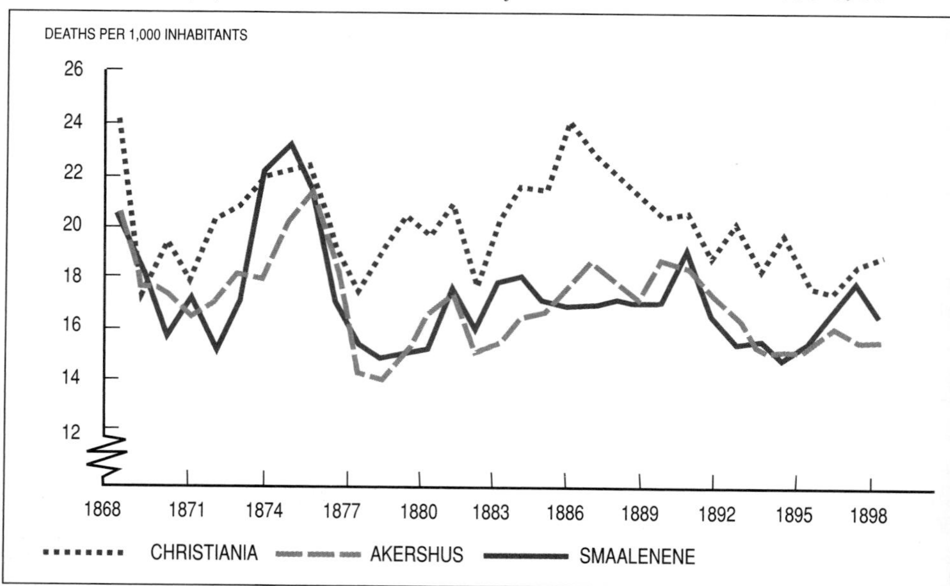

rate in the three areas shows much variation, often associated with major epidemics.

An overview in the Medical Reports for 1868–1872 shows that common causes of death in Kristiania were tuberculosis, acute and chronic bronchitis, meningitis (both viral and tuberculoid), and diarrhea and cholera. Cancer was a minor cause of death. These were still important causes of death at the turn of the century, but cancers accounted for a slightly higher proportion of deaths.

Important causes of death mentioned in the Medical Reports for both Akershus and Smaalenene include tuberculosis, pneumonia, scarlet fever, typhoid fever, and meningitis.

References

Bull, E. *Nordmenn før oss*. Oslo: Tanum Norli, 1976.

Emblem, T, T. Syvertsen and Ø. Stenersen. *Cappelens historieverk*. Oslo: Cappelens Forlag, 1983.

Hansen, L.I.K. *Koleraen i Christiania i 1853*. Oslo: Seksjon for medisinsk historie, Universitetet i Oslo, 1985.

Holst, PM. *Våre akutte sykdommers epidemiologi og klinikk*. Oslo: Aschehoug, 1954.

Kjær, A-Th. *Akershus amt 1814-1914*. Christiania: Steenske boktrykkeri Johannes Bjørnstad, 1921.

Myhre, JE. *Oslo bys historie, bind 3*. Oslo: 1990.

CHAPTER 9.9

Diseases, Geography, and the Medical Profession

ØIVIND LARSEN

Do our studies of the development in health conditions and of the changes in the social situation of the Norwegian population in the latter half of the nineteenth century, tell us anything of interest pertaining to the shaping of the medical profession?

The main sources for our considerations are the annual reports submitted by the district physicians. Of course they pose some questions as to their reliability as historical sources about the medical profession. The reports are written by members of the profession, so they are not by any means independent sources. On the other hand, this assures the medical competence which is required to be able to assess the health situation.

The reports which have been used in most cases for our studies are the printed ones that were compiled at the county level. We have argued that a possible bias caused by this fact should be only diminutive if the evaluations which we aim at also mostly refer to an agglomerate level.

A certain bias may also exist because the reports usually concentrate on what was bad and wrong. But, for the general history of Norway, other sources are at hand; writing a comprehensive annual survey of what had been going on in the communities was not the purpose of the district physicians' reports. And the given format of course gave a framework for the writing that could be regarded as a constraint; but seen from another perspective, it was a guarantee against omissions.

A key point, also mentioned and discussed by several of our authors, is the impact of an eventual under-registration of disease: that the figures for the incidence of diseases might be too low in periods. This would, among other things, influence the calculations of lethality and also of the health concern index. But some diseases increase and others decrease during the period (Diagram 9.52), making it unlikely that a failure in the sources is universal. If one assumes that the doctors' coverage increased over time, and that the registration gradually becomes more complete, at least for a shorter period, especially at the end of the century, this error should be negligible. And the data should allow for geographical comparisons at given points in time, without any problems (Diagram 9.53).

It is therefore assumed that a possible registration bias does not disturb the reasoning, if due caution is exercised in making

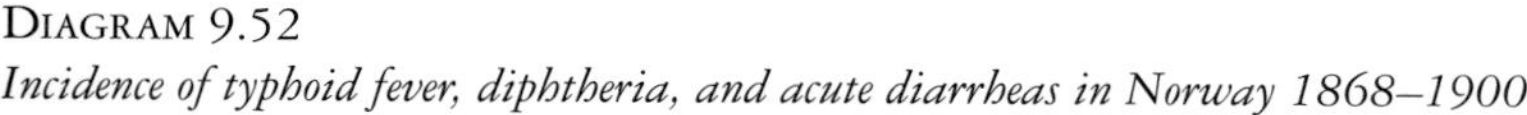

DIAGRAM 9.52
Incidence of typhoid fever, diphtheria, and acute diarrheas in Norway 1868–1900

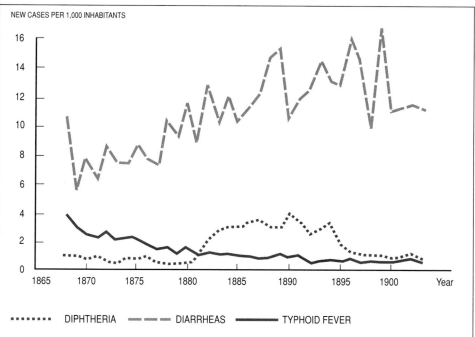

the considerations, if conclusions are drawn only on a long-term scale, and if the indications are interpreted as trends.

As sources to Norwegian medical history, the district physicians' reports concentrate on health problems as they were experienced in primary health care. Achievements in hospital medicine, for example in the surgical departments, do not appear clearly. On the other hand, at this time primary care medicine was the quantitatively most important; as described, the number of hospital doctors was still low. But the reports contain a large variety of information, as pointed out by our various authors, who have approached the reports from different angles and have used them for different purposes.

How does the picture of the health situation of Norway emerge from the information that can be extracted from the reports? It seems quite clear that the general standards of living, except for those of a few wealthy people, were austere and low. Poverty was common; sometimes life touched on the limits of subsistence. Hygienic conditions were simple and poor, often not because of lack of knowledge, but because of lack of resources to do something about them. On the other hand, it has to be remembered that a rather low hygienic standard, tolerated by a small and stable population living on scattered farms, did not necessarily lead to disease; problems with infections arose only when this relative stability was disturbed, or when an infection entered from outside. Standards tolerable in the countryside were unacceptable when transferred to the growing cities. That means that the motivation for accepting changes in the name of hygiene was not necessarily very strong.

Diagram 9.52 illustrates the course of three important diseases. Typhoid fever diminished in incidence, mainly because of social changes and improved hygiene. Diphtheria took its toll on an unprotected population. It easily infected mainly children in crowded urban dwellings, and possibly spread rapidly because it was an especially virulent form of the bacteria. But the acute diarrheas – often called the domestic cholera, cholera nostra – increased in incidence. For this less dangerous disease, a certain underregistration might have occurred, but nevertheless an increase is what could be expected when mobility increases. Diagram 9.53 clearly indicates the connection between migration and infections; the pattern of incidence for acute diarrheas matches the pattern for demographic activity.

Social modernization, however, did take place. The tight connection between living conditions and health was clearly observed, and an inprovement of the living standards obviously had an important influence on the progress in health. Urbanization was an ambiguous process, as far as health was concerned, but it is important to keep in mind that much of the economic progress that formed a base for the improvement of standards originated in the new cities.

The rural districts also changed. During the latter half of the nineteenth century, the traditional cottar system began to be phased out. In 1885, 65,060 cottars were registered in Norway; in 1910 there were only 19,763 left. New opportunities that promised a bright future tempted many people to move to the cities, and letters from the United

Diagram 9.53
Incidence of acute diarrheas in cases per 1,000 inhabitants in 1882 (Larsen 1991).

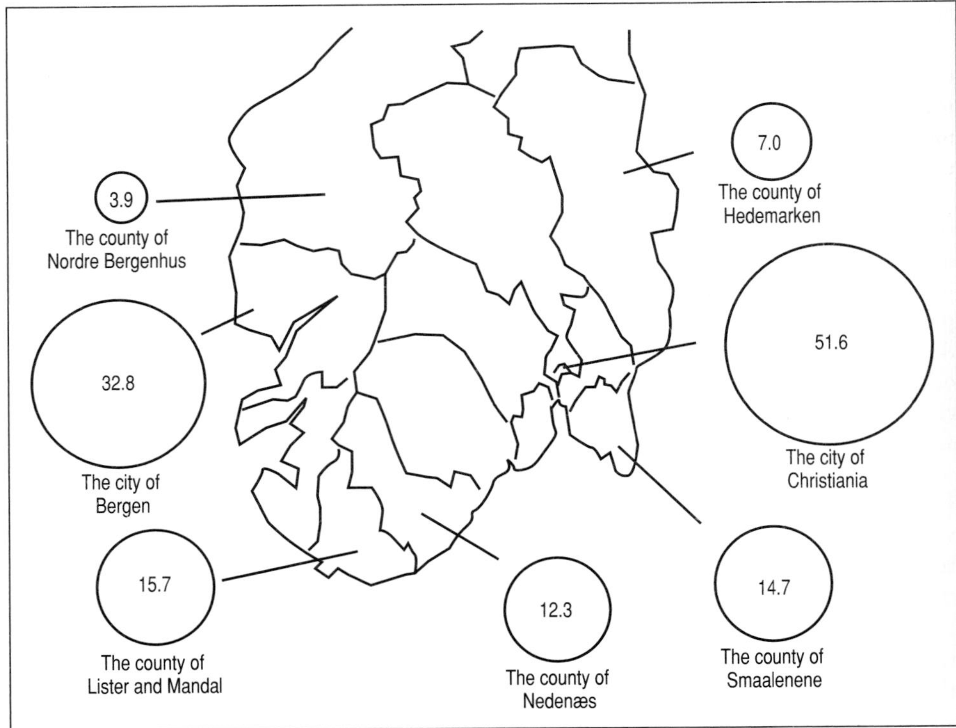

described how prosperity could be attained overseas. The impressive waves of internal migration and of emigration document the importance of this process. But new techniques in agriculture also had diminished the need for manpower. Such social changes also influenced the health situation, and altered the soil in which infections took root.

In some places in Norway, for example in Western Norway, farming was hampered by a very inpractical subdivision of fields, which had taken place over a long time (Skre 1991). The farmhouses were clustered in a very densely populated small village, and small fields with different ownerships or with different types of access for the individual farmers were distributed over a large area. A sort of severance system had been established to clear this up, in order to establish individual farms. The hygienic advantages that occurred, when crowded villages were split up were obvious.

The last decades of the nineteenth century were years of scientific achievements in international medicine. But medical treatment of the common diseases did not change as dramatically. Thus, important years of shaping of the new Norwegian medical profession occurred during a phase when hygiene and public health measures were the most important on a nationwide scale. The concern about health was increasing, as also indicated here by means of the health concern index, and the doctors had to supply the population with information. The sanitary act of 1860, which entitled the doctors to take on a paternalistic role in health matters, without doubt played an important part not only in the practical work of medicine, but also in forming the general image of the doctor in society.

It might be concluded that this image of a doctor at the turn of the century included a large share of public responsibility and social consciousness. The reasons for this are given in the medical and social development which appears through the medical reports of the district physicians.

References

Larsen, Ø. "Vekst i byen og helse på landet." *Jord og Gjerning*, 5(1991):66-78.

Skre, B.G. "Garden Havrå på Osterøy." *Jord og Gjerning* ,5(1991):88-105.

CHAPTER 10

A Day in the Life of a Country Doctor – Occupational Hazards in General Practice in the Nineteenth Century

ELIN OLAUG ROSVOLD

10.1. "There are few who know how much danger Norwegian physicians are exposed to in the course of their daily excursions."

The above quotation is taken from the biography of Doctor Julius Anton Sand (1844–1916), and is reproduced in the second edition of *Norges Læger (The Physicians of Norway)* (Kiær 1888). In the same book, we also find the biography of his colleague, Dr. Johan Ludvig Møinichen (1838–1915), which gives us insight into the life of an ordinary physician during the second half of the nineteenth century. Møinichen was born in Trondheim in 1838, and graduated as a physician in Christiania in 1868. He was an intern for one year at "Fødselsstiftelsen" (The Childbirth Foundation) and in the main ward at Rikshospitalet (the National Hospital). During the same period he also functioned as a fishery physician in Lofoten in Northern Norway. In 1870, he became district physician in Lurøy in Northern Norway, and in 1876 he took over the post of district physician in Lærdal in Western Norway. He married in 1871. By 1886 he had fathered ten children, eight sons and two daughters, of whom one son was stillborn and another died at the age of one of pneumonia and convulsions associated with whooping cough.

In the biography in Norges Læger we can read the following:

> In February 1871, after several journeys to places where diphtheria was prevalent, he himself was infected with the disease, though no other members of the family became infected. In March 1872, his wife caught scarlet fever, probably from a patient who had visited the physician. In the spring of 1877, he probably had scarlet fever himself, without exanthema, but with subsequent oedema and long-lasting weakness. In the winter of 1877–1878, three of the children, and in the spring of 1886 at least three of the children, caught whooping cough. In July 1876, he pricked himself with a needle, while carrying out a post-mortem, and subsequently got lymphangitis in the wounded arm, and later, for a couple of months, recurrent abscesses, similar to carbuncles. In 1885, during a journey, he crushed his right leg between a stone and a sled, and fractured his fibula. In 1874, he had to send his family to Christiania for the winter, since his house in Lurøy was in a poor condition, and no other comfortable family accommodation could be obtained.

This quotation from *Norges Læger* is a good illustration of the life and practice of

Norwegian physicians in the second half of the nineteenth century. Their practice was characterized by a continuous battle against infectious diseases for which there was no effective treatment (Reichborn-Kjennerud et al. 1936), and the physician himself was in danger of being infected when he treated his patients. In addition, he often had responsibility for a large health district, which involved long, tiring, and sometimes dangerous journeys to visit the sick. The physician's family was also in danger of being infected because of his work, and they were not spared from losing a child in the first years of life. Despite the fact that physicians were senior government officials, the passage quoted above shows that the accommodations that they were offered in the districts could be quite wretched.

10.2. A Risky Profession?

Are Dr. Møinichen's experiences representative of the life of Norwegian physicians in the second half of the last century? It does not seem unlikely that the physician was exposed to infection, since he visited or was visited by infectious persons every day. The physician's home was often his office, and at times served as a hospital ward (Løken 1974), and some physicians had their living quarters in the same building as the hospital. These conditions made it possible for his wife and children to come in contact with the patients. On the other hand, there is reason to believe that the physician's knowledge about the danger of infection and about hygiene, in addition to the better living conditions which the physician's family had compared to those of most people (Holst 1955), led to less exposure to infection.

Based on data from the biographical work *Norges Læger*, this chapter will take a look more closely at the life and health of Norwegian physicians in the second half of the nineteenth century to find out what kind of diseases the physician and his family suffered from, whether the diseases were fatal, and whether the physicians or their families were exposed to infections that could be traced back to the physicians' profession.

10.3. Data Collection

Dr. Frantz Caspar Kiær (1835–1893) was the editor of the first two editions of *Norges Læger* (Kiær 1873 and 1888). He was interested in epidemiology and statistics, and among other things, he was concerned about whether physicians exposed themselves or their families to the risk of disease because of their profession. While he was collecting information for the second edition of the book, he sent an appeal to the physicians through *Norsk Magazin for Lægevidenskaben* (*the Norwegian Magazine for Medical Sciences*) (Kiær 1886). In addition to demographical information on marital status, children, employment and offices held, the physicians were asked to give information about the most important diseases from which either they or their families had suffered. Furthermore, they were requested to specify whether any of these diseases could be regarded as a consequence of the physician's profession. Kiær specified that he was particularly interested in exanthemic typhus, typhoid fever, smallpox, scarlet fever, diphtheria, Asiatic cholera, and dysentery, as well as infections caught while carrying out operations and post-mortems. He also wished to obtain information about dangers and accidents while traveling on duty. In regard to the wives, he was particularly concerned about puerperal fever.

Kiær received answers from 647 physicians. In addition, biographies on 629 more physicians are to be found in the book. The information in these biographies partly comes from the first edition of *Norges Læger* (Kiær 1873), and partly from information sent in by others. In the preface to *Norges Læger*, Kiær mentioned that he wished to work further with the material. Unfortunately, he died in 1893, before he managed to publish any results. However, all the information is to be found in print in the biographies of the individual physicians in *Norges Læger*.

For this study, biographies of physicians born between 1835 and 1854, included in the second edition of *Norges Læger*, were selected. This means that physicians who were born during this interval, but who had not yet finished their medical education when the book was published, are not included in this study. The material comprises 398 physicians, all men. For each physician, date of death (year and month), cause of death, place, post held, and age at the time of death were registered. The same information was collected for each episode of disease and for each accident in which the physician was involved. Corresponding information was collected for deaths and diseases of the physicians' wives and children.

In order to describe length of life and cause of death of physicians and their wives, information on year and cause of death was collected from later editions of *Norges Læger* (Kobro 1915 and 1944). A detailed description of the data collection has been published earlier, together with the main findings from the study (Rosvold and Larsen 1996).

10.4. The Material

The 398 physicians in the study were born between 1835 and 1854. Sixty percent of them were born in the second half of this period (Table 10.1). The physicians graduated between 1858 and 1884. They all qualified at the University of Christiania, with one exception, a Norwegian who graduated in Copenhagen. The physicians' mean age at graduation was 26.8 years; the youngest was

TABLE 10.1
Year of birth for the physicians in the study (n=398)

1835 – 1839	65	16,3%
1840 – 1844	93	23,4%
1845 – 1849	123	30,9%
1850 – 1854	117	29,4%
Total	398	100%

23, the oldest was 35. In 1889, the physicians had practiced for an average of 15.3 years, ranging from one to 31 years. Five physicians had ceased to practice by this time – two had become pharmacists, two were farmers, and one had become chief inspector in a prison. It is difficult to find out how long the physicians continued to practice after 1889, since for many of the physicians, the time of retirement is not stated.

The physicians were averaged 31.2 years of age when they married for the first time. Their first wives were, on average, seven years younger than they were (mean age 24.2 years of age). In other words, most of the physicians got married after they had completed their studies, when they were in a position to support a family. By the end of 1889, 83 percent (330) of the physicians were married. Fourteen percent (54) gave their marital status as single; while data are missing for four percent (14). Twenty-two physicians got married for the first time after 1889. Altogether 88 percent of the physicians got married. Forty-one physicians married twice, and two physicians were married three times.

By 1890, two-thirds of the physicians (267) reported being fathers. Five percent (20) said that they were childless. For the other 28 percent (111), data on the number of children is lacking, but 54 of these were single and 15 were married only a short time before the registration. In all, 1,133 children, born before 1890, were registered.

10.5. What Did the Physicians Die of in the Nineteenth Century?

Causes of death for Norwegian physicians born in the nineteenth century have previously been studied by Hjort (Hjort 1983). He analyzed the biographies of all physicians born between 1791 and 1860. This means that his analyses include the material which is described here. After having divided his material into three groups (physicians born in 1791–1820, 1821–1850, and 1851–1860) Hjort found that infectious diseases were the most important cause of death in the first group, while cancer and heart and circulatory diseases dominated in the second and third groups.

From Sweden, data is available on the cause of death for 92 Swedish district physicians between 1840 and 1879. In this group, infectious diseases were the most common causes of death, followed by heart and circulatory diseases (Nilsson and Persson 1995).

The distribution of the causes of death in different age groups in our material has been published previously (Rosvold and Larsen 1996). Sudden death by a disease accounted for the largest group of deaths, followed by chronic diseases, and infections. Heart and circulatory diseases were the most important causes of sudden death. One hundred nineteen (37 percent) of the 322 physicians with a diagnosis that could be categorized according to Hjort, died of heart and circulatory diseases (including those with apoplexy and heart infections such as pericarditis). Among physicians who died while they were still young (25–54 years of age), infectious diseases were the most important causes of death, while sudden death became more important in the older groups.

The average length of life for the whole study group was 65.0 years (median 68 years). The youngest physician who died was only 25 years old; the oldest lived to be 95. Forty-seven physicians died before 1890, while eight lived until the first half of the 1940s.

10.6. Death and Disease among the Physicians before 1890 – Infectious Diseases Dominated

In the following description of this material, only the deaths and diseases that occurred from the time when the physicians were students and up until the year 1890 will be discussed, since this is the period in which we have the most detailed knowledge. In 1890, the physicians were between 36 and 55 years old. Altogether, 189 physicians (47 percent) reported that they had been struck down by one or more diseases. Of these, 47 (12 percent of the 398 physicians in the total material) had died. Their mean age at death was 37.0 years (range: 25–50 years).

Altogether, we have information about 278 cases of disease. One-third of the 189 physicians who had been sick, had had two or more diseases. Table 10.2 shows that infections accounted for 85 percent of the diseases and 59 percent of the deaths. Many of the diseases shown in Table 10.2 are unusual today. Diphtheria was the most common of the airborne infections, with 41 cases of which two led to death. Smallpox came next with 12 cases, then scarlet fever with 11 cases and, among these, one death. We have information about six cases of tuberculosis, and all of these physicians died before 1890. Thus, during this period, tuberculosis was responsible for 14 percent of the 44 deaths for which we have an excact diagnosis.

Typhoid fever (nervefeber), which probably was caused by salmonella typhi and paratyphi, was the most important disease that was transmitted through water or food. As many as 45 cases are registered, of which five cases ended in death.

Another important water-borne infection was Asiatic cholera. However, the physicians in the study began to practice after the end of the large cholera epidemics (there were two smaller epidemics in Norway in 1866 and 1873) (Hansen 1985). Only one physician reported to have had cholera, and he

TABLE 10.2
Diseases among the physicians

(278 cases, of which 47 resulted in death)

	Cases	Deaths among the cases		Cases	Deaths among the cases
Air-borne infections 35%			Injuries and accidents 5%		
- diphtheria	41	2	- fracture	3	0
- smallpox	12	0	- contusion	3	0
- scarlet fever	11	1	- cut on the head	2	0
- tuberculosis	6	6	- rupture of a muscle	1	0
- pneumonia	6	2	- shot wound	2	1
- whooping cough	5	0	- violent haemorrhage after an accident	1	0
- measles	4	0	- drowning	2	2
- throat infections	4	0			
- bronchitis	2	0			
- rheumatic fever	2	0			
- influenza	1	0	Other diseases 10%		
- lung abscess	1	0	- kidney disease	5	4
- common cold	1	0	- cancer	2	2
			- gall stones	2	1
Food and water-borne infections 19%			- liver disease	1	1
- typhoid fever	45	5	- pancreatitis	1	1
- dysentery/diarrhea	6	0	- encephalitis	1	1
- cholera	1	0	- organic brain disease	1	1
			- mental illness	1	1
Vector-borne infections 8%			- organic heart disease	1	1
- exanthemic typhus	23	8	- anaemia	1	1
			- chronic lung disease	1	0
Contact infections 1%			- abdominal abscess	1	0
- syphilis	2	1	- slipped disc	1	0
			- rheumatism	1	0
Wound and skin infections 22%			- impaired hearing (after typhoid fever)	1	0
- lymphangitis	27	0	- disease of the retina	1	0
- erysipelas, abscess	12	0	- exhaustion	4	1
- boils, infections from corpses	20	1	- unknown diseases*	5	3
- anthrax pustule	1	0			
			Total 100%	278	47

* Unknown diseases have been excluded from the table when percentages were calculated. Thus, in the calculation, n= 273.

had caught the disease abroad. Exanthemic typhus (spotted fever), caused by rickettsiae and transmitted by lice, accounted for 23 cases, of which eight led to death. Thus, along with tuberculosis, typhoid fever and exanthemic typhus were the most important causes of death among physicians before 1890.

The figures for typhoid fever and exanthemic typhus are rather uncertain, since the term "typhus" is used in 16 cases of disease. In Norway the term "typhus" was for a long time also used for typhoid fever (nervefeber, abdominal typhus), while the term was reserved for exanthemic typhus in other countries. In addition, for a long time these diseases were regarded as two variations of the same disease. It was not until 1870 that these two diseases began to be distinguished in the district physicians' reports (Holst 1954). In this study, "typhus" is classified as exanthemic typhus. This has possibly led to some cases of typhoid fever being placed in the group with exanthemic typhus.

Two cases of syphilis are reported, of which one resulted in death. However, it is very likely that one death which was reported as insanity, was really tertiary syphilis the general paralysis of the insane. Among skin or wound infections, lymphangitis accounted for the largest group. Several physicians contracted local skin infections, boils, and abscesses after pricking themselves with instruments while carrying out post-mortems or operations. One physician died of such an infection. He developed blood poisoning through a cut in his hand after bandaging a patient.

10.7. Were Disease Caused by the Physicians' Profession?

10.7.1 Risk of Infection

If all the cases of disease are studied, it becomes apparent that the physicians in more than half of the cases caught the diseases as a result of their practice (Table 10.3). However, the number could be greater, since information on the cause of the disease is lacking in 42 percent of the cases, and it is possible that diseases transmitted from patients could be hidden in this group. On the other hand, it is also possible that the physicians were more conscientious about giving information about diseases that they assumed were connected with their profession. These diseases could therefore be overrepresented in the material.

Skin and wound infections (54 cases) make up the largest group of diseases where infection was transferred through the physician's practice. Other diseases frequently transmitted during practice were diphtheria, typhoid fever, smallpox, exanthemic typhus, and scarlet fever.

We know with certainty that nine physicians died as a result of being infected through their practice. Four caught exanthemic typhus, two typhoid fever, two diphtheria, and one died from a wound infection. Dr. Johannes Anthonius Holmboe Ruth (1848-1884) is a typical example. He graduated in December 1876 and practiced mainly as a hospital physician and as a temporary district physician before he took the post of district physician in Sortland in Northern Norway in August 1883. In his biography (Kiær 1888), it is written that he died "in Sortland on June the 9th 1884 of typhus (probably exanthemic typhus). He himself believed that he was infected at the cottage hospital which he had established in Sortland, or perhaps from a pillow which he had lent a patient. His disease became worse after an exhausting journey to Øksnes." Thus he died when he was only 36 years old, just one year after he had started in his first permanent job.

In 38 of the cases in this study, the physicians had been infected while carrying out a post-mortem or an operation (Table 10.3). Usually this involved skin or wound infections. But diphtheria was also transmitted during operations; there was an obvious risk of infection in such cases: Eight physicians were infected while carrying out tracheotomies. In order to help the patient to breathe, they cut open the wind pipe in the throat. Then they placed a silver pipe in the opening, through which they sucked out the pus. This treatment was not unusual, and several physicians mentioned that they had carried out such operations without being infected. Dr. Kiær therefore saw the necessity of asking specifically about infections after carrying out tracheotomies.

In *Norsk Magazin for Lægevidenskaben*, the hospital physician D.G. Martens described, in 1858, a case of croup that he had treated successfully with tracheotomy. He maintained that this type of operation had rarely been carried out in Norway before this time, and had only been carried out two times

TABLE 10.3
Causes of disease among the physicians

(278 cases of disease, of which 47 resulted in death)

	Cases	Deaths among the cases
Causes associated with profession 56%		
- treating a patient	94	9
- operation	20	0
- post-mortem	18	0
- accident	12	2
- overworking/tiring journeys	11	1
Causes not associated with profession 2%		
- infected by family members	2	0
- accident	3	1
- infected while traveling	1	0
Cause not given 42%	117	34
Total 100%	278	47

previously in his home town of Bergen (Martens 1858). In an article written in 1864 on the infectiousness of diphtheria, district physician S. Høegh refers to two cases at the National Hospital, where two physicians caught diphtheria after sucking pus through a cannula that was placed in the throat of a patient with croup (Høegh 1864). In 1888, chief physician C. Kahrs reported on 122 tracheotomies, that were carried out in cases of diphtheria. In the description of the method, he describes the use of a quill that, in order to induce coughing, was placed into the opening made in the patient's throat. In the article he writes:

> This part of the operation is not particularly pleasant for the surgeon. Blood and slime and diphtherous membranes often hurl straight into his face. Making this even more unpleasant by sucking these substances up by mouth with or without the use of a tube, is, in my view, completely unnecessary. It is just as well, better in fact, to tickle with a quill, and thus making the patient cough. (Kahrs 1888).

So, sucking out secretions was not a recommended method in this operation, but since Dr. Kahrs felt that it was necessary to warn against such an action, there must have still been some physicians who were carrying out tracheotomies in this dangerous way.

In the biography of Dr. Hermann Cappelen (1837–1892), it is reported that in 1861, when he was a deputy house surgeon in the surgery department at the National Hospital, he caught diphtheria of the throat. This happened just after he had used a silver pipe to suck out the secretions from the windpipe of a patient who had been operated on for diphtherous infection of the throat. During the same event, another physician (Dr. Føyn) also caught the disease. This could be the episode mentioned in Høegh's article, which is referred above. One may wonder whether it was the idealism of youth that drove physicians to carry out this kind of treatment that was so hazardous to their own health. Six out of eight physicians who were infected from tracheotomies caught diphtheria while they were voluntary helpers at the hospital when they were still students or house officers. Such was the case with Dr. Paul Christian Føyn (1835–1872), mentioned above, who was a house officer when he became infected at the National Hospital.

10.7.2 Dangerous Journeys to Visit the Sick

During the nineteenth century, it was common for the physician to come to the patient, and not the other way around. This meant that physicians spent much time, up to several days at a time, on journeys to patients in remote districts, often under extreme weather conditions. They often had to travel by both boat and horse and carriage on the journey. Such journeys could be a serious occupational hazard.

Before 1890, we have information about 27 physicians who were involved in accidents during their journeys to visit the sick. Ten physicians had been involved in several accidents. Thus, altogether there are reports of 41 accidents. Fourteen were capsizes, and in seven other accidents the physicians had fallen through the ice while driving their sleighs on frozen lakes or rivers. Furthermore, 19 accidents with horse and carriage on country roads are reported, as well as one attack by a patient's relatives. In addition, 15 physicians reported that they had been in danger several times during journeys at sea, while four physicians stated that they had experienced dangerous situations while traveling on land.

Not all the accidents resulted in injuries, but we have information about nine injuries and one case of disease resulting from accidents on journeys to the sick, while one physician was injured when he was attacked by a patient. In addition, two physicians drowned on sea journeys, one of them with the rest of the crew. Two physicians were injured in accidents not associated with their work, and one physician died in a hunting accident.

Exhaustion resulting from tiring journeys to the sick as well as a heavy work load is given as the reason for ten cases of disease and one death.

Dr. Didrik Ferdinand Schumacher (1842–1899) provides an example of how journeys could wear down a physician's health. He was district physician in Lofoten in Northern Norway from 1874 until 1888. In the biography dated November 19th 1887, the following is stated (Kiær, 1888):

> As a physician in Lofoten, he has often been in danger during journeys. During journeys it was not uncommon that he had to walk for part of the journey, then travel by boat, then walk again or ride a horse, or the other way round, on the same trip. His traveling clothes were very often unsuitable for the variable weather, and as a result of this he caught severe colds and frequently recurring bronchitis.

Dr. Thorvald Charles Egeberg (1846-1885) was district physician in Kistrand in Northern Norway when, in 1882, in an application for a job, he wrote that:

> Throughout the winter, journeys have to be made either by open boat, on skis, or with reindeer. In most cases, several different means of transportation must be used on the same journey, which often lasts several days and not uncommonly several weeks, during which time one often has to spend days and nights out in bad weather or else in terrible lodgings or barns with both people and cattle (Kiær 1888).

His application must have been impressive, because one month later he got a new job as district physician in Tranøy, also in Northern Norway. There he died of typhoid fever during an epidemic in 1885. He was confined to bed after having traveled "a tough 30 kilometers journey by sea" to attend to a woman during childbirth.

Some physicians did not want to over-dramatize their everyday life. Thus, Dr. Hjalmar Ingjald Frithjof Blütecher (1849–1891) wrote that, as a physician in Lardal in Telemark, in Southern Norway, he was in danger many times during his journeys because of snowstorms and thin ice, "but had gone through the ice only twice" (Kiær 1888).

10.8. Diseases in the Physician's Family

Up until 1890, 73 physicians (18 percent) reported that neither they nor their families had suffered from any epidemic diseases. However, this information is somewhat uncertain. Among other things, some physicians reported that they had not suffered from any *serious* epidemic diseases. We can therefore not exclude the possibility that the family had suffered from minor diseases (for example, childhood diseases), which the physician did not think it necessary to mention. On the other hand, these diseases were included in the district physicians' reports (*Medicinalberetningene*), so it is to be expected that the physicians were well acquainted with the need to register all cases of epidemic disease.

10.8.1 Diseases Among the Wives – Diseases and Infections Associated with Childbirth

In all, we have information about 105 cases of disease among the physicians' wives (Table 10.4). This includes 42 deaths, of which the cause of death is missing for 18. Seven wives are registered as having had two diseases and one is registered as having had three. The diseases are therefore divided between 96 women. The mean age of the 42 wives who died before 1890 was 30.1 years.

For the wives as well as for their husbands, infectious diseases make up a large group, 42 cases (48 percent of the 87 cases for which we have a diagnosis). Another important group consisted of the diseases of childbirth, with 40 cases (46 percent), of which 13 ended in death. Thirty women suffered from puerperal fever, and eight of them died as a consequence. Two women had suffered from puerperal fever twice. The figures for puerperal fever might be higher, since the other cases of diseases of childbirth include diagnoses such as puerperal peritonitis and perimetritis, and phlegmasia alba dolens (phlebitis) or the diagnoses "death during childbirth." Several of these diagnoses should probably have been categorized as puerperal fever (Kjærheim 1980). In addition, one wife died of an infection after retention of the placenta. Of the 42 cases of infections other than puerperal fever, diphtheria, scarlet fever, typhoid fever, and tuberculosis were the most frequent. Six of the wives died of tuberculosis before 1890. In addition, two cases of mental illness are mentioned: insomnia and melancholy. According to the descriptions given by the two physicians, these cases were seen as connected to their working and living conditions (Kiær 1988).

TABLE 10.4
Diseases among the wives
(105 cases of disease, of which 42 resulted in death)

	Cases	Deaths among the cases
Air-borne infections 37%		
- diphtheria	10	0
- scarlet fever	9	0
- tuberculosis	6	6
- whooping cough	2	0
- measles	1	0
- smallpox	1	0
- pneumonia	1	1
- bronchitis	1	0
- pleurisy	1	1
Food and water-borne infections 7%		
- typhoid fever	5	0
- dysentery	1	0
Vector-borne infections 2%		
- exanthemic typhus	2	0
Wound and skin infections 2%		
- erysipelas	2	0
Diseases of childbirth 46%		
- puerperal fever	30	8
- other diseases of childbirth	10	5
Other diseases 6%		
- insomnia/melancholy	2	0
- peritonitis/periyphlitis	2	2
- gastric ulcer	1	1
Unknown causes of death *	18	18
Total 100%	105	42

* Unknown causes of death were excluded when the percentages were calculated. In the calculations n=87

Dr. Franz Oscar Carlsen (1845–1915), who was district physician in Lødingen and later in Bodø in Northern Norway, related the following incident about his wife:

> Right after his wife gave birth for the first time, he had to travel by sea to Tysfjorden in terrible weather. Because of this, his wife became terribly frightened, and she was

depressed for several weeks.

Dr. Ole Bornemann Bull (1842–1916), who was an eye and ear specialist in Christiania, married twice before 1890, and both of his wives became ill during childbirth.

> His first wife died (in 1884) of a puerperal infection after partial retention of the placenta. In November 1886, his second wife caught severe puerperal fever. At the same time, two of his sons had typhoid fever, which they had contracted in Horten (Kiær 1888).

There is information about the cause and mode of infection for 21 of the cases of disease among the wives. None of these cases led to death. In nine of the cases, it is reported that the wife was infected by the physician, and in two cases by the physician's patients (in one of these cases, the wife was an assistant to the physician while he was treating patients). In two cases of puerperal fever, the women were probably infected by the midwife. Three cases of disease are ascribed to living conditions or climate (one case of bronchitis in addition to the two cases of depression mentioned above), while two cases were associated with an epidemic. In three cases, it is reported that the wife was infected at home, by sick children.

10.8.2 Diseases Among the Children – Whooping Cough, Measles, and Scarlet Fever

Of the 1,133 children in the material, 214 died before 1890. One hundred and forty-eight physicians reported that all of their children were alive, while 119 physicians had lost at least one child. One physician had lost nine children, 92 physicians had lost one. For two physicians, it is unclear whether the child died before or after 1890. These children were therefore assumed to have been alive in 1890. Altogether 991 cases of disease are registered, including the deaths (Table 10.5). If we exclude the 122

TABLE 10.5
Diseases among the children

(991 cases, of which 214 resulted in death)

	Cases	Deaths among the cases
Air-borne infections 90%		
- whooping cough	227	12
- scarlet fever	221	10
- measles	213	2
- diphtheria	58	11
- chickenpox	16	0
- mumps	9	0
- German measles	9	0
- "all childhood diseases"	9	0
- pneumonia	12	10
- bronchitis	1	1
- tuberculosis	8	8
Food and water-borne infections 5%		
- typhoid fever	23	0
- dysentery/diarrhea	20	8
Vector-borne infections 1%		
- exanthemic typhus	8	0
Wound and skin infections 1%		
- erysipelas	8	4
- infection in the navel/ other wounds	3	2
Injuries 0.1%		
- foreign body in the throat	1	1
Other diseases 3%		
- meningitis	4	4
- peritonitis	2	2
- kidney disease	2	2
- sepsis	1	1
- unknown infection	1	1
- leukemia	1	1
- convulsions	1	1
- diabetes	1	1
- spina bifida	1	1
- still-born	7	7
- dead in the first day of life	2	2
Unknown causes of death *	122	122
Total 100,1%	991	214

* Unknown causes of death have been excluded when the percentages were calculated. In the calculations n=869.

cases in which the cause of death is unknown, we are left with the diagnosis in 869 cases of disease among the children. Whooping cough, measles, and scarlet fever together account for 76 percent of the cases. Other commonly reported diseases were diphtheria, typhoid fever, diarrhea, and different childhood diseases.

Eight children died of tuberculosis, most of them of tuberculous meningitis or miliary tuberculosis. Diphtheria, diarrhea, and pneumonia, along with whooping cough and scarlet fever, were also common causes of death.

We have information on age at the time of death for 89 of the 214 children (42 percent). Two-thirds of these children died before they had reached the age of one. (Nine of them were stillborn or else died during the first day of life, and yet another ten died during the first month of life). An additional 26 died before they were six years old. Three died when they were of school-age and one died at 19 years of age.

In 110 of the 991 cases of disease, there is information on the probable mode of infection. Table 10.6 shows that it was suspected that infection was associated with the physician's practice in 35 percent of cases. In addition, in 17 percent of cases, the child was infected during an epidemic, without the physician having stated the origion of the infection.

Dr. Cato Andreas Christian Holmsen (1843–1923), medical officer for the poor in Enebakk, brought an infection home with him and it was caught by his children:

> In January 1876, 2 of his 4 surviving children and a servant girl had scarlet fever. They had been contracted from him, one day when he came home ill from patients with scarlet fever, and was unable to take the normal precautions (Kiær 1888).

Work in hospitals was also associated with the risk of infection for the family members, as Dr. Johan Vilhelm Midelfart (1835–1898) stated:

> In June 1887, one daughter and one servant girl in his house were infected with typhoid fever, probably infected through himself from a patient admitted to the County Hospital (Kiær 1888).

Dr. Jacob von der Lippe Parelius (1852–1890), medical officer for the poor in Støren and later district physician in Lyngen, and his family were infected several times:

> During an epidemic in Støren in February 1879, he himself was infected with typhoid fever, from which he did not recover until the end of April of the same year. During her last childbirth in January 1886, his wife caught puerperal fever with subsequent parametritis. The night before she gave birth, her husband was called out to visit two patients, suffering from septicemia. In the spring of 1884, his son in Lyngen was very ill with diphtheria in the throat. He had probably been infected by children who, during the present epidemic, had been brought to the physician's house (Kiær 1988.

TABLE 10.6
Causes of disease among the children

(110 cases of disease, of which 10 resulted in death)

	Cases	Deaths among the cases
Infection caught from the physician's practice 35%		
- from a healthy physician	17	1
- from a sick physician	14	1
- from a patient	7	0
Infection caught from elsewhere 48%		
- from family members/servants	14	4
- outside the home	37	0
- while traveling	2	0
Infected during an epidemic (from an unknown person) 17%	19	4
Total 100%	110	10

10.9. Discussion

The descriptions above show that the risk of death and disease in the nineteenth century was also a part of life for physicians and their families. However, the way in which the data were collected makes it difficult to produce any figures on the incidence of disease that can be compared directly with public statistics on diseases within the population, such as those found in the district physicians' reports. One reason for the uncertainty is associated with the way in which the actual data were collected. The answers are probably influenced by the editor's request for information on specific diseases. Less serious diseases could therefore have been underdiagnosed. For example, skin or wound infections were so common that many physicians probably did not think them worth mentioning. There are also some physicians from whom there is no information about diseases, although they had not reported that they had not been sick. There are also most probably some occurrences of disease which have been forgotten, since the registration was done retrospectively. There is reason to believe that under-reporting of children's diseases was especially common. This is because it probably was difficult to remember several years later exactly when the children were sick and how many of them were sick. Also, some physicians have simply reported that their children had had the "usual childhood diseases," without giving additional information on which diseases they had had, or on how many children had been sick. Taking into account these reservations, the figures in the tables should probably be regarded as minimum figures.

In addition, some diseases have probably been wrongly diagnosed, though we must assume that registration carried out by physicians themselves is much more reliable than if the same information had been collected from lay people.

Another problem that makes it difficult to compare the figures with the general population is that there are no data on the exact number of individuals in the physicians' families at any given time. Neither are there any exact data on the time at which many of the diseases occurred. With regard to diseases of childbirth, it is possibile to make a cautious comparison with the general population. Diseases of childbirth, puerperal fever being the most frequent, were important causes of death and disease among women of fertile age. Among all women between 15 and 50 years of age, death during childbirth accounted for 10 percent of the mortality in the period 1866-1880 (Drejer 1907). Of the physicians' wives who died between 1862-1889, 13 of them died from diseases of childbirth. (This is 31 percent of all the 42 deaths, or 54 percent if we exclude the 18 unknown causes of death among the wives). In connection with the data collection, Kiær writes:

> I have gained the impression that physicians' wives are at a greater risk of contracting puerperal fever than others, and regard it to be of interest to collect material for solving this problem (Kiær 1886).

Although the data cannot be compared directly, it does appear as though death during childbirth had an abnormally high prevalence among physicians' wives. The reason for this, however, is unknown.

The information about the mode of infection is also a possible source of error. The physicians had a limited knowledge of the mode of transmission of different diseases, and many of the causal connections seem to be mere assumptions. At the same time, the physicians knew that diseases could be transmitted through contact with the sick. During the period when the diseases were registered, more and more knowledge about micro-organisms was gained (Reichborn-Kjennerud et al. 1936). In the cases where the biographies give more detailed information about the transmission of a disease, it is usually in accordance with what we today know about the mode of transmission, incubation period, and course of diseases. An example is the previously mentioned Dr. Ruth, who died of typhus, probably exanthemic typhus. He himself believed that the disease could have been transmitted through a pillow which he had lent to a patient. This theory is plausible, since this disease is transmitted via lice.

The results show that physicians had a risky profession. However, we have no overview of mortality and morbidity in other comparable professional groups in Norway from the same period. It is therefore difficult to say whether the medical profession involved greater health risks than other professions.

Despite uncertainties in the data collection and the problem of comparing physicians with the general population, the material that Kiær collected provides important documentation on the lives and health of physicians and their families during the nineteenth century. It gives us an insight into the everyday lives of physicians, lives that were quite different from those of physicians today. From this material, the conclusion can be drawn that more than half of the cases of disease experienced by physicians seems to have been related to their professional practice. In addition to the danger of infection, exhausting journeys involving the danger of accidents were a professional hazard. The wives and children of physicians were also at risk of being infected as a result of the physician's practice, either by being infected by the physician himself or by patients who visited him.

References

Drejer, P.M. "Om dødelighet på barselseng i Norge," *Norsk Magazin for Lægevidenskaben*,(1907):600–627.

Hansen, L.I.K. *Koleraen i Christiania i 1853. Thesis*, Oslo: Seksjon for medisinsk historie, Universitetet i Oslo, 1985.

Hjort, E.F. "Rekruttering av Norges leger på 1800-tallet," *Tidsskrift for Den norske lægeforening*,14(1983):1149–1154.

Holst, P.M. *Våre akute folkesykdommers epidemiologi og klinikk.* Oslo: H. Aschehoug & Co. 1954.

Holst, P.M. "Helseforholdene i Norge omkring 1880," *Tidsskrift for Den norske lægeforening*, Jubileumsnummer (1955).

Høegh, S. "Iagttagelser under en Epidemie af Diphteritis faucium," *Norsk Magazin for Lægevidenskaben*,(1864):120–149.

Kahrs, C. "122 Trakeotomier i Difterit," *Norsk Magazin for Lægevidenskaben*, (1888):441–462.

Kiær, F.C. (ed.) *Norges Læger i det nittende Aarhundrede (1800–1871).* Christiania: A. Cammermeyer, 1873.

Kiær, F.C. "Opfordring til Kolleger i Anledning af en ny Udgave af 'Norges Læger'," *Norsk Magazin for Lægevidenskaben* April Heftet (1886):303–306.

Kiær, F.C. ed. *Norges Læger i det nittende Aarhundrede (1800–1886). Anden betydeligt forøgede Udgave.* Christiania: A. Cammermeyer, Bind I (Aa-K) 1888, Bind II (L-Ø) 1890.

Kjærheim, K. *Mellom kloke koner og hvitkledte menn. Det norske jordmorvesen på 1800-tallet.* Oslo: Seksjon for medisinsk historie, Universitetet i Oslo, 1980.

Kobro, I ed. *Norges Læger 1800–1908.* Kristiania: H.Aschehoug & Co, Bind I (Aa-K) 1908-1912, Bind II (L-Ø) 1915.

Kobro, I ed. *Tillegg til Norges læger 1800–1908.* Oslo: H. Aschehoug & Co. 1944.

Løken, K. *Karjol-dokter'n.* Oslo: J.W. Cappelens forlag A.S, 1974.

Martens, D.G. "Tracheotomie mod Croup foretaget med heldigt Udfald," *Norsk Magazin for Lægevidenskaben*,(1858):560-568.

Medicinalberetningene. (The district phy-

medisinaldirektoratet 1932. Medicinalberetningen og innberetninger om epidemiske sykdommer, kolera etc. 1835–1921," Riksarkivet i Oslo.

Nilsson, P. and B. Persson. "Dödsorsaker bland svenska provinsalläkare 1840–1879," *Allmänmedicin*,1(1995):30–31.

Reichborn-Kjennerud, I., F. Grøn and I. Kobro. *Medisinens historie i Norge*. Oslo: Grøndahl & Søns Forlag, 1936.

Rosvold, E.O. and Ø. Larsen. "Krankheiten im Arztberuf. Die Gesundheit norwegischer Ärzte und ihrer Angehörigen im ausgehenden 19. Jahrhundert," *Medizinhistorisches Journal*,1–2(1996):167–180.

CHAPTER 11

Norwegian Dentistry

KAI HUNSTADBRÅTEN

11.1 The Professionalization of Dentists

During the nineteenth century, there was a gradual formalization of the discipline of dentistry. The professionalization of dentists took place at a somewhat slower pace than it did for the physicians.

The necessity of a formalization and regulation of the dentist's work was a result of the development within both medicine and dentistry. Althoug earlier his main task was to extract teeth, during the last decades of the nineteenth century the dentist became responsible for a magnitude of new tasks, such as implanting artificial teeth, filling cavities, performing dental surgery with the use of anaesthetics, prescribing medicine, and instituting prophylactic measures.

Prior to 1852, dentists' activities were regulated by the same laws that applied to doctors and quacks. As early as 1844, a proposal for a new law to organize the health system was put forward. This law contained specific regulations on who was entitled to practice as a dentist; no formal examination was required, but an authorization could be received if the applicant could document his abilities. A specific examination for dentists was introduced in 1852. The first candidate, Conrad Christopher Schive (1821–1883), was examined in 1860, according to regulations given by Order in Council September 9th 1857.

Until 1893 there were no formal educational requirements for dentists; neither did the first regulations say anything about practical training. During the examination, the candidate was supposed to prove his insight and ability in the art of dentistry. For the first couple of decades the jury consisted of two professors from the Medical Faculty and one authorized dentist. Practical and theoretical training were performed under the supervision of other dentists, but the regulations did not contain any specific demands pertaining to the duration and the topics covered by this training until 1881, when the duration of the practical training was set at two years by Order in Council November 5th 1881. In addition to their education in Norway, many dentists traveled abroad for further training and to acquire further knowledge.

In 1893, a dental policlinic run by the state opened in Kristiania, and in 1905 the Norwegian Dentists Association opened their Technical Institute, where Ministry of Church Affairs approved the teachers and a university professor was in charge. This institute was transformed into the State Institute of Dentistry in 1909, and four professors taught the main topics: dental surgery, prosthetics, conservative treatment, and orthodontics. The education given here was a three-year program. In 1928 the institute became the National School of Dentistry, and was regulated by a new law of 1938. The education was extended to a four-year period. The college was incorporated in the University of Oslo in 1959, as the Faculty of Odontology, and the duration of the education was set at five years. In 1962 an Institute of Odontology was established at the University of Bergen, with part of the education to be conducted by the Faculty of Medicine.

11.2 Dentists in Norway 1860–1900

Prior to 1860, dentistry was performed by a few foreign dentists, medical doctors, and surgeons, but also by watchmakers, goldsmiths, and pharmacists. After receiving an authorization, the dentist had to report to the official medical doctor about his activity. For instance, C.C. Schive received the following (in translation): "Permission to clean, fill and pull out teeth on condition that he is under the control of the Regional doctor and that the permission can be withdrawn should he infringe the conditions under which the permission was granted."

According to the official list, there were six certified dentists in Norway in 1860, four of whom practiced in Kristiania. Ten years later, the number increased to 21, 10 of whom practiced in Kristiania, that is, there was one dentist per about 82,000 inhabitants for the country as a whole. In 1900 there were 201 dentists, about one per 11,000 inhabitants.

Information on the dentists' daily activities can be found in the annual medical reports from the mid-1860s. The dentists' reports were not mandatory, as were the medical reports of the physicians, therefore they vary both in contents and number. Some dentists reported only the number of patients treated, whereas others delivered elaborate reports of diagnosis and remedy, and long descriptions of cases thought to be of interest. In spite of their shortcomings and weaknesses, in their variety they render a picture of the condition of dental health in Norway at the time.

11.3 Some Examples From the Reports

The medical reports from dentists all over Norway also teach us about several central elements in the process of professionalization. Indirectly they tell about how knowledge was diffused by mentioning the treatment given in different places in Norway at various times, about salaries, and about the consolidation of dentists as a group.

The dentists themselves express concern over payment and propose ways of paying dentists that will improve dental health in Norway by offering treatment to selected groups, for instance, the poor or the school children.

Dentist David Eilertsen (1852–1887) of Tromsø perhaps could be called the father of Norway's public dental care. Among other things, he wrote the following in his report for the year 1886:

> "I take the liberty of drawing the mighty ministry's attention to the unfortunate relationship between the poor and the dentist. Either the dentist has to treat them free of charge, which is something our dentists, who are usually unsalaried by State or County, naturally cannot do if they are to survive, or these many poor creatures do not get an adequate treatment. None other than that which the doctor for the poor renders."

He suggested that it should be the government's duty to correct this situation by giving an appropriate salary to dentists for the treatment of the poor. The district physicians' salaries were based on this principle, he writes further, and it was specified that the regional doctor should live at a specified place and first and foremost treat the poor. The counties were not in a position to manage this matter in a satisfactory way, he noted, since their budgets were already overburdened.

Other examples from the medical reports show how the dentists look upon themselves as a professional group, and in these examples the dentists also propose cooperation with another defined professional group, the physicians, to improve general dental health.

In his report for Trondheim for 1868, dentist Chr. Jahn (1837–1914) wrote, among other things: "Tooth care has actually a very low priority here in comparison to other parts of the country. The filling of decayed teeth is not as common as it should be. It would be desirable if doctors involved themselves in this matter more than they do, and recommend treatment; the public would then probably be more watchful than they are at present."

The dentist Georg Moe (1826–1877) in Arendal expressed the same opinion in his medical report for 1867, where, among other things, he wrote:

> "But since something should be done, it would certainly be of great importance if this matter was presented to the doctors, so that they could use their influence to turn the public's attention towards the necessity of a better and more frequent cleaning of the mouth, and also towards the help that the art of dentistry, in its presently developed stage, could offer, to anyone who seeks its help in time."

The distress of dentist Ole Eskild Sørum (1871–1932) in Northern Aurdal in Valdres in 1890 is apparent in the follwing comment:

> "According to my comparatively short experience, the state of teeth here in Valdres is very bad. It is sad to see how the majority of the young here live with such sick gums, bad breath, teeth covered in tartar, and not offer a little time to the care of their mouth and seek timely help, before it becomes a necessity."

In the medical reports of other dentists, however, there are detailed statements of the number of patients and executed treatments. The numbers vary greatly. Carl Opsahl (1831–1903) in Hamar reports that he treated approximately 1,300, 1,500 and 1,400 patients in 1872, 1873, and 1874, respectively. Other dentists treated between 300 and 400 patients annually.

References

Hunstadbråten, K. *Tannleger i trekvart århundre. Norsk odontologi 1800–1875.* Vikersund: Thesis, 1970.

Hunstadbråten, K. *Odontologiens utvikling.* Oslo: Folkets Brevskole, Norsk kommuneforbund, Universitetsforlaget, 1979.

Hunstadbråten, K."Fra våre kollegers praksis for 100 år siden." *Norsk Tannlegeforenings Tidsskrift*,100(1990):596–599.

CHAPTER 12

Do Physicians, Lawyers, and Theologians Have Comparable Careers?

ELIN OLAUG ROSVOLD

12.1 Three Professions, Different Careers?

In Norway, as in other countries, medicine, theology, and law are among the oldest academic disciplines (Aubert 1960). Even though the study of the three disciplines leads to three very different professions, they all have in common that human problems are an essential part of their theoretical basis. In all three professions, one not only has to take the fates of other people into consideration, but also often has to intervene in other people's lives. In addition, they have in common the kind of academic education that in itself throughout history has made it possible to attain positions that imply a certain status, as well as the reward of financial benefits to a greater or lesser extent.

The question is: Do the three professions resemble each other when it comes to the professional careers themselves, or to the possibilities that present themselves after one has completed the degree? In this chapter two cohorts of physicians, lawyers, and theologians will be analyzed. The first cohort began their professional careers towards the end of the nineteenth century, while the others began their careers fifty years later. We shall investigate whether the physicians stand out from the lawyers and the theologians when it comes to background, family conditions, career possibilities, and mobility.

12.2 The Material

The information about the careers is collected from the 25th anniversary yearbooks for two cohorts of students who passed the examen artium (the student qualifying exam for the university), namely, students having passed between 1890 and 1894 (Studentene fra 1890, 1891, 1892, 1893, 1894) and students having passed in 1943 (Møller 1968). The anniversary yearbooks were published in 1915–19 and in 1968. According to these books, about 1,220 students passed the examen artium between 1890 and 1894. The numbers are somewhat uncertain, since several students took their exams more than once. Out of the 1,220 students, 636 (52 percent) attained a degree in one of the three disciplines in question. More than half of them chose to study law. In 1943, there were, according to the yearbook, about 3,500 students who passed the examen artium, 359 (about ten percent) of whom completed a degree in one of the three disci-

TABLE 12.1
The number of lawyers, physicians, and theologians among the examen artium students of 1890–94 and 1943.

Degree	1890–94 Cohort				1943 Cohort			
	n	%	Men	Women	n	%	Men	Women
Lawyers	346	54	342	4	212	59	197	15
Physicians	216	34	203	13	113	31	111	2
Theologians	74	12	73	1	34	9	31	3
Total	636	100	618	18	359	99	339	20

plines. The distribution of the students can be seen in Table 12.1.

12.3 Social Backgrounds

12.3.1 The 1890–94 Cohort

Table 12.2 shows the occupations of the fathers of the students who passed the examen artium between 1890 and 1894. Many of the candidates chose the same profession as their fathers. The representation of the theologians in this case was significantly higher than the representation of both physicians (p=0.02) and lawyers (p=0.02). There is, however, reason to believe that the percentage of lawyer-fathers among the lawyers is higher than shown in the table, since there are probably some lawyers in the businessmen or high-ranking employees groups as well (Palmstrøm 1935). In Torgersen (1972) a survey shows that, among the students qualifying for their degree in one of the three disciplines in 1889, the theologians and the lawyers with fathers in the same profession were represented almost equally (21 percent and 20 percent, respectively), while the physicians had a lower percentage (14 percent). Twenty years later, in 1909, 21 percent of the theologians, 16 percent of the lawyers, and nine percent of the physicians had fathers in the same profession. Adopting their father's profession therefore seems to have been less common among physicians than among lawyers and theologians.

Except for adopting their father's profession, the physicians and the lawyers in the 1890-94 cohort had quite similar backgrounds. Especially the business community had produced many candidates in law and medicine. Significantly more physicians than theologians had fathers in the business community (p=0.01). The theologians, on the other hand, had a higher percentage of farmers' sons that both the physicians and the lawyers (p=0.001).

The distribution of the fathers' professions in our material corresponds with Aubert and his colleagues' survey on the backgrounds of the theological, medical, and law candidates in the time-span 1890–1909, shown in their survey on Norwegian candidates in the period 1800–1950 (Aubert et al. 1960). According to Aubert et al., the great amount of recruiting from the business community reflects the fact that in Norway, in contrast to many other countries in the 1800s, there was very little distance between the business community and people with university education. The businessmen and the university graduates together made up one social circle, with mutual visits and family relations. The result was that businessmen's sons were recruited to pursue academic studies, and businessmen's daughters were married to university graduates and government officials.

The large percentage of farmers' sons

TABLE 12.2
The examen artium students of the period 1890–94 divided according to their university degrees and their fathers' occupations. Number (percent).

	University degree					
Fathers' occupations	Lawyers n=344*		Physicians n=214*		Theologians n=74	
Lawyers	44	(13)	3	(1)	1	(1)
Physicians	14	(4)	25	(12)	1	(1)
Theologians	29	(8)	21	(10)	17	(23)
Other University Graduates	12	(3)	3	(1)	2	(3)
Engineers	2	(1)	1	(1)	1	(1)
Military Officers	18	(5)	14	(7)	6	(8)
Teachers	14	(4)	10	(5)	7	(9)
Businessmen	79	(23)	63	(29)	11	(15)
Farmers	39	(11)	21	(10)	19	(26)
Shipmasters	13	(4)	14	(7)	1	(1)
High-ranking Employees	20	(6)	9	(4)	2	(3)
Low-ranking Employees	40	(12)	20	(9)	5	(7)
Craftsmen	16	(5)	10	(5)	1	(1)
Laborers	2	(1)	0	–	0	–
Musicians	2	(1)	0	–	0	–
Total	344	(101)	214	(101)	74	(99)

* The occupations of the fathers of two lawyers and two physicians are unknown

among the theologians was, according to Aubert et al., due to the fact that the sons of businessmen and university graduates showed less and less interest in theology at the end of the nineteenth century. This is supposedly a symptom of the secularization in the higher strata of the town societies. In our material, the lawyers and physicians had a smaller percentage of farmers among their fathers than the theologians did. But, at the same time, we can see from Table 12.2 that there was a rather large percentage of the lawyers and physicians who had fathers who were theologians. This could be the result of the fact that social mobility from the agricultural population to academic professions can take several generations; a farmer's son becomes a teacher, the teacher's son becomes a theologian, and the theologian's son becomes a physician or a lawyer (Aubert et al. 1960).

12.3.2. The 1943 Cohort

Fifty years later, among the students who passed the examen artium in 1943, the law and theology candidates showed less of a tendency to choose the same profession that their fathers chose (Table 12.3). The percentages in the three groups were therefore fairly similar. This corresponds with the tendency in the aforementioned survey in Torgersen 1972 that also gives figures from 1949. In our study, we also found that the percentage of lawyers and physicians with theologian fathers had decreased. Engineers at the same time made up a large group among the

TABLE 12.3
The examen artium students of 1943 divided according to their university degrees and their fathers' occupations. Number (percent).

	University degree		
Fathers' occupation	Lawyers n=197*	Physicians n=111*	Theologians n=32*
Lawyers	17 (8)	1 (1)	0 –
Physicians	7 (4)	11 (10)	0 –
Theologians	5 (3)	4 (4)	3 (9)
Other University Graduates	4 (2)	14 (13)	4 (13)
Engineers	8 (4)	12 (11)	2 (6)
Military Officers	9 (5)	1 (1)	0 –
Teachers	8 (4)	5 (5)	2 (6)
Businessmen	44 (21)	20 (18)	4 (13)
Farmers	14 (7)	7 (6)	6 (19)
Shipmasters	5 (3)	1 (1)	1 (3)
High-ranking Employees	21 (11)	7 (6)	3 (9)
Low-ranking Employees	38 (19)	16 (14)	5 (16)
Craftsmen	6 (3)	6 (5)	2 (6)
Laborers	5 (3)	1 (1)	0 –
Others	6 (3)	5 (5)	0 –
Total	197 (100)	111 (101)	32 (100)

* The occupations of the fathers of 15 lawyers, two physicians and two theologians are unknown.

fathers, especially when it came to the physicians. Compared to the lawyers, the physicians had a significantly higher percentage of engineers among their fathers (p=0.02). The percentage of fathers with an university degree can be found by combining the top four categories in Table 12.3. The lawyers in the 1943 cohort seem to have had a lower percentage of fathers with an university degree than physicians and theologians, although we here, as earlier, must consider the fact that some of the fathers among the businessmen and high-ranking employees could also have been lawyers. The group of fathers who were low-ranking employees increased during the 50-year span between the two cohorts in the material.

The fact that there are so few theologians in the material makes it difficult to say whether there were obvious differences between them and the other candidates. However, it does seem as though the theologians were still recruited more from the agricultural population than was the case for the physicians and the lawyers.

12.4 Period of Study

2.4.1. The 1890–94 Cohort

Table 12.4 shows the average age of the three groups of candidates when they passed the examen artium, when they finished their degrees, and when they were married for the

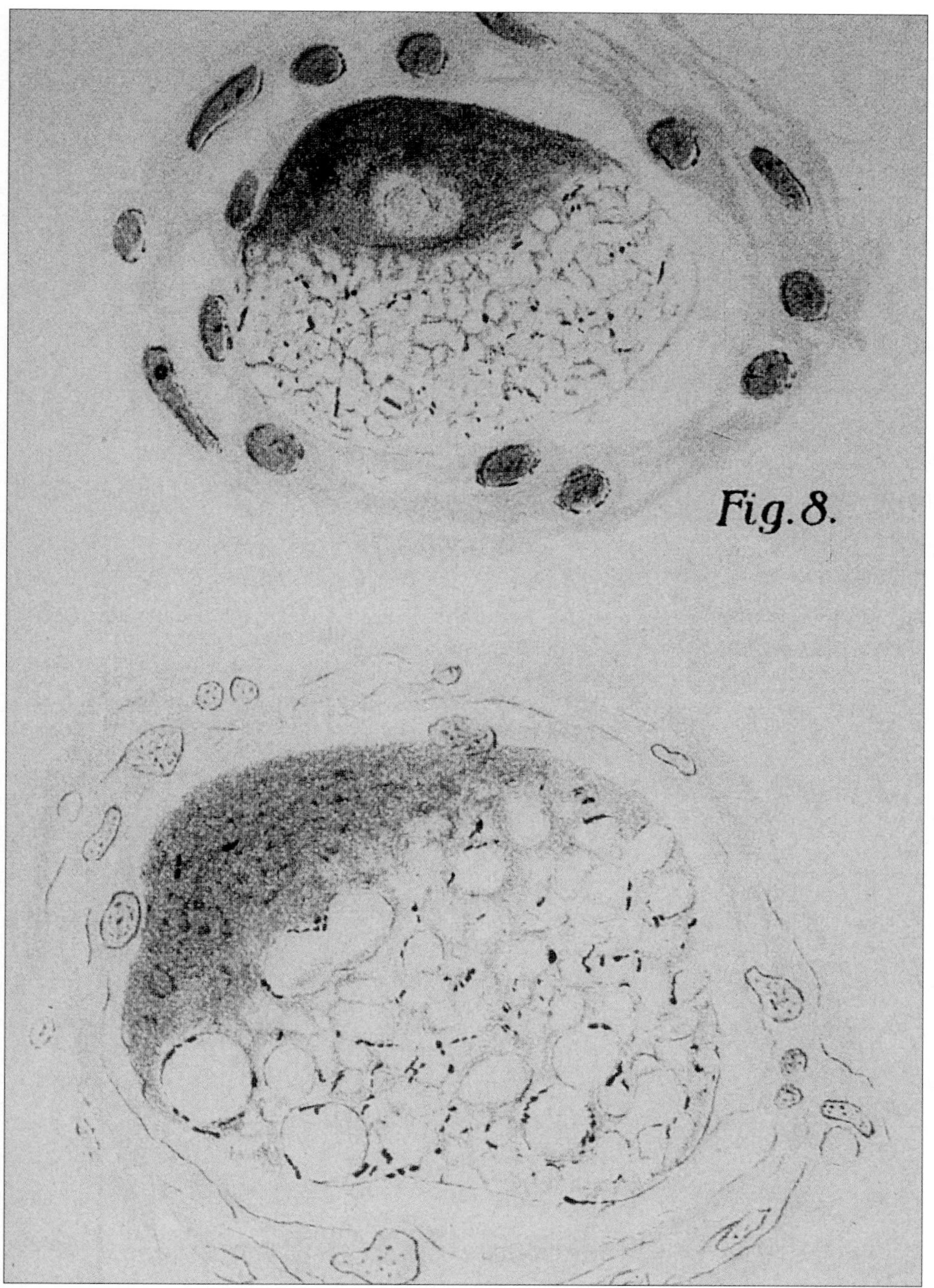

Figure 28: Leprosy was a quite frequent disease in Noway in the nineteenth century, especially in the coastal districts. In Bergen, advanced research was performed, and Gerhard Henrik Armauer Hansen (1841-1912) discovered the leprosy bacillus in 1873. But there were other researchers, too. This illustration shows leprous changes in nervous tissue, and was published by Hans Peter Lie (1862-1945) in 1905.

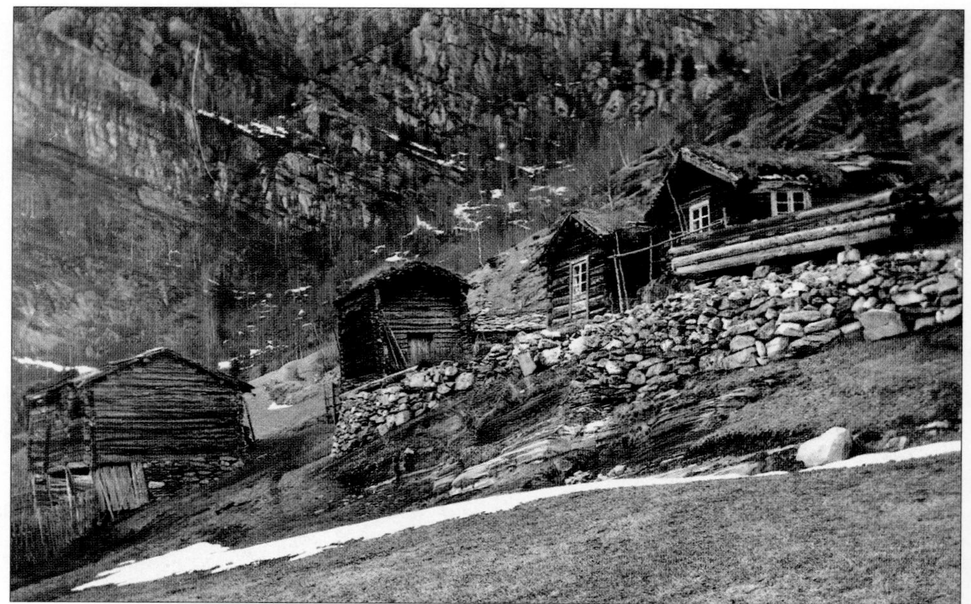

Figure 29: The abandoned cottar's farm Skar in Fron, the Gudbrandsdalen valley (Photo: Pål Kluften. Courtesy De Sandvigske Samlinger, Lillehammer).

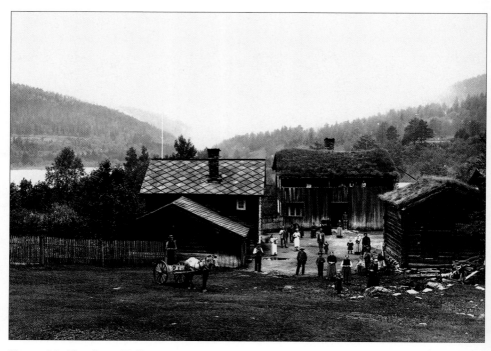

Figure 30: The farm Kolloen, Sjoa, the Gudbrandsdalen valley (Photo: Hans H. Lie 1896. Courtesy De Sandvigske Samlinger, Lillehammer).

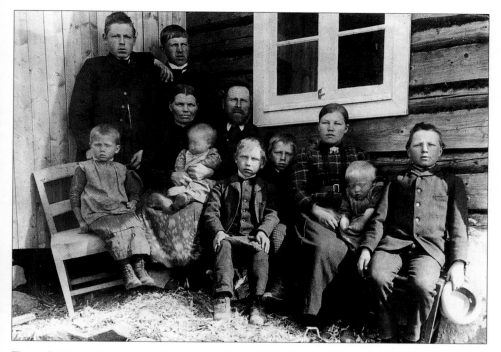

Figure 31: Outside the cottar farm Samuelstuen 1893 (Courtesy Hedmarksmuseet).

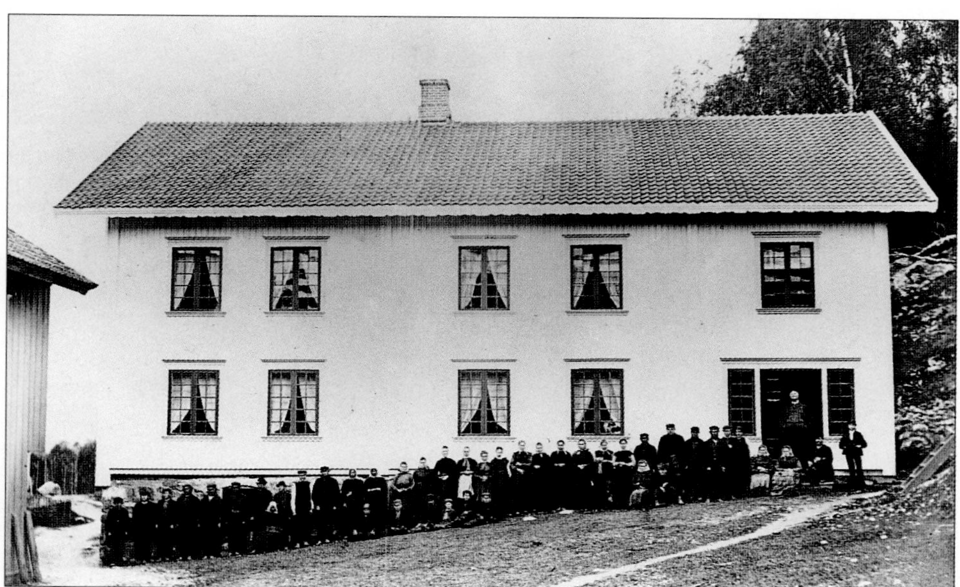

Figure 32: Social conditions could be very different in rural Eastern Norway. The working team for the potato harvest at the farm Berg in 1876 (Courtesy Hedmarksmuseet).

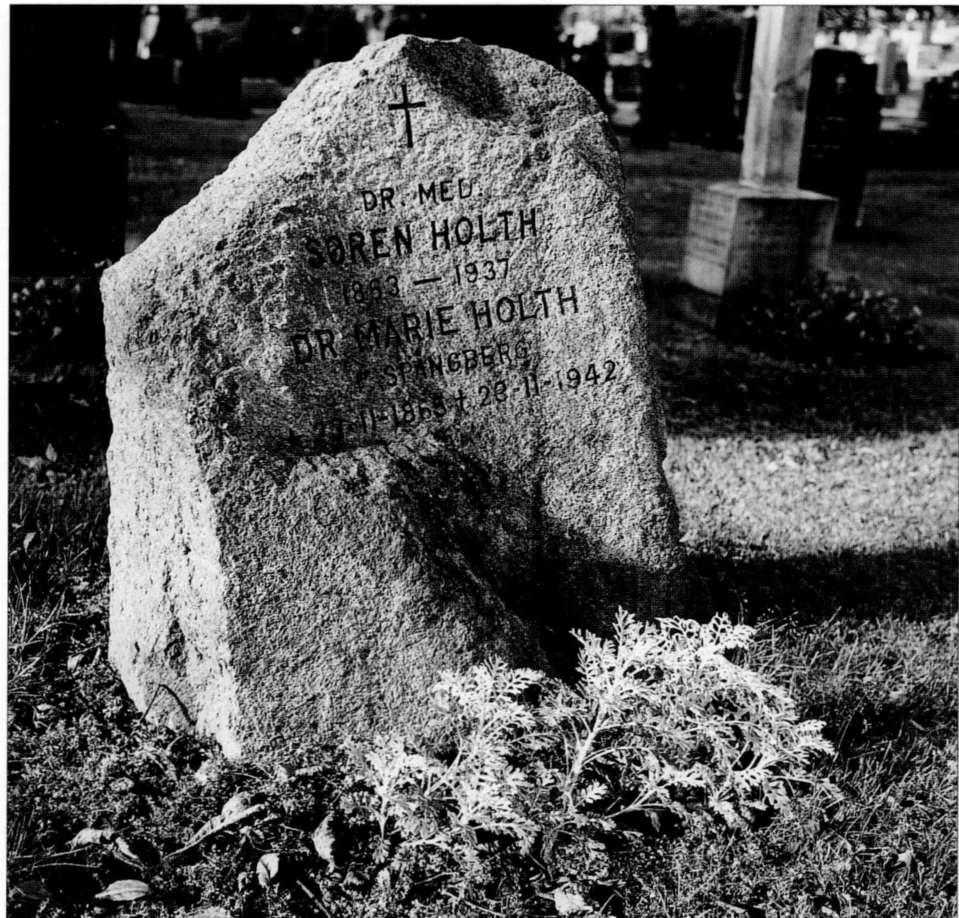

Figure 33: Marie Spångberg (1865-1942) was the first woman to graduate as a physician in Norway (1893). Like many of her later female colleagues, she married a male doctor. Søren Holth (1863-1937) was an ophthalmologist (Tombstone at the Cemetery of Our Saviour [Vår Frelsers gravlund] in Oslo. Photo: Øivind Larsen 1996).

TABLE 12.4
Year of birth and year of university graduation for the examen artium students of 1890–94 and 1943. The table also shows the students' mean age at the time of examen artium, graduation, and first marriage.

	1890–94 Cohort			1943 Cohort		
	Lawyers n=346	Physicians n=216	Theologians n=74	Lawyers n=212	Physicians n=113	Theologians n=34
Year of birth	1859–77	1866–78	1860–76	1911–25	1913–26	1910–25
Year of graduation	1894–10	1896–06	1894–08	1946–64	1946–62	1947–57
Mean age at the time of:						
- Examen artium	18.9	18.7	20.0	20.6	19.8	20.7
- Graduation	24.9	26.9	26.6	27.9	29.3	28.1
- First marriage	30.4	30.6	31.1	29.6	29.4	28.3

first time. In the 1890–94 cohort, the average age for passing the examen artium was 18.9 years. The theologians were, however, significantly older than both the physicians and the lawyers when they passed the examen artium. Palmstrøm (1935) has shown earlier that there was a tendency that students with an agricultural background had a higher mean age when passing the examen artium than other students. This may have been because they, to a greater extent, had to pay for their own education. Among the students in our study, theologians had the highest percentage of students who came from the agricultural population, and this could explain some of the age differences.

At the time of receiving their degree, the lawyers in the 1890-94 cohort were significantly younger than both the physicians and the theologians ($p<0.001$). This was probably due to the fact that law studies were fairly unrestrained; one could study on one's own and take the final exam within only a few years. Six lawyers graduated as early as three years after the examen artium, and after four years 11 percent of the lawyers had received their degree. In all, 52 percent had finished their degrees five years after the examen artium, while almost 90 percent graduated within seven years. In comparison, the physician who was quickest to finish his degree, received it after five years, while 27 percent finished after seven years and 90 percent after nine years. Among the theologians, the shortest study period was three years, while it took eight years before almost 90 percent had received their degree. Theology and medicine were studies with more structure than the law study, and it was difficult, especially for the physicians (Larsen 1989), to reduce their study period. The capacity to accommodate students in the obligatory training courses in different medical subjects was restricted and the medical students therefore often had waiting periods during their time of study (Larsen 1989).

This prolonged the study period for the physicians. For theologians who wished to be ordained as pastors, their obligatory practical training (the practical theological seminary) was additional to all the studying they had done for their degree. (In Table 12.4, the age for finished education is calculated from the year of the degree.)

The figures above do not give an exact illustration of how long each individual student took to complete his education, since we do not know when students started on their studies. Palmstrøm (1935) found that the completion of a normal profession study in the period 1911–1931 took four years for law students, four to five years for theologians, and seven to seven and a half years for medical students. In our material, the law students used an average of six years from passing the examen artium till they had finished their degree, while the theologians used 6.6 years and the physicians used 8.2 years. There were, however, large variations in the time spent on attaining a degree: One lawyer received his degree 18 years after he had passed the examen artium, while one theologian used 14 years and three physicians used 13 years. According to the biographies, several students had to take breaks both before and during their studies so as to earn a living. While studying, the students often found part-time work within their field: the physicians as interns at hospitals, the lawyers as clerks for attorneys, and the theologians as substitute teachers. Some of the students had started their careers in the military: 11 percent of the physicians and the lawyers, and five percent of the theologians, had completed, or partially completed, military school before commencing their studies. Moreover, five of the lawyers had tried studying medicine before switching to law. Two physicians took a degree in law after having practiced medicine for about ten years. They both continued to practice medicine afterwards.

12.4.2 The 1943 Cohort

The careers of the students who passed the examen artium in 1943 got off to a belated start. This was due to the war and the closing of the University of Oslo in the fall of 1943. When they passed the examen artium in 1943, the mean age for the future physicians was significantly lower than that of the future theologians ($p=0.01$) and the future lawyers ($p=0.002$) (Table 12.4). After receiving their degrees, there was still a significant age gap, but this time the physicians were the oldest. Seven years after the examen artium, almost two-thirds of both the lawyers and the theologians had finished their studies, while only seven percent of the physicians had graduated. Ninety-two percent of the theologians had passed their exams after nine years, and 92 percent of the lawyers passed theirs after ten years. For the physicians, it took 13 years after passing the examen artium before 92 percent had received their university degree. The longest time spent on attaining a degree after having passed the examen artium was by the lawyers 21 years, the physicians 19 years, and the theologians 14 years.

Many of the students who passed the examen artium in 1943 spent the time they couldn't use on studying, working in occupations that would be relevant for their later studies. Forty-three (20 percent) of the future lawyers had given the information in the yearbook that they had gone to a commercial school after passing the examen artium, and 29 (14 percent) had gained experience in the police troops in Sweden during the war, or in the police in Norway after the war. Twelve (11 percent) of the future physicians gave the information that they had taken the examen artium once more, or they had taken some other form of education. Possibly they did this to make it easier to be accepted into medical school, since the discipline had been numerus clausus since 1940 (Larsen 1989). Three of the theologians reported that they had worked as teachers, and two had worked in professions connected to religion, while waiting to start their studies. Obviously, the information in the yearbook about work during war time is incomplete. Although only some have given information, most of the students probably had some kind of work while waiting for the war to end.

While the candidates in the 1890–94 cohort, with few exceptions, took their degrees in Oslo, the physicians among the students from 1943 did not follow this pattern. More than 1/4 of the physicians received their education abroad, 23 in Denmark, two in Sweden (out of which one completed his degree as early as 1946), three in Switzerland, two in England, and two in the United States. The large number of physicians educated in Denmark is due to the fact that the Danes opened their universities for Norwegian students because the University in Oslo did not have room for all the medical students after the war. One theologian attained his degree abroad as well; he studied to become a catholic priest in France. Some of the other students in the 1943 cohort received their degrees at the University of Bergen.

12.5 Marriage

In the 1890–94 cohort there was no significant difference in the mean age at the time of the first marriage (Table 12.4), or in the percentage of those who married, between the lawyers, physicians, and theologians. Twenty-five years after passing the examen artium, 77 percent of the lawyers, 82 percent of the physicians, and 84 percent of the theologians had married. Of those who were married, most of them (more than 90 percent) waited to marry until after they had completed their education and secured their position.

Among the students in the 1943 cohort, there were less theologians (83 percent) than physicians (98 percent) and lawyers (95 percent) that married. The figures here are, however, somewhat uncertain, owing to the fact that we do not have information about the maritial status of 43 of the 359 candidates. There was no significant difference in age concerning the first marriage for the three groups of candidates (Table 12.4). In contrast with the students 50 years earlier, many of the students from 1943 did not wait to finish their degrees before marrying. This was especially the case concerning the physicians, among whom 37 percent had already married by the time they received their degree. Corresponding figures for the theologians and the lawyers were 27 percent and 25 percent, respectively. The difference between them and the physicians is significant.

12.6 Careers

12.6.1. The Physicians Became Physicians

The candidates' first position after receiving their degrees, along with their position 25 years after having passed the examen artium, are shown in Tables 12.5, 12.6, and 12.7. Among the physicians in the 1890–94 cohort, close to half of them started their career in a hospital as an intern or a junior resident, while one-third of them had their first job as an assistant in a doctor's office outside of the hospital, or as a substitute for district physicians or physicians in private practice (Table 12.5). Twenty-six physicians (12 percent) opened their own practice directly after having attained their degree. In the period 1915–19, 25 years after having passed the examen artium, 12 percent of the physicians were deceased. Among the remaining physicians, more than 80 percent of them were in positions outside the hospitals, as district physicians or in other public posts, or as private practitioners. Six physicians (three percent) had university positions.

TABLE 12.5
The physicians' first position after graduation, and their position 25 years after the examen artium. Absolute figures.

Position	1890-94 Cohort First	1890-94 Cohort After 25 years	1943 Cohort First	1943 Cohort After 25 years
In the public sector				
– District physicians	9*	31	3	6
– Other publicly appointed physicians	12	28	0	1
In hospitals:				
– Hospital superintendents	0	4	0	0
– Chief physicians	0	7	0	24
– Specialists	0	0	0	8
– Residents	11	7	9	13
– Interns	77	0	23	0
– Other hospital physicians	6	9	22	1
Private practice:				
– General practitioners	26	62	5	13
– Specialists	0	20	0	5
Substitutes	17	0	2	0
Assistant physicians in primary care	48	0	3	0
At the University:				
– Professors, Associate professors	0	4	0	11
– Researchers, Research fellows	1	2	3	2
– Further studies in medicine	2	0	0	0
– Further studies in other subjects	1	0	0	0
Military physicians	2	2	16	1
Other physicians	0	8	5	3
Other professions	0	1	0	0
Without position	1	2	0	1
Unknown position	3	3	22	20
Dead	0	26	0	4
Total	216	216	113	113

* Substitutes

TABLE 12.6
The theologians' first position after graduation, and their position 25 years after the examen artium. Absolute figures.

Position	1890-94 Cohort First	1890-94 Cohort After 25 years	1943 Cohort First	1943 Cohort After 25 years
In the church, missions, etc.				
– Rural dean, Parish pastor	0	29	0	6
– Pastors, Assistant pastors	24	19	5	9
– Missionaires, Seamen's pastors	1	3	2	3
– Catechists, Deacons	5	0	0	0
– Employed in Christian associations	2	4	13	2
In the school system:				
– Principals	6	0	0	2
– Lecturers, Head teachers	0	6	0	8
– Teachers	26	6	2	0
At the University:				
– Professors, Associate professors	0	2	0	0
– Researchers, Research fellows	0	0	0	2
– Further studies in theology	5	0	6	0
– Further studies in other subjects	1	0	1	0
Editors	1	1	1	0
Other professions	1	1	0	1
Without position	0	1	0	0
Unknown position	2	0	4	1
Dead	0	2	0	0
Total	74	74	34	34

For the physicians in the 1943 cohort, information on the first positions is missing for 22 (19 percent), and information on the positions 25 years after the examen artium is missing for 20 (18 percent). Of the remaining, almost 60 percent started off as interns or junior residents at a hospital. As a consequence of the development in the public health service, there were far more physicians in the 1943 cohort who chose a hospital career than had been the case in the cohort 50 years earlier. In 1968, 25 years after the examen artium, more than half of the physicians were working as chief physicians, specialists, or senior residents in hospitals. Many of the physicians also went into scientific careers, and 13 (15 percent of the physicians who gave information on their positions) were in university positions in 1968.

12.6.2. The Theologians Became Pastors or Teachers

When they had finished their degree, the theologians in the 1890-94 cohort had the choice between a career in the church or in the school system, and in choosing their first position, they were quite evenly distributed in both fields (Table 12.6) The school system, however, was seen as only a temporary position by many of the theologians. They committed themselves only to shorter contracts, and then, later, went back to the university to take the practical theological seminary so that they could be ordained as pastors. The fact that many of the theologians went to work in the school system could also be due to the difficult labor market for pastors around the turn of the century. Until the year 1912, it could be difficult to get a position in the Norwegian Church (Palmstrøm 1935). However, in 1915–19, 25 years after the examen artium, three-quarters of the theologians held positions in the church or in a Christian association, and only 17 percent were in the school system. As was the case among the physicians, three percent of the theologians had university positions 25 years after the examen artium.

Among the theologians who passed the examen artium 50 years later, there was a larger percentage (two-thirds) who started off in a position in the church or in a Christian association right away. The number of theologians in the school system increased with time, and 25 years after the examen artium about 30 percent of them were appointed in the school system. Two theologians (six percent) were in university positions.

12.6.3. The Lawyers Became Attorneys, Businessmen, or Government Officials

The lawyers who completed their degrees around the turn of the century had more positions to choose from than their fellow-students in medicine and theology had. Fifty-six percent of those who gave information on their first position started their careers as an assistant for a district stipendary magistrate or a bailiff (Table 12.7). Another nine percent started off in other positions in the public sector. With the exception of those who continued their studies, or who joined the military, the remaining new lawyers started up in positions in the private sector of the economy (8 percent) or as attorneys' assistants (16 percent) or public attorneys (7 percent).

Twenty-five years after the examen artium, 48 lawyers (14 percent) were dead, and 13 were in unknown positions. Among the remaining lawyers, almost two-thirds of them were in private positions, either as attorneys or as businessmen. The rest of the lawyers were to be found in the public sector, most of them in government appointed positions. Only two lawyers (less that one percent) were in university positions 25 years after the examen artium.

In the 1943 cohort, information about the first position is missing for 41 (19 percent) of the lawyers. Among the remaining lawyers, the percentage that started in the public sector was somewhat lower than 50 years earlier. But still, almost half of all the lawyers started their career there. The ministries provided for a large number of the work places. Twenty percent of the lawyers started in the private sector of the economy, and 23 percent started in a private practice; either as assistants, or owning their own practice. No lawyers were working for the press, which 50 years earlier had been a place of work for several lawyers.

In 1968, 25 years after the examen artium, the lawyers were fairly evenly apportioned between the public sector (47 percent) and the private sector (45 percent). An university career, on the other hand, does not seem to have been a very popular choice. Even though ten lawyers continued their studies after having completed their degrees, none of them were to be found in

TABLE 12.7
The lawyers' first position after graduation, and their position 25 years after the examen artium. Absolute figures.

	1890–94 Cohort		1943 Cohort	
Position	First	After 25 years	First	After 25 years
The public sector				
– Deputy secretaries, Undersecretaries, Assistant secretaries	0	21	0	11
– Other positions in the Ministry	7	15	40	25
– Lawyers in other government institutions	6	9	7	17
– Regional commisionaires, District stipendiary magistrates, Bailiffs	1	8	0	1
– Assistants at the office of the district stipendiary magistrate or the bailiffs office	181	1	0	0
– County and township administration	6	6	11	22
– Judges	1	10	0	2
– Registrars	0	0	17	2
– Chief of police	0	11	0	0
– Police inspectors, State attorneys	4	11	6	10
– Employed at Norwegian embassies	4	4	0	2
Private practice				
– Solicitors, Attorneys	21	132	9	34
– Assistants of solicitors and attorneys	51	0	31	1
In the private sector of the economy:				
– Directors, Presidents	3	15	2	16
– Lawyers in private companies	11	19	30	26
– Lawyers in employers' associations	1	0	2	12
– Editors, Owners of newspapers	3	10	0	0
– Editorial secretaries, Journalists	7	4	0	0
At the University:				
– Professors, Associate professors	0	1	0	0
– Researchers, Research fellows	0	1	1	0
– Further studies in law	2	0	6	0
– Further studies in other subjects	4	0	3	0
Other lawyers	2	0	1	4
Military officers	5	3	5	4
Other professions	0	4	0	6
Without position	1	0	0	1
Unknown position	25	13	41	13
Dead	0	48	0	3
Total	346	346	212	212

university positions 25 years after the examen artium.

12.6.4. A Comparison Of the Three Professions' Careers

This survey of the careers of physicians, lawyers, and theologians shows that the physicians stood out from both the theologians and the lawyers by having such a small dispersion of positions. Almost all of the medical students started working as physicians when they had finished their degree, and they were still to be found in medical positions 25 years after the examen artium. In contrast to the physicians, who could only choose between various medical positions, and the theologians, who could choose between positions in the church or in the school system, the lawyers had far more positions to choose from. In the public sector, it was possible for the lawyers to find work in the public administration, in the county and community administrations, in the courts or in the police. In the private sector of the economy, they found positions in the business world or in the press, or else they became attorneys.

All three of the professions had their career ladders. The physicians started off as interns, and later on became district physicians or opened their own private practice. In the cohort from 1943, the position as a chief physician also had become a quite widely held position. The theologians became parish pastors or rural deans, while those who entered the school system, became head teachers or principals. (There were also some theologians who started off as principals, but only in small elementary schools in sparsely populated areas). The lawyers became chiefs of police or were placed in high-ranking positions in the ministries. Others pursued their careers in their own private practices or in high-ranking positions in the business world.

All of the three professions had the possibility of finding positions in both the public and the private sectors, although the private sector had rather few positions to offer the theologians. Some of them worked as secretaries in Christian associations. In the 1890-94 cohort, there was a tendency for physicians and lawyers to start off in the public sector, and then switch over to the private sector later on. Fifty years later, there was still a large percentage of the two professions which started off in the public sector. But, at the same time, there was now a larger percentage of those who decided to stay on in the public sector. The physicians continued as hospital physicians, while the lawyers worked in the county administrations or in the government departments.

Thirteen of the students who passed the examen artium in the period 1890–94 had defended their academic thesis 25 years later. Out of these, six were physicians, five were lawyers and two were theologians. One of the theologians, however, did not defend his academic thesis in theology, but in linguistics. Among the students who passed the examen artium in 1943, the doctorates were less widespread. Eighteen out of the 19 thesis were done by physicians, while the remaining one was completed by a theologian. One explanation for the large amount of theses among the physicians could be that their clinical activity – the practical part of the profession – as well as the research, were often closely linked. This meant that the university professor could, for example, also be a chief physician in a clinical ward. In the other two professions, a university career could mean giving up the practical part of their profession

12.7 The Careers of the Female Candidates

The female candidates are included in the description above. Still, it might be of interest to take a closer look at their careers.

Among the students who passed the examen artium between 1890 and 1894, there were 73 women (about six percent), out of which 18 (25 percent) took their degree in law, medicine, or theology (Studenterne fra 1890, 1891, 1892, 1893, 1894). In 1943, the percentage of females among the students who passed the examen artium had risen to about 34 percent, but of these only about two percent took a degree in one of the three disciplines (Møller 1968). The decline in the percentage of women with the examen artium completing a higher education is also shown by Palmstrøm (1935). The percentage of women among the graduates in law, theology, and medicine, however, doubled in the 50-year-period. Among the students in the 1890–94 cohort, three percent were women, while the percentage had increased to six percent in the 1943 cohort. Among the female candidates in the 1890-94 cohort, there were mainly physicians (13 out of 18), while lawyers made up the largest group (15 out of 20) in the 1943 cohort (Table 12.1).

Of the 18 women in the 1890-94 cohort, one physician chose not to practice, and one physician and one lawyer continued their studies, while the rest started to work in their profession. Twenty-five years after the examen artium, one lawyer had died, two physicians had limited practices, and one physician was not practicing. Only seven out of the eighteen women who completed their degrees got married. The three physicians who were not working full-time belonged to this group.

Diagram 12.1

The examen artium students of 1890–94. The region[1] of birth for lawyers (n=344), physicians (n=215), and theologians (n=74). Percent.

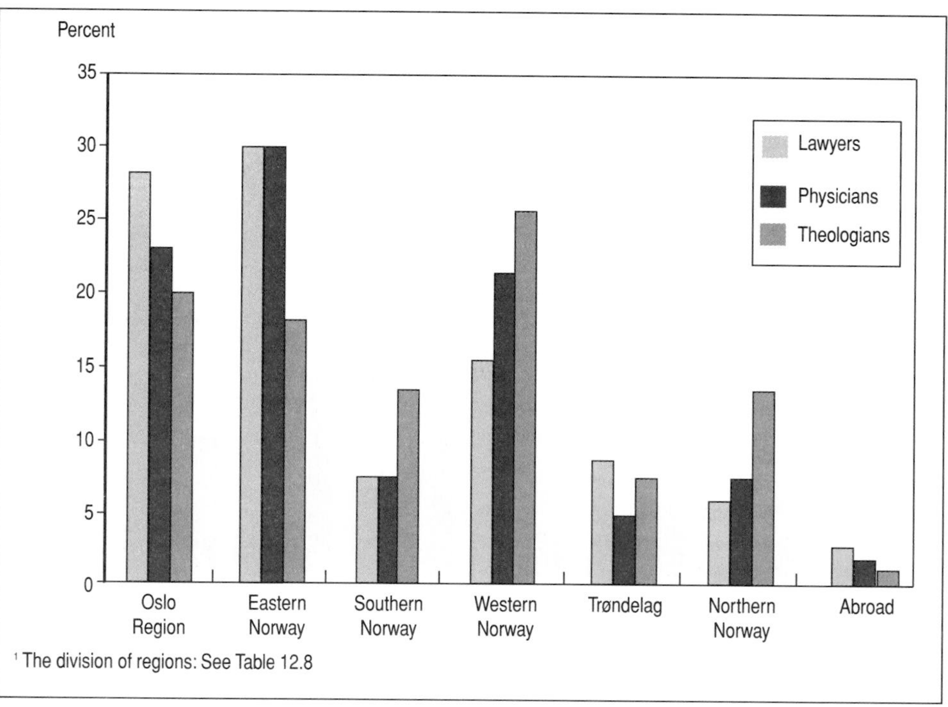

[1] The division of regions: See Table 12.8

Out of the 20 women in the 1943 cohort, we have information on the first position of 16 of them. They all started off in positions that were relevant to their educations. Twenty-five years after the examen artium, 15 of the women were working within their line of work, while two of them, a lawyer and a physician, were housewives. Two lawyers and one theologian were in unknown positions. The percentage of married women in the 1943 cohort was greater than it had been 50 years earlier. Fourteen of the 20 women had married and three remained unmarried. We do not have information on the marital status for the three remaining women.

12.8 Mobility

12.8.1 The 1890–94 Cohort

Diagram 12.1 shows the region of birth for the students in the 1890-94 cohort. The theologians stood out from the physicians and the lawyers by having a larger percentage born outside of the Oslo and Eastern Norway regions. The difference is significant ($p<0.02$).

The location of the first position after graduation is shown in Diagram 12.2. A large percentage of the theologians (38 percent) stayed on in the Oslo region after having completed their degrees. The reason for this is probably that many of the theolo-

DIAGRAM 12.2

The examen artium students of 1890–94. The region[1] of the first residence after graduation for lawyers (n=311), physicians (n=202), and theologians (n=68). Percent.

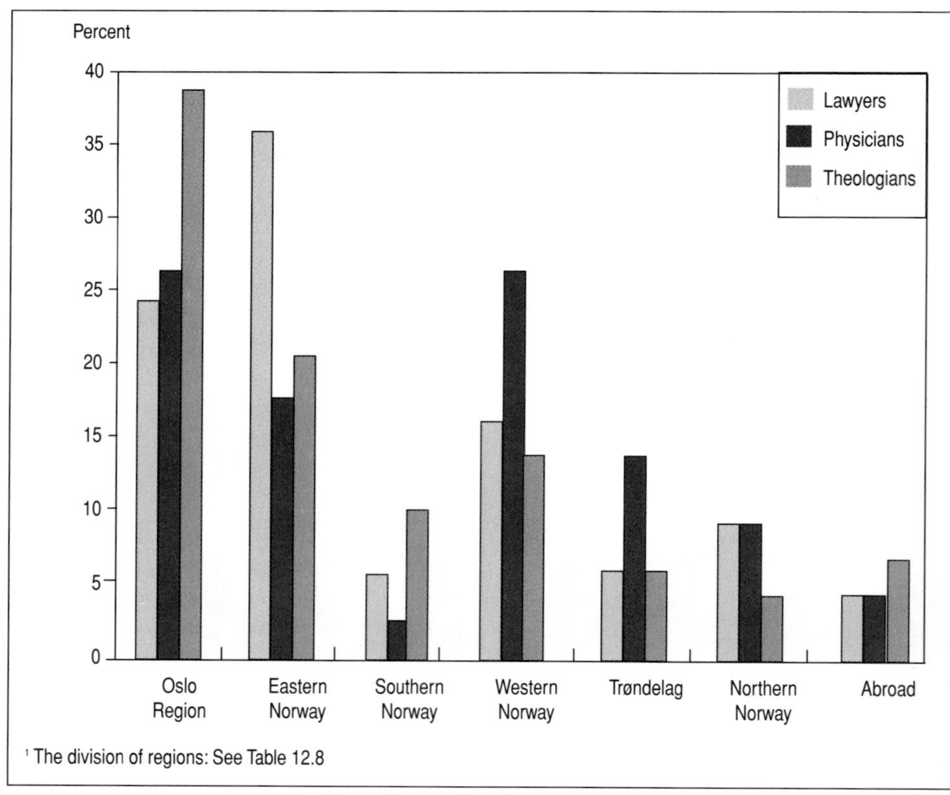

[1] The division of regions: See Table 12.8

TABLE 12.8

The lawyers in the 1890–94 cohort. Region[1] of birth and region of residence 25 years after the examen artium (n=286, 60 missing). Percent.

Region of residence 25 years after the examen artium	Region of birth								
	Oslo Region	Eastern Norway	Southern Norway	Western Norway	Trøndelag	Northern Norway	Abroad	Total %	n=
Oslo Region	74	45	42	32	32	32	83	50	143
Eastern Norway	4	39	8	9	14	11	0	17	49
Southern Norway	0	1	33	0	0	0	0	3	9
Western Norway	6	4	0	41	9	16	17	12	33
Trøndelag	4	3	4	2	32	0	0	5	15
Northern Norway	5	4	8	7	9	32	0	7	21
Abroad	7	2	4	9	5	11	0	6	16
Total %	100	98	99	100	101	102	100	100	
n=	82	89	24	44	22	19	6		286

[1] The division of regions: The counties are categorized as follows: The Oslo Region consists of Oslo and Akershus; the Eastern Norway consists of Østfold, Hedemark, Oppland, Buskerud, Vestfold, and Telemark; the Southern part of Norway is Aust-Agder and Vest-Agder; the Western Norway is Rogaland, Hordaland, Sogn og Fjordane, and Møre og Romsdal; Trøndelag consists of Sør-Trøndelag and Nord-Trøndelag; while Northern Norway refers to Nordland, Troms, and Finnmark.

Diagram 12.3

The examen artium students of 1943. The region[1] of birth for lawyers (n=209), physicians (n=112), and theologians (n=33). Percent.

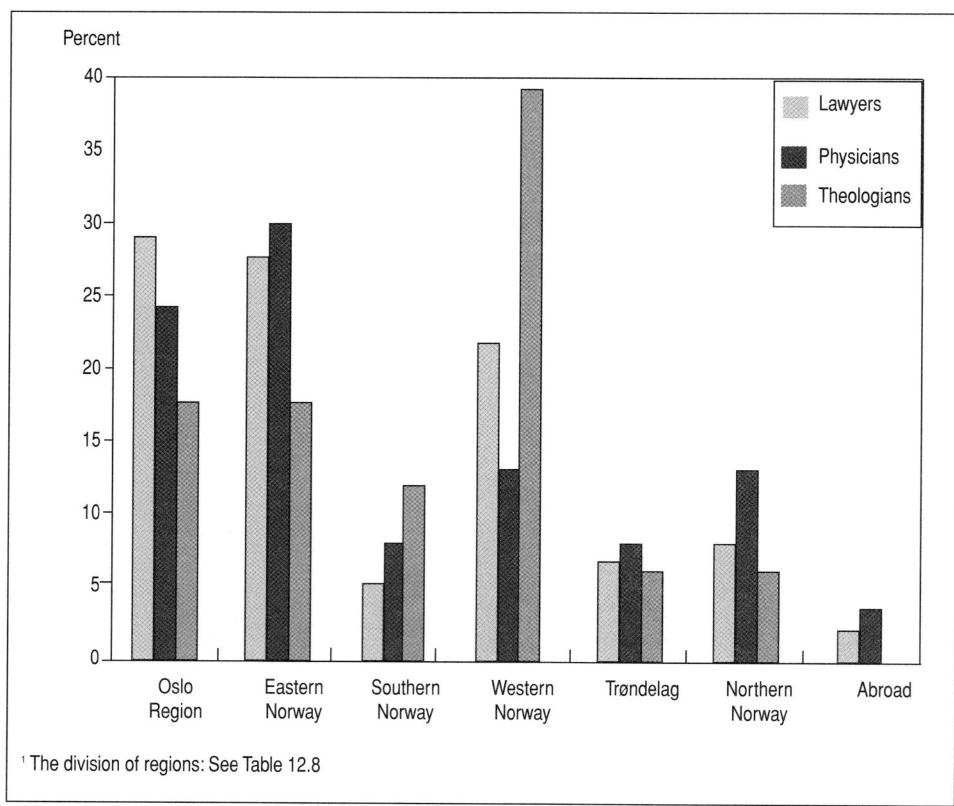

[1] The division of regions: See Table 12.8

gians were substitute teachers in Oslo for shorter periods before their enrolement in the practical theological seminary; 16 out of the 26 theologians who had their first position in the Oslo region were teachers, and they all lived in the capital. Diagram 12.2 also shows that the newly educated physicians left the Oslo and the Eastern Norway regions to a greater extent than both the lawyers and the theologians did. The number of physicians who went to the Western Norway region was especially high. As earlier shown in Table 12.5, many of the physicians found their first position as an assistant physician for a district physician or for a private practitioner. And, even though most of the intern positions were situated in hospitals in the Oslo region, there were also medical interns located in hospitals in other parts of the country.

It was, however, not completly coincidental where the new university graduates ended up in the country. Nineteen percent of the physicians in the 1890–94 cohort had their first job in the exact same place as they were born, while the corresponding percentage for lawyers was 16 percent and for theologians nine percent. More than half of these graduates were from Oslo, and they remained in the town. Among those who went back to their place of birth outside of Oslo, there were some physicians who had

TABLE 12.9

The physicians in the 1890–94 cohort. Region[1] of birth and region of residence 25 years after the examen artium (n=186, 30 missing). Percent.

	Region of birth								
Region of residence 25 years after the examen artium	Oslo Region	Eastern Norway	Southern Norway	Western Norway	Trøndelag	Northern Norway	Abroad	Total %	n=
Oslo Region	57	25	19	21	11	29	40	31	57
Eastern Norway	21	43	13	5	11	7	40	23	43
Southern Norway	5	3	25	5	0	0	0	5	10
Western Norway	7	11	13	56	11	14	0	20	37
Trøndelag	0	3	13	3	55	7	0	6	11
Northern Norway	2	5	6	8	11	29	20	8	14
Abroad	7	10	13	3	0	14	0	8	14
Total %	99	100	102	101	99	100	100	101	
n=	42	61	16	39	9	14	5		186

[1] The division of regions: See table 12.8

DIAGRAM 12.4

The examen artium students of 1943. The region[1] of the first residence after graduation for lawyers (n=148), physicians (n=86), and theologians (n=25). Percent.

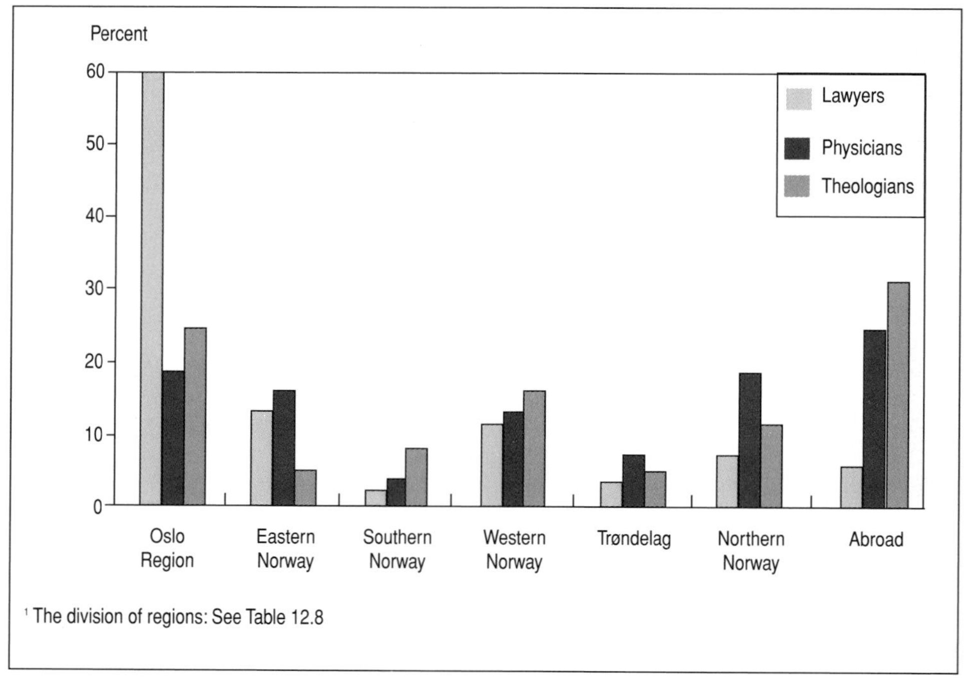

[1] The division of regions: See Table 12.8

their first job working as an assistant physician for their fathers, who also were physicians. In some cases, a physician or a theologian is mentioned to have had his first position working for his father, but that the latter at the time was living in a different location than where his son had been born.

Norwegians have the tendency to move back to the region in which they were born, or to the Oslo or the Eastern Norway regions (Østby 1970, SSB 1975). Tables 12.8, 12.9, and 12.10, show the location of residence 25 years after the examen artium, as well as the place of birth, for the students in the 1890-94 cohort. The tables confirms the tendencies shown for Norwegians in general, namely that the candidates either settled down in the region where they were born, or they took up residence in the Oslo or Eastern Norway regions. There was a significantly larger percentage (67 percent) of lawyers that settled down in the Oslo or Eastern Norway regions, compared to the physicians (54 percent) and the theologians (53 percent).

12.8.2. The 1943 Cohort

When it comes to the students who passed the examen artium in 1943, Diagram 12.3 shows that there still were a higher percentage of the theologians than the physicians and lawyers who were born outside of the Oslo and Eastern Norway regions. There were especially many theologians from the Western part of the country (39 percent). However, our material contains only 34 theologians, so the figures should be analyzed with care. As had been the case 50 years earlier, more than half of the physicians and the lawyers were from the Oslo or Eastern Norway regions.

TABLE 12.10

The theologians in the 1890–94 cohort. Region[1] of birth and region of residence 25 years after the examen artium (n=69, 5 missing). Percent.

	Region of birth								
Region of residence 25 years after the examen artium	Oslo Region	Eastern Norway	Southern Norway	Western Norway	Trøndelag	Northern Norway	Abroad	Total %	n=
Oslo Region	38	38	20	24	0	33	0	28	19
Eastern Norway	31	31	10	18	50	22	0	25	17
Southern Norway	8	8	10	6	0	0	0	6	4
Western Norway	0	0	60	47	33	11	0	25	17
Trøndelag	0	8	0	6	17	0	0	4	3
Northern Norway	8	15	0	0	0	22	0	7	5
Abroad	15	0	0	0	0	11	100	6	4
Total %	100	100	100	101	100	99	100	101	
n=	13	13	10	17	6	9	1		69

[1] The division of regions: See table 12.8

Diagram 12.4 shows the first location of residence after having completed their degree for the students in the 1943 cohort. A significantly higher percentage of the lawyers than the physicians and theologians settled down in Oslo and the Eastern Norway regions. As a result of the fact that a large percentage of the lawyers in question held their first positions in a ministry, almost 60 percent of them ended up in the Oslo region after receiving their degree. The physicians were distributed fairly evenly throughout the country, as well as abroad. Tweny-one physicians held their first position outside of Norway. Out of these, 14 were in Sweden or Denmark, where some of them had completed their education. Four physicians had their first positions as military physicians abroad, out of which three served in the Norwegian brigade posted in Germany. Among the theologians, there was also quite a large percentage that traveled abroad after finishing their degree; two took positions in the seaman's mission, while six others continued their studies abroad.

The connection between the place of birth and the location of residence 25 years after the examen artium have also been analyzed for the 1943 cohort. As was the case for the students 50 years earlier, most of them could be found in the region where they were born, or in the Oslo and Eastern Norway regions. And, as was the case for the 1890-94 cohort, there was a significantly larger percentage of lawyers (74 percent) than theologians (56 percent) and physicians (54 percent) that lived in the Oslo and Eastern Norway regions.

12.9 Summary

This comparison between two cohorts of physicians, lawyers, and theologians from the turn of the century and then 50 years later, shows that the physicians and the lawyers had fairly similar backgrounds: the largest group was from the business community. The theologians, on the other hand, had a larger percentage with backgrounds in the agricultural population. In both cohorts, the physicians had the lowest mean age at the time they passed the examen artium, but they were, on an average, older than the other candidates when they received their degree. This was primarily due to the fact that medicine was a restricted study that permitted few liberties, and therefore made it difficult for the students to shorten the time spent on it. When it comes to their careers, the physicians stood out from the theologians and the lawyers in terms of the dispersion of their positions. Almost all of the physicians started off working in the medical profession when they had completed their studies, and they stayed there. The theologians had two main choices: to become clergymen or teachers. As for the lawyers, there was wide range of professional possibilities that was open to them, everything from various public positions, to business and private practice as attorneys. It seems that the physicians chose, to a larger extent than the theologians and the lawyers, to pursue an university career, something that led to a larger number of academic theses being produced by the physicians.

Among the students who passed the examen artium in the period 1890–94, only a few got married before they had finished their degrees. This was not so much the situation 50 years later. Among the students in the 1943 cohort, there was an especially large number of physicians who married before they had attained their degrees.

Even though the percentage of female students with examen artium who took a higher education decreased during the 50 years between 1890–94 and 1943, the percentage of women among the candidates who received their degrees doubled during the same period. However, when it came to selecting studies, their choices had changed.

Among the female candidates in the 1890–94 cohort, most were physicians, while lawyers were in the majority 50 years later. Most of the women who took a degree went into positions that had relevance to their educations. The percentage of female candidates who married was largest in the 1943 cohort.

A survey done on the mobility patterns showed that the physicians in the 1890-94 cohort, to a larger extent than was the case for the lawyers and theologians, found their first post outside of the Oslo and Estern Norway regions. Fifty years later, the physicians were still being posted all over the country when they first started their careers, while the lawyers mainly settled down in the Oslo region after having attained their degree. Twenty-five years after the examen artium, all the groups in the two cohorts showed clear tendencies towards following the Norwegian migration pattern: they were either living in the region in which they were born, or in the Oslo and Eastern Norway regions.

References

Aubert, T., U. Torgersen, T. Lindbekk and S. Pollan. "Akademikere i norsk samfunnsstruktur 1850-1950," *Tidsskrift for samfunnsforskning*,1,4(1960):185–248.

Larsen, Ø. *Mangfoldig medisin*. Oslo: Universitetet i Oslo, Det medisinske fakultet, 1989.

Møller, D.J. *Studentene fra 1943*. Oslo: Oscar Andersens Boktrykkeri, 1968.

Palmstrøm, H. "Om en befolkningsgruppes utvikling gjennom de siste 100 år," *Statsøkonomisk tidsskrift*,49(1935):161–370.

SSB. *Flyttingene i Norge 1971 og 1949–1973*. Rapport nr. 3 fra Flyttemotivundersøkelsen 1972. Oslo: Statistisk Sentralbyrå, 1975.

Studenterne fra 1890. Kristiania: Grøndahl og Søns boktrykkeri, 1915.

Studenterne fra 1891. Kristiania: Grøndahl og Søns boktrykkeri, 1916.

Studenterne fra 1892. Kristiania: Grøndahl og Søns boktrykkeri, 1917.

Studenterne fra 1893. Kristiania: Grøndahl og Søns boktrykkeri, 1918.

Studenterne fra 1894. Kristiania: Grøndahl og Søns boktrykkeri, 1919.

Torgersen, U. *Profesjonssosiologi*. Oslo-Bergen-Tromsø: Universitetsforlaget, 1972.

Østby, L. *Geografisk mobilitet. En gjennomgåelse av dens teoretiske grunnlag, og behandling av flyttingene i Norge 1966–1967*. 1–2, Oslo: Meddelelser fra Geografisk Institutt, Universitetet i Oslo, Kulturgeografisk serie nr. 4, 1970.

CHAPTER 13

Knowledge and Implications - Information Diffusion Among Norwegian Doctors

CHAPTER 13.1

Scientific Literature and the Shaping of a Medical Profession in Norway

MAGNE NYLENNA

13.1.1. Introduction

Scientific journals and medical literature are crucial elements in the shaping of the medical profession.

Journals keep doctors united by giving them a sense of identity and making them share common values. Journals develop a common language that is only partly understood by outsiders. Journals contribute to the training of doctors, the setting of standards and limits for medical activities, and the definition of a professional role. Through journals, the professional "masters" can even exercise power over the members. All these features are fundamental parts of a sociological definition of a profession (Table 13.1) (Goode 1957).

But none of these qualities was the reason for establishing the early scientific and medical journals. Their main purpose was to communicate information, enabling scientists to bring their work before the public and doctors to share their experience and theories with colleagues.

Analyzing the impact of scientific literature on the shaping of a medical profession

TABLE 13.1
Sociological characteristics of a profession (Goode 1957)

- Its members are bound by a sense of identity.
- Once in it, few leave, so that, for the most part, it is a terminal or continuing status.
- Its members share values in common.
- Its role definitions vis-à-vis both members and non-members are agreed upon and are the same for all the members.
- Within the areas of communal action there is a common language that is understood only partially by outsiders.
- The community has power over its members.
- Its limits are reasonably clear, though they are not physical and geographical, but social.
- Though it does not produce the next generation biologically, it does so socially. Through its control over the selection of professional trainees, and through its training processes, it sends these recruits through an adult socialisation process.

is no easy matter. No real history of medical journalism has been written so far, and few records exist other than the published articles and books themselves (Burnham 1990). While libraries and data bases provide a good overview of what has been authored and printed over the years, our knowledge of what has actually been read and used of the published literature is limited. Neither the number of books printed, nor the circulation of the various journals, nor the citation rates of the papers themselves are valid indicators of their importance. And the significance of the medical literature as a whole and of medical journalism as a historic phenomenon is another thing altogether, and quite different from the meaning of individual articles and published works. The development of a profession is a complex process, and it is hard to separate and define the influence and impact of one single factor, such as scientific literature.

13.1.2 The History of Medical Publication

The story of medical publication reflects the history of medical practice and science. A chronological review of the most important works in medicine and related sciences reveals not only the progress of medical science, but also developments in medical publishing. A bibliography of almost 9,000 major contributions to the medical literature shows when and how the various discoveries and breakthroughs were made public, and shows the development of organizations of health care (Norman 1991).

The oldest known medical work, the code of Hammurabi, King of Babylon about 2000 b.c., mentions the fees payable to a physician following successful treatment, and the punishment if an operation was a failure (Norman (ed) 1991). Documents on medicine and other sciences are found in the papyrus libraries of Ancient Egypt. Later on, parchment, made from the skin of sheep or goats, was used for medical writing, a practice that continued throughout the Middle Ages, mainly in the scriptoria of monasteries (Warren 1991). Paper replaced parchment in the thirteenth and fourteenth centuries, and the invention of printing in the fifteenth century led to many more books of scientific relevance for medicine being published over the following centuries, stimulated by the scientific revolution during the same period. Medical papers were published mainly in the proceedings of the learned societies (Booth 1982).

Up to the end of the Middle Ages, there was no clear distinction between medical literature for the lay public and scientific publications written for physicians and scientists. Medical books and herbals for example, from the School of Salerno reflect the medical knowledge and accepted treatments and remedies at that time, and indicate the advice to be given to patients. During the seventeeth and eighteenth centuries, the medical literature became divided into two branches: scientific literature intended for professionals and the popular literature intended for the general public. The latter became further divided into two categories: publications on preventive medicine and publications on treatment of specific symptoms and diseases (Larsen 1966a, Larsen 1966b).

The scientific journal was invented in the seventeenth century. The first independent scientific journal, Journal des savants, was published by the French Academy in Paris on January 5, 1665, and the Philosophical Transactions of the Royal Society in London came out a few months later. These were followed by similar publications by other national academies. The standards were variable and the contents covered a wide field of interests.

During the late seventeenth and the eighteenth centuries the natural sciences advanced on a broad front. Many more specific and scientific medical journals appeared, based mainly on papers read before medical societies. Most of these journals did not last for long, like the Acta of the Royal Medical and Philosophical Society in Copenhagen, which was established in 1681, and the first medical journal in Britain, which appeared in Edinburgh in 1731 and was called Medicinal Essays and Observations (Booth 1982).

An example of a medical publication from the Age of Enlightenment is found in the educational and public-oriented journal Sundhetstidende, published in Copenhagen from 1778 to 1781 by Johann Clemens Tode (1736–1806) (Larsen 1991). Modeled on French publications, Tode founded a journal of preventive medicine that was aimed at educating the public about medical topics. This was the first popular medical journal to be published in the Nordic countries, and Tode introduced a new literary genre in his publication, in which he emphasized reports and abstracts based on foreign dissertations and research and the popularization of scientific progress.

Scientific medical journals as we know them today with a mixed content of original research, reviews, comments, and debate, date back to the early nineteenth century (Lock 1992). Not until then were any medical journals of a high quality established on a permanent basis. These were general medical journals covering the entire universe of medicine and including not only clinical topics but a wide variety of topics related to medical practice, social affairs, and health politics. The oldest of these journals still in existence are Bibliothek for Læger, established in Denmark by Det Classenske Literatur Selskab in 1809, the Transactions of the Medical Society of London (now the Journal of the Royal Society of Medicine) (established in 1810), the New England Journal of Medicine (1812), and the Lancet (1823). By the turn of the century most developed countries had general medical journals of their own.

By the mid-nineteenth century both the content and the structure of each article, and of the journal as a whole, had come to resemble the articles and medical journals as we know them today. Compared with today's articles, the ones published in the nineteenth century were more personal in style and often much longer. Even though the so-called IMRAD-structure of scientific papers (an introduction stating the background for the study, a methods section describing how the study was performed, a results section presenting the findings, and a separate discussion section interpreting these findings) was first identified specifically by Sir Austin Bradford Hill in the 1960s (Bradford Hill 1965), research articles had included the elements of this structure for more than 100 years.

According to Stephen Lock, former editor of the British Medical Journal, medical journals had three striking features up to the end of the Second World War: there was a preponderance of printed orations and lectures by the great medical names, most clinical reports were of an anecdotal nature, and many contributions that would now be signed were then anonymous (Lock 1991).

The growth in the number of scientific journals has remained stable at around seven percent a year since the seventeenth century, giving a doubling time of approximately ten years (de Solla Price 1961, de Solla Price 1981). This corresponds with the growth of the sciences during the same period.

In 1840 there were probably no more than 300 scientific journals in the whole world. In 1990 the total was about 100,000, some 25,000 of which were devoted to the biomedical field. The National Library of Medicine now records about 600 new journals annually in the field of medicine alone (Lock 1990).

Peer review, the evaluation of papers by the author's "peers," was a feature of the first scientific journals in the seventeenth century. For the next 300 years this system was used intermittently to improve the quality of scientific reports. After the Second World War, peer review was introduced in most medical journals as a replacement for or supplement to the personal judgments made by the editor alone. Editorial peer reviewing appeared independently of grant peer reviewing, and has been taken up by different journals, if somewhat unsystematically. One reason for introducing peer review may be to improve quality assurance; another may be problems in handling an increasing number of submitted manuscripts and meeting the demands of an increasingly specialized world (Burnham 1990). Today three out of four western scientific journals use peer review for assessment of original articles before publication (Lock 1991). The use of external referees to assess the quality of the submitted papers and advise editors on the priority of publication is now a characteristic of scientific journals, and makes publishing an integral part of the research process, not merely a matter of printing and distributing manuscripts. Most referees do their work without payment or compensation, as a part of their general academic duties, thus underlining the integrated role of publishing in the medical community. The referee is seen as a specialist adviser to the editor, not a decisionmaker. The editor will normally tell the author the reason why a paper was rejected, and the referee will likewise be informed of the fate of the paper, including any reasons why his or her advice was not followed (Lock 1985).

Another main characteristic of a scientific journal is that it is usually indexed in international data bases, thereby making its articles searchable and retrievable for researchers and clinicians. The National Library of Medicine, Bethesda, Maryland, which is the largest medical library in the world, has indexed scientific literature since 1879. Its main data base, Index Medicus, available as Medline and searchable online in Norway since 1973, is the single most important collection of articles of relevance to physicians.

13.1.3 Medical Publication in Norway

The first printing machine in Norway was introduced in Christiania (the former name for Oslo) in 1643, later than in any other European country. Another 78 years passed before the second printing office was established, this time in Bergen, the largest Norwegian city at that time (Høyer 1995).

The birth of the Norwegian press is normally dated to May 25, 1763, with the launching of the newspaper Norske Intelligenz-Seddeler. It is hard to distinguish between the different kinds of periodicals, such as newspapers and journals, that were published before 1800. Several Norwegian publications were established in the late eighteenth century (Høyer 1995).

After more than 400 years of Danish rule, Norway acquired its own Constitution in 1814. The first Norwegian university, Universitas regia Fredericiana, was established by Royal Decree of September 2, 1811, and the Medical School was established with three professors and three students in 1814 (Larsen 1989). Rikshospitalet, the National Hospital of Norway, was opened in 1826. Before then, there had been hardly any scientific production by Norwegian doctors, and Norwegian medical publications were few and far between.

13.1.3.1 Books

Medical books in Norway from the Middle Ages are all translations and compilations, mainly from Denmark. The most famous Nordic physician at that time, the Dane Henrik Harpestreng (1164–1244), has left behind several herbals and manuscripts based on the traditions from the School of Salerno (Reichborn-Kjennerud 1924). Fragments of an Old Norwegian translation from the last part of the fourteenth century has been found (Larsen 1989). Later on, the medical books of great importance in all Nordic countries were those by a Dane, Christiern Pedersen (dead 1554), and especially another Dane, Henrik Smid (1495–1563) (Larsen 1966b, Reichborn-Kjennerud 1924).

In a review of the history of medical books in Norway, Reichborn-Kjennerud (1865–1949) underlines the importance of the Harpestreng manuscripts, the Dublin manuscript (a hand-written manuscript found in the Royal Irish Academy in Dublin and probably written by an Icelander in a monastery in Bergen in the fifteenth century) and medical books from Iceland and Denmark (Reichborn-Kjennerud 1936).

The first medical publication printed in Norway in the Norwegian language is said to be the pamphlet "Kongs-Kildevands Beskrivelse" by City Medical Officer Johan Christopher Lincke (dead 1761) from 1745 (Reichborn-Kjennerud 1936). "Radesygen" (probably a kind of endemic syphilis) was the topic of a few publications in the early nineteenth century, notably the dissertation by Frederik Holst (1791–1871), defended in Christiania in 1817.

As medical publication developed, and a clearer distinction was made between information for the lay public and professional literature for doctors, it became a more common practice in all countries to publish original research in scientific periodicals rather than in books.

Medical books for professionals fall into four main categories: general textbooks, specialized textbooks, monographs on specific topics, and updated review series (Oldershaw 1992). In addition, there are catalogues and reference books of a more or less authorized nature (e.g., on pharmaceutical preparations, classification of diseases, institutions, etc.). Owing to the small number of physicians in Norway, the market for medical books in Norwegian has always been limited. Books intended exclusively for Norwegian doctors have been produced, but the majority of textbooks used by medical students and doctors in training have been in foreign languages. In the 1990s, it is estimated that 80 percent of the literature read by medical students is in English, and the proportion of such reading in the Norwegian language is declining (Kallevik 1993). The medical journals have always had, and still have, a common Nordic marketplace, but Norwegian physicians turn to international textbooks, German ones in the beginning of this century, and later mainly British and American. A survey of reading habits among Norwegian doctors in 1990 showed that all categories of physicians reported spending approximately one hour reading material other than journals and articles, mainly textbooks and reference works, out of a total reading time of 3 to 4 hours a week (Nylenna 1991).

During the nineteenth century, most Norwegian literature of all kinds was published by Danish publishers. Even though some Norwegian publishing houses were established earlier (John Grieg 1721, Grøndahl & Søn 1812, J. W. Cappelen 1829, N.W. Damm & Søn 1843, Fabritius & Sønner 1844, Alb. Cammermeyer 1867, H. Aschehoug & Co. 1872), it was not until Gyldendal Norsk Forlag was bought from Denmark by Norwegians in 1925 that the national publishing industry started to flourish.

Based on the students' welfare organization at the University of Oslo, an organization for the purpose of publishing and distributing textbooks and teaching material for students was established in 1935 (Universitetets studentkontor). This led to the founding of the publishing house Akademisk Forlag in 1950, which has been called Universitetsforlaget (the Norwegian University Press) since 1956. In the 1950s the regulations for academic dissertations in

Norway required that doctoral theses should be published in the form of a book, which created a significant market for scientific literature. Close cooperation between the Norwegian University Press and the Norwegian Research Council resulted in a "service office" for scientific authors in 1957, and the same year the Norwegian University Press published 50 scientific books and 20 journals (Egeland 1996). Over the years, the selection of topics for Norwegian medical books seems to be more or less coincidental, but one guiding principle has been to produce books on national, specific issues and in fields where the international literature is not very relevant for medical students and physicians in Norway. One of the best examples is the book "Veileder i praktisk sosialmedisin" (Guide in practical social medicine), by Arne Marthinsen (born 1926), Eva Koren, and Axel Strøm (1901–1985), first published in 1955. Since 1975 Rolf Hanoa (born 1942) has been author of this book, of which the 14th edition was published in 1990. In some fields of medicine there have never existed any literature in the Norwegian language. But for example in psychiatry, there have been two comprehensive textbooks by Norwegian authors since early 1970s (Egeland 1996).

The Norwegian University Press now publishes 15 to 20 medical books in Norwegian annually, with an average circulation of 2,000 copies (Kallevik 1993). The production of major textbooks for the Norwegian market alone is too costly for such textbooks to be able to compete with international literature.

After taking over the Swedish publishing house Almqvist & Wiksell in 1991 and in cooperation with the Danish publisher Akademisk Forlag, the Norwegian University Press formed Scandinavian University Press, the largest publisher of scientific and scholarly journals in Scandinavia. Scandinavian University Press publishes (1996) more than 110 journals, about 30 of them medical ones.

13.1.3.2 Journals

According to a survey of journals and periodicals in Norway up to 1920 (Table 13.2), few journals in medicine and related fields were established until the last decades of the nineteenth century. By the turn of the century, most health professions (pharmacists, midwives, dentists, etc.) had their own journals (Tveterås 1984).

In 1823 the first Norwegian general science journal, Magazin for Naturvidenskaberne, was founded, and a few medical articles were included during the following years.

The first Norwegian medical journal Eyr (named after Eir, a medical goddess in the Nordic mythology) was established in 1826 by Michael Skjelderup (1769–1852), the first professor in medicine at the new university, and Frederik Holst. Eleven volumes

TABLE 13.2
Growth of journals and periodicals in Norway up to 1920 (Tveterås 1984)

Year of foundation	Journals in medicine and related fields	All journals
Before 1800	–	37
1800–10	–	13
1811–20	–	14
1821–30	1	35
1831–40	–	53
1841–50	2	79
1851–60	1	75
1861–70	–	87
1871–80	1	152
1881–90	8	234
1891–1900	9	314
1901–10	6	493
1911–20	18	646
Total	*46*	*2,232*

of four issues each were published until the journal ceased to exist in 1837, mainly due to a shortage of contributors.

The first reading club for doctors was established in Christiania in 1826, and the Norwegian Medical Society (Det norske medicinske Selskab) was founded in its wake in 1833. In 1840 the Society established Norsk Magazin for Lægevidenskaben (The Norwegian Magazine for Medical Science). The mandate of the journal reads as follows: "Its principal aim is, partly to establish an outlet for our own doctors' literary works, and partly to report on the most important foreign literature; consequently, it is these two items which constitute the foundation of the journal." Once again, the supply of original contributions was scarce, which led to some irregularities during the early years and a short interruption in 1846. The financial status of the journal was difficult and the the Medical Society saw the publication as an economic burden. A slight decrease in subscribers in 1910, when the circulation was down to 570, almost caused the journal to cease to exist, but it was published regularly until it became a part of the journal Nordisk Medicin in 1939. In 1933 the circulation was about 1,100. From 1845 to 1881 Norsk Magazin was the only medical journal in Norway, and it played an important role in promoting Norwegian medical research during its 100 years of existence (Grøn 1933).

Another journal, Ugeskrift for Medicin og Pharmacie, which published papers on both medicine and pharmacology, was established in 1842 by Johan Heiberg (1805–1883), but ceased to appear after only four years.

The journal Medicinsk Revue, which aimed mainly at presenting reports and abstracts from internationally published research, was established in Bergen in 1884. Through its first 15 years this journal was published as a private enterprise, but from 1899 on by the Medical Society in Bergen (founded in 1831). Medicinsk Revue also merged with Nordisk Medicin in 1939.

On January 1, 1881, the three Norwegian physicians Michael Skjelderup (1834–1902), Fredrik Nicolai Stabell (1832–1899), and Cæsar Peter Møller Boeck (1845–1917) launched Tidsskrift for praktisk Medicin (the Journal of Practical Medicine) in Christiania. Norsk Magazin was the leading scientific journal at this time, and the founders of the new journal did not intend to challenge its position. They planned a journal with a more clinical approach for practicing physicians, and hoped to succeed through contributions from doctors all around Norway. However, a certain tension between the two journals rapidly evolved, and the editor of Norsk Magazin, Edvard Bull (1845–1925), accused Tidsskrift for praktisk Medicin of lack of scientific quality: "... all literary medical activity must either be scientific or non-scientific, it is not possible to construct something in between and call it "practical"; regarding philosophy, stringency and shape, every medical product must be scientific, also when it comes to that grain of medicine that is described as medical art." This dispute over scientific versus practical medicine in 1881 reflected a growing conflict between the more conservative, philosophical and theoretical medicine of the past and an incipient experimentally based medicine of the future (Berg 1986).

Tidsskrift for praktisk Medicin was taken over by the Norwegian Medical Association in 1888.

The small number of physicians in Norway in the nineteenth century must have made it financially very hard to produce medical journals. In 1816, when the first statistics of Norwegian doctors appeared, there were 99 physicians in Norway as a whole. The number rose to 129 in 1833. In 1886, when the Norwegian Medical Association was founded, there were three medical journals (Norsk Magazin, Medicinsk Revue and Tidsskrift for praktisk Medicin) and only 581 doctors in Norway. The new medical association saw no economic possibility of launching another journal.

In December 1886 the founders of Tidsskrift for praktisk Medicin offered the Norwegian Medical Association a takeover. In a letter to the Association they wrote that "The Journal has built up a satisfactory financial position in the past six years." By then they had accumulated a reserve of 750 Norwegian kroner (NOK). The subscription rate had been NOK 6 per year, but was reduced to NOK 2.50 beginning in 1888. The Norwegian Medical Association had 472 members by then, and the circulation of the Journal was 450. The economic situation deteriorated rapidly after the takeover. In June 1888, the Board of the Norwegian Medical Association decided to apply for a governmental grant of NOK 1,200 "considering that the Journal's main purpose is to deal with topics regarding public health care." The Ministry of Justice could not support the journal directly, but the Association received a yearly grant of NOK 1,200 from the Government from 1894 to 1904. From 1893 on, all members of the Norwegian Medical Association received the Journal free of charge as a membership benefit, but the membership fee was raised from NOK 5 to NOK 10 per year (Berner 1936).

Since 1881, no new medical, scientific journal has been launched that is peer reviewed and indexed in international data bases, is published in the Norwegian language, and is still in existence. Several specialist journals have been established as joint Nordic enterprises published in international languages, but in general, readers and authors alike have turned to international channels of communication. The new publications and newsletters established in Norway, such as the 12 journals published by the specialist branches of the Norwegian Medical Association (Nicolaysen 1994), focus mainly on organizational and collegial issues.

13.1.3.3 Academic Dissertations

The publication of doctoral theses in medicine in Norway started with Frederik Holst's dissertation, written in Latin in 1817. This was the first academic dissertation in Norway. The three following dissertations (1829, 1830, and 1842) were all medical, and were written and defended in Latin. After a pause of more than 30 years, the next medical dissertation was defended in 1875. From then until the turn of the century, all dissertations were written in Norwegian. An increasing number of dissertations were written in German during the first two decades of the twentieth century, and after the First World War Norwegian and German were the prevalent academic languages. A few dissertations were published in English, but until the Second World War, German was the dominant language of international scientific communication in the Scandinavian countries and Central Europe. After the Second World War English rapidly became predominant. Until the 1960s dissertations were published as books or monographs, frequently as a supplement to one of the Nordic specialist journals. Since the mid-1970s the vast majority of medical dissertations in Norway have consisted of compilations of articles published in scientific journals. Approximately one-fourth of all Norwegian academic dissertations have been medical. After a steady increase, the yearly number of dissertations has remained stable at about 100 since the late 1980s. By the end of 1993 a total of 1,589 medical dissertations had been published in Norway (Olsen 1994).

13.1.4. The General Journal

13.1.4.1. The National General Journal

While the first medical journals were general in every sense of the word, the specialization of medicine has left general medical journals as a tiny minority among current publications. Only one or two journals in each country have retained a general orientation. Of the more than 20,000 medical journals in the world, only a few can be named national, general journals (1988).

A national medical journal is a generalist journal with a wide readership within a nation or a region. It covers all specialties of medicine and is issued frequently, often weekly or biweekly. Such journals are often membership journals published by national medical associations; some are published by local societies (e.g., the New England Journal of Medicine) or independent commercial publishers (e.g., the Lancet). They are primarily characterized by a wide variety of articles consisting of a mixture of original research, reviews, debate, and news items. Four main elements of a general journal have been identified: information, instruction, comment, and amusement (Lock 1987). While electronic data bases are constructed ideally for problem-oriented reading and the search for an answer to a specific question, general journals present unasked for, even unexpected and sometimes surprising, information to their readers.

National medical journals constitute one of the most visible links that unite the medical profession within a country, despite specialties and types of employment. In smaller countries these journals have special tasks as regards the national professional environment and culture. English has become the international language of medical communication, and about 80 percent of all scientific medical papers in Norway were published in English in 1979-1981 (Kyvik 1991). It is important, however, both for doctor-patient communication and for cultural identity, to maintain and develop a national professional terminology in the non-English-speaking countries. In this context, the national journals play an important role. It is not by mere chance that all the national journals in the Scandinavian countries have specific and regular columns for language and national medical terminology (Nylenna 1990).

With a greater diversity of interests and specialities among doctors and increasing professional challenges, the general medical journals are steadily broadening their acitivities, adding health economics, management, decision making, legal affairs, and ethics to the long list of topical issues.

13.1.4.2. The Journal of the Norwegian Medical Association

Tidsskrift for Den norske lægeforening (The Journal of the Norwegian Medical Association), commonly called Tidsskriftet (the Journal), is a typical national, general journal. To repeat: it was founded in 1881 as a private enterprise called Tidsskrift for praktisk Medicin and has been a journal for members of the Norwegian Medical Association since 1888. On January 1, 1890, the journal was named Tidsskrift for Den norske lægeforening (the Journal of the Norwegian Medical Association).

For a hundred years it has been the most important single medical journal in Norway, serving the scientific community, meeting readers' demands for updated and continuing education, and acting as a forum for the professional organization regarding "trade union" politics and information to members. In 1900 Axel Holst (1860–1931) was appointed its first scientific editor. Most of the time thereafter Tidsskriftet has had two editors: a scientific editor responsible for the medical-scientific content, and the Secretary General of the Norwegian Medical Association, who has edited the part of the Journal covering "professional interest and association issues." During an interregnum from 1938 to 1945, the Secretary General was even responsible for the scientific part of the Journal (Bjercke 1961). Since 1992, as a provisional arrangement, one single editor, this time the scientific editor, has again been responsible for the complete journal.

The periodic updating of the aims and objectives of the journal (Table 13.3) shows a shift from individual-oriented clinical medicine from the start in 1881 to a more community-based policy when the Medical Association took over in 1888, and a new shift back to practical, clinical medicine after the Second World War (1945) (Harlem 1986). The present aims of the journal, ratified in 1987 (Nylenna 1987), also reflect the changing role of the general medical journal as compared with other sources of medical information, as well as a steadily broader approach that includes the ethical, cultural, and political aspects of medicine. The aim is no longer to keep all doctors updated, but to stimulate them to maintain their professional competence as a personal responsibility.

When the Norwegian Medical Association took over Tidsskriftet in 1888, there was a shift from it being a practical journal of clinical medicine (as opposed to the more scientific Norsk Magazin) to one concerned more with social medicine, preventive medicine, and political issues. The editors of the medical-scientific part of the Journal were recruited mainly from Norway's epidemiologists and doctors engaged in preventive medicine (Storm-Mathisen 1981).

During the first part of the twentieth century, clinical medicine was covered by Norsk Magazin for Lægevidenskaben, a journal intended mainly for hospital physicians in different specialties. General practitioners felt an increasing need for their own journal with a more clinical and practical approach than that of Tidsskrift for Den norske lægeforening. In 1941 the General Practitioners Association (Alment praktiserende lægers forening; founded 1938) launched a new journal, Den praktiserende læge (the Practicing Physician). This journal had a difficult time during the Second World War, and in 1945 it merged with Tidsskrift for Den norske lægeforening. The new editor, Jens Bjørneboe (1908–1963),

TABLE 13.3
Changing aims and objectives of Tidsskrift for Den norske lægeforening (The Journal of the Norwegian Medical Association)

1881
«The articles written in this Journal will contribute to the common instruction and benefit»
«...that this periodical which is based entirely on practical scientific interest... will fulfil the decision... to strengthen and revive our Brothers' mutual loyal sympathies and common medical interests»

1888
«... the editors will emphasize the treatment of topics relating to hygiene and through discussion of the various social questions presently in focus, to find a solution to which doctors' co-operation is required...»

1945
«– give professional guidance so that the readers are constantly in touch with medical progress
– promote the output of Norwegian medical works
– be a membership journal for The Norwegian Medical Association and its bodies, as well as the Society of General Practitioners»

1987
«– be a body for medical education which stimulates the doctor as a general clinician to professional upkeep and renewal
– stimulate medical research and profes sional development
– contribute towards professional conduct in doctors by the further development of ethical and cultural ideals in the medical tradition
– promote the debate on health politics
– be a membership journal for The Norwegian Medical Association»

developed Tidsskriftet further. Its basic content became a mixture of scientific papers and instructive articles of special relevance to primary care physicians. Tidsskriftet became a widely read journal, with increasing authority. From 1962 to 1987 Ole K. Harlem (1917–) continued this strategy, as his successor Magne Nylenna (1952–) has done since taking over in 1987.

The subtitle Tidsskrift for praktisk medisin (Journal for Practical Medicine) was replaced by the English The Journal of the Norwegian Medical Association in 1985, even though the language of the publication continues to be Norwegian. This has been seen as a symbol of Tidsskriftet now becoming more than a journal for practical medicine. In the 1980s new columns were introduced, for example, for health politics. Simultaneously there was a shift toward more active editing, with increasing emphasis on commissioned papers, thematic series of articles, more editorials, more news reports, and so on. Full color photographs were introduced on the front page and the lay-out was gradually updated. All these changes were adjustments to the needs and demands of a new generation of readers.

A readers' survey in 1990 showed a high degree of satisfaction with the content and presentation of Tidsskriftet. The average reader spent 47 minutes on each issue. The 1980s saw a significant increase in the proportion of readers who found the journal topical and easy to read, and a drop in the number who thought the journal uninteresting (Nylenna 1990).

The Journal was published every other week until the early 1970s. Since then it has been published every ten days. Table 13.4 shows the circulation and the number of pages.

TABLE 13.4
Circulation and yearly number of pages of Tidsskrift for Den norske lægeforening from 1881 to 1990

Year	Circulation[1]	Total number of pages
1881	450	376
1890	530	576
1900	800	1,218
1910	1,060	1,320
1920	1,140	1,046
1930	1,610	1,450
1940	2,460	1,114
1950	3,260	867[2]
1960	4,190	1,244
1970	5,640	2,306
1980	11,400	2,125
1990	15,700	4,006

[1] The circulation from 1890 to 1970 is estimated as the total membership of the Norwegian Medical Association plus ten percent

[2] The journal changed format in 1945

13.1.5 Specialization and Internationalization

A profession as such exists when a specific, long-term education is acquired by individuals whose main intention is to achieve a specific occupation which, by social norms, cannot be held by persons other than those possessing this education (Torgersen 1972). According to this definition the medical profession has been said to be the most representative of all professions (Torgersen 1972). A distinguishing characteristic of modern professions is a high degree of autonomy (Freidson 1970).

In the shaping of the medical profession, the main criteria have been knowledge, ethics, and institutional organization. The shift of medical knowledge and power from the patients' control to control by the physicians has been crucial in this process (Gelfand 1993).

In the development of medical practitioners' authority and control over their work and over the organization of their professional lives, medical journals have played a significant role. Scientific journals, more than other institutions, have been "closed circuits" within the medical community. Not only have authors and readers belonged to the same profession, but so have editors and referees, and many journals have even been published by the profession itself through its associations and societies.

13.1.5.1 Specialization

Specialization is the most striking feature of the changes in the medical profession in the twentieth century. Scientific progress is the strongest force behind this specialization, which started in the late nineteenth century and has accelerated since the Second World War. New knowledge and technology have led to new services. The demand for these services has created what resembles a marketplace, making it possible for doctors to specialize in different fields and later develop new professions. This can be seen as a stepwise process: scientific progress followed by market expansion and subsequent professionalization (Hofoss 1980). Medical journals have played an important role in this development. Editors and publishers have identified professional trends, and journals focusing on new areas of medicine have normally been established at an early stage in the specialization process. Sometimes, enthusiastic and dedicated physicians, who have invested much time and often money of their own in their mission, have become editors of specialist journals even before the specialty, or sub-specialty, has been formally recognized. Such individual editors, with support of small groups of front-line professionals, have made up the core of many new medical specialties.

Publications have had an active impact on the developments by accelerating the shaping of specialties and sub-specialties. Medical journals have not only been "mirrors of medicine," as reads the title of the book produced on the 150th anniversary of the British Medical Journal (Bartrip 1990), but also "supporters of specialization."

The traditional and historical division between medicine and surgery can be said to be the basis for the specialization of the medical profession. There is no systematic pattern in the structure of this process, however. Some medical specialties are based on organ systems (like gynecology and ophthalmology), others on the etiology of diseases (like infectious diseases and occupational medicine), others on technology and methods of treatment (like radiology and surgery), and some even on the age of the patient (like pediatrics and geriatric medicine) or the organization of the health care system (like family medicine and community medicine).

Since specializiation can also be a threat to professions because it can undermine the profession as a whole, specialization is a controversial issue within any established profession (Torgersen 1972). Extreme "specialism" will eventually lead to fragmentation and deterioration of the original profession. This may end up with the old, basic part of the profession itself becoming a speciality. General practice as a recognized medical specialty can be regarded as an example of this development (Torgersen 1972).

The first medical specialists in Norway were certified in 1918. Thirteen specialties were established, increasing to 23 by World War II, and to 43 recognized specialties in 1990. When the first 115 specialists were certified in 1918, they comprised 9 percent of all Norwegian doctors (Berg 1986). In 1990, 58 percent of all Norwegian doctors held specialist certificates. Table 13.5 shows the number of specialties and certified specialists in Norway, from 1920 to 1990.

Sub-specialties have developed within the broader specialties, especially within surgery and internal medicine. Even though the number of recognized specialties with board certificates is more limited in Norway than in other countries, there is a trend

TABLE 13.5
Number of medical specialties and certified specialists in Norway (based on statistics from the Norwegian Medical Association)

Year	Number of medical specialties	Number of certified specialists[1]	Total number of physicians in Norway	Population in Norway (millions)
1920	13	115	1,346	2.65
1930	20	333	1,770	2.82
1940	23	616	2,357	2.98
1950	31	1,046	3,330	3.28
1960	32	1,536	4,066	3.57
1970	35	2,520	5,665	3.86
1980	38	3,882	8,663	4.08
1990	43	7,497[2]	12,952	4.23

[1] Actually number of specialist certificates, which means that (the few) physicians holding more than one specialty are counted according to number of specialties

[2] The large increase in number of specialists from 1980 to 1990 is partly caused by the new specialties general practice (962 specialists certified from 1985 to 1989) and community medicine (323 specialists certified from 1984 to 1989)

toward a less formalized specialization, with individual doctors specializing in one particular disease or even one diagnostic or therapeutic procedure.

This specialization is strongly reflected in the development of specialist journals, which restrict their content to one specialty and often publish mainly technical articles. Internationally, a few of these specialist journals were established as early as in the first half of the nineteenth century, for example, Annales d'Hygiene (established 1828), Archiv für Anatomie (1834), the Pharmaceutical Journal (1841), and the British Journal of Psychiatry (1853). Most of the medical journals established in the twentieth century are specialist journals, and by the Second World War the vast majority of the new journals were specialized. Over the last decades, journals have been established that are dedicated not only to one sub-specialty, but perhaps even to a single disease. Just like medicine itself, journals have branched out from general to specialist, and then even further to sub-specialist and sub-sub-specialist. A theoretical sequence of journals may be defined in several tiers: the general science journal, the general medical journal, the specialist journal e.g., in geriatric medicine, the sub-specialist journal e.g., a journal of geriatric neurology, a journal of a specific disease e.g., dementia, a journal solely for the treatment of this disease, and lastly perhaps a journal for research into this treatment, which could eventually lead to a hypothetical sub-sub-specialist journal such as the imaginary Journal of Dementia Treatment Research.

In recent years, even specialist review journals have been founded. The idea behind these activities is to guide potential readers within a field with rapidly increasing publication rates. It is extremely difficult to catch up and keep updated on the specific specialties and sub-specialties. Textbooks are to some extent outdated on publication, so journals publishing review papers are intended to cover the gap between journals based on original reports and the traditional books.

Journals covering several traditional specialties and sub-specialties but based on a specific methodology could also be named specialist journals. An example of such a journal, which combines the review perspective with a truly scientific approach, is the newly established journal Evidence Based Medicine, publishing meta analyses and critical reviews within all fields of medicine.

13.1.5.2. Internationalization

The specialization of medicine is closely related to its internationalization. The increase in exchange of professional information and scientific cooperation across national borders, together with the growth in international travel and communication systems in general during the present century, have made medicine a truly international field. Combined with a specialization that made it more natural for many doctors, especially researchers, to keep in touch with specialist colleagues abroad than to work with local physicians in other specialties, the modern journals have created a new means of scientific communication. Most new journals established in the twentieth century are not only specialist journals, but also international journals.

International communication is dependent on a common language. Until the end of the eighteenth century, Latin was the language of medical and other scientific publications, both nationally and internationally. When mother tongue-based academic communication was accepted, a need for alternatives emerged. French, and especially German, became the new international languages, reflecting the importance of Paris, Vienna, Berlin, and other European cities for nineteenth-century medicine. German was the most important language for international publications until the 1930s, when it was gradually replaced by English. Since the Second World War English has become the lingua franca.

13.1.5.2.1 Internationalization Through Nordic Cooperation

On the way to internationalism, Norwegian medical publishing has gone through a long period of Nordic cooperation. Owing to the limited number of physicians, and especially of specialists in the different fields of medicine, Norwegian doctors have sought professional cooperation abroad. Since the Nordic countries have a common political, cultural and linguistic background, the justification for joint Nordic journals is obvious.

A joint Nordic journal was discussed as early as 1844 (Grøn 1933). However, another 25 years were to pass before the first Nordic journal was established at Karolinska Institutet in Stockholm as Nordiskt Medicinskt Arkiv, a continuation of Medicinskt Arkiv, founded by Axel Key (1832 1901) in 1863 (Ljunggren 1970). The articles were published in Danish, Norwegian, or Swedish, with a summary in French. The supply of scientific contributions was scarce, however, and many Scandinavian scientists preferred to publish in international languages, mainly in German journals. In 1901, the journal was divided into two sections, one medical and the other surgical, and it was made known that original articles should preferably be written in German, English, or French. Articles in the Scandinavian languages were now given a German summary. By the end of the First World War, no papers were published in the Scandinavian languages, and the two journals were renamed Acta Medica Scandinavica and Acta Chirurgica Scandinavica in 1919. These names were later changed. Acta Medica Scandinavica became the Journal of Internal Medicine in 1989, and Acta Chirurgica Scandinavica became the European Journal of Surgery in 1992.

Nordic collaboration in the nineteenth century was not limited to clinical medicine. In 1848, C.P. Boeck (1798 1877) became professor of physiology in Oslo, and

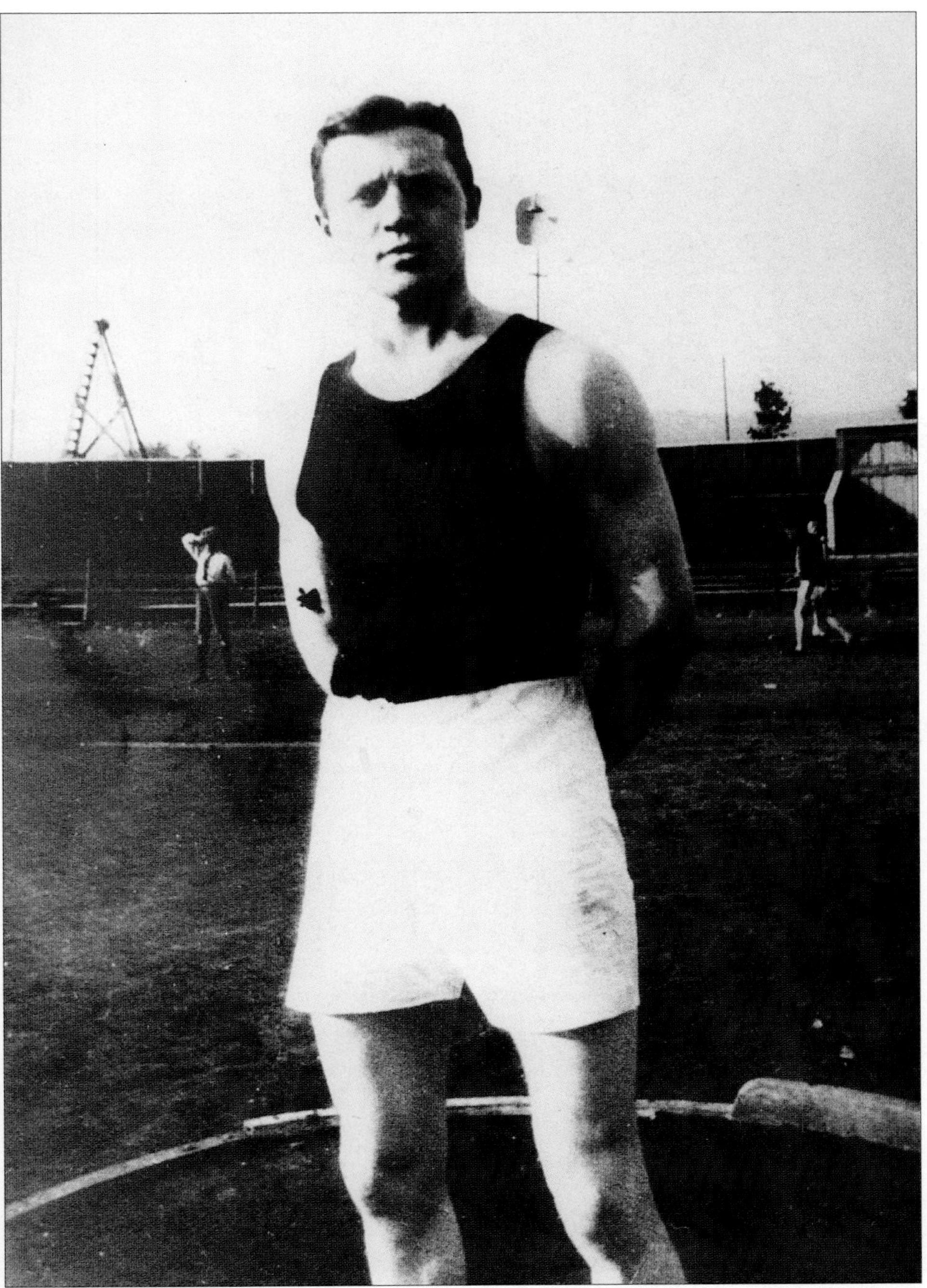

Figure 34: Although many times it is not mentioned in their autobiographies, many physicians also have remarkable achievements outside their professional work. Here, as an example, is the young student Sverre Sørsdal (1900-1996) performing athletics in 1920. He won a silver medal in boxing in the Olympic games of 1920, a bronze medal in the Olympics of 1924, and was number four in the Olympic games of 1928 (Courtesy Randi Sørsdal).

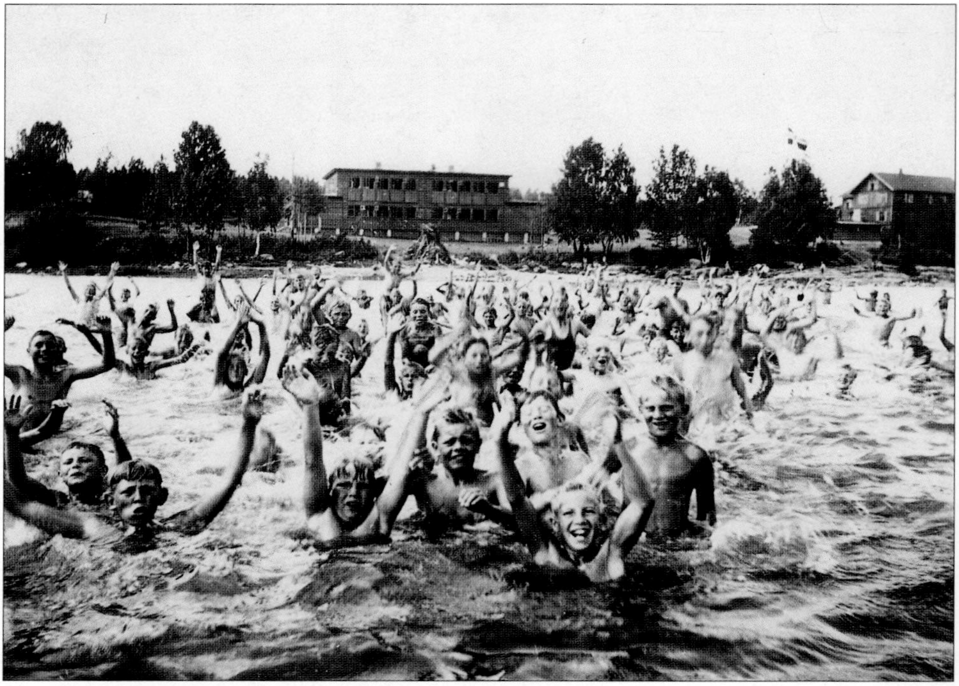

Figures 35 and 36: Sun, fresh air, adequate nutrition - and fun, were important elements in the preventive work for children in the hygiene era of the 1920s and 1930s. These pictures are probably from ca. 1935 and show children on a vacation camp in the countryside and in a nursery in Åkebergveien in Oslo (Photos from the archives of the School Health Board in Oslo).

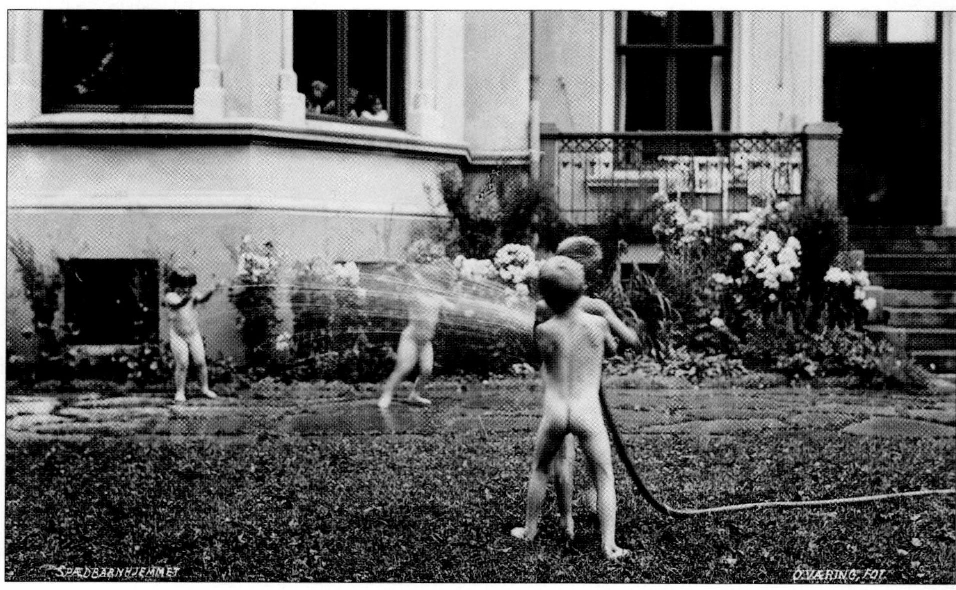

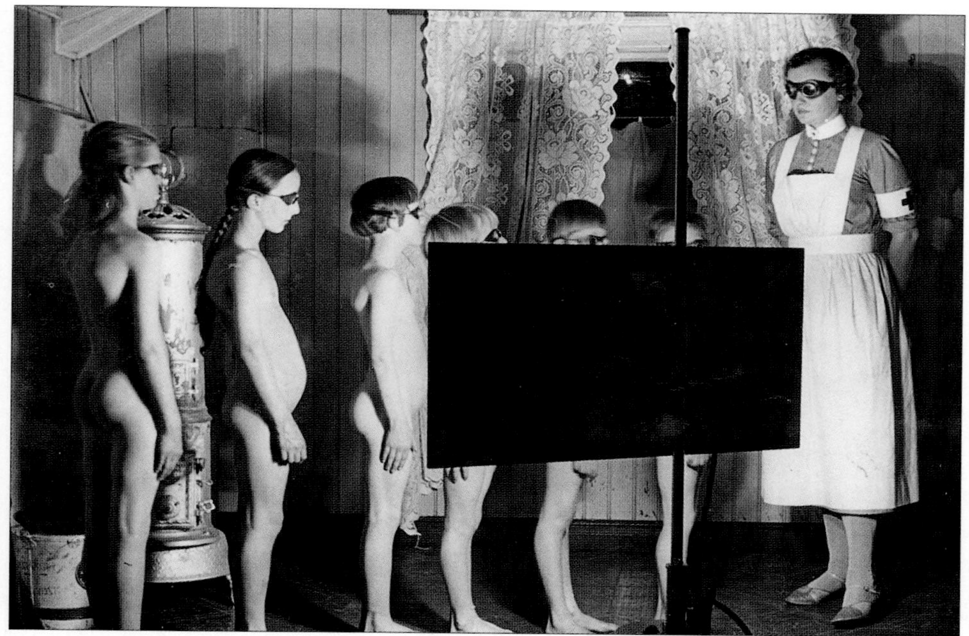

Figure 37: Prevention of rachitis by means of artificial light in the Red Cross cottage hospital in Kjøllefjord in the arctic region of Finnmark 1938-1939 (Photo: Dr. Knut A. Schrøder).

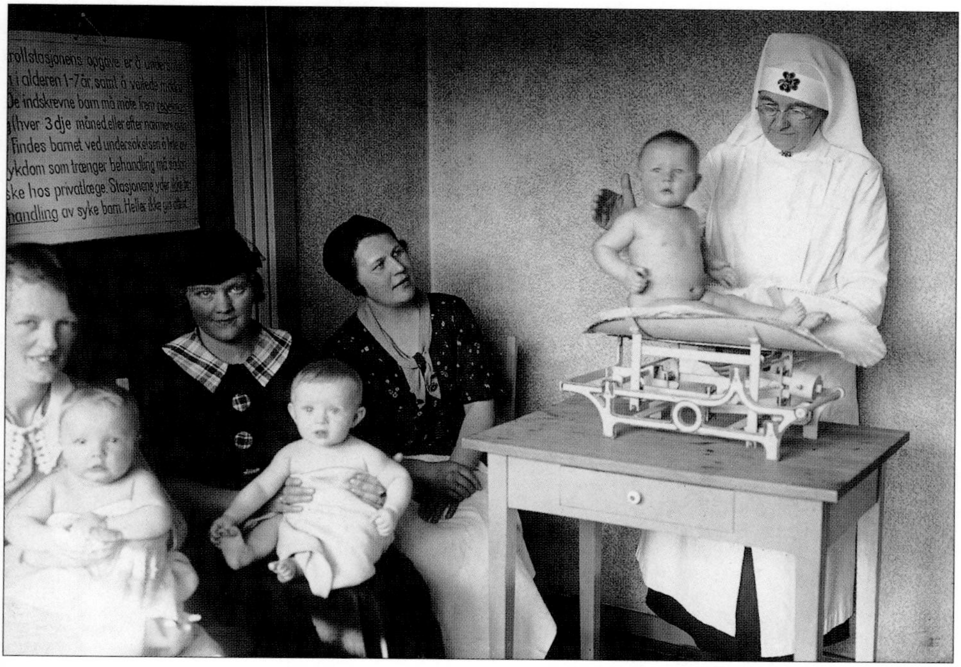

Figure 38: Health checkups for infants and children gained in importance in the years between the two World Wars, as a preventive and diagnostic measure (Photograph from the archives of the Oslo School Health Board).

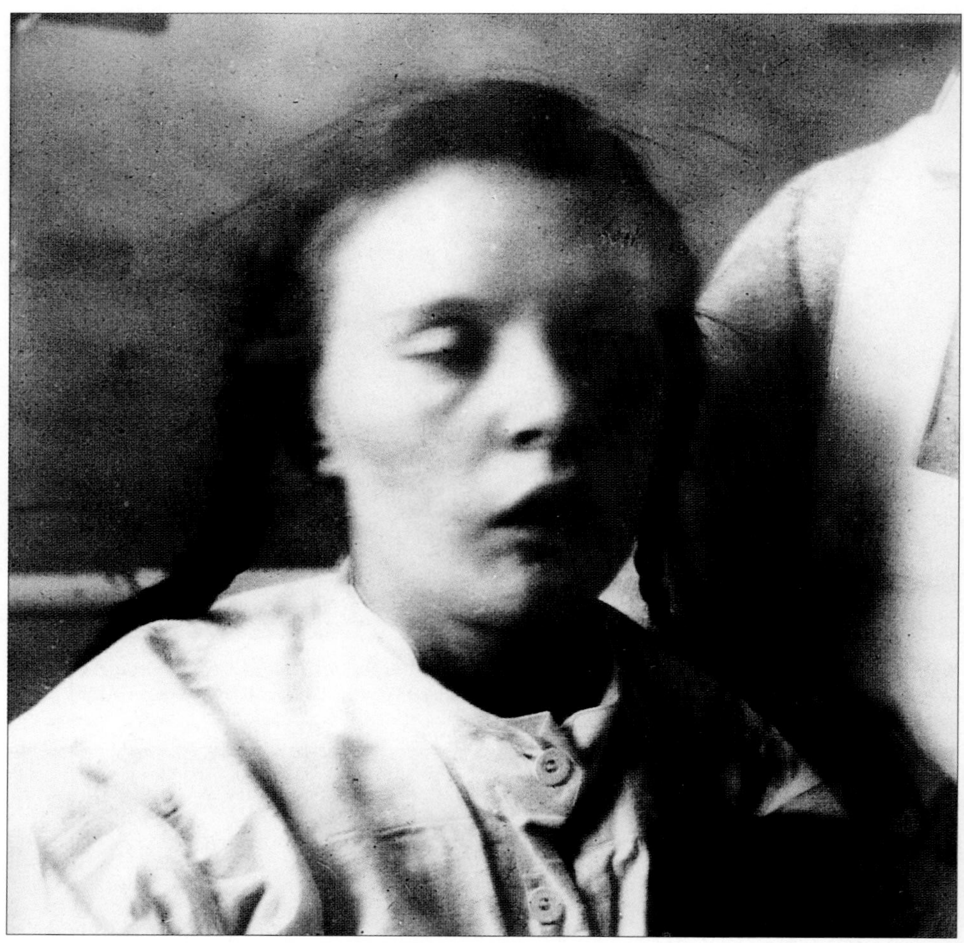

Figure 39: A mysterious, but frightening disease: Encephalitis lethargica (von Economo's disease) ravaged as a pandemic disease in the years 1915-1925. Also Norway experienced several cases in the early twenties. Lethality was high, and more than twenty years later survivors still suffered from Parkinsonism originating from this disease (Photograph from Ullevål Hospital in Oslo 1920, courtesy prof. Erik Enger).

as chairs and research institutes in physiology were established in all the Nordic countries, a need arose for a joint journal. In 1889 Danish, Swedish, and Norwegian physiologists launched Skandinavisches Archiv für Physiologie almost 40 years before the Nordic Physiological Society was established. The strong influence of German physiology was reflected not only in the name of the journal. Up to the 1930s the vast majority of papers were written in German and until the Second World War the journal was printed in Germany. For easily-understandable reasons, the journal was renamed Acta Physiologica Scandinavica in 1940 (Folkow 1990).

After the First World War, there were additional political motives for combined Nordic effort, and several specialist journals were established around 1920, most of them named Acta, a link to the Latin tradition that still prevailed in continental Europe. One of the earliest was Acta Gynecologica Scandinavica (now Acta Obstetrica et Gynecologica Scandinavica), which was started in 1921. Like the other medical specialties, gynecologists also needed a common Nordic journal. The main obstacle was lack of funding. In this case, the Swedish tycoon Ivar Kreuger (1880–1932) helped to overcome that particular problem and offered economic backing for the journal (Bergjsø 1991).

Nordisk Hygienisk Tidskrift was established in 1920 by a merger of the Swedish and Danish journals of hygiene and public health, and also became an organ for Norsk Hygienisk Forening (The Norwegian Association of Hygiene). The journal merged with Work Environment Health and became Scandinavian Journal of Work, Environment and Health in 1975 (Natvig 1974).

The joint Nordic journals established after the Second World War were often called Scandinavian Journals, reflecting the shift toward an Anglo-American tradition. Several such journals were established in the 1960s, and an example of this kind of journal with Norwegian roots is the Scandinavian Journal of Gastroenterology. This journal was founded in 1966 by Johannes Myren (1915–1996), Egil Gjone (1925–) and Lars S. Semb (1933–1980) with support from the Norwegian University Press and with co-editors in all Nordic countries. The circulation increased from 600 in 1966 to 3,000 in 1995. At the start, four issues of 90 pages were published yearly, increasing to 12 issues of 96 pages in 1995. In 1983 a Spanish edition and in 1986 a Chinese edition were established. It is estimated that 80 percent of all clinical research in gastroenterology in Norway is published in the Scandinavian Journal of Gastroenterology (Myren 1995).

The process of internationalization of Nordic scientific publication has been studied by Gunnar Sivertsen (Sivertsen 1991). Out of 128 scientific and scholarly journals in this study that were published in an international language and edited in a Nordic country, 54 were medical journals (including pharmacy, dental research and veterinary medicine). On average, these 54 journals were published more often than bimonthly, with 96 articles per year, each of 6.5 pages, and an average circulation of 1,384. The study shows a clear trend toward true internationalization of these journals, which were founded as Nordic enterprises based on articles authored by Nordic researchers and intended for Nordic readers. Over the years the journals have had an increasing number of authors and subscribers from outside the Nordic countries, especially from the United States, the United Kingdom, and Japan. In the period 1988-1990 a total of 44 percent of the articles were written by non-Nordic authors. Many of the Nordic journals have openly changed to an international editorial policy; they invite authors from all over the world to publish in them and have established international editorial boards.

Table 13.6 is a chronological summary of medical journals that were established as, or have developed into, Actas or Scandinavian Journals. More than half of the 33 journals were established in the two peak decades, the twenties and the sixties. The circulation of the joint Nordic specialist journals is fairly low, with an average of 2,400 (range: 300 to 8,500). The changing names of the journals seven have deleted Acta or Scandinavian Journal from the name reflect the shift from a Nordic foundation toward a more international orientation.

During the last decades, journals aiming at international authorship and readership from the very start have been established in Norway. Some of these journals have no specific Nordic basis and therefore no history as Actas or Scandinavian Journals. An example is Cephalalgia, devoted to headache research and founded in 1981. Cephalalgia was founded by professor Ottar Sjaastad (1928-) and the Norwegian Migraine Society and is published by the Scandinavian University Press. It is now the official journal of the International Headache Society. The editor-in-chief is located in the United States and the circulation has increased from 500 in 1981 to 1,600 in 1996.

13.1.5.2.2 Increasing Internationalism and Growing Nationalism: a Cultural Paradox

At the same time as a true internationalism, in society in general and in science in particular, has been developing through trade, travel, and communications, a new kind of nationalism has been emerging all over the world. This has been identified by John Naisbitt and Patricia Aburdene in their book Megatrends 2000 as "global lifestyles and cultural nationalism" (Naisbitt 1990). It may be regarded as a paradox that two seemingly contradictory trends are being experienced simultaneously, but the more homogeneous and universal our lifestyle becomes, the more understandable it becomes that people are keeping traditional languages and cultures alive. This has to do with people's need to preserve their identity, be it national, local, religious, linguistic, or racial. Since English has become the first truly universal language and the language of the information age, it challenges other national languages and thereby national cultural identities. Naisbitt and Aburdene put it this way: "... an economically integrated Europe will be accompanied by an outbreak of cultural assertiveness for the rest of the 1990s. It will inflame and enhance the global renaissance in the arts and literature, in poetry and dance and song" (Naisbitt 1990).

This paradox of increasing internationalism on the one hand and cultural nationalism on the other is reflected even in medicine and the medical journals. Smaller nations and cultures, like Norway, are more vulnerable than larger countries are, but the retreat from the international system of physical units, SI-units, by some major American medical journals, which still insist on the so-called conventional units of gallons, inches, and yards, can be viewed as an example of the very same thing (Nylenna and Smith 1992).

A national medical culture in Norwegian publication has been defended and maintained by the national, medical publications, first and foremost the Journal of the Norwegian Medical Association, Tidsskriftet. But just as a Norwegian national identity during the nineteenth century developed in close interaction with our Scandinavian neighbors (Sørensen 1994), a Norwegian medical identity during the twentieth century has developed as a result of a comprehensive Nordic cooperation. All the Nordic countries have had more or less the same need to protect their national medical iden-

TABLE 13.6
Nordic medical journals established as, or changed into, Actas or Scandinavian Journals (year of foundation or change of name)

Original name	Later names			Circulation 1996
Medicinskt Arkiv (1863)	Nordisk Medicinskt Arkiv (1869)	Acta Medica Scandinavica (1919)	Journal of Internal Medicine (1989)	1,800
		Acta Chirurgica Scandinavica (1919)	European Journal of Surgery (1992)	4,500
Skandinavisches Archiv für Physiologie (1889)	Acta Physiologica Scandinavica (1940)			1,700 (1991)
Acta Oto-Laryngologica (1918)				2,000
Acta Dermato-Venerologica (1920)				1,100
Nordisk Hygienisk Tidsskrift (1920)	Scandinavian Journal of Work, Environment & Health (1975)			1,400
Acta Gynecologica Scandinavica (1921)	Acta Obstetrica et Gynecologica Scandinavica (1925)			4,800
Acta Paediatrica (1921)	Acta Paediatrica Scandinavica (1965)	Acta Paediatrica an International Journal of Paediatrics (1991)		2,000
Acta Radiologica Diagnosis (1921)	Acta Radiologica (1987)			3,400
Acta Radiologica Oncology (1921)	Acta Oncologica (1987)			1,400
Acta Ophthalmologica (1923)				1,700 (1991)

Original name	Later names		Circulation 1996
Scandinavian Journal of Respiratory Diseases (1924)	The European Respiratory Journal (1989)		5,200
Acta Pathologica et Microbiologica Scandinavica (1926)	Acta Pathologica, Microbiologica et Immunologica Scandinavica (1982)	APMIS (1988)	1,100
Acta Psychiatrica Scandinavica (1926)			1,800
Acta Orthopaedica Scandinavica (1930)			4,000
Acta Odontologica Scandinavia (1939)			500
Acta Allergologica	Allergy (1978)		2,700
Acta Endocrino-logica (1948)	European Journal of Endocrinology (1993)		1,300
Scandinavian Journal of Clinical & Laboratory Investigations (1949)			1,800
Acta Rheumato-logica Scandinavica (1955)	Scandinavian Journal of Rheumatology (1972)		1,800
Acta Anaesthesiologica Scandinavia (1957)			3,500
Acta Neurologica Scandinavica (1961)			1,300
Scandinavian Journal of Haema-tology (1964)	European Journal of Haematology (1988)		1,150

Original name	Later names	Circulation 1996
Scandinavian Journal of Gastroenterology (1966)		3,000
Scandinavian Journal of Plastic & Reconstructive Surgery (1966)	Scandinavian Journal of Plastic and Reconstructive and Hand Surgery (1987)	4,600
Scandinavian Journal of Thoracic and Cardiovascular Surgery (1966)		300
Scandinavian Journal of Urology and Nephrology (1966)		1,100
Scandinavian Journal of Infectious Diseases (1969)		1,200
Scandinavian Journal of Rehabilitation Medicine (1969)		1,200
Scandinavian Journal of Immunology (1972)		1,600
Acta Socio-Medica Scandinavica (1973)	Scandinavian Journal of Social Medicine (1980)	800
Scandinavian Journal of Sports Sciences (1979)	Scandinavian Journal of Medicine & Science in Sports (1990)	4,000
Scandinavian Journal of Primary Health Care (1983)		8,500

tity, and the editors and editorial staff of the national medical journals in the five Nordic countries have met yearly or every other year since 1973 to discuss common problems in this connection. A more informal network among the editors of the general medical journals in Sweden, Denmark, and Norway has also been established.

Joint Nordic journals have been used not only to achieve internationalization, but also to take care of the national cultural aspects of medicine. An example is Nordisk Medicinsk Tidskrift, which was launched on January 5, 1929, as a general Nordic journal founded by the Swedish professor Gunnar Holmgren (1875–1954) with a national editor in each of the five Nordic countries. The program of this journal was "to give a general view of medicine's present level in Nordic languages, and with mainly Nordic authors, and development through publication of short articles on such topics as are of common interest to readers." In 1939 it was time to broaden the Nordic cooperation by merging Nordisk Medicinsk Tidskrift with seven Nordic national journals (including the Norwegian Norsk Magazin for Lægevidenskapen and Medicinsk Revue) to become Nordisk Medicin. After the Second World War, the circulation was approximately 8,000, and almost 40 percent of all physicians in the Nordic countries subscribed to the journal (Bonnevie 1980). In the 1940s and 1950s Nordisk Medicin published original research and proceedings from the medical societies in the Nordic countries. The journal played an important role in the exchange of medical research and clinical experience among the Nordic countries. Members of the Medical Societies in Oslo and Bergen paid a reduced subscription fee. Beginning in 1962 members of all the medical societies in Norway (Oslo, Bergen, Drammen, Kristiansand, Rogaland, and Trøndelag) received the journal free; the subscription was included in their membership fee. In 1972 Nordisk Medicin was taken over by the national medical associations in the Nordic countries and has since been a monthly journal for members (Bonnevie 1972). From that time the journal has changed. The emphasis has shifted from research to medical education and ethics and issues of common interest to the Nordic medical associations. While most other joint Nordic journals have become international and have introduced English as their language of publication, Nordisk Medicin has held onto the Nordic languages and limited its themes to Nordic issues. In terms of circulation 62,000 in 1996, the journal is among the biggest medical journals in Europe.

Thus, Nordic cooperation has been an important factor both in the trend toward internationalism of Norwegian medicine and in the countertrend toward national cultural assertion.

13.1.6 Knowledge, Identity and Merits

The publication of medical journals and scientific literature serves several functions for the groups involved. For scientists and authors, it is a way of getting papers assessed and with luck published, of communicating with other researchers and clinicians, and even of receiving merit and honor. For editors, it is a means of realizing well-defined goals, and for publishers a possible profitable source of income, or a way to advertise the existence of a medical society or association. For its readers, the medical literature is a source of information that can be used to update and maintain professional knowledge. Medical journals also serve as a means of communication with colleagues and as a symbol of being a member of a college (Nylenna 1994).

Over time an evolution in the tasks of medical journals has taken place; from being more or less exclusively channels for professional information, the journals have become important elements in the professionalization of medicine and in shaping the identity of specialties and subgroups. Last, but not least, increasing emphasis has been placed on journals as tools in the qualification process and for bringing credits to authors. This evolution can also be described as a shift from a main focus on the reader as the recipient of information (reader-orientation), via the group, or the "tribe," often represented by the publisher, to more emphasis on the author, who gains recognition by publishing scientific papers (author-orientation).

13.1.6.1 Dissemination of Knowledge

One of the main forces behind the creation of medical societies in the nineteenth century was the desire for knowledge, and the professional literature was the most important instrument for satisfying that desire. Apart from making study visits from the peripherally located Nordic countries mainly to Germany and France, reading was the only way to obtain professional information.

In Christiania, a medical reading club was founded in 1826, and at the very first meeting of the Medical Society of Trøndelag on November 17, 1842, it was decided to subscribe to four medical journals, two in German, one in French, and one in Swedish (Leira 1993).

The desire for education and factual information was strong among Norwegians in general in the nineteenth century, and there was no strict distinction between factual prose and fictional literature. The famous Norwegian authors Henrik Wergeland (1808-1845) and Bjørnstjerne Bjørnson (1832-1910) became central figures in Norwegian society and in the political debate, not because of their poems, but because of their high-quality factual prose (Johnsen 1995). In a Norwegian textbook on the history of literature published in 1896, non-fictional literature was awarded much attention and 130 pages were devoted to medical literature alone, mainly articles in medical journals (Schønberg 1896). During the twentieth century, non-fictional literature, which comprises some four-fifths of all literature published, has gradually become distinct from fiction. A research program (Norwegian Non-fictional Writing) has just been launched to study the influence of specialized literature in general on political and cultural developments in Norway during the last 200 years (Johnsen 1995). The aim of this project is to uncover the contents, genres, and usages of non-fictional writing through a number of approaches, for example theoretical analyses, chronological surveys, and thematic studies.

As other channels of information have developed, the relative importance of the scientific journals for the dissemination of professional knowledge has been reduced. The traditional scientific journal is challenged by an explosive development in information technology during the twentieth century, extensive traveling by doctors and scientists, an enormous increase in personal ways of information exchange, and a tremendous increase in the number of congresses, seminars, and other professional meetings, both nationally and internationally. It has been shown that even physicians and medical researchers frequently use reports in the lay press as a gateway to the scientific literature (Philips 1991). Nevertheless, reading medical literature, and medical journals in particular, is still regarded as one of the most important means of staying updated professionally (Richards 1986). An American study from the 1970s revealed that medical literature was the most important source of information for physicians (Stinson 1980). Reading peer-reviewed journals is the best approach to coping with the growing body of medical knowledge (Arndt 1992).

A survey among Norwegian physicians in 1993 showed that attending medical courses, meetings, and congresses was regarded as the most important source of information, closely followed by reading medical literature (Nylenna 1996). Physicians who give such activities a high priority are more likely to regard themselves as sufficiently updated compared with others who do not value this activities (Nylenna).

Nine out of ten Norwegian physicians read Tidsskrift for Den norske lægeforening regularly, and two out of three read Nordisk Medicin. Every fifth doctor reads at least one of the four largest general medical journals (the British Medical Journal, the Lancet, the New England Journal of Medicine, and the Journal of the American Medical Association (JAMA)), while only one out of fifteen reads the Swedish or Danish national journal regularly (Nylenna 1991).

13.1.6.2 Identity Shaping

In the nineteenth century, the traditional apprenticeship system of medical education lost ground, and a more centralized system of medical schools developed. Medical practitioners extended their control over several aspects of medical work. An important part of this process was the elaboration and the more effective enforcement of a code of medical ethics. At that time, medical ethics was not concerned primarily with regulating the behavior of doctors toward their patients, but the behavior of doctors toward their fellow practitioners (Waddington 1990).

Many articles on ethical subjects were published in the medical journals of the nineteenth century. In an editorial in the first issue of the Tidsskrift for praktisk Medisin after the Norwegian Medical Association took over in 1888, it was declared that "apart from the social questions, the journal will deal with the various questions regarding professional loyalty, e.g. the Code of ethics." To the Norwegian Medical Association, the membership journal has always been an important means of realizing its main objectives, "to secure the doctors' influence on various social matters, to protect their interests within and outside the profession, and promote scientific work" (Bjerke 1961).

With the specialization of medicine, the identity-shaping function of the journals became more visible and important. The fragmentation of medicine into subdisciplines created a need for each of these groups to professionalize and produce objects of identification of their own. The smaller the group, the stronger the need. Journals, often published by specialist societies or organizations, frequently became such objects.

According to Derek de Solla Price, research is based on a series of "invisible colleges" formed to serve the needs of new disciplines. Every ten years or so, a group of the members of one discipline will form a new invisible college and this college will need a journal of its own. At this stage, members of the college write mostly for one another. The authorship is the same as the readership (deSolla Price 1961). After another decade or so, a new subdiscipline will be established and will contain enough members for another breakout, forming a new invisible college with a need for a new journal. A recent international example of this development is provided by the journals devoted to AIDS. In the early 1980s it was obvious that at least one sub-specialist journal devoted to the subject would be needed. In fact, there are now scores of them focusing on different aspects of HIV-infection, and new titles are still appearing (Lock 1992).

To many Norwegian doctors, the several Nordic Actas and Scandinavian Journals, and other international specialist journals as well, have served as unifying and identity-shaping objects within a medical speciality. On a less academic and scientific level, the economic prosperity of the 1980s and 1990s, combined with modern publishing technology, has opened opportunities for establishing journals and newsletters for a number of subgroups of Norwegian physicians. These publications mainly carry information on organizational matters; normally they do not use peer review and are not indexed in international data bases. Their main objectives are the formation of a common identity and the maintenance of a team spirit within the group. Over the last years, however, some national specialist journals with higher academic ambitions have been launched. An example is the journal Norsk Epidemiologi (Norwegian Journal of Epidemiology) established by the Norwegian Society of Epidemiology in 1991. This journal has a circulation of 500 (1995) and publishes scientific papers in epidemiology both in Norwegian and in English. The journal publishes 3 or 4 issues yearly, often theme issues, and doctoral theses as supplements.

Four out of seven professional branches within the Norwegian Medical Association now produce their own journals. The oldest and largest of these journals is Ylf-Forum, a journal for younger doctors established in 1986, published ten times per year and with a circulation of 3,600 (1995). A number of the local, geographically based departments of the associations also publish their own journals or newsletters, as does the Medical Students Association (Nicolaysen 1994).

13.1.6.3 Merit Award

"Publish or perish" is one of the most commonly used slogans among medical researchers. Scientific publication has become the most qualifying activity that an aspiring doctor can engage in, and the productivity and quality of a scientist is almost exclusively evaluated on the basis of the articles he or she has authored. At the same time, the practitioner-author in medical journals has gradually been replaced by the academician-author (Fye 1990).

One hundred years ago, medical journals had already replaced books as a medium for presenting original research. The merit or credit aspect of medical journals has become increasingly visible during the last decades along with the development of the so-called bibliometric methods of scientific evaluation. Such methods, like the citation frequency of a paper or the journal impact factor, emphasize the medical journals' new role as a marketplace for the qualification of scientists. In the publication process, this aspect of medical journals turns the focus from the reader as the main target of an article to the author as the producer of information.

As mentioned above, specialization and internationalization are characteristic trends as regards medicine and medical journals in the twentieth century. This international shift is connected with increasing international cooperation among researchers, but also with the status of journals in relation to the evaluation of the individual researcher's publications. Among academic bodies, international journals have a higher prestige than regional journals, and regional journals have a higher prestige than national journals. Papers appearing in high-prestige journals bring the author greater credit than papers published in journals with lower prestige. For authors aiming at high-ranking academic positions, this leads to a desire to publish internationally. After the Second World War, this meant publishing in English, and in most fields of medicine American journals with an international approach have the highest status.

Even though citation frequencies have been shown to correlate poorly with the scientific quality of individual papers (Seglen 1989), this measure is still frequently used as a means of evaluating individual researchers. The Science Citation Index, a data base recording how often each published paper is cited, is also used for national and international comparisons concerning both the quantity and quality of Norwegian medical research. Norwegian publishing activity in clinical medicine is high, approximately 200 articles per 1 million inhabitants, and the citation frequency for Norwegian papers is about the average for the OECD countries (Olsen et al. 1994). During the period 1979-1981, faculty members in Norwegian medical schools produced an average of 8.2 publications, of which 7.6 were journal articles (Kyvik 1991).

The "impact factor" of a journal has become important to authors. This factor is defined as the average number of citations per paper published in a single journal. However, in individual medical specialities or geographic areas, this is not always correlated with the clinical importance of a journal, defined as the influence of a journal on the clinical practice of medicine. High-impact journals are much more important to researchers and academicians than to practicing doctors. In non-English-speaking countries, like Norway, this is especially relevant, since the whole system of citation analyses is based on papers published in English. The combination of internationalization and prestige, which has its origin in the basic sciences and biomedicine, also causes special problems in some fields of medical publishing. Clinical medicine, and even more so community medicine, has strong ties to local culture, and even in a world of more or less universal molecular biology, different and historical interpretations of symptoms and signs will lead to different diagnostic and therapeutic decisions (Payer 1988). The closer one gets to the molecular level of medicine, the easier it is to generalize from the results and the more international research and publishing become. The closer one gets to the community level of medicine, the harder it is to generalize and the more national or local the research and publishing become. Evaluating research by level of "internationalization" is therefore biased in favor of the basic sciences.

One obvious side effect of the focus on productivity of publication and the pressure to publish is an inflation of the authorship concept. To most scientists, it is important to have a long list of publications, which is one of the reasons for an increase in the average number of authors per paper. The average number of authors per paper in the Annals of Internal Medicine increased from 1.3 to 4.7 from 1930 to 1979, and in the New England Journal of Medicine from 1.2 to 5.2 during the same period (Burman 1982). To stop this development, initiatives have been taken to base professional evaluation of applicants to academic positions on a limited number of papers (Riis 1992). Specific criteria for authorship of scientific papers have also been produced (International Committee of Medical Journal Editors 1985).

From an historical point of view, the proliferation of multi-author papers has been seen as a threat to the integrity of the scientific article, and it has been stated that this integrity can only be restored by returning to a more traditional definition of authorship (Benson 1991).

13.1.6.4 An Example

The three different tasks of medical journals described above dissemination of information, identity-shaping, and merit producing can exist side by side in one, single journal. In the case of the major international general journals especially, which receive a grat many papers and have a high rejection rate, most of the papers published are original, topical, and relevant to a broad group of readers, and also bring high credits to the author.

In many scientific journals, the shift from reader-orientation to author-orientation is reflected by a changing emphasis on each of these qualities over time.

Sometimes, and in some fields, a distinct shift from one aspect to the other can be seen in the establishing of new journals.

A pertinent example is the old, but formally young, specialty of general practice in Norway. Traditionally, Norwegian general practitioners (GPs) have obtained their professional information from Tidsskrift for Den norske lægeforening. More than other physicians in Norway, GPs have always based their reading and continuing medical education on Tidsskriftet. On the way to becoming a recognized and certified speciality in 1985, however, Tidsskriftet, which covers all medical specialties as a general membership journal, was unsuitable as an identity-shaping journal for general practitioners. For this ideological purpose, a new "underground" journal, Utposten, was established in 1971. Soon Utposten became a symbol of professional identity among primary care physicians and a tool to be used in the fight for a certified specialty. But, neither Tidsskriftet nor Utposten were suitable for the publication of narrow scientific articles in this field written by GPs as a means of furthering their academic qualifications. Consequently, and according to a long tradition of Nordic cooperation, the Scandinavian Journal of Primary Health Care was established in 1983. This is a journal devoted mainly to orginal research, and more than in the other GP journals, the authors write for other researchers or for evaluation committees (in the Nordic countries normally set up to assess applicants for academic positions), making the merit aspect of the journal more visible.

Thus three separate journals highly relevant for the same medical specialty, in this case general practice/family medicine, have come to serve three very different purposes.

13.1.7 The Future

"The death of biomedical journals" was the title of a recently published article, describing the challenges from new information technology to the traditional paper journal system. According to an international group of futurologists, Internet, electronic mail, and other means of rapid exchange of information will soon make the printing technology of scientific publishing obsolete (LaPorte 1995).

By the end of 1995, Internet included about 100 peer-reviewed science journals, and the number of such journals is increasing very fast. Some journals now only exist in electronic form. As compared with paper journals, electronic versions add search functions, links to related articles, automatic notification and alerting of readers and discussion forums. Some electronic journals, such as the Journal of Image Guided Surgery, even include videofilms (Taubes 1996).

However, the total number of medical journals seems to have reached a plateau, since the scientific world is converting from an era of growth to an era of steady state activity (Varmhus 1995).

At the same time, physicians are exposed to a threat of deprofessionalization. As doctors lose clinical autonomy and simply become employees and health care providers, the medical profession is being deprofessionalized (Armstrong 1990). The physician's influence on the content of his or her work has been reduced, and numerous market forces challenge the unity of the profession. Unhappy doctors all over the world are discussing how to reorganize the different health care systems. Medicine is a profession in trouble (1990).

Medical journals are no longer the "closed communication circuits" of the profession. In the general medical journals the number of non-medical authors is increasing, now that the journals are covering a wider range of issues and are including articles by economists, philosophers, historians, and so on. On the other hand, scientific journals of various kinds are no longer read only by members of the different professions or specialties. More coverage of research results in the lay press and the new electronic media is giving wider groups of constantly better educated people access to more or less the same information as physicians get. Thus, the information gap between the public and the profession is narrowing and the advantage of the professionals based on their exclusive ownership of information is diminishing.

People have complained about the information overload for several hundred years. So far, however, the means of coping seem to have increased faster than the mass of information. In a report from the first reading club in Christiania published in Eyr in 1827, medical journals were discussed in general, and it was stated "... their importance in medical science, in which the literature is so voluminous that a doctor devoting his whole time to it, would not possibly be able to read ... even a tenth of it." At that time, the library of the young University of Christiania subscribed to 18 medical journals, 16 German and two Danish (1933).

Two thirds of Norwegian physicians report that they are able to obtain sufficient information to keep updated. They are able to do this by attending meetings and conferences and reading medical literature (Nylenna 1996). Obviously, electronic publication is a challenge to medical journals, but up to now, no new medium has ever eliminated an old one. Paper journals are likely to survive for a long time, and to play an important role in concert with the new electronic information systems, just as daily newspapers do in today's era of radio and television. To prosper, however, journals must become more reader-oriented and the focus must shift from the author and back to the reader. Whatever technology is used for information dissemination, the message and the needs and demands of the reader will always be the most important, not the channel of communication.

The seemingly bleak prospects for both medical journals and the medical profession might be turned into a common opportunity for prosperity and renewal for both. Journals should continue to select papers for their originality, scientific value, and relevance to clinical practice, but more attention must be paid to ethics and collegial matters, and the democratization of medicine and patients' rights and demands. General medical journals will probably become increasingly general, as will the first tier of specialist journals. Future journals will be marked by health politics, health economics, law, cost effectivness, and focus on patient satisfaction. The professionalization of medical journals and editing will continue, and it is hoped that the journals will even contribute to confidence about the future among physicians (Nylenna 1994, Smith 1991).

In this way medical journals can contribute to the reprofessionalization of medicine, not by turning back the clock a hundred years, but by taking the responsibility of being self-governing in today's society seriously. Medical journals may again become a link between society and medicine. With the help of medical journals "doctors will have to learn that a satisfied patient is as important as a medically improved one. The implication of these changes for traditional medical education and practice, which have always implicitly emphasized the importance of professional dominance, are considerable but reflect a historical transformation to the environment in which professions now operate" (Armstrong 1990).

References

Armstrong, D. "Medicine as a profession: Times of change," *British Medical Journal*,301(1990):691–3.

Arndt, K.A. "Information excess in medicine," *Arch Dermatol*,128(1992):1249–56.

Bartrip, P.W.J. *Mirror of medicine*. Oxford: Clarendon, 1990.

Benson, K.R. "Science and the single author: Historical reflection on the problem of authorship," *Cancer Bull*, 43(1991): 324–31.

Berg, O. "Verdier og interesser – Den norske lægeforenings fremvekst og utvikling," in: *Legene og samfunnet*, eds. Larsen, Ø., O. Berg and F. Hodne. Oslo: Den norske lægeforening, 1986.

Bergsjø, P. "Acta seventy years ago," *Acta Obstet Gynecol Scand*,70(1991):5–7.

Bergsjø, P. "Tidsskrift for Den norske lægeforening status presens og veien videre," in: *Kunnskap er makt og bør deles med andre*, eds. Fugelli, P. and M. Nylenna. Oslo: Universitetsforlaget, 1987.

Berner, J.H. red. *Den norske lægeforening 1886 1936*. Oslo: Centraltrykkeriet, 1936.

Bjercke, O. "Lægeforeningens sekretariat gjennom 75 år," *Tidsskrift for Den norske lægeforening*,81(1961):646–58.

Bonnevie, P. and H. Theorell. "Nordisk Medicin historia och nutid," *Nord Med*, 87(1972):1.

Bonnevie, P. "Nordisk Medicin 50 år. En epoke er endt, men den videnskabelige kontinuitet sikret," *Nord Med*,95(1980): 26–8.

Booth, C.C. "Medical communication: The old and the new," *British Medical Journal*,285(1982):105–8.

Bradford Hill, A. "The reasons for writing," *British Medical Journal*,2(1965):870–2.

Burman, K.D. "'Hanging from the masthead': Reflections on authorship," *Ann Intern Med*, 97(1982):602.

Burnham, J.C. "The evolution of editorial peer review," *JAMA*,263(1990):1323–9.

deSolla Price, D.J. "The development and structure of the biomedical literature." In: *Coping with the biomedical literature*. Warren K.S., ed. New York: Praeger, 1981:3–16.

deSolla Price, D.J. *Science since Babylon*. New Haven, Connecticut: Yale University Press, 1961.

Egeland, *M. Med kunnskap skal landet bygges. Universitetsforlaget 1950–1990*. Oslo: Universitetsforlaget, 1996.

Folkow, B. "History of physiology in Scandinavia," *Acta Physiol Scand*, 138(1990):5-12.

Freidson, E. *Profession of medicine: A study of the Sociology of Applied Knowledge*. New York: Dodd Mead, 1970:71.

Fye, W.B. "Medical authorship: Traditions, trends, and tribulations," *Ann Intern Med*, 113(1990):317–325.

Gelfand, T. "The history of the medical profession," in: *Companion encyclopedia of the history of medicine*, eds. Bynum, W. F. and R. Porter. London: Routledge, 1993.

Goode, W.J. "Community within a community: The professions," *American Sociological Review*,22(1957):194–200.

Grøn, F. D*et norske medicinske Selskab 1833 1933*. Oslo: Steenske boktrykkeri Johannes Bjørnstad a/s, 1933.

Harlem, O.K. "Tidsskriftet. En målsettingskavalkade," *Tidsskrift for Den norske lægeforening*,106(1986):1269–71.

Hofoss, D. *Spesialisering av helsepersonell hvorfor og hvordan? Rapport nr. 3 1980*. Oslo: Norges allmennvitenskapelige forskningsråds gruppe for helsetjenesteforskning, 1980.

Høyer, S. *Pressen mellom teknologi og samfunn. Norske og internasjonale perspektiver på pressehistorien fra Gutenberg til vår tid*. Oslo: Universitetsforlaget, 1995.

International Committee of Medical Journal Editors. "Guidelines on authorship," *BMJ*, 291(1985):722.

Johnsen, E.B. *Den andre litteraturen. Hva sakprosa er*. Oslo: Cappelen, 1995.

Johnsen, E.B., ed. *Virkelighetens forvaltere*. Oslo: Universitetsforlaget, 1995.

Kallevik, S.A. "Utenlandske bøker foretrekkes," *Tidsskrift for Den norske lægeforening,* 113(1993):2455.

Kallevik, S.A. "Ønsker medisinske fagbøker på norsk," *Tidsskrift for Den norske lægeforening*,113(1993):2454.

Kyvik, S. *Productivity in science. Scientific publishing at Norwegian Universities*. Oslo: Norwegian University Press, 1991.

LaPorte, R.E., E. Marler, S. Akazawa, F. Sauer, C. Gamboa, C. Shanton et al. "The death of biomedical journals," *British Medical Journal*,310(1995):1387–90.

Larsen, Ø. and B.I. Lindskog. *Sundhedstidende 1778-1781. Johann Clemens Tode*. Oslo: Seksjon for medisinsk historie, Universitetet i Oslo, 1991.

Larsen, Ø. "Gamle trykk. Legebøker i Danmark og Norge," *Liv og Helse*,33(1966): 231–4, 237.

Larsen, Ø *Mangfoldig medisin*. Oslo: Det medisinske fakultet, Universitetet i Oslo, 1989.

Larsen, Ø. "Urtebøkene," *Liv og Helse*,33 (1966):181–4.

Leira, H. *Trøndelag Medisinske Selskap 150 år.* Trondheim: Tapir, 1993.

Ljunggren, E. "Nordiskt Medicinskt Arkiv och dess båda Acta. Ett hundreårsminne. I. Kirurgi." In: *Yearbook of the Museum of Medical History Stockholm*. Växsjö: Smålandspostens Boktryckeri AB, 1970.

Lock, S. *A difficult balance. Editorial peer review in medicine*. London: The Nuffield Provincial Hospitals Trust, 1985.

Lock, S. "As things really were?" In: *The future of medical journals*. Lock, S. ed. London: British Medical Journal, 1991.

Lock, S. "Journalology: Evolution of medical journals and some current problems," *J Int Med*,232(1992):199–205.

Lock, S. "One hand clapping," *British Medical Journal*, 301(1990):677–8.

Lock, S. "The medical journal how?" in: *Kunnskap er makt og bør deles med andre*, eds: Fugelli, P. and M. Nylenna. Oslo: Universitetsforlaget,(1987):115–8.

Lundberg, G.D. "Countdown to millennium – Balancing professionalism and business of medicine," *Journal of the American Medical Association*, 263(1990):86.

Myren, J. and C.W. Janssen. *Fra gastroenterologiens historie i Norge*. Oslo: Norsk Gastroenterologisk Forening, 1995.

Naisbitt, J. and P. Aburdene. *Megatrends 2000*. London: Pan Books, 1990.

Natvig, H. "Refleksjoner ved opphøret av Nordisk Hygienisk Tidsskrift," *Nordisk Hygienisk Tidsskrift*,55(1974):129–37.

Nicolaysen, K.G. "Er egne medlemsblad løsningen?," *Tidsskrift for Den norske lægeforening*,114(1994):2176–7, 2304–5, 2432–3.

Norman, J.M. (ed.). *Morton's medical bibliography*. 5th edition. Aldershot: Scolar Press, 1991.

Nylenna, M. and R. Smith. "American retreat on SI units," *British Medical Journal*,305(1992):268.

Nylenna, M. and H.M. Svabø. "Tidsskriftets målsetting," *Tidsskrift for Den norske lægeforening*,107(1987):3003.

Nylenna, M., O.G. Aasland and E. Falkum. "Keeping professionally updated: Percieved coping and CME-profiles among physicians," *The Journal of Continuing Education in Health Professions*, 1996: in press.

Nylenna, M. "Det nasjonale medisinske tidsskrift – hvorfor?" *Ugeskrift for Læger*, 152(1990):3761–5.

Nylenna, M. "Norske Legers lesevaner," *Nord Med*,106(1991):53–5.

Nylenna, M. "The future of medical journals: An editor's view," *Croatian Medical Journal*, 35(1994):195–8.

Nylenna, M. "Tidsskriftets leserundersøkelse 1990," *Tidsskrift for Den norske lægeforening*,110(1990):3912–3.

Oldershaw, J. "Accessing the literature," *British Journal of Hospital Medicine*,47(1992): 433–7.

Olsen, T.B., H.F. Hansen, T. Luukonen, O. Persson, and G.Sivertsen. *Nordisk forskning i internasjonal sammenheng – en bibliometrisk beskrivelse av publisering og siteringer i naturvitenskapelig og medisinsk forskning, Temanord*,(1994):618. Copenhagen: Nordisk Ministerråd, 1994.

Olsen, T.B. *Norske doktorgrader i tall – med særlig vekt på tiårsperioden 1984-93. Rapport 9/94*. Oslo: Utredningsinstituttet for forskning og høyere utdanning, 1994.

Payer, L. *Medicine and culture: Varieties of treatment in the United States, England, West Germany, and France*. New York: H. Holt, 1988.

Phillips, D.P., E.J. Kanter, B. Bednarczyk and P.L. Tastad. "Importance of the lay press in the transmission of medical knowledge to the scientific community," *New England Journal of Medicine*,325 (1991):1180–3.

Reichborn-Kjennerud, I. "En oversigt over og karakteristik av de gamle nordiske lægebøker," *Tidsskrift for Den norske lægeforening*,44(1924):381–6,424–9.

Reichborn-Kjennerud, I. "Lægebøker." in: *Medisinens historie i Norge*, eds: Reichborn-Kjennerud, I., F. Grøn and I. Kobro. Oslo: Grøndahl, 1936.

Relman, A.R. "The purpose and prospects of the general medical journal," *Bull NY Acad Med*,64(1988):875–80.

Richards, R.K. "Physicians' self-directed learning. A new perspective for continuing medical education I. Reading," *Möbius*, 6(2)(1986):1–13.

Riis, P. "New paradigms in journalology," *J Int Med*,232(1992):207–13.

Schønberg, E. "Medicin." In: Jæger, H. *Illustreret Norsk Litteraturhistorie*. Kristiania: Hjalmar Bieglers forlag, 1896.

Seglen, P. "Bruk av siteringsanalyse og andre bibliometriske metoder i evaluering av forskningskvalitet," *Tidsskrift for Den norske lægeforening*,109(1989):3229–34.

Sivertsen, G. *Internationalization via Journals Scientific and scholarly journals edited in the Nordic countries*. NORD 1991:49. Copenhagen: Nordic Council of Ministers, 1991.

Smith, R. "Through the crystal ball darkly," in: *The future of medical journals*, ed: Lock, S. London: British Medical Journal, 1991.

Stinson, E.R. and D.A. Mueller. "Survey of health professionals' information habits and needs," *Journal of the American Medical Association*,243(1980):140–3.

Storm-Mathisen, H. "Hvilken betydning har 'Tidsskriftet' hatt for den praktiserende lege og for sykehuslegen?" *Tidsskrift for Den norske lægeforening*,101(1981):43-6.

Sørensen, Ø., ed. *Nordic paths to national identity in the nineteenth century*. KULTs skriftserie nr. 22. Oslo: The Research Council of Norway, 1994.

Taubes, G. "Science journals go wired," *Science*,271(1996):764–6.

Torgersen, U. *Profesjonssosiologi*. Oslo-Bergen-Tromsø: Universitetsforlaget, 1972.

Tveterås, H.L. *Norske tidsskrifter. Bibliografi over periodiske tidsskrifter i Norge inntil 1920*. Oslo: Universitetsforlaget, 1984.

Varmus, H. "Shattuck lecture – Biomedical research enters the steady state," *New England Journal of Medicine*,333(1995): 811–5.

Waddington, I. "The movement towards the professionalisation of medicine," *British Medical Journal*, 301(1990):688–90.

Warren, K.S. "From papyrus to parchment to paper to pixels: Information technology and the future of medical publishing," in: *The future of medical journals*, ed: Lock, S., London: *British Medical Journal*, 1991.

CHAPTER 13.2

Recreation or Professional Necessity – The Study Tours of Nineteenth Century Norwegian Physicians

BENT OLAV OLSEN

13.2.1 Introducing the Physicians on Study Tours

In the history of travels and tourism one thing remains stable, the fact that people travel. There are individual differences in preferences and in the rationale behind peoples' travels. And there are also structural differences, which change according to time and place. The impact of travels also varies considerably.

There have been waves of travelers, each with different characteristics: pilgrims, English gentlemen on "the Grand Tour," twentieth-century masstourism, and so on. Each wave is the result of a complex mix of factors.

Because of the interesting combination of leisure and work, the traveling academics are an important group, and this chapter takes a closer look at one part of this group: Norwegian physicians.

In the nineteenth century, an increasing number of Norwegian physicians traveled. These physicians belonged to the first wave of academic-related travels that originated in Norway. The increase in the number of physicians going abroad can partly be explained by the journeys of a pioneering group of physicians who acquired basic knowledge, paved the way, published information, and functioned as role-models.

Three groups of physicians have been chosen to represent the travels of Norwegian physicians. The first group was born between 1810 and 1815, the second between 1840 and 1845, and the third between 1870 and 1875.

13.2.1.1 What is a Study Tour?

A study tour can be defined as a journey undertaken in order to learn something about one or more academic disciplines.

For practical reasons, due to the source material available, our definition of a study tour includes naval expeditions, physicians on emigrant ships, physicians on whaling expeditions, journeys to combat zones, other journeys connected with military service, house physician posts abroad, and travels in Norway and abroad when such travels have been described as scientific.

Travels not included are emigration and other permanent relocation, missionary travels, and travels with leisure as the only given purpose for the journey.

"Study tour" can be widely interpreted, and we do not wish to put too much stress on the formal educational aspect. Many of the central tasks of the physician are learned by doing. This is the main reason why some types of journeys that were undertaken in order to engage in paid work are defined as study tours. For example, military physicians gained new knowledge about medicine as a result of journeys to combat zones or of other journeys connected to military service.

13.2.1.2 Motivation

For the Norwegian physicians there could be a wide range of professional reasons for undertaking a journey: to gain new knowledge purely for their own academic benefit, to gain new knowledge and skills for the good of their patients, to gain knowledge for the development and establishment of a national medicine, and to improve their position vis-à-vis other physicians.

The traveler's motivation is a mixture of factors. In each of the aforementioned four groups, recreational reasons for travel might contribute to the decision to undertake a journey. Or it might be the main reason for the journey. Study tours were often combined with recreational travel, and the journey was often a pleasure in itself. Study tours today most often involve activities other than purely academic ones. Attending a congress often involves an academic/professional element and a more leisure/tourist-related element. For the nineteenth-century physicians, the contrast to everyday life and the anticipated experiences in the great cities of Europe contributed to their decision to travel. In accounts of the history of tourism, travels of a more leisurely type are often justified as "study tours."

13.2.1.3 Some Limitations in the Source Material

The main source of our knowledge of the extent of study tours undertaken by Norwegian physicians in the nineteenth century is the biographies in the books "Norges Læger" (The Physicians of Norway). In the first books (1873, 1888, 1890, 1908–1912, and 1915) there are many records of the travels of Norwegian physicians, because the editor Frantz C Kiær (1835–1893) specifically asked Norwegian physicians for them in Norsk Magazin for Lægevidenskaben (Kiær 1871). However, the questions Kiær asked led the physicians to give standardized answers. Furthermore, Kiær edited the answers to make them even more uniform. So only a few accounts represent the physicians' own story, in their own words.

Another source is the numerous travel letters written by Norwegian physicians to magazines and newspapers and a few travel accounts which appeared in books. In this part of the chapter, these letters are used to exemplify some general problems and findings. Travel letters in magazines are systematically discussed in the next chapter. These letters are more often the physicians' own story, in contrast to the accounts that we find in the biographies. These reports, however, are influenced by a particular purpose as well, as they were often written with a professional objective in mind, for a specific audience, following standardized patterns for writing scientific articles, or to give an account of travels to committees that awarded grants. (For the number of tours for the three groups of physicians, see Table 13.7.)

In later editions of "Norges Læger" and later volumes of "Norsk Magazin for Lægevidenskaben," records of physicians' travels became less frequent, though this does not necessarily mean that the physicians traveled less. There is reason to believe that as traveling became more common, physicians' colleagues and the general public became less interested in travel accounts and travel letters.

13.2.1.4 Travelers' Tales or Travelers' Fairy-tales?

We have little direct information from other sources that we can use to check the reliability of the physicians as informants. But pre-

TABLE 13.7
Number of tours for the three groups of physicians

Number of tours	Born 1810-15	%	Born 1840-45	%	Born 1870-75	%
0	63	54.8	49	41.5	114	44.0
1	18	15.7	23	19.5	64	24.7
2	20	17.4	9	7.6	29	11.2
3	4	3.5	13	11.0	14	5.4
4	4	3.5	6	5.1	11	4.2
5 or more	5	4.3	18	15.3	21	8.1
Unknown	1	0.9	0	–	6	2.3
Total	115	100.1	118	100.0	259	99.9

sumably we have a sort of internal professional control. The editor of the "Norges Læger" had various ways of checking the accuracy of the information. And, furthermore, the physicians had no strong motive for giving false statements. It is also possible that some journeys have been forgotten, or have deliberately not been mentioned. But travelers' tales could be travelers' fairy-tales. There may well have been a tendency to exaggerate, dramatize, or embellish what happened (Helk 1991, p. 147).

13.2.2 Changes in Types of Travelers and their Destinations

13.2.2.1 No Grand Tour

All the physicians' journeys examined here were undertaken in the period 1831-1938. On an international scale, the first part of this period was the end of the Grand Tour era. A Grand Tour was the conclusion of the education of the young gentlemen from the landed gentry. In the course of time this changed, and beginning in the late eighteenth century the middle classes came to be the dominant group undertaking such tours (Towner, 1985, p. 310). The Grand Tour, in the strict sense, was an infrequent type of journey among the Norwegian upper and middle classes. It was primarily a phenomenon connected to Great Britain, and was one of the first major epochs in the history of tourism. However, it also had its parallel in the Nordic countries. The aim of long journeys to continental Europe, which often lasted for 2 or 3 years, was to gain cultural refinement. Educational motives, in the strict sense, were mainly found during the period from the middle of the seventeenth to the middle of the eighteenth century (ibid., p. 311). From the recent work of the Danish historian Vello Helk, we have solid information on the study tours of people from the Danish-Norwegian Kingdom in the years 1536–1813 (Helk 1987, 1991). The Grand Tour period is generally regarded as having come to an end some time before the middle of the nineteenth century. One reason for this is that duration is one of the factors in the definition of the Grand Tour, and shorter trips for example, to summer courses became more and more common. This development also seen among the Norwegian physicians in the three groups.

In an international perspective, the journeys of these physicians were undertaken in a travel-transition period. This transition started from a combination of luxury journeys of upper-class travelers on the one hand, and their counterparts of necessity travelers on the other. It seems reasonable to group religiously motivated travels as a third group. In this period, journeys themselves began to have a value for large parts of society, and not just as a means to an end. This transition is a process that is still going on, a process whereby traveling is becoming more and more common.

13.2.2.2 Little Material on Non-travelers
After these general statements and introductory figures, let us start with the physicians who did not report having traveled, and define them as non-travelers. This is obviously an uncertain assumption. An analysis of the information we have on these physicians does not help to explain why they did not travel abroad. This is also a general problem for the analysis of tourism and travel motivation today (Haukeland, 1990). While many physicians provided information, although partial, on why they traveled, none of them gave reasons for staying at home and just doing their work. What we can try to do is see if there are any differences between those who traveled and those who did not.

If we start with the assumption that each physician had the opportunity to travel, a health element might have been of importance in whether a physician chose to travel, and a possible explanation could have been that non-travelers died earlier than those who traveled. There is a difference between the three groups in this respect (Table 13.8). To a large extent this difference can be accounted for by one of the problems with using "Norges Læger" as a source. The first books in what came to be the "Norges Læger" series, are based on both autobiographies and information from other sources. Some of the "non-travelers" were in fact "non-responders," their biographies being compiled from other available sources by the editor. One group of "non-responders" comprised physicians who were deceased at the time the book was written, so that information on traveling

TABLE 13.8
Age at death for non-travelers and travelers

Age at death	Born 1810–15 (n=115)		Born 1840–45 (n=118)		Born 1870–75 (n=259)	
	non-traveler	traveler	non-traveler	traveler	non-traveler	traveler
unknown	3 (4.8%)	–	3 (6.1%)	–	7 (6.1%)	5 (3.4%)
<50 years	24 (38.1%)	7 (13.7%)	17 (34.7%)	8 (11.6%)	28 (24.6%)	17 (11.7%)
>50 years	36 (57.1%)	45 (86.5%)	29 (59.2%)	61 (88.4%)	79 (69.3%)	123 (84.8%)
Total	63 (100.0%)	52 (100.0%)	49 (100.0%)	69 (100.0%)	114 (100.0%)	145 (99.9%)

would be more limited for these physicians. In our 1840–1845 group, this is not a major problem, since the first book was published in 1873; the 1810–15 group is more influenced by this possible bias.

One of the factors that determines whether one travels or not is of course finances. "Despite past fictions that the professions were communities of equals, they have always been stratified" (Freidson, 1983 p. 287). It is a myth nurtured by the medical profession in Norway as well, but this has little resemblance to reality. Could it be that those who did not travel could not afford it? For those who did travel, many of the tours were undertaken when the physicians were young, and for some of them economic support from their families might have been necessary. However, the information available in our sources does not suggest that family status, as indicated by father's occupation, was an explanatory factor. This is not to say that this was of no importance, but only that our material is not good enough for any examination of this theory.

13.2.2.3 A Universal Urge to Travel?

Is it the case that given the opportunity, every doctor would be a traveler? The American historian, Daniel J. Boorstin, writes: "When we say that men climb the highest mountain `simply because it's there' we think we are describing changeless human nature. In fact, we are expressing a peculiarly modern point of view" (Boorstin, 1975, p. 4). Although there is some evidence for the positive evaluation of travel as a means of gathering knowledge, for the sake of science or the sake of the nation, and although there has been a long tradition for this, I would like to close the discussion of reasons for not traveling with a reflection on the normality of traveling. Is it legitimate to view travel, the will to travel, the urge to travel, or the opportunity to travel as the normal for physicians, or is this also a peculiarly modern point of view?

13.2.2.4 Better Information on those who Traveled

The information we have concerning those who did travel is, in spite of its limitations, better suited for an analysis.

TABLE 13.9
When did the physicians undertake their first journey?

Number of travelers: (in % of those who traveled)	Born 1810-15 (n=52*)	Born 1840-45 (n=69)	Born 1870-75 (n=145*)
Before medical examination	4 (7.7%)	9 (13.0%)	8 (5.5%)
Same year or the year after medical examination	12 (23.1%)	16 (23.2%)	21 (14.5%)
Within 5 years after medical examination	28 (53.8%)	52 (75.4%)	70 (48.3%)

*including those with vague statements

In the three cohorts, there was little difference in their age when they finished their medical education. We will see later, that of the three groups, those who were born between 1840 and 1845 were those with the most registered study tours. In Table 13.9, we see that, in this cohort, 75 percent of those who traveled had done so within 5 years after they had taken their medical examinations. For those born between 1840 and 1845, the high proportion of physicians who had traveled within 5 years of taking their medical examination can partly be explained by the need to travel abroad in order to specialize. For those born between 1870 and 1875, this reason for going abroad was less important because of the development of the Norwegian university, clinics, and hospitals. Further, the development of the labor market, with a slight over-production of physicians at the end of the nineteenth century, might have reduced the willingness to travel for those physicians who had no steady employment. Studytours could, however, have been a way of indicating special qualifications when competing for jobs.

13.2.2.4.1 Influencing their Careers?

Did the traveling have any influence on the physicians' future careers? In the first place, we can consider their journeys in relation to their last known occupation before they traveled. We have information on the occupation immediately before the first journey for most of the physicians. Public medical officers are over-represented in the non-travelers group, and those public medical officers who did travel, traveled less often than physicians in the other groups. Many of these public medical officers were district medical officers, and many of their journeys were to conferences held for them in Norway.

Does some sort of correlation exist between physicians' journeys and their final main occupation? We know that several of those who traveled later in their career worked on topics related to their travels. But whether their travels influenced the direction of their careers, or whether their careers influenced their travels, remains an open question.

Taking all groups of physicians together, we can say that those who traveled most were that small group of physicians who ended up in what we might call high-ranking medical positions.

13.2.2.4.2 Where did they Travel?

To find out where the physicians traveled can be used as a basis for analyzing the structure of their travels, in order to find out more about their preferences. It may also tell us about changes in where scientific progress was believed to be found.

To find out where they went, each destination is counted once each time it is mentioned in the biographies. If a doctor traveled to Denmark, France, Paris, the English baths, and Africa during the same tour, then each of these places is registered as one visit to that destination.

13.2.2.4.3 The Destinations

Vello Helk writes about the study tours of inhabitants of the Danish-Norwegian Kingdom during the period 1661–1813. In general, those who traveled went to Germany, the Netherlands, England and Scotland, France, Switzerland, and Italy. Helk found that what we might call basic university studies were undertaken in Germany. Those who traveled to Paris, London, Rome, and Vienna traveled as specialists or tourists. This was a view held by some Norwegian physicians in the late nineteenth century as well. Holland, and especially Leiden and Utrecht, was the main destination for physicians or medical students from Denmark and Norway in the first part of the period

TABLE 13.10
Journeys with one or more destinations in the six most frequently visited countries (as a % of all journeys).

	Born 1810-15	Born 1840-45	Born 1870-75
Sweden	22 (17.2 %)	43 (17.6 %)	40 (11.7 %)
Denmark	39 (30.5 %)	60 (24.6 %)	86 (25.2 %)
Germany	43 (33.6 %)	74 (30.3 %)	144 (42.2 %)
France	30 (23.4 %)	24 (9.8 %)	31 (9.1 %)
Great Britain	20 (15.6 %)	26 (10.7 %)	23 (6.7 %)
Austria	11 (8.6 %)	62 (25.4 %)	31 (9.1 %)

1661–1813. Later the German educational institutions, especially those in Halle and Berlin, became more important. Physicians went to different places to study different branches of medicine. Surgeons and anatomists preferred Paris during its most important period in the middle of the eighteenth century. Strasbourg was also important. For the general Norwegian travelers, the orientation had been towards England and Scotland (Helk 1991, p. 124). And for the physicians and medical students of the Danish-Norwegian kingdom, London and especially the opportunity to study with the Hunter brothers there and also Edinburgh were important destinations. Although the data is not directly comparable, we see in our groups that this had changed drastically.

Some of the study-tours mentioned were to Norwegian destinations only. It is more than possible that the small number of such journeys does not give a correct picture of Norwegian physicians traveling in Norway. However, we must remember that we are discussing study tours, not journeys for private reasons, to take over a new job, and so on.

Germany is the country that was visited most often by Norwegian physicians in all of our three groups, but especially by the physicians born between 1870-75. The reduced importance of French medicine, and the importance of Austria for physicians born between 1840–45 is also striking. See Table 13.10.

Another interesting way to indicate the importance of a country is to look at the number of registered destinations in each country. Here again Germany is the most important country. One of the reasons for this is the well-developed health and university system, with organized courses and a diversity of possibilities for the academic tourist.

The ranking of cities as destinations also gives us an interesting picture of the development of Norwegian physicians' study tours. Alb. Kolstad (1861–1928) exclaims "Ah Paris! The whole world is going to Paris, and the whole world ends up going there again" (Kolstad 1898), but Norwegian physicians had other favorite places. Table 13.11 gives the ranking of the cities, with the number of times the city is mentioned as

TABLE 13.11
Most frequently visited destinations

Born 1810-15	Born 1840-45	Born 1870-75
Copenhagen (32)	Vienna (53)	Berlin (81)
Paris (21)	Berlin (43)	Copenhagen (55)
Berlin (14)	Copenhagen (31)	Hamburg (25)
Stockholm (8)	Stockholm (29)	Paris (25)
London (8)	Paris (19)	Stockholm (23)
	London (16)	Oslo (21)
		Vienna (20)

a destination in parentheses. The growth, and later on, the decline of Vienna as a destination, the ever increasing importance of Berlin, and the relative decline in the importance of Paris, which had been an important destination for physicians and surgeons in the eighteenth century, partly reflects the scientific development during those years. But it is also a reflection of the orientation of Norwegian medicine.

The journeys of Norwegian physicians are part of what can be viewed as a traditional Central European orientation in some parts of Norwegian society. In this respect, the journeys to Denmark are interesting. First of all, for the Norwegian physicians, Denmark is on the route to the most important country during this period, Germany. But Denmark is also traditionally important, since in 1814 the Norwegian union with Denmark was dissolved and Norway was forced into a union with Sweden. Earlier, most physicians in Norway were either educated in Denmark or they were Danish citizens. Despite the union with Sweden, Swedish cities and universities had a slightly weaker attraction than Danish destinations. There is another possibility, though hardly likely, that journeys to Sweden are not registered as going abroad because of the union.

Until now we have only briefly touched on the problem of why destinations were chosen. The attraction of a place, which is the result of many interrelated factors, both physical and mental, will be one of the main themes in the next chapter.

13.2.2.5 Many Types of Information Diffusion

Information is one essential concept for approaching the journeys of Norwegian physicians. It is reasonable to assume that their journeys were planned in advance, at least to some extent. Therefore, in order to find out something about why physicians chose their destinations, we need to consider what they knew about these destinations in advance of their journey. There are two interconnected categories of information, which the physicians could have been aiming to acquire: travel information and information on the latest inventions, scientific findings, and so on.

13.2.2.5.1 Physicians and the Attractions of Places and People

When the physicians went abroad, they went to see tourist attractions. "Tourist attraction" is one of the key concepts in tourist studies, and this concept can be used when discussing the journeys of Norwegian physicians.

There is almost no limit to what can be regarded as a tourist attraction. For the Norwegian physicians, a sight might be a social institution such as a hospital, a library, an infirmary, the sewer or a museum, just as it might be for ordinary tourists (see, for instance, Helk 1991, p. 184; MacCannel 1989, pp. 62–76).

The sight could often be a person and the activities related to his profession, viewed by the visitors in order to learn and to admire and sometimes at a price.

People and their activities not only continuously modify places, but are also part of what a place is, and therefore part of the attraction of the place. Some people who personified the scientific attractions of the eighteenth century were Hermann Boerhaave (1668–1738) and Bernhard Sigfried Albinus (1697–1770) in Holland, Friedrich Hoffmann (1660–1742) in Halle, Albrecht von Haller (1709–1777) in Göttingen, and the famous anatomists in Berlin, Johann Nathanael Lieberkühn (1711–56) and Johann Friedrich Meckel (1717–1774) (Helk, 1991, p. 165).

In 1899, among others, the professors Ludwig Lichtheim (1845–1928), Ernst Neumann (1834–1918), and Richard Pfeiffer (1858–1945) were essential attractions in Königsberg for the Norwegian doctor Olaf Frich (1863–1935) when he went there that year financed by Dr. Roll's grant (Frich 1900). It is not clear whether he had heard of these professors before he decided to go there, but it is probable that he had. From an article in a Norwegian medical journal, we know that one of the main purposes senior registrar C. Budde (1825–1888) had for traveling to Berlin was to attend courses given by B. von Langenbeck (1810–1887), Albrecht Graefe (1828–1870), and later Virchow (Budde 1859, p. 889). It comes as no surprise that Rudolph Virchow (1821–1902) is mentioned in several articles by Norwegian physicians (for instance, C.T. Kierulf, 1853 and J.A. Voss, 1851). Virchow, who is described by Lyons and Petrucelli as the dominant figure in European medicine in the second half of the nineteenth century and who is considered to have been one of its greatest pathologists (Lyons and Petrucelli 1987, p. 508), was probably one of the greatest scientific attractions of the nineteenth century. Some of the other famous scientists who are mentioned in Norwegian accounts of travels are Armand Troussau (1801–1867) (Kierulf 1853, Faye 1855, Preus 1847) and Joseph Skoda (1805-1881) (Gjör 1859, Kierulf 1853).

13.2.2.5.2 Experience and Information

Our former experiences and the information we have about places contribute to our picture of other journeys and shape our preferences for later journeys. Frich's aforementioned travel can be used as an illustration. Frich traveled to Germany several times. In the autumn of 1891 he studied internal medicine and surgery in Berlin, Vienna and Copenhagen, and in the spring of 1894 in Berlin. But in 1899, he wanted to visit the smaller university cities. The reason for this, in his own words, was that during his preceding visits "the so-called courses in Berlin one was regarded as a person whose main justification for existence as a participant was that one had paid one's 30-40 Marks; besides, there were always too many participants on the courses given by the most proficient teachers" (Frich 1900, p. 1273, my translation).

In Frich's account, Königsberg was a desirable destination because it had one of the smaller universities, and this was presumed to be conducive to learning. No general conclusion can be reached from this. What we have is one person's evaluation of German universities, based on his own unfavorable experiences. It is well known that giving official and private lectures had been an important source of income for professors and lecturers for a long time, and that this had been practiced in Germany as a trade (Helk 1991, p. 74).

When this system was utilized properly, it could strengthen the position of a university. Because of the popularity of the university, in the later half of the eighteenth century, Göttingen could continue to attract proficient teachers, because of their higher salaries and the potential for additional "popularity" income (Helk, ibid.). Helk calls this Göttingen system academic mercantilism (Helk, ibid., p. 97). The Norwegian doctor Alb. Kolstad wrote in 1898 that the Germans' economic sense had not been renounced for science, since this is employed to good purpose through paid courses, which make up the most general form for the acquisition of medical knowledge in Germany's large university towns. This is a practical arrangement, particularly for young general physicians and for beginners in a specialist branch (Kolstad 1898, p. 801).

13.2.2.5.3 Guidebooks

Frich wrote his article in order to share with other physicians the benefit of his experiences. By so doing, he was an un-official and detatched guide to German universities, and in that respect he partly fulfilled the function of "Let's Go," "Baedeker," and other guidebooks. August Laurentius Koren (1833–1929), then a company surgeon, did the same when he wrote in a way that resembles the text of a guidebook: "If you come to Berlin, do not miss visiting the magnificent `Allgemeines Städtisches Krankenhaus' on Friederichs Hain ..."(Koren 1875). However, such accounts only partly fulfill the function of a guidebook, because they mainly provide their readers with information on the medical attractions of different cities. Frich also gave information on the cultural milieu of the city and mentions the theater, the opera, and famous artists who have visited the city. But he did not provide information on different routes or accommodations. Others did that in their travel accounts, but whether they did so or not largely depends on the reason for writing the account.

The importance of this is not to emphasize the similarity between travel letters and guidebooks, but to make it explicit that in order to get information on other travel-related matters, physicians had to look to a variety of sources. Some information could be obtained from guidebooks and published travel letters and diaries. Neither of these was new (on early guidebooks, see for instance De Beer, 1952). To take a Nordic example, in 1674 Thomas Bartholin (1616–1680) had published a guide for young physicians so that they could undertake their medical study tour in the right fashion (Bartholin 1674).

Information necessary to the traveler could also be obtained at meetings of medical societies. For instance, Lecturer J. A. Voss (1815–1897) gave two lectures at the Norwegian Medical Society in Christiania based on his experiences from travels abroad (Voss 1851, p. 834). Travelers could also ask physicians who had been abroad for information, as Chief County Medical Officer Ole Sandberg (1811–1883) did. He traveled to Christiania in 1850 to confer with colleagues who had traveled abroad and became more convinced to make Paris his main destination (Sandberg 1851, p. 613–614; Winge 1848, p. 84 on Prague).

13.2.2.5.4 Publication

One way of using the biographies to study the information impact of the journeys is to see whether the journeys resulted in a publication, such as an article or a book. New knowledge might also have been published without mentioning the journey. Many physicians, many of whom had obtained a grant to travel, wrote such articles. Of course we do not know to what extent these articles were read, or if the information provided was of any use to the readers. Some articles start with a "reply" to the editor: "Dear friend. In your last kind letter you forward your wish that I provide information on the understanding and treatment of these diseases..." (see, for instance, Koren 1875, p. 272 and premier lieutenant E. Klaveness 1901, p. 236). So these travel accounts were at least of interest to the editors, who were in regular contact with many of the Norwegian physicians.

13.2.2.5.5 Were Travelers Accounts "Scientific Enough"?

In 1869, Doctor of Medicine Professor F. C. Faye (1806–1890) gave his opinion on the scientific value of travel letters. Faye tells us that travel letters in medical journals seldom were read critically, although they could be a source of amusement and reflection, especially for those who were unfamiliar with foreign countries (Faye 1869, p. 109). But on the other hand, some travelers' accounts were consistent with travel letters written by other physicians (for instance Kierulf 1853, p. 392). Faye's purpose in the article was to correct the views of a young graduate who had traveled to Prague to study obstetrics at a summer course given by Professor Seyfert.

One problem with some of these travelers was that they were inexperienced. Did they have the knowledge required to distinguish between what was important and what was worthless in all the new things they learned? As Thomas Bartholin wrote in 1674: "Not all the learned ought to be approached, nor all that is being taught listened to" (Bartholin 1674, p. 55). This problem is of some importance to us as well.

But Faye did not deny the usefulness of traveling abroad. On the contrary, he strongly recommended study tours to the main educational institutions and hospitals abroad. Choice of destination and lecturers should be carefully considered, he said. So he helped the young graduate, and gave him letters of introduction for a new study tour.

Letters of introduction and the use of diplomats certainly gave access to places which otherwise could have been inaccessible to the traveler (Faye 1855, p. 4). Such letters of introduction were important in the period 1661–1813 (Helk 1991, p. 39), and still are in the nineteenth century. Travelers took letters with them, and could obtain additional letters when traveling (for instance, Voss 1851, p. 579). In terms of acquiring new knowledge, letters of introduction were perhaps not only advantageous, but could also direct travelers to people who were already well known, to safe places, and to scientific milieus that corresponded with the writer's views.

13.2.2.5.6 Manifestations of Information Diffusion?

The building of asylums, garden cities, baths, clinics, and prisons may all be manifestations of some sort of information diffusion. The entire structure of courses at universities and schools could be imported from abroad.

In Norway, international influence was strong, as can been seen in the building of baths, even though this was the work of a few enthusiasts and entrepreneurs. Information about baths in other countries, gathered from visits abroad or from international articles (especially German), was used in the development of local baths (Ebbesen 1856; Thaulow 1866; Mellbye 1903; and several articles in NMFL by Professor Doctor F. C. Faye).

13.2.2.6 Time and Money

Let's return to the three cohorts in order to see how much time was used on their travels. The duration of the journeys was given for approximately half of the journeys in all three groups. As already mentioned, as time progressed more physicians traveled, they

TABLE 13.12
The duration of the physicians' journeys (in % of all journeys)

	Born 1810–15	Born 1840–45	Born 1870–75
Journeys with a stated duration	65 (50.8%)	123 (50.4%)	158 (46.3%)
2 months or less	6 (4.7%)	18 (7.4%)	28 (8.2%)
6 months or less	23 (18.0%)	64 (26.2%)	91 (26.6%)
12 months or less	37 (28.9%)	85 (34.8%)	101 (29.6%)
Seasons etc.	19 (14.8%)	32 (13.1%)	49 (14.4%)

traveled more often, and, even though Table 13.12 shows no drastic development in this respect, their journeys became shorter as well.

For many of those who only vaguely referred to the duration of the journey, there is reason to believe that their journey was short. For example, in some biographies it is stated that in the spring a particular physician went to participate in a medical congress. And many of those who did not mention the duration of their travel mentioned activities such as conferences as their main reason for travel, indicating a short-time study tour.

However, many journeys lasted longer than one month. All journeys, even though they were mainly to Europe, required much effort. They involved being away from family and forgoing income and involved problems and expense. The financial burden could have been eased if grants had been available. When Norway was part of the Danish-Norwegian Kingdom, few Norwegian travelers were given a grant (Helk 1991, p. 25). Although the situation was gradually improved during the nineteenth century, still, for most journeys no financial assistance was available (Table 13.13).

For most of the physicians, study tours abroad were self-financed projects, although in addition to grants, some of them might have had some financial assistance from their employers. Meanwhile, the fact that

TABLE 13.13
Journeys financed by grants

	Born 1810–15	Born 1840–45	Born 1870–75
Journeys financed by a grant (as a % of all journeys)	7 (5.5%)	25 (10.2%)	46 (13.5%)
Physicians traveling on a grant (as a % of all travelers*)	6 (11.5%)	20 (29.0%)	39 (26.9%)

*all, including vague references

grants were available indicates that there was a political will to send practitioners abroad for further education and that it was regarded as necessary.

There was another category of governmental grant that was given, not for study, but for gathering information on an important problem. Physicians and medical students received such grants to investigate quarantine institutions, military barracks, the building of hospitals, mental asylums, prisons, and so on.

13.2.2.7 The Scandinavian Meetings of Natural Scientists, Tours to Meetings of National or International Scientific Associations

In the period discussed here, the Scandinavian meetings of natural scientists were an important regular opportuning to meet other scientists and get an update on scientific developments (Table 13.14 summarizes these meetings). In 1838, the Norwegian physician C. A. Egeberg (1809–1874) issued an invitation, signed by a number of Scandinavian scientists, to Danish, Norwegian, and Swedish natural scientists and physicians to attend a meeting in Gothenburg on July 16, 1839. Sixty-one Swedes, 21 Danes, and 10 Norwegians participated in this first meeting in a series which continued until 1929.

Politics of course interfere with science. Finns were invited to attend the third meeting in Stockholm. In 1902, a meeting was scheduled to be held in Helsingfors. However, due to the conditions, Russian scientists had to be invited. This meeting was named the Nordic meeting of natural scientists and physicians (Nordiskt naturforskar- och läkarmöte) and was not included as one of the series of Scandinavian meetings. There were 1,069 participants. In 1907, a meeting was planned in Kristiania. Due to the political crisis between Norway and Sweden, the meeting was postponed.

There was also another reason to postponing the meeting: It was discussed whether science had split up into separate disciplines so that the time had passed for holding such joint meetings. It was noted that there existed many purely medical congresses. The Swedish committee was dissolved. At the initiative of the Norwegians, the series of meetings were resumed, and the next meeting took place in 1916.

The function of conventions is to serve as a job market, as a place to meet colleagues and make useful contacts, and as an "opportunity for ritualized whoopee" (Roth 1974, p. 8). In the nineteenth century, for some physicians, short, organized journeys to meetings of scientific associations provided their main contact with colleagues abroad and was their way of gaining first-hand

TABLE 13.14
The Scandinavian Meeting of Natural Scientists

Number in the row	Year	Location	Number of participants
1	1839	Gothenburg	92
2	1840	Copenhagen	303
3	1842	Stockholm	436
4	1844	Christiania	176
5	1847	Copenhagen	472
6	1851	Stockholm	362
7	1856	Christiania	246
8	1860	Copenhagen	451
9	1863	Stockholm	713
10	1868	Christiania	368
11	1873	Copenhagen	418
12	1880	Stockholm	734
13	1886	Kristiania	450
14	1892	Copenhagen	563
15	1898	Stockholm	585
16	1916	Kristiania	503
17	1923	Gothenburg	526
18	1929	Copenhagen	740

Source: Nordisk familjebok. Reprint of 1923–1937 edition. Malmö 1946.

information on new directions in medical studies. 31.8 percent of the journeys undertaken by the 1840–45 group were made for these purposes.

As we have seen from the Scandinavian Meetings of Natural Scientists, these meetings often had many participants. In 1873, when the British Medical Association held its 41st yearly meeting, there were 3,000 members and 400 guests (Virchow, Langenbeck and others are mentioned in a short note in NMFL, 1873, p. 550–551).

The journeys that have been the main theme of this chapter so far are those of individual physicians in the nineteenth and early twentieth centuries. The study tour of the individual traveler is typical of this period. During the twentieth century, journeys became more and more organized. This was primarily an important aspect of leisure travel, with the development of the packagetour and other types of mass tourism. But as leisure travel became more organized and routine, so did work-related travel.

Organization of travel can be divided into two categories. First we have organization of travel in general, such as hotel development and ticket booking by travel agencies. Second, and in this respect, more interesting, we have organization of courses and congresses, predominantly aiming to profit from the demand for further education. Such courses and congresses were developed early in Germany, which contributes to the explanation of the strong position of German destinations. Another aspect that may have influenced travel patterns was language. Traditionally, German was familiar to Norwegian physicians, but we have several examples of lack of knowledge of English being a problem (Stang 1873, p. 184; Bugge 1943, p. 15).

TABLE 13.15
*Number of journeys according to reason for the journey**

Group	Born 1810–15		Born 1840–45		Born 1870–75	
Reason given		%		%		%
To study	25	19.5	41	16.8	76	22.3
To study one or more subjects, institutions or services	31	24.2	63	25.8	191	56.0
Attend meetings, conferences, congresses or courses	35	27.3	80	32.8	57	16.7
Military purposes	13	10.2	26	10.7	2	0.6
Recreation, official tasks, scientific expeditions, other	8	6.25	14	5.7	6	1.8
Unknown	16	12.5	20	8.2	9	2.6
Total	128	100.0	244	100.0	341	100.0

* Each journey can be placed in several groups, since we had up to four reasons for traveling. If «meeting» was mentioned first, the journey was placed in the meeting group. If «subject» was mentioned first, the journey was placed in the study group. All journeys with a military purpose were placed in the military group, irrespective of other business.

13.2.3 So, Why did They do It?

In his study of the period 1536-1813, Helk states that medically oriented travelers were the most stable group of travelers, since physicians were eager to acquire new knowledge and reacted quickly to present trends (Helk 1991, p. 165). So, why did they travel, and why did the numbers of physicians traveling increase?

13.2.3.1 Stated Reasons

Physicians' own statements about the field they studied abroad provide one type of answer to this question. First-time travelers were older in the 1870–75 group. Older and more experienced physicians may have had more scientific or professional intentions for their journeys, and they may have gained more from them. The increasing number of journeys to study specific fields of medicine, institutions, and so forth might indicate this (For the number of journeys according to the reason for which the journeys were taken, see Table 13.15). On the other hand, the apparent reduction in attendance at meetings, congresses, and the like may represent a failure to mention such journeys in their biographies, as travel became more commonplace.

In eighteenth-century Denmark the universities did not develop proportional with demand. One reason for going abroad was to study a variety of subjects. In Norway in the nineteenth and early twentieth century, there was a clear parallel to this in the situation. The study tours of Norwegian physicians reflect the fact that Norwegian physicians were in many ways dependent on obtaining medical knowledge abroad. In a substantially rural country, one could hardly expect to have access to the concentration of educational resources that could be found for example in the great city of Vienna.

One of the reasons for traveling to European cities and hospitals was the availability of diseases that could be seen in some hospitals, as pointed out by the then recently graduated Peter E. Winge (1818-1902). A sufficient number of less common operations also could be seen only in the large hospitals in Europe (Winge 1848, p. 84).

13.2.3.2 Changing Traveling Conditions

Traveling in the nineteenth century was more difficult than it is today. Generally, travel-related technology was slow and undeveloped in the nineteenth century. The revolution in communication made traveling and other forms of communication easier and faster. Changes in the infrastructure and superstructure of travel partly explain why the number of physicians going on study tours abroad increased. With the development of better roads, coaches, railways, and ferries, access to foreign places was made easier. Extraneous factors, such as Germany being united, which reduced border problems, could be important. On the other hand, the desire to travel must exist or be created, if new possibilities are to be taken advantage of.

Although travel conditions improved, lack of speedy and safe transport was not necessarily a barrier to physicians, since many of them were used to facing the hazards of travel in their everyday work.

There were other problems, though, such as being quarantined due to the outbreak of disease (see Geirsvold, 1900). In 1831 Andreas Christian Conradi (1809–1868), then a company surgeon, later professor of pathology and therapy, traveled to Hamburg to gain information on Asiatic cholera. The journey to Hamburg took 22 days. The disease was then declining and he stayed in Hamburg for two months. But due to quarantine in Rendsburg and Sweden, the journey back to Norway took a full month (Kiær 1888).

These problems with nineteenth-century and early twentieth-century communications should not be exaggerated. From the lecturer J. A. Voss (1815–1897), we learn that the journey by steamer from Christiania (Oslo) to Hull took four days (Voss 1858, p. 835). This was probably a steamer belonging to the British company Wilson & Co., which had established a route between Christiania and Hull in 1852. When Frich traveled to Königsberg in 1899, his route was from southern Norway to Copenhagen-Gedser-Warnemünde-Königsberg, a journey which took approximately 50 hours (Frich 1900). Frich preferred not to travel by sea, which made the journey more expensive and longer.

The development of European railways improved communication, so that from the middle of the nineteenth century the most frequently visited destinations in Central Europe could be reached by train. By 1870 almost all parts of Europe were accessible by train, although for a long time the Mediterranean was reached by horse (on the development of the European railways see G. Freeman Allen 1982, p. 38–39). Railways were primarily constructed for the transportation of goods, but as early as the late nineteenth century, lines were constructed exclusively for tourists (Lepowitz 1992, p. 127).

In our first two groups, all the physicians were men, and the number of women physicians in our last group is so limited that there is no basis for analyzing differences between male and female physicians. Meanwhile, the female physicians had special reasons for traveling, and therefore their journeys are of special interest. Due to resistance from the professors, they were not appointed to training positions in hospitals, which made their journeys essential. The fact that they all studied obstetrics and female diseases reflects both the general ideology in Norwegian society and perhaps their own ideology as well.

13.2.4 Conclusion

The study tours of Norwegian physicians had numerous effects, effects that can be arranged on a continuum ranging from personal factors to factors of benefit to society. Some of the effects are intended, while others are more in the category of "unanticipated consequences of purposive social action" (Merton 1936). There is reason to believe that the work of the profession has been influenced by some of the study tours. In addition, the fact that so many physicians traveled, and the use of physicians as "delegates " must have contributed to the development of Norwegian medicine. As specialist training was not available in Norway (a fact noted above), some of the study tours abroad might have functioned as, and been regarded as unofficial specialization.

It is safe to say that most of the journeys mentioned in the biographies are mostly "real" study tours, and not "camouflaged" recreation. Although it is possible that more tourist considerations might have influenced their travels.

Since Norwegian medicine and physicians were placed on the periphery of international medicine in the nineteenth century, and were in many ways dependent on European development, it is almost self-evident that the journeys of nineteenth-century physicians have contributed to the shaping of their profession. A secondary effect was that their travels influenced the building of Norwegian society. But, for the last time, these general effects need, of course, not be intended effects.

References

Allen, G. F. *Railways. Past, Present & Future*, London: Orbis Publishing, 1982.

Bartholin, Thomas. *On the Burning Of His Library*, Copenhagen: Petrus Haubold, 1670, and *On Medical Travel*, Copenhagen: Daniel Paulli, 1674. *On the Burning of His Library and On Medical Travel*, translated by Charles D. O'Malley, 1961.

Boorstin, D.J. *The Exploring Spirit*, New

York: Random House, 1975.

Budde, C. "Beretning om en med Stipendium foretagen videnskabelig Reise," *Norsk Magazin for Lægevidenskaben* (1859):-889–914.

Bugge, J. *På tokt med korvetten Nordstjernen 1869/70*, Oslo: J. Johan Grundt Tanum, 1943.

De Beer, E.S. "The development of the guide-book until the early nineteenth century," *Journal of the British Archaelogical Society* 15(1952):35–46.

Ebbesen, J. "Om en Høsten 1855 foretagen videnskabelig Reise til en Deel af Tysklands Bade samt en Sammenstilling mellem disse og Sandefjords Bad," *Norsk Magazin for Lægevidenskaben* (1856):217–249.

Faye, F.C. "Om Forholdene ved flere af Udlandets Hospitals-Indretninger, hovedsagelige dem for Qvinder og Børn," *Norsk Magazin for Lægevidenskaben* (1855):1–43.

Faye, F.C. "Nogle Bemærkninger i Anledning af et i Magazinets Novemberhefte f. A. optaget Brev fra Udlandet vedkommende Læren om Fødsel og Fødselshjelp," *Norsk Magazin for Lægevidenskaben* (1869):109–124.

Freidson, E. "The Reorganization of the Professions by Regulation," *Law and Human Behavior* 7(1983):279–290.

Frich, O. "Fra et studieopphold i Kønigsberg in/Pr," *Norsk Magazin for Lægevidenskaben* (1900):1273–1283.

Geirsvold, M. "Europeiske kvarantæneanstalter," *Norsk Magazin for Lægevidenskaben* (1900):1248–1272.

Gjør. "Beretning om en med Stipendium foretagen videnskabelig Reise," *Norsk Magazin for Lægevidenskaben* (1859):857–889.

Haukeland, J.V. "Non-Travellers. The Flip Side of Motivation," *Annals of Tourism Research*, 17(1990):172–184.

Helk, V. *Dansk-norske studierejser fra reformationen til enevælden 1536–1660: med en matrikel over studerende i udlandet*, Odense: Odense Universitetsforlag, 1987.

Helk, V. *Dansk-norske studierejser 1661–1813 bd I*, Odense: Odense Universitetsforlag, 1991.

Helk, V. *Dansk-norske studierejser 1661–1813 bd II Matrikel over studerende i udlandet*, Odense: Odense Universitetsforlag, 1991.

Kierulf, C.T. "Indberetning om en med Stipendium foretagen videnskabelig Reise i Udlandet," *Norsk Magazin for Lægevidenskaben* (1853):361–401.

Kiær, F.C. "Opfordring til Landets Læger," *Norsk Magazin for Lægevidenskaben* (1871):271–272.

Kiær, F.C. *Norges Læger i det nittende Aarhundrede (1800–1871)*, Christiania: A. Cammermeyer, 1873.

Kiær, F.C. *Norges Læger i det nittende Aarhundrede (1800–1886) Anden betydeligt forøgede Udgave bd I*, Christiania: A. Cammermeyer, 1888.

Kiær, F.C. *Norges Læger i det nittende Aarhundrede (1800–1886) Anden betydeligt forøgede Udgave bd II*, Christiania: A. Cammermeyer, 1890.

Klaveness, E. "'Elida's' vintertogt 1900/1901," *Norsk Magazin for Lægevidenskaben* (1901):-236–241.

Kobro, I. *Norges Læger 1800-1908 bd I*, Kristiania: H. Aschehoug & Co. (W. Nygaard), 1908–1912.

Kobro, I. *Norges Læger 1800-1908 bd II*, Kristiania: H. Aschehoug & Co. (W. Nygaard), 1915.

Kolstad, A. "Korrespondance," *Norsk Magazin for Lægevidenskaben* (1898):800–805.

Koren, A. "Nogle Optegnelser fra en Udenlandsreise væsentlig vedkommende veneriske Sygdomme," *Norsk Magazin for Lægevidenskaben* (1875):273–283.

Lepowitz, H.W. "Pilgrims, Patients, and Painters: The Formation of a Tourist Culture in Bavaria," *Historical Reflections*, 18(1992):121–145.

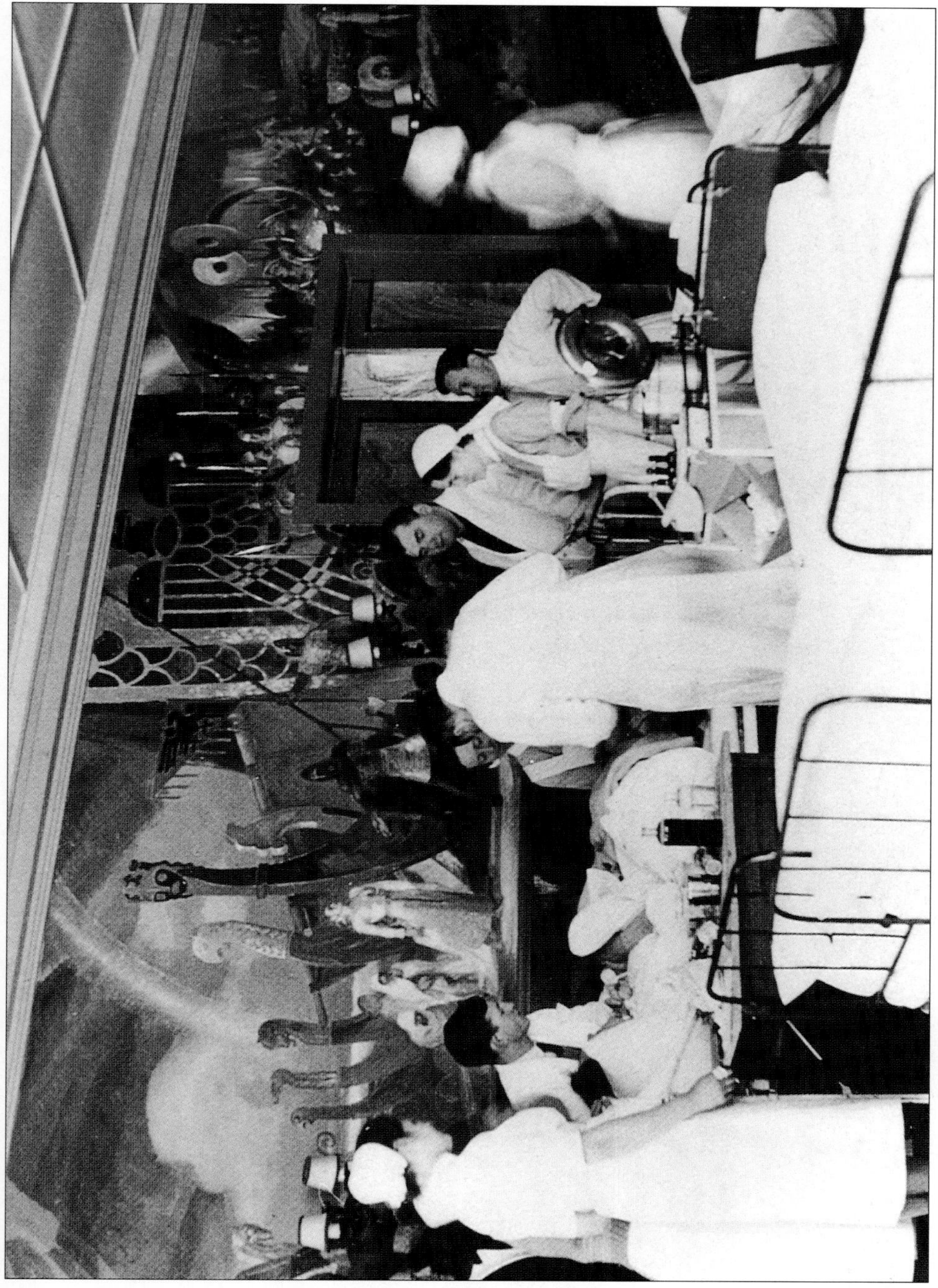

Figure 40: When German forces attacked Norway on April 9, 1940, the hospital at the Horten Naval Base was evacuated and moved to a nearby summer hotel in the village of Åsgårdstrand, where Norwegian and German casualties were admitted. Doctors in charge were Johan Hagen (1908-1989) and Kristian Haugseth (1885-1948). The photo was taken by Dr. Johs. Hagtvet (1904-1989). (Courtesy Dept. of Medical History, University of Oslo.)

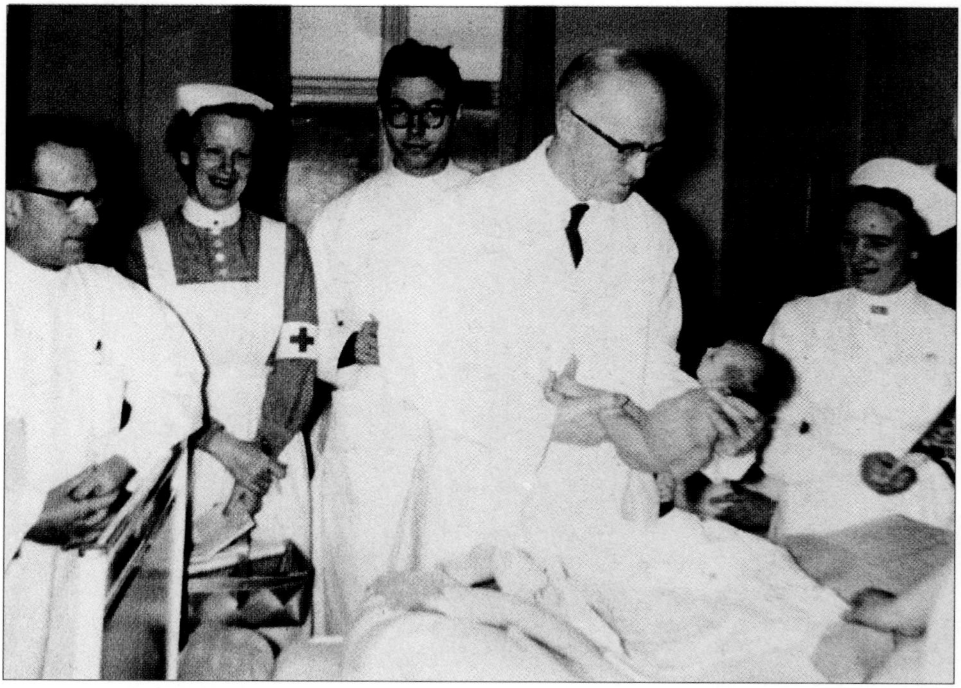

Figure 41: Dr. Sverre Sørsdal (1900-1996) examining a newborn baby in the Søndre Land hospital in the 1950s (Courtesy Randi Sørsdal).

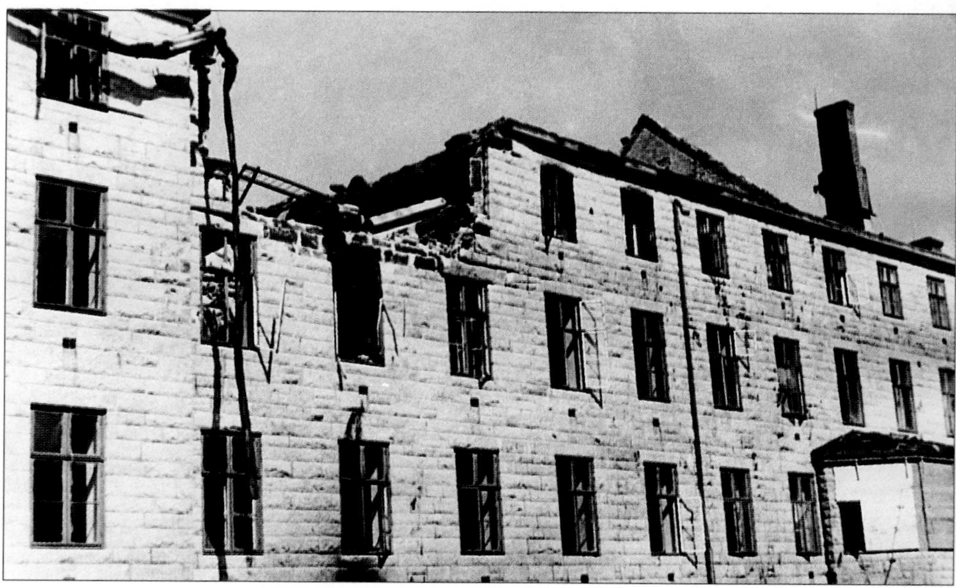

Figure 42: The hospital in Bodø after the bombing in 1940 (Courtesy Randi Sørsdal).

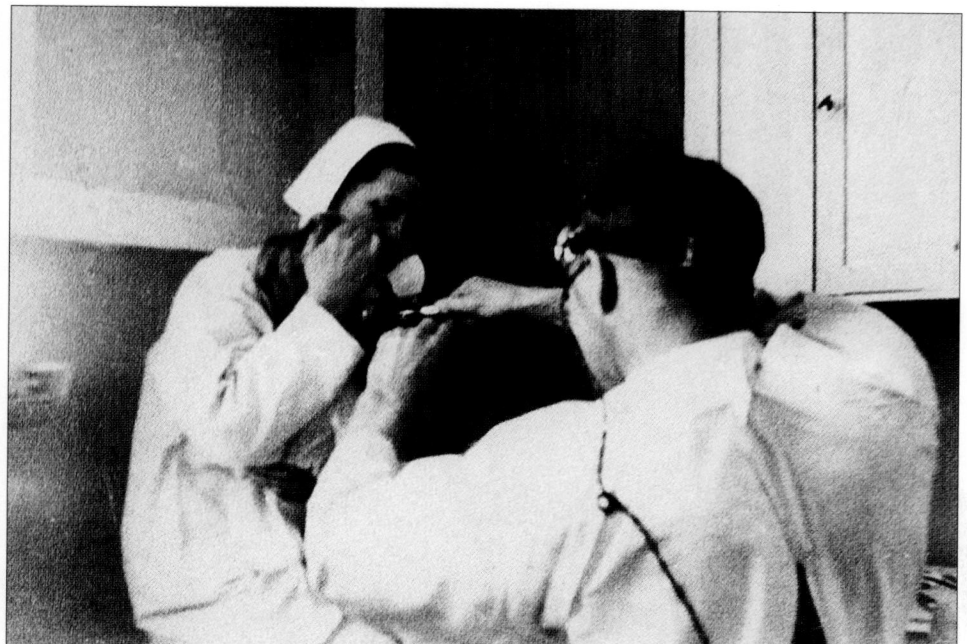

Figure 43: Chief physician Sverre Sørsdal (1900-1996) performing otolaryngology, assisted by head of the nursing staff Martha Ekman, at the Vardø hospital during World War II (Courtesy Randi Sørsdal).

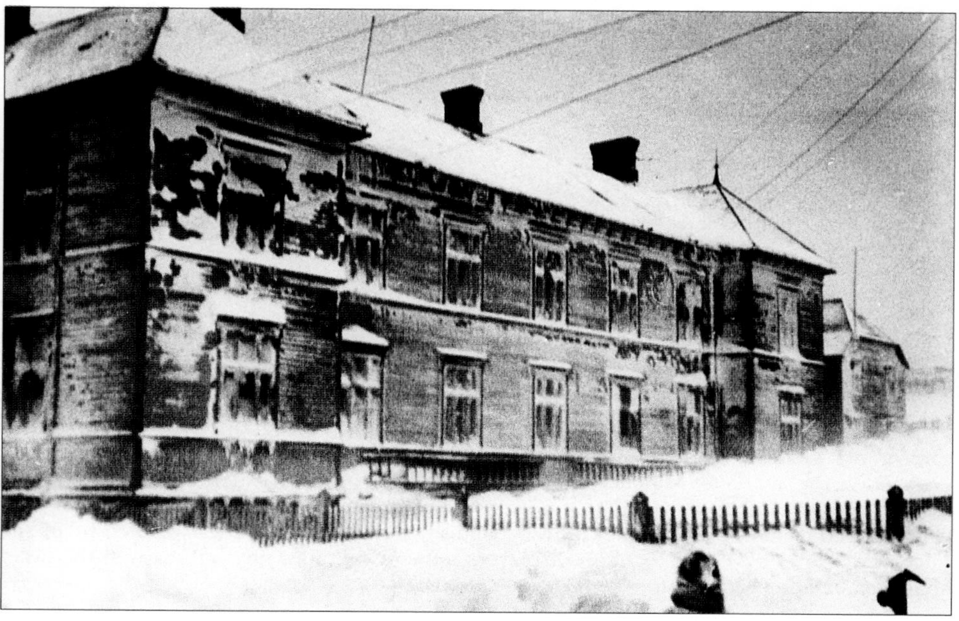

Figure 44: The Vardø hospital in Northern Norway after a winter storm in the 1930s. This hospital was totally destroyed in a bombing raid on March 1, 1942 (Courtesy Randi Sørsdal).

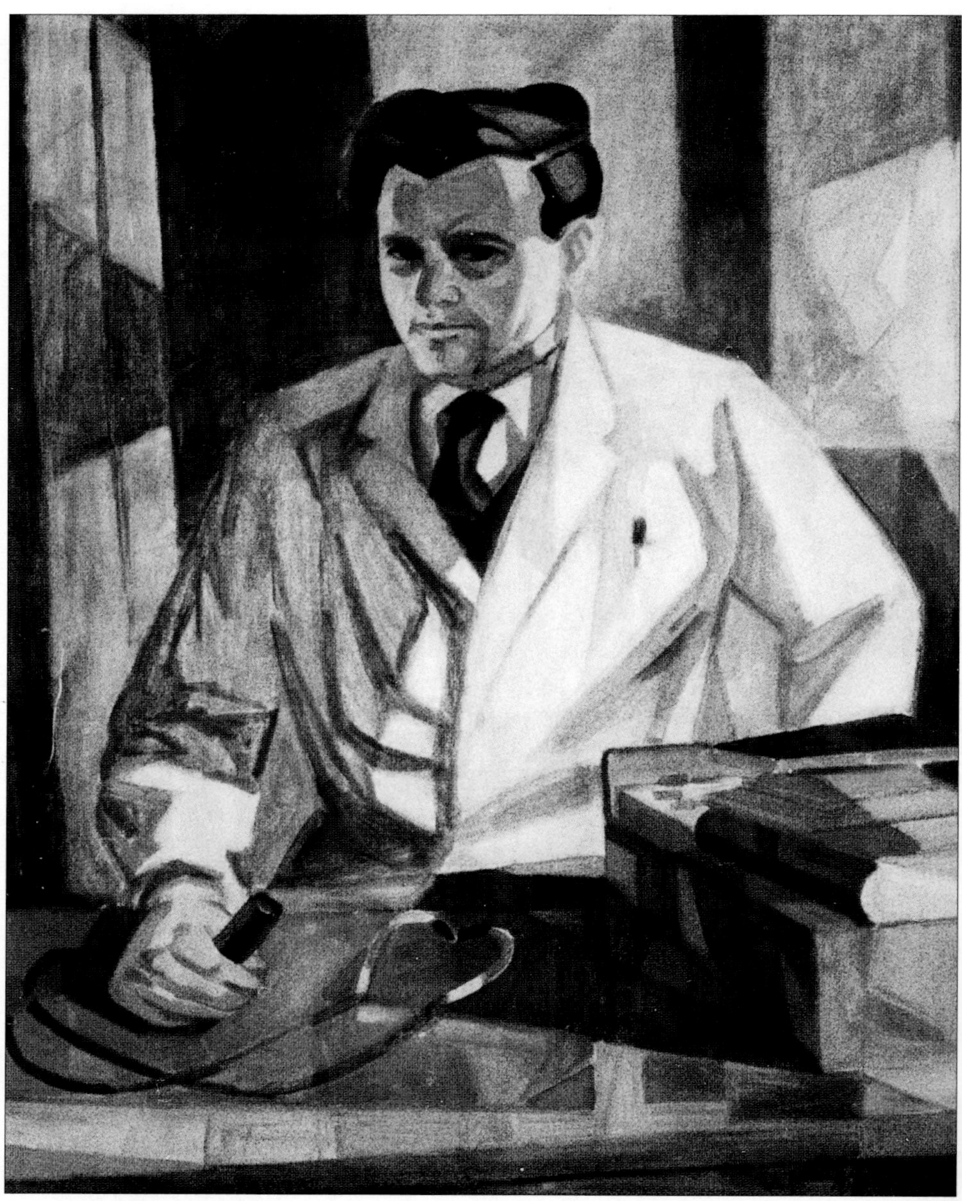

Figure 45: World War II also took its toll among Norwegian physicians. The picture shows one of the victims, Dr. Ingvar Martinius Hansen (1907-1944). Since 1934 he had been engaged in the Workers' Athletics' Organization in Oslo (Oslo arbeideridrettskrets). He lost his life on September 8, 1944 as a prisoner on board the German transportation ship "Westphalen" when it went under off the Swedish coast. His portrait was painted by Bjarne Engebret (1905-1985) in 1950 and is displayed in the institute for physiotherapy at the Bislet sports stadium in Oslo (Photo: Øivind Larsen 1996).

Lyons, A. S. and R. J. Petrucelli. *Medicine, An Illustrated History*, Gyldendal Norsk Forlag, 1987.

MacCannel, D. *The Tourist. A New Theory of the Leisure Class*, New York: Schocken Books, 1989.

Mellbye, P.A.M. *Norges kursteder og deres kurmidler*, Kristiania: Alb. Cammermeyers forlag, 1903.

Merton, R.K. "The Unanticipated Consequences of Purposive Social Action," *American Sociological Review* (1936):894–904.

Preus, J.K.K. "Indberetning til Kirke-Underviisnings-Departementet om en med Stipendium foretagen videnskabelig Reise i Udlandet," *Norsk Magazin for Lægevidenskaben* (1847):434-451.

Roth, J.A. "Professionalism: The sociologists decoy," *Sociology of Work and Occupations*, 1(1974):6-23.

Sandberg, O. "Indberetning til Kirke- og Underviisnings-Departementet om en med Stipendium foretagen videnskabelig Reise i Udlandet," *Norsk Magazin for Lægevidenskaben* (1851):613–663.

Stang, J. "Indberetning til det akademiske Kollegium om en med offentligt Stipendium i 1871 foretagen Udenlandsreise,"

Norsk Magazin for Lægevidenskaben (1873): 171–197.

Thaulow. "Beretning om Reiser til tydske Bade, foretagne i Aarene 1863 og 65," *Norsk Magazin for Lægevidenskaben* (1866):312–330.

Towner, J. "The Grand Tour. A Key Phase in the History of Tourism," *Annals of Tourism Research*, 12(1985):297–333.

Voss, J.A. "Indberetning til Kirke- og Underviisnings-Departementet om en med Stipendium foretagen videnskabelig reise i Udlandet," *Norsk Magazin for Lægevidenskaben* (1851):566–585.

Voss, J.A. "Optegnelser fra en Reise i de forenede Stater i Nord-amerika i sommeren 1857," *Norsk Magazin for Lægevidenskaben* (1858):834–854.

Winge, P.E. "Beretning om en ved Stipendium foretagen Reise i Udlandet," *Norsk Magazin for Lægevidenskaben* (1848):81–104.

CHAPTER 13.3

Travel Accounts in the Norsk Magazin for Lægevidenskaben, 1840–1880

HANNE WINGE KVARENES

13.3.1 Why So Many Articles on Traveling?

About 50 percent of the Norwegian physicians working during the period 1840–1880 had been on study trips abroad, something that led to many experiences in the foreign country they had visited. The journal "Norsk Magazin for Lægevidenskaben" published a total of 78 travel reports from this period, giving the readers an opportunity to update their knowledge on the scientific developments taking place in medicine in Europe.

One explanation of why the journal contained so many travel accounts from abroad may be that the editors lacked contributions from the readers and had easy access to travel accounts, since they already existed as written reports to the physician's employer. In fact, the journal had to be discontinued for a short period in 1846 because of the lack of contributions.

13.3.2. The Characteristics of a Travel Account

The majority of the accounts are easily recognized by their headings. The account from company surgeon J.J.K. Preus (1813–1853)was titled "Report to the Academy Collegium about a scientific journey abroad made on a travel grant" and is a typical example. The author had made a study trip financed by a grant. In return, he was obliged to write a report about the journey.

The report, however, did not necessarily always end up with the people who had given the grant. Reports were usually addressed to the Senate, but in some cases they were also addressed to the government ministries, for example, the Ministry of Education and Church Affairs, the Ministry of the Interior, and the Ministry for Labor.

Such accounts were often long, exhaustive, and contained reports about the entire journey, along with elaborate discussions on professional subjects.

Some employers gave the travelers detailed instructions before the journey. An illustration of this is the journey on royal command made by corps physician C.T. Schiøtt (1811–1890) and battery surgeon C.A. Egeberg (1809–1874). They traveled to the Military Camp Assembly near Stockholm in 1843. They were given particularly detailed instructions from General Surgeon M. Thulstrup (1769–1844), who asked them to gather information on the Swedish army's dietary regulations and rules for the composition of menus. They were also to find out if the food was delivered from the house economist according to a fixed amount per capita, calculated according to a full portion or a half portion, if the provisions were delivered as raw materials and prepared by the cook, and if the latter was paid on a certain weekly, monthly, or yearly basis.

Another group of travel accounts are minutes from the professional debates, the so-called negotiations, in the Medical Society and the Medical Association. Typically, a physician gave a speech at a Society meeting, after he had been abroad. Minutes were written and later published in the journal. These minutes on the trips taken, only deal with a few places, people, and subjects. In some of these minutes, it is somewhat difficult to decide whether they should be considered as travel accounts at all. The reports from the negotiations are therefore left out in many of the analyses in this chapter, when that was considered appropriate.

There is also a third group of travel accounts, which contains all the material that does not fit into the first two categories. The length and content of these travel accounts vary.

Some of the accounts resemble the reports written by the physicians who had received grants, but seem somewhat incomplete in this respect. Others are short notes on topics such as a health resort that was visited on a journey abroad, or on the lectures of professor Skoda (1805–1881) in Vienna. The journey itself is of lesser importance in these reports, and many of the circumstances of the journey are not described. (For the number of accounts in each of the groups, and the average number of pages, see Table 13.16.)

TABLE 13.16
The number of accounts in each of the groups, and the average number of pages

	Group		
	1	2	3
Number	10	13	42
%	29.5	16.7	53.8
Pages, average	53	6	28
Pages, median	46	3	16

The amount, as well as the different types of material on the travels varied throughout this forty-year period.

In Table 13.17, the 78 travel accounts have been organized in ten-year periods.

The travel reports from the minutes of the meetings, Group 2, in this case are less interesting, because they probably cannot be used as information on editorial policies concerning travel accounts.

In the last ten-year period, 1870 to 1879, the large amounts of material from journeys abroad is represented almost solely by the third group. The shorter reports in Group 3 may have been more in line with the preferences of the readers, as they were more spe-

TABLE 13.17
Travel accounts organized in ten-year periods

Period	Number	Gr 1	Gr 2	Gr 3	Gr 1+3
1840–49	(10)	5	1	4	9
1850–59	(25)	11	1	13	13
1860–69	(19)	5	7	7	12
1870–79	(24)	2	4	18	20

cialized and topical, and less focused on the journey itself. This happened in the period just before the launching of the more specialized and practically orientated "Tidsskrift for Praktisk Medisin" (Journal of Practical Medicine) in 1881. In fact, when the editorial staff of "Norsk Magazin for Lægevitenskapen" (The Norwegian Magazine for Medical Sciences) was enlarged in 1866, Ole R. Aa. Sandberg (1811–1883) claimed that this was done in order to enable them to present the more specialized subjects (F. Grøn 1933).

13.3.3. The Physicians who had their Travel Accounts Published

About 50 percent of the travel accounts were written by authors under the age of 40, the youngest being 23 and the oldest 72. The mean age of the authors at the time that their first travel account was published was 34, the minutes from the society meetings being left out.

In the period between 1860 and 1866, 22 percent of the Norwegian physicians lived in Christiania(Larsen, Berg, Hodne 1986). About 70 percent of the authors of the accounts lived in Christiania before their first trip abroad. Physicians with more than one account are registered each time. Bergen and Trondheim are represented with one author each; the others usually resided in smaller townships and rural districts.

Table 13.8 shows the different positions held by the 47 authors of the travel accounts.

Forty-seven percent of the authors had already been abroad prior to the journey in question. 81 percent of the authors had worked as candidates at Rikshospitalet (the National Hospital) in Christiania.

TABLE 13.18
Positions held by authors of travel accounts

Position	Number
Professor	22
Corps physician	11
Candidate	6
Cand.med.	5
District physician	5
Chief physician	5

(persons with more than one account are counted for each article)

13.3.4. Grants

We have information on the financing for 31 of the journeys, and on two of these the authors traveled at their own expense. Virtually all the journeys made with grants were of the reporting type in Group 1. Nineteen of the authors had public or royal grants and commissions as the source of pecuniary contributions; eleven of them state that they had received another type of scholarship or grant.

The Schytt grant and the count Hjelmstjerne-Rosencron grant were the most common sponsors for the authors. Both funds were administered by the University, and grants were awarded by Royal resolution. The recipients had to send their reports to the Academic Collegium on return.

The obligation to write reports was discharged with a varying sense of duty. Some gave a painstaiking account of everything they had seen, and tried to justify every little deviation from the journey plan, while others only described parts of the journey.

The material indicates that the sums that the travelers received varied between 200 and 800 Speciedaler (Spd). As a comparison, in 1886, a candidate at the National Hospital had an annual income of Spd 400, while a chief physician earned Spd 1200 (Larsen, Berg, Hodne 1986).

Professor and corps physician were the most commonly registered positions among the grant recipients. Hospital employees was the group of physicians where most had received a grant, but there was no difference between higher and lower positions, neither for hospitals nor for university employees. Some said that they had been on several journeys that were financed "externally."

13.3.5. The Types of Studies that were Grant Funded

The travelers write about 29 different fields of study, types of institutions, and so on, of which surgery, dermatology, and pediatrics occur most frequenly.

Usually, a wide variety of medical topics were studied on each study tour. When he was thirty years old, A.F. Grøn (1819–1905) went to Paris and Vienna on a grant to study pediatrics, obstetrics, dermatology, surgery, pathology, and pathological anatomy. An explanation for this professional dispersion may be the nineteenth-century ideal of the "multi-scientific" physician, who not only mastered most areas within medicine, but also engaged himself in several other scientific subjects.

The accounts were written in a period when a considerable number of institutions were built in Norway. At that time, discussions were widespread in Norway on the development of psychiatric health care, and mental hospitals are the institutions which are mentioned most often.

Only one of the physicians received support for more than one year. Six months and twelve months were the most common periods of support. Prolongations sometimes occurred; one of the travelers extended an extra 18 months. There are also examples of authors who applied for, and actually received, additional support while they were still out traveling.

13.3.6. The Destinations of the Physicians who Wrote for the Journal

The traveling pattern which emerges from the accounts turned out to deviate from the analysis made by Olsen, where the biographies are the sources of information. He shows, among other things, that Germany was the most frequently visited country in every one of the four decades, that it was the country with the highest number of visited places, and that the importance of Berlin was great, and increasing, throughout the period. The pattern in the travel accounts in "Norsk Magazin for Lægevitenskapen" is shown in Table 13.19. Here, France and Austria top the list.

Does this show the actual traveling pattern, or is it just an expression of what places the authors thought it worthwhile to write about? Were France and Austria regarded as more strange and exotic than Germany, and therefore more interesting to write about? Do we sense an editorial policy of the journal? It has been implied above that the accounts in Group 1 (reports) to a great extent listed the whole course of a journey, and within this group the traveling pattern turned out to be exactly as in Table 13.19. In other words, there are indications that the authors in Group 1 might have had a traveling pattern different from other traveling physicians.

In Group 3, the circumstances were turned upside-down concerning the most important destinations: in this group, Berlin and Vienna were the dominating ones.

What could be the reason that the traveling patterns analyzed by B.O. Olsen and the ones found in "Norsk Magazin for Lægevidenskapen" do not agree? It has been shown above that a great many of the authors had already undertaken several journeys abroad before they had their first account published in the journal. In addition, many of them had written several accounts during the

TABLE 13.19
Number of accounts that report to have visited:

Paris	25
Vienna	19
Berlin	13
London	12
Prague	11
Copenhagen	8
Hamburg	8

period. Consequently, many of the authors contributing to "Norsk Magazin for Lægevidenskapen" were experienced travelers who might, for exactly this reason, visit other places than those chosen by traveling physicians in general.

Overall, Paris as a destination clearly dominates in the accounts; Rouen is also mentioned by one of the authors.

In comparison, more than twenty places in Germany were registered; included here are only destinations within the borders of Germany today. In addition, a great number of spas are mentioned. These have been classified as educational institutions, and thus do not occur in the table of visited destinations. This means that even though Berlin as a destination seems to be less important to the travelers who were published in the magazine, Germany was frequently visited and had a great number of interesting destinations.

Visits to Paris are most frequently mentioned in the published reports from the period 1840–1880. Berlin is mentioned only a few times in the first ten-year period, but then becomes increasingly important. When we look at London, we find the opposite tendency. Vienna and Prague are relatively well represented in all the periods. The United States does not play an important part in the accounts until the 1850s.

13.3.7. Reasons for Choice of Destination

None of the physicians state that their skill with a particular language was of any vital importance to their choice of destination. There are, however, examples of there being a need for language instruction. For instance, Joh. Stang (1829–1877) went to Christiania for a fortnight to learn English before he left for Edinburgh to study Lister's antiseptic treatment.

The location of the different hospitals, universities, collections, and so forth, within a city was important to the traveler. Great distances between them meant a lot of time spent on commuting, difficulties of combining different interests, and as a result a smaller gain. Favorable cities as regards this were Vienna and Edinburgh. In Vienna, most of the university education took place at the Allgemeines Krankenhaus. Many of the authors recommended the city to other travelers for this very reason. This kind of geographic concentration of educational institutions was important particularly to the newly trained physicians, who traveled abroad to strengthen their basic education within a broad spectrum of specialities. The material shows that Vienna was the most visited destination among the authors under 30 years of age.

Many of the older physicians concentrated on a limited range of topics; for example F.C. Faye (1806–1890) devoted himself increasingly to obstetrics, and accordingly he was primarily interested in visiting maternity hospitals and similar institutions at the different destinations. The dispersion of educational institutions was of little importance to travelers like Faye. Big cities with many medical institutions, such as Paris and London, were no hindrance to receiving good professional benefits, and offered a greater amount of relevant and interesting cases to the more seasoned travelers.

The great names in contemporary medicine, professional authorities such as Rudolf Ludwig Carl Virchow (1821–1902), Joseph Lister (1827–1912), Carl Friedrich Schröder (1838–1887), and others, constituted in themselves good reasons for choosing a destination. Many physicians went to Utrecht to study the latter's theories in psychiatry, and spoke of him with enthusiasm. In Paris, Armand Trousseau (1801–1867) and the syphilodologist Philippe Ricord (1799–1889), among others, were recognized and frequently sought after.

Many authors write that they would have profited more from their stay if the universities had not been closed for the holidays, a fact which leads to the suspicion that the authors were badly informed, or that they might have used this as an excuse to give themselves some alleviation from the professional studies. Two of the accounts in the material are written as if they were travelers' guides, and perhaps were written to prevent problems of this kind.

13.3.8. Evaluations of the Different Places

13.3.8.1. Paris

The main impression of Paris was that the conditions for visitors were difficult. The lectures and courses were given in different parts of the town and the courses were long. This made it difficult to participate for shorter periods. On the other hand, the courses were free of charge. Most of the travelers stated that the standards in several specialties were very satisfactory, especially concerning surgery, ophthalmology, and dermatology.

Still, some institutions are given scathing assessments. F.C. Faye commented on the "Hospice des enfants trouvés et orphelins," and stated that it looked more like a churchyard than a hospital, and that he was not sure whether the charitable work done there was not in reality barbaric. The conditions, he stated, could in no way be justified.

13.3.8.2. Vienna

The study possibilities at Vienna were characterized as good, but this appraisal applies mostly to the organization of the studies. The professional status of Vienna seems to have been disputed, and changed during the period: in 1840, an author writes about the "disinclination of the Viennese to serious pursuits," and describes the university system as being inflexible and virtually closed to new knowledge; he is critical about the fact that the lectures were given in Latin, that foreign literature was censored, that there were too few teachers, the curriculum was strict, and so on.

In 1879, another physician writes that Vienna is the place in Europe which is best organized for studies, and praises the city. A third author proclaims that the Viennese treatment is symptom oriented, and praises the more "cause oriented" treatments in Berlin. A fourth uses the term "the nihilism of the school of Vienna".

13.3.8.3. Other Places of Study

According to the authors, anatomy and chemistry were fields of study in which Berlin held its own. However, many of the hospitals were harshly criticized, especially the old Charité.

Many of the authors laud London for its good hospitals, especially mental institutions. They often comment on the special financing systems of these hospitals (private charities both ran and funded them). The museums of London for example, Hunter's Museum were also popular and were rated above the French ones.

The best features of Prague seem to have been the concentration of its educational institutions within a small area, and the fact that the university was open when others were closed. Many are impressed with the professional standards of this university.

13.3.9 Subjects Studied

Table 13.20 shows what subjects were generally studied, that is, in how many accounts the author mentions having studied the individual subjects.

A recurring and noticeable trait of the travel accounts in "Norsk Magazin for Lægevidenskaben" is the strong focus on the conditions at universities and institutions, something that probably can be attributed to the extensive constructing of institutions in Norway in this period. This includes the position, architecture, soil, and surroundings of the spas, institutions, and hospitals. Many of the authors also take an interest in

TABLE 13.20
Subjects studied by the authors of travel accounts

Subject	Number of accounts
Surgery	22
Dermatology	17
Obstetrics	15
Pediatrics	15
Gynecology	14
Ophthalmology	14
Pathological anatomy	12
Anatomy	10
Military medical service	10
Other subjects studied:	
Institutions, interior	21
Collections, ex. anatomy	16
Institutions, administration	16
Syphilis studies	14
Institutions, exterior	13
Institutions, hygiene	12
Spas	10
Education, curriculum	10

administrative and financial conditions, but it seems that most interesting to them are the arrangement of rooms, furnishing, equipment, and hygiene. There are detailed discussions of room size, headroom, sanitary installations, kitchens, number of patients per room, number of nurses per patient, and ventilation devices.

13.3.10 What the Travel Accounts can Tell About the Consequences and Significance of Journeys Abroad

The journeys have clearly given the individual traveler new knowledge of various kinds. Some of the authors state that they have learned new methods of treatment, some tell about new implements and equipment, while others tell about the unusual cases they have observed.

There are also examples of Norwegian physicians having an influence on foreign conditions. Joh. Stang went to Edinburgh in 1871 to study Lister's antiseptic treatment. He taught Lister about boracic acid as an antiseptic remedy, and sent a sample from Christiania after his return. Lister wrote in his letter of thanks that this was "a great addition to our resources."

The story of F.C. Faye's journey to Europe in 1849 holds a unique position. He undertook it to study the conditions at maternal and children's hospitals. He wanted to get information on the mortality of women in confinememt in Paris, but the general managers of the respective hospitals "had considered it neither useful nor advisable to publish the mortality rates." He finally received the information he wanted under the condition that the results were not made public in France. The report that Faye later wrote to the journal was snatched up by a French medical journal. The numbers were later used several times, for example, in the discussion on puerperal fever in Academie de Medicine. Faye himself wrote that "From that time, one has considered open accounts of all conditions which are relevant to this kind of hospital activity, as the correct way to prepare for desirable reforms."

References

Grøn, F. *Det norske medicinske Selskab 1833–1933*. Oslo: Steenske boktrykkeri Johannes Bjørnstad A/S, 1933.

Larsen, Ø., O. Berg and F. Hodne. *Legene og samfunnet*. Oslo: Universitetet i Oslo, Den norske lægeforening, 1986.

References to the travel accounts by J.J. Preus, C.T. Shiøtt, C.A. Egeberg, A.F. Grøn, F.C. Faye, and Joh. Stang in Norsk Magazin for Lægevidenskaben, can be found in the Bibliography, chapter 33.

CHAPTER 13.4

Physicians Who Remained Abroad – Doctors in Norse America

ØIVIND LARSEN

13.4.1. Those Who Left and Stayed

Is there an urge to travel? A sort of force of nature within us, an inborn unrest, paired with curiosity, general interest, and a sense of adventure? Some geographers suggest so. That hypothesis may be supported when we look at the vivid traveling activity undertaken by the Norwegian physicians. The frequent moving by the members of the profession may be part of the same, but this is more difficult to assess, because of the social pressure from career expectations, established career patterns, the setup of the health services, family life, personal economy, etc.

Among the physicians there is a group which stands out as something special in this respect: Those who left Norway and chose to spend their lives abroad. And a group among these physicians took part in an extensive general migration that involved large numbers of Norwegians who emigrated. The number of emigrants who went to America was by far greater than the number who went to other places outside of Norway. Therefore it is sensible to concentrate on what happened among the Norwegians in America.

However, the number of Norwegian physicians who emigrated to the United States of America up to the Second World War, 126 according to Klaveness (1943), was quite diminutive in relation to the masses of their countrymen who broke away from their homes. In the century following the landing of the emigrant sloop Restauration in New York on October 9, 1825, nearby 800,000 Norwegians moved to America, a number which is even more impressive when we compare it to the population of Norway at the census in 1801: 883,487 (Lovoll 1988).

This emigration has been covered in depth in historical literature (e.g., Semmingsen 1941, 1950; Blegen 1931, 1940). What started as a decision to break away and set out for a new world for reasons that contained religious elements, a sincere step to take for traditionally stable Norwegians, developed into a mass movement in which persuasive letters from overseas and clever agents had an easy task. Attractive prospects of money and adventure pulled many a young man or woman away from home (Blegen 1955, Jenswold 1986). Over the years a variety of factors took part in propelling the emigration. B. Lindsay Lowell (1989) discusses the different theories dealing with the forces behind the emigration, based on sociological and statistical analyses, and concludes that with its roots in the upheaval of tradition-bound society, mass emigration was driven, paradoxically, by itself.

DIAGRAM 13.1
Early Norwegian settlements in the United States (after Gjerset & Hektoen).

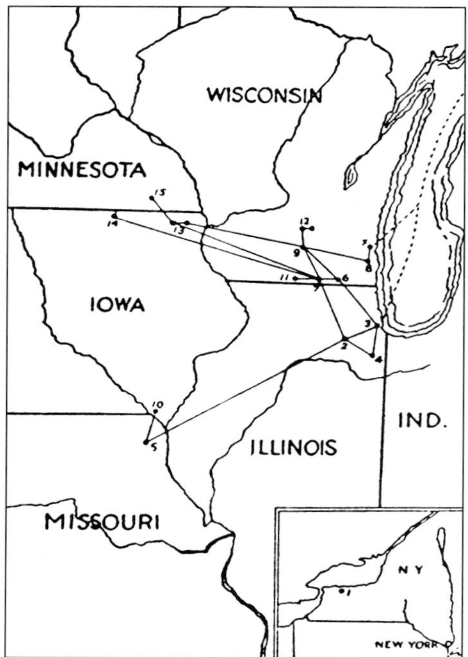

Key to Map
1. Kendall, Orleans County, New York 1825
2. Fox River, La Sallc County, Illinois 1834
3. Chicago, Illinois 1836
4. Beaver Creek, Iroquois County, Illinois 1837
5. Shelby County, Missouri 1837
6. Jefferson Prairie, Rock County, Wisconsin 1838
7. Rock Prairie (Luther Valley), Rock County, Wisconsin 1839
8. Muskego, Wisconsin 1839
9. Koshkonong, Dane County, Wisconsin 1840
10. Sugar Creek, Lee County, Iowa 1840
11. Wiota, La Fayette County, Wisconsin 1841
12. Spring Prairie and Bonnet Prairie, Columbia County, Wisconsin 1845
13. Washington Prairie, Winneshiek County, Iowa 1850
14. St. Ansgar, Mitchell County, Iowa 1853
15. Filmore County, Minnestota 1853
x. Milwaukee, Wisconsin

Two waves of emigration from Norway to the United States may be identified: one mainly agrarian migration in the years 1846–1865 comprising around 71,000 people (Diagram 13.1), and the emigration which took place from the 1860s until the great depression of 1929, including more than ninety percent of the total number in the great emigration period. Most people in this group went to urban areas in the New World.

No wonder that physicians also joined the westward stream. It is quite natural that doctors also contracted the so-called America fever. What sort of people were they? What were the medical conditions among the emigrants, and to what extent did these call for the services of Norwegian physicians?

But there is another aspect, too: Did the emigrant physicians influence American medicine, and did they contribute to the contacts between Norwegian and American medicine in the years to come? And how did their emigration influence Norwegian medicine?

At least the first group of settlers arrived in a country where everything had to be started anew. The new settlements in a way were subject to a repetition of the development in the Old World, so that the changes in attitudes towards health and disease, the priorities given to health care, the sanitary conditions and the understanding of hygiene, and so forth played over the screen again.

And as for the physicians who settled and stayed: Did they feel that the conditions they encountered in the New World were a constraint or a challenge?

13.4.2. The Very First

It is not clear where the Trondheim-born doctor Johan Martin Kalberlahn (1722–1759) (Hans Morten Kelberlade) got his medical training, but it seems like it was in his home town, perhaps as an apprentice. At the time there was no formal medical or surgical teaching available in Norway. In 1743 he went on a tour to Bergen, Hamburg, and Lübeck. The next year he went to Copenhagen and Slagelse. He stayed in Copenhagen, joined the religious movement of the Brethren (the Moravians), and got a position as a physician there. In 1753 he went to London and then moved on to America. On arrival, he went to Bethlehem in Pennsylvania, but proceeded to serve as a physician to the new Moravian colony called Bethabara in North Carolina. He had married in Bethlehem in 1758, but back again in Bethabara in 1759 he fell victim to a feverish epidemic which hit the colony.

On September 9, 1904, the Norse-American newspaper Decorah-Posten published a rather detailed article on Kalberlahn. His work as a physician is described as strenuous and lonely; making house calls could include traveling up to one hundred miles by foot through the forests. For preparing medicines he collected plants, and at home he had arranged a garden for medical herbs, a pharmacy, and a laboratory. One day his house caught fire. During the rescue work he got severe burns. In spite of that, he managed to nurse a fellow congregation member, who had been badly injured by a falling tree, back to health. Patient and physician healed together, according to the biographer.

Dr. Kalberlahn was probably the first of the Norwegian emigrant doctors. A liking for travel may be noted; not unusal for young people training for skilled work. In olden times, years of wandering were part of the education in many vocations, trades, and crafts. Perhaps the persisting and traditional mobility of the professions is a remnant of such old habits, and has to be discussed as such. Therefore, it is not astonishing to learn about the travels of Dr. Kalberlahn. On the other hand, the congregation which Dr. Kalberlahn joined and was committed to, fled Europe for reasons of religious persecution. We must therefore assume that his motives probably were more to follow the group to which he belonged, than an intention to set up a medical practice abroad as an objective in itself.

But when emigration really started in 1825, religion still was a motive.

13.4.3. Health Conditions in Rural Norse America

In 1926 the Norwegian-American Historical Association published its first volume of a series of books on the Norwegian immigration and the history of the Norwegian element in the United States. The opening chapter was written by Knut Gjerset and Ludvig Hektoen and dealt in rather complete detail with the health conditions and the practice of medicine among the early Norwegian settlers, that is, in the years 1825–1865 (Gjerset & Hektoen 1926).

For obvious reasons, the immigrants usually brought only a few belongings with them to the United States. When they arrived at the place where they would stay, houses had to be built. Often these were very crowded, and the economy was bad. Lack of essential utensils for work and household is also mentioned as a problem that added to the hardships for the newcomers. Several settlers also broke away again from the place they had initially chosen, and started over again in another place. Although there were advisors who recommended to the immigrants where to go to find a place to settle, there were often several reasons why the first choice of land did not become the final one. The soil or the climate could be unsuitable, economic prospects might have proved disappointing, or perhaps rumors about better conditions elsewhere exerted their influence.

Some of the settlements were situated in rather unhealthy regions, where marshland and moisture made malaria and cholera scourges that led to a large death toll. The hygienic conditions, for example, concerning drinking water and housing are generally described as so bad that the ravages by infectious diseases must have been inevitable. For a long time, easily polluted shallow ponds and creeks were used for their water supply, saving the settlers the effort of digging wells. Privies were not usual in the early settlements, and the human discharges out in the open was a special problem when gastrointestinal diseases were prevalent.

Some of the infectious diseases had been contracted during the voyage from Norway, and the conditions at the destination made them spread even further. In addition, hostile Native Americans (Indians) at times were a life-threatening nuisance to the settlers. Alcoholic beverages, which were readily available, perhaps served as an escape from the stress of everyday life. Excessive use of liquor is mentioned as a problem among many of the Norwegian settlers.

Under such conditions, there was no place where a doctor could set up a medical practice and make a living from fees. Mostly, the settlers had to make do with the knowledge and the remedies which were at hand. From Rushford in Minnesota there are stories from the early days of immigration about two practicing Norwegian "doctors" named Holm and Frøken; the medical training of one of them was based on his service as a drug-store clerk in Norway. Among others practicing medicine, were two Norwegian farmers, Romøringen and Hallingen, living at North Prairie, who offered blood-letting and cupping and administered medical remedies. And the market for patent medicines, which allegedly could cure a wide variety of ailments, was open and active.

However, it would be unjust to leave an impression that the more or less lay practitioners were only exploitative quacks; midwives and also doctors' wives are mentioned, who did a good job for their fellow settlers, together with self-educated doctors.

13.4.4. Emigrant Physicians – Some Examples

Hans Christian Brandt (1814–1893) passed his medical examination at the University in Christiania in 1838. Allegedly because of an unhappy love affair, he emigrated in 1840 to practice among Norwegians in Illinois. Later he lived and worked in Iowa and Indiana, until he settled in Missouri, where he stayed until his death, having gained a substantial reputation as a medical practitioner and having acquired a fortune as well.

Brandt was the first of the Norwegian-trained physicians who followed the emigration wave, and perhaps his reasons for doing so were not so different from the motives turning the eyes of many other young and unsettled people towards the west. A dissatisfaction with how things had turned out at home was probably the main reason why people left Norway.

The career of his contemporary colleague Theodor Alexander Schytte (1812–1849), who graduated in Christiania in 1840, turned out quite differently. After hospital work and general practice in Norway, he went to America as a physician on an emigrant ship in 1843 and settled as a practicing physician among the Norwegians in Koshkonong, Wisconsin. However, we learn that he found the work among poor immigrants unsatisfactory. He returned to Norway in the winter of 1847–1848, took over an appointment as a district physician in Finnmark, and died at Vardø in 1849. In the same year he published a guide for emigrants (Schytte 1849).

If the prospects of earning money was the prime motive for going west, medical work turned out to be disappointing; it was too early. The market for medicine had not developed yet, at least not in those parts of America where the Norwegians lived.

The world had changed half a century later when Adolf Gundersen (1865–1938) arrived in La Crosse, Wisconsin in 1891. The Solør-born Norwegian with a medical degree from the University in Kristiania in 1890 had celebrated his graduation from the University by setting out on adventurous travel together with two comrades from the medical school, Peder Hafsal (1864–1934) and Karl Borge (1862–1892) (Hessel 1991). On board a Jamaica-bound fruit steamer, he came across a newspaper advertisment, in which the Norwegian physician Christian Christensen (1852–1919), an M.D. graduate from Kristiania in 1879, and a previous industrial medical officer in Bamble 1880–1888, sought an assistant for the medical practice he had set up in La Crosse, Wisconsin. Gundersen responded and agreed to work there for one year to earn money to cover his debts. His two mates also started to work as physicians in America; however, Dr. Borge died after a short time, and Dr. Hafsal later returned to Norway.

When Adolf Gundersen came to La Crosse, the city on the banks of the Mississippi River probably looked like many other outposts. It had a colorful mixture of industry, hotels, riverboats coming and going, and a frontier culture. Thirty-three physicians of different brands supplied by four homeopaths opened their doors to patients. But they experienced a heavy competition from quacks and other people offering their sorts of cures. The biographer stresses that Dr. Gundersen felt uncomfortable with the situation. He nevertheless chose to stay; among the reasons were that in spite of everything, he considered the prospects for a medical practice were better here than back in the homeland.

The Gundersen practice in La Crosse developed over the years into the prestigious Gundersen Clinic, Ltd. of today, with more than 300 physicians on staff. Together with his descendants Dr. Gundersen founded a medical family dynasty with a notable impact on American medicine; one of his sons, Dr. Gunnar Gundersen (1897–1979) even was elected president of the influential American Medical Association (AMA) in 1958 and held the post for ten years.

In an article in the Journal of the Norwegian Medical Association in 1955 on Norwegian doctors in America, Dr. Gunnar Gundersen points out the fact that the Norwegian doctors were able to compete in terms of medical quality because of their good medical training in Norway (Gundersen 1955). High standards in American medical education were not obtained until after the work of the Flexner Commission on medical training had been implemented well into the twentieth century (Flexner 1910, 1912).

These differences in medical training and competence in nineteenth-century America, or more generally speaking the lack of established requirements for qualifications, caused internal problems among the physicians. For example, in 1898 the Norse-American newspaper Skandinaven reflected through a series of articles a heated argument between European-trained physicians and those who had been taught medicine in the United States. There was competition among physicians for patients, and to have the right credentials was an important asset when it came to building a practice.

At the Gundersen Clinic, practice, teaching, and research went hand in hand. Dr. Adolf Gundersen was a highly esteemed specialist on open prostate surgery; his son, Dr. Alf Gundersen (1898–1986) later enjoyed a corresponding reputation in the transurethral resection of prostatic tissue.

The Gundersen example is by and large a history of a continuous medical success. The American society provided the opportunity to establish and develop an independent medical institution. On the other hand, this opportunity also included a vulnerability to the fluctuations in the surrounding economy, a fact which also makes up a part of the history of private medical practice. The decision made by Dr. Adolf Gundersen in the 1890s to extend his planned one-year money-raising venture into something more permanent was probably one of the wisest choices he ever made.

When medical schools and centers in America attained international prestige, they attracted young doctors from abroad. So also the Gundersen Clinic. For example, Dr. Kaare Kristian Nygaard (1903–1989) went to La Crosse in 1930, shortly after his graduation in Oslo in 1929. In 1931 he moved on to another famous medical center, the nearby Mayo Clinic in Rochester, Minnesota, where he worked until 1937. After a few years back in Oslo he started a surgical practice in White Plains New York in 1940. Dr. Nygaard also enjoyed a high standing as a visual artist because of his impressive sculptures.

The Gundersen Clinic in a way seems to have served as an extension of Norwegian medical professionalism, and has knit lasting ties between Norwegian and American medicine. Effective as of 1996, an agreement allows medical students from the University of Oslo to complete part of their in-service practical training in family medicine at the Gundersen Clinic.

But could it be that the waves of emigration also attracted the more outstanding personalities, that the prospects of going to America attracted Norwegians who felt unrest inside their chests and who were adventurous of mind and prolific in deed?

An example of this type of person from the earliest emigration years could be Johan Christian Brotkorb Dundas (Dass) (1812–1883), a merchant's son from Lurøy in Northern Norway. He studied medicine in Christiania for three years, but then went to Copenhagen, and later on to Germany to continue his studies. He worked for two years at a Bergen hospital, then went abroad again and pursued studies at universities in Sweden, Finland, Germany, and Switzerland.

He got a job as a ship's doctor on board a Dutch warship sailing to Java. There he practiced medicine for three years. Again he went to sea, this time as doctor on board an emigrant ship heading for America, where he arrived in 1847.

In New York, Dr. Dundas was asked to go to the Norwegian settlement of Koshkonong in Wisconsin, where malaria was ravaging. He agreed to go, and there he achieved a solid reputation because of some successful cures. But later on he left for Chicago and St. Louis to assist in fighting cholera epidemics there.

For two years Dr. Dundas was out traveling again, this time to China, Japan, and London, then he resumed practice in Koshkonong, before he finally settled in Cambridge, Wisconsin. Had he "an urge to travel"?

The fame of Dr. Dundas as an able doctor seems to have been substantial. He was said to have performed major surgery even before anaesthetics came into ordinary use. However, he must have possessed a very special personality. His biographers used quite impressing phrasings: ... (He was) very eccentric, rough, and possibly conceited. He treated his colleagues with the greatest contempt. ... He seems to have possessed a fearlessness and a practical judgment which enabled him to act with great success in critical situations. But because of his impressive personality, his haughty bearing, and the hard-handed way in which he treated many, the people stood in awe and fear of him and called him only in very serious cases...

It adds to a complex picture that this man was a dedicated poet who published verse in the Norse-American newspapers.

Among the emigrant physicians were many with impressive endurance. Søren Johan Hanssen (1820–1885) of Skien in Southern Norway made his way to the university by means of working in an office from the age of fifteen on and working as a teacher. He received his medical degree in Christiania in December 1855. In 1856 he went to Copenhagen to work there during the cholera epidemic. The same year he went to Koshkonong, Wisconsin, for economic reasons, and he established a flourishing practice. In 1861, when the Civil War had broke out, a Norwegian Volunteer regiment was established. Dr. Hanssen served as a surgeon in this cruel and bloody war with his wife assisting as a nurse. However, he contracted malaria, had to resign in 1862, and went back to his Wisconsin practice, severely suffering from fever and dysentery. For health reasons he returned to Norway in 1866, was appointed district physician in Romsdal, from which post he resigned in 1883. Dr. Hanssen is said to have had a somewhat odd personality, could have a violent temper, and had so many skirmishes with the men of the church that many patients thought that they could not be saved if they were treated by Dr. Hanssen.

13.4.5. The physicians' Emigration Wave

In 1943, Eivind Klaveness (1870–1952) published a survey of 126 Norwegian-trained physicians who had emigrated to the United States. The last doctor included in his book arrived in 1938. It seems reasonable to base the considerations on the emigrant physicians on this pre-World War II period, as the increase in travel activities and the more extensive contacts across the Atlantic in the period to come blur the distinctions between study travels, short-time occupational commitments, and emigration.

As seen from Table 13.21, the major part of the Norwegian physicians went to the United States from 1880 onwards and in the next thirty years. Explanations for this clustering may be found in the history of emigration, but also have to be considered in light of the market for work for young doctors in Norway.

Table 13.22, which has also been calculated on the basis of the Klaveness material, indicates the geographical preferences of the emigrating physicians. Wisconsin was the most preferred destination, followed by the other Mid-West States of Minnesota, North Dakota, South Dakota, and Iowa. The importance of Chicago is also reflected in the numbers for Illinois. Among the Norwegian physicians there is a certain migration within the United States. In Table 13.22, the last sites of practice or residence are noted. The concentration in Minnesota, Wisconsin, and North Dakota is remarkable.

By and large, the Norwegian-educated physicians chose to go to the regions in America where they found their countrymen and where their first colleagues already had settled.

As pointed out by several authors (e.g., Lovoll 1988), apart from the pioneer years, the lion's share of the general Norwegian emigration went to a New World where structures already were established. It was mainly an urban emigration, and the city of Chicago played a special part for the Norwegians. This overall shift to an urban migration over the years is not reflected in this material of physicians. However, even the earliest physicians already might be said to belong to an urban culture, and their desti-

TABLE 13.21
Norwegian physicians in the United States, arrived 1753–1938. Year of first arrival.

≥1839	1
1840–1849	4
1850–1859	2
1860–1869	3
1870–1879	4
1880–1889	30
1890–1899	34
1900–1909	28
1910–1919	9
1920–1929	2
1930–1939	4
Missing data	5
	126

nations were the early urban dwellings, albeit in the traditional rural districts.

What about other professions? Did they feel attracted by the prospects of the New World as much as the physicians were?

Ore (1956) has studied the careers of some of the emigrants who had an academic background when they left Norway. They were few, as compared to the total number of emigrants. One obvious reason was that the percentage of Norwegians with an academic background was generally low in the nineteenth century, another reason that people with higher education might feel that there were few possibilities for suitable work in America, and some of them belonged to affluent families where there was no need for going abroad to earn money for a better living. However, Ore mentions a reason which perhaps should be underscored: Patriotism and social responsibility in Norway gave emigration a certain flavor of treason.

Table 13.23 is compiled from the material of Ore. He found only 186 emigrants among people taking their Norwegian student examinations in the years 1830-1880. Twenty-six of these had no academic training exceeding student examination when leaving Norway. Theology, medicine, and law were the dominating groups, so the doctors were not alone. The other professions had a similar demographic behavior when it came to emigration.

TABLE 13.22
Norwegian physicians in the United States, arrived in 1753–1938. Sites of settling.

	First place of practice	Last place of practice/ residence
Michigan	1	1
Wisconsin	41	30
Minesota	17	31
North Dakota	16	19
South Dakota	11	6
Iowa	9	6
Missouri	1	2
Illinois	12	8
New York	10	7
Washington	2	3
Oregon	3	1
«West Coast» (unspecified)	0	1
British Columbia	0	1
California	0	2
Alaska	0	1
North Carolina	0	1
Nebraska	0	1
Montana	1	2
Florida	0	2
Unspecified/unclear	2	1
	126	126

13.4.6. The Next Generation

Because the early Norwegian population in the United States had such strong ties to the homeland culture, it makes sense to mention some of the physicians of the second generation. A detailed study of this group would have been a valuable supplement to our knowledge on the health services for the Norwegians and on the mutual relationship between Norwegian and American medicine, but such a study lies beyond the scope of this book.

Some doctors belonging to what we here call the second generation were born in Norway and accompanied their parents westwards, or they left Norway as grown-ups, but got their medical qualifications elsewhere. Others were born in the United States to Norwegian emigrants, and had their medical training in America.

An example: Stephen Oliver Himoe (1832–1904) emigrated to the United States as a boy and received his medical education at a medical college in St. Louis, Missouri. Dr. Himoe served as a surgeon during the Civil War, and had to resign because of ill health.

An example of physicians of the second generation who made a career in the field of medical science: Ludvig Hektoen (b. 1863), Wisconsin-born, but of Norwegian parents, became a distinguished professor of pathology in Chicago.

Beatty (1983) has looked at the medical services for Norwegians in the Chicago region in detail, and has partly based his investigation on hospital records. He concludes that the Norwegians had the same access to a variety of health services as had most of the other citizens there. Poor housing and dangerous working conditions created medical problems for the poor Norwegians just as they did for other poor immigrants. However, he concluded his article by pointing out that thanks to their positive and cooperative efforts, the Norwegians in some cases had even better care than the others.

In Chicago the Norwegian-American Hospital was founded in 1894, and a Norwegian Lutheran-Deaconess hospital was opened in 1897. However, internal controversies among the immigrants, often with religious overtones, also seem to have influenced, perhaps hampered, the organizing of health services.

In 1887 the Scandinavian-American Medical Society had been established in Chicago, organized like the medical societies in Scandinavia (Lovoll 1988); for example, they offered meetings and lectures. One of the ten physicians who established this society was the Trondheim-born Gerhard Paoli (1815–1898) (Klaveness 1943). Paoli had started his medical studies in Christiania, but he did not pass the examinations and had to complete his education in Stockholm in Sweden. In 1846 he embarked on a sailing ship for America, settled at first in Madison, Wisconsin, and then proceeded after six months to Springfield, Ohio, where he set up a practice. Paoli is described as being an extroverted person, and in Springfield, he participated actively in political work in connection with the presidential elections in 1852. He also took an active part when the Republican Party was established in 1856, writing articles and giving political speeches. He was afterwards appointed city medical officer in Chicago, allegedly as a reward for his politi-

TABLE 13.23
Norwegian students or graduates who emigrated 1830–1880.

Not exceeding examen artium at the time of emigration	26
2.examination	48
Theology	40
Law	31
Medicine	32
Science	2
Dentistry	1
Philology	3
Mining	1
Pharmacy	1
Music	1
	186

cal efforts, and was elected president of the Chicago Medical Society two times.

Many of the physicians whom we have described here as second generation Norwegian physicians, received their medical training in Chicago. Rush Medical College is often mentioned. Dr. Paoli was awarded a medical doctorate *honoris causae* here in 1866. Dr. Paoli had, however, strong non-medical interests which had ties to Rush Medical College. As a boy of fourteen he had been taken in as an apprentice in a pharmacy, and until 1839, when he entered the medical school in Christiania, he had been engaged in pharmaceutical work. Chemistry was one of his main interests. And in America, he got a medal at the Crystal Palace Exhibition in New York in 1853 for an invention, a method for removing fusel oils from alcohol. Professor J.V.Z. Blaney at Rush Medical College persuaded him to come to Chicago, and the two doctors established a company which built a refinery based on the Paoli process. When the plant caught fire after two years, insurance coverage proved to be insufficient. The factory was never rebuilt and the two colleagues suffered severe losses. This event forced Dr. Paoli to concentrate more energetically on his work as a physician, Klaveness states.

The length of the studies at Rush could be short: probably the influential Niles Theodore Quales (b. 1831) from Kinsarvik drew on his previous vocational experiences and education in agriculture and as a veterinarian, when he entered Rush in 1864 after resigning as a leader of a veterinarian hospital in the Civil War. He received his medical degree in 1866 after only two years of study.

While the first Norwegian female doctor graduated in Oslo in 1893, there seem to have been slightly fewer prejudices against women entering medical schools in the West, although female doctors still had to endure such nicknames as "hen medics" (Lovoll 1988). In 1870 the Woman's Medical School in Chicago opened its doors and became part of Northwestern University in 1892. Again Dr. Paoli was on the stage as one of the founders, and he also worked for women's liberation and voting rights. He served on the first teaching staff of the school. The Kongsberg-born Dr. Helga Ruud graduated from the school in 1889, followed by Dr. Marie Olsen from Kristiania in 1891.

Dr. Ingeborg Rasmussen, born in Bergen in 1855, emigrated in 1887, and graduated as a physician in Chicago in 1892. She had a background as an actress at the Christiania Theatre in Norway, and in the United States she pursued cultural and feminist interests and edited the Women's Page in the Norse-American newspaper Skandinaven. She became the first female member of the Scandinavian-American Medical Society in 1893.

Dr. Helga Ruud, Dr. Marie Olsen, and Dr. Ingeborg Rasmussen became cornerstones of the activity at the Norwegian-American Hospital for a long time. The hospital had a nursing school from the beginning, graduating the first nurses in 1896. The Norwegian Lutheran Deaconess Home and Hospital had a nursing school with a marked religious profile, and the first nurses graduated in 1900.

13.4.7. Emigrant Physicians: Entrepreneurs, Unstable Personalities, or People Fleeing Domestic Difficulties?

Among the emigrant physicians and their descendants, a wide variety of human beings are found. The general impression, however, is that many of the medical professionals found opportunities to exploit their talents in the New World in an easier way than they perhaps had been able to at home. But generalizations may be misleading.

At least it can be noted that the group of Norwegian physicians who left for the United States in the emigration period, and their professional descendants, became a visible and active element in the new society they became part of, and many of them exerted a lasting impact on it, with repercussions that were also felt in the homeland.

References

Beatty, W.K. "Medical care for Norwegian immigrants in the Chicago area," *Proc Inst Me. Chgo* 36(1983):147–150.

Blegen, T.C. *Norwegian migration to America 1825–1860*. Northfield, Minn.: The Norwegian-American Historical Association, 1931.

Blegen, T.C. *Norwegian migration to America. The American transition*. Northfield, Minn.: The Norwegian-American Historical Association, 1940.

Blegen, T.C. (ed.) *Land of their choice. The immigrants write home*. St. Paul, Minn.: The University of Minnesota Press, 1955.

Flexner, A. *Medical Education in the United States and Canada*. New York: Carnegie Foundation, 1910. (Bulletin No. 4)

Flexner, A. *Medical Education in Europe*. New York: Carnegie Foundation, 1912. (Bulletin No. 6)

Gjerset, K., and L. Hektoen. "Health conditions and the practice of medicine among the early Norwegian settlers, 1825–1865," *The Norwegian-American Historical Association: Studies and Records*. Vol. I (1926):1–59.

Hessel, S.T. *Medicine: The Gundersen Experience 1891-1991*. La Crosse, Wisc: Gundersen Clinic, 1991.

Jenswold, J.R. "'I live well, but'; Letters from Norwegians in Industrial America," *Norwegian-American Studies*, 31 (1986):113–29.

Klaveness, E. *Norske Læger i Amerika 1840-1942*. St. Paul, Minn.: 1943.

Lovoll, O.S. *A Century of Urban Life – The Norwegians in Chicago before 1930*. The Norwegian-American Historical Association, University of Illinois Press, Champaign, Ill., 1988.

Lowell, B.L. "Sociological Theories and the Great Emigration," *Norwegian-American Studies* 32(1989):53–69.

Ore, O. "Norwegian emigrants with university training 1830- 1880," *Norwegian-American Studies and Records, Vol. XIX, pp. 160–88*. Northfield, Minn.: Norwegian-American Historical Association, 1956.

Schytte, T. *Vägledning för emigranter. En kort framställning av utvandringarnes svårigheter och fördelar, jemte en skildring af de skandinaviska koloniernas ekonomiska, politiska och religiösa tillstånd i Nordamerika. Med ett bihang om de år 1847 utvandrade Erik Janssons anhängares sorgliga öde*. Stockholm: Joh. Beckman, 1849. (Reprint: Stockholm: Bokförlaget Rediviva, 1970.)

Semmingsen, I. *Veien mot vest. Utvandringen fra Norge til Amerika 1825–1865*. Oslo: Aschehoug, 1941.

Semmingsen, I. *Veien mot vest. Utvandringen fra Norge til Amerika 1865–1915*. Oslo: Aschehoug, 1950.

C H A P T E R 1 4

1900–1940: Increasing Numbers and Increasing Expectations – Doctors Recruiting for Medical Progress

ØIVIND LARSEN

As we have discussed earlier in this book, Norway changed and modernized profoundly in the course of the nineteenth century. A population which had experienced a rapid growth, and which had been redistributed through an intense migration, presented a series of new problems for preventive and curative medicine which awaited a solution. Medicine as a science had broadened and deepened, and had much more to offer than it had had only decades earlier. A corps of well-educated physicians had a professional obligation to deal with these problems. But, it was not clear in what direction the development would head.

In 1904 there were 1,210 physicians in Norway. The number ninety years earlier, in 1814, was 100, if one only counts those with strict academic qualifications. The figure of 160 is often used, which includes some additional medical practitioners, and this figure probably gives a more pragmatic description of the situation. This means that there was one doctor for every 5,634 inhabitants in Norway, but the doctors were not evenly distributed. By the turn of the century, the number of physicians had increased around tenfold, but the doctor/population ratio had only doubled (1:2,025), due to the rapid increase in the number of inhabitants. And physicians as a group had changed into a defined and rather homogenous profession.

At the turn of the century, this profession, led by the Norwegian Medical Association, which had been founded in 1886, directed its attention beyond the mere patient-doctor relationship and the working situation of doctors toward important public health issues. The work being done on the causes and treatment of tuberculosis and cancer was a main concern of the Association over many years (Falkum & Larsen 1981) (Larsen, Berg, Hodne 1986).

The fact that the interests of the profession was to go in this direction, was not something to be taken for granted. Hospitals had been established in the newly expanded cities, especially in Kristiania, where the new National Hospital (1883) and the large municipality-owned Ullevål Hospital (1887) were evidence of the public responsibility that had developed toward the numerous therapeutic challenges of the time, and of course supplied positions for new physicians.

A shift in attitudes toward disease increased the demand for health services, and at least for a part of the population, it became within reach of the private economy to meet these demands on a private base. Thus, prospects could seem promising for those Norwegian physicians who wanted to set up a private practice. And that was just what some of the emigrant doctors of the time did when they arrived in America. They set up practices in the New World, some of which soon became successful. In Norway, general practice, either as a private or as a district physician, was also usually the only choice given to physicians. At the turn of the century, only about one out of seven physicians were employed in hospitals or in research. When medicine gradually was split up into specialized fields, a private specialist practice also became an option.

An outstanding example of a successful private practice was that of the surgeon Alexander Malthe (1845–1928). He graduated as an M.D. from the University in Christiania in 1875. After some years of private practice, hospital work, and extensive study traveling, he established a private hospital in 1886 with 15–20 beds. He was a daring surgeon and got a reputation for performing advanced operations: Malthe was a pioneer in performing abdominal surgery, which was still considered dangerous to patients at the end of the century. As a private surgeon, without being a hospital or university staff member or head of a department, he combined his role as one of the leading professionals in his specialty with success as a businessman; at his death he left behind a remarkable fortune that he had earned from his flourishing practice. Being a bachelor who was dedicated to his work and his profession, he made substantial bequests in his will that would benefit the medical profession.

Of course there were other well-off and professionally esteemed practitioners too. But in spite of Malthe's obvious success, few followed his example. Neither his American-style private practice nor private hospitals established a strong foothold in Norway.

The orientation toward health as a matter that concerned the general population, and not just individual patients, for a long time had been reflected in the interests of many physicians. Carl Schiøtz (1877–1938), who was a later professor of hygiene at the University of Oslo, defended a doctoral thesis in 1918 based upon the examination of 10,000 school children. Such large-scale studies revealed shortcomings in health care and nutrition. Health education and follow-up measures could make use of new scientific achievements in fields such as vitamin research, in which Norway had attained a special reputation through the studies on beri-beri and scurvy performed by Axel Holst (1860–1931), Theodor Frølich (1870–1947), and Valentin Fürst (1870–1961).

Schiøtz organized a school health system in the capital of Oslo in the years after 1918. A medical surveillance system was established for the pupils, and a school meal was offered. Important side effects of these efforts of course was a general promotion of interest in health and an increased level of health education among the population.

Carl Schiøtz also introduced a new type of occupational health services in Norway, a system which attained a great degree of popularity. Previously, mining companies and later some factories had engaged physicians to look after their workers when there were accidents or cases of disease, but the new brand of health services introduced by Schiøtz had a preventive profile. He had been appointed as an industrial physician in the Freia chocolate factory in Kristiania (Oslo). Because of his work there, 1917 is regarded as the year of birth of the new occupational health services. Health examinations, workplace inspections, and counselling both individuals, and factory leaders were the main objectives of the services; medical practice was only a minor and supplementary part of the activity. The growing system experienced some resistance from parts of the medical profession, mainly from private practitioners who were afraid of the competition, as the occupational health services by and large were free of charge to the individual employees. Pupils, collaborators, and successors of Schiøtz, such as Axel Strøm (1901–85), Haakon Natvig (1905–), Eivind Thiis-Evensen (1906–), and Arne Bruusgaard (1906–1992), were instrumental in consolidating the system.

In 1943, when wartime conditions had made the need for collaboration and practical solutions even more visible, a provisional agreement was settled between the employers, the trade unions, and the physicians on the scope and arrangement of the industrial health services. Because of the German occupation, this agreement had to be officially confirmed in 1946, when normal conditions had been restored and the organizations of the parties involved were functioning again.

Since 1977, when the occupational health services were somewhat changed as a result of new legislation, the lion's share of Norway's workforce has been covered by the system. At the individual level, the effect of this service is difficult to assess, but the indirect impact in terms of imposing preventive measures and promoting the understanding of the importance of approaching health problems on a group level, not only among the general population, but among the doctors as well, probably cannot be underestimated.

But, in spite of its many positive sides, which have been experienced by most parties involved in the services, the approach to health problems through a work-place-based system of industrial physicians still was controversial, and it has remained so. Why?

It might be said that the first half of the twentieth century reflected a deep commitment to a social medicine which originally relied on the ideas of a medical, political science, the "medicinische Polizey," developed by the Enlightenment Viennese physician and counseller to the Austrian Emperor, Johann Peter Frank (1745–1821). This medical policy had later been further elaborated into a modern social medicine by German social hygienists in the years between the two World Wars. Heavy obligations as to the health of the population were placed on society as a whole. Alfred Grotjahn (1869–1931), Alfons Fischer (1873–1936), and Adolf Gottstein (1857–1941) were ideologists for a comprehensive discipline called social hygiene, a direction followed with interest in Norway (Larsen 1975, Larsen & al. 1992). Many of the most active Norwegian physicians interested in the field of social medicine belonged to the leftist side in politics and had social responsibility as one of their main commitments.

And in addition: Many of the prominent physicians of the time accepted as true the old saying that the health of the people should be the superior law, a motto used on the cover page of the health promotion periodical Liv og Helse (Life and Health), which was launched by Carl Schiøtz in 1934. The reasons for the discontinuation of this journal in 1972, instead of modernizing it and adapting it to the actual situation, is another story, but also an important symptom of the general interest in health promotion and preventive medicine.

But in the 1930s something important happened for the development of the health services and the medical profession in Norway: the appearance of Karl Evang.

References

Falkum, E., and Ø. Larsen. *Helseomsorgens vilkår*. Oslo: Universitetsforlaget, 1981.

Larsen, Ø. ed. *Forebyggende medisin*. Oslo: Universitetsforlaget, 1975.

Larsen, Ø, D. Brekke, K. Hagestad, A.T. Høstmark and O.D. Vellar eds. *Samfunnsmedisin i Norge teori og anvendelse*. Oslo: Universitetsforlaget, 1992.

Larsen, Ø., O. Berg, F. Hodne and F. Hodne. *Legene og samfunnet*. Oslo: Den norske lægeforening, 1986.

C H A P T E R 15

Between Crises and War. District Medical Services between the Wars

AINA SCHIØTZ

15.1. Into a New Situation "One gains an attachment to that which is poor and stripped, for that which is simple and grand – matched with a kind of satisfaction and a kind of pride at having been able to master the situation."

The 31-year-old district physician, Knut A. Schrøder (1905-1988), sent this statement from Kjøllefjord in June 1936. Schrøder qualified as a physician in 1931, and had five years' practice as a hospital staff member and as assistant district physician before he took over the post as district physician in Lebesby municipality in March 1936.

Lebesby is situated in the county of Finnmark, which is in the very north of Norway. Schrøder was educated at a time when the country struggled with enormous economic and social problems, and he became a doctor at a time when there was a surplus of doctors. He was one of the many candidates who fought for a post as district physician. Possibilities for obtaining a post were primarily at hand in the northern counties, where the toughest working conditions and the greatest challenges also were to be found.

The young doctor came to experience how the people in this part of the country, more than any others, had felt the great difficulties that the country had struggled with during the previous 15 to 20 years (Bull, 1979: 177 ff).

From the dissolution of the Union with Sweden in 1905, and up until the outbreak of the First World War in 1914, Norway experienced an exceptional period of prosperity. The country was undergoing an industrial revolution – production in industry increased by over 80 percent – and new technology was introduced in nearly all branches of industry. Electricity became commonplace, while steamships, new road networks and the telephone contributed to binding the people and the nation more closely together. Significant changes in settlement patterns occurred, as did changes in class structure and in public and private economy. Last but not least, since Norway became more of a part of the international society, the country's economy became subject to international economic fluctuations (Furre, 1972: 13 ff).

When the war ended in 1918, the authorities had lost control of the economic development. The export industry was in the process of collapsing, and during a large part of the time between the wars Norway struggled with the debt which had built up during the war years (Hodne, 1986: 133). The economy became steadily worse, and during the next two decades the country went into the worst economic crises of the century. The 1920s and 1930s were characterized by long and hard labor disputes, strong political contentiousness, continually shifting governments ten in all, and public poverty.

The crisis came to a head for the first time in 1921, with general strikes and lock-outs; then in 1926–27, and again in the period 1931–34, the people were severly affected and poverty was widespread. 156,000 breadwinners received public assistance for the poor in 1935. This meant that almost 300,000 people – or about 11 percent of the population – had to rely on poor relief that year (Seip, 1987: 278).

Just as in other sectors of society, the health services also were affected by the economic problems. After a strong expansion in public health expenditure before and during the First World War, the 1920s and the beginning of the 1930s were a time of contraction. A significant increase in the health budget did not occur again until after 1936 and up until the outbreak of the Second World War (Hodne, 1986: 132–33).

In this chapter we shall look more closely at how public physicians – primarily district physicians – developed as a professional group during the turbulent time between the wars. We shall explore how the fluctuations within society influenced doctors, and how the profession itself contributed to forming the medical profession – through responding to external pressure, but also by taking the initiative itself. In the last part of the chapter, we shall describe what it was like to be a district physician in those times – the role, the professional challenges, trials, and rewards.

15.2 The Districts and Public Physicians – How Many?

The most obvious change which occurred during the period 1918-1940 was a relatively large increase in the number of districts and public physicians. In order to find the background for the changes, we must go back to the so-called Royal Commission for Doctors of 1898, which was charged with proposing a thorough revision of public medical services. The work of the Commission later resulted in the Public Medical Services Act of 1912. The report contained a recommendation for a comprehensive and carefully prepared plan for expanding the public medical services. The plan involved the step-wise and hierarchical expansion and establishment of a series of new health districts. According to the earlier medical system, Norway was divided into rural medical districts and city medical districts. In addition, there was a chief county physician in some counties, with special responsibilities for lepra and psychiatry. In 1900 there were 161 public physicians in the country. The proposal in the new plan was for an additional 194 new posts making a total of 323 district physician posts, 26 city physician posts and in the 6 largest cities, city physician posts (stadsfysici)).

When the plan was initiated in 1914, the number of district physician posts was further increased to 372. The Ministry of Justice and the county councils had recommended this increase. The plan involved a formidable expansion of the public medical services, and clearly reflected having come into existence at a time when public economy was good (Box 151). In 1923, there were 400 public physicians, who made up about one-third of all the doctors in the country (Bjørnsson, 1965: 34–35).

The proportion of females among district physicians was relatively low. Among the candidates who took final medical exams in the period from 1893 to 1920, 7.1 percent of the women (7 out of 99) became district physicians, compared to 17.3 percent of the men (102 of 593). In comparison, 35.4 percent of the women became private practitioners, compared to 21.8 percent of the men (Larsen, 1986: 364).

By 1914, there was no longer a shortage of vacant districts; instead there was a shortage of available doctors. In the following decade, the lack of doctors was critical, and conditions in the north were particularly difficult. In 1919, over 40 district physician posts were vacant. As early as 1916, the Director of Public Health had discussed the problem in a note to the Ministry of Health and Social Affairs, and had stated that the lack of applicants was partly due to the low number of newly qualified candidates. The number of students should therefore be increased, and foreign doctors should perhaps be brought into the country. But the lack of newly qualified candidates was not the only reason for lack of applicants for district posts. The war and the boom period had greatly intensified the problems.

> "That the situation has steadily become worse – in spite of 22 newly qualified doctors in June of this year – is undoubtedly due to the abnormal conditions which have developed as a result of the World War. The flow of money, which has accrued so abundantly to certain groups of the population such as in the large towns, has created a higher standard of living for precisely these young doctors in the most favorable areas of the country, and has thus further increased their reluctance to settle in the less favorable areas. At the same time, the marked fall in the value of money has created a situation where a permanent post with a fixed income, which previously played a fairly important role in the household, now counts for proportionately much less." (Box 197)

In addition to suggestions about compulsory service in remote districts and importing foreign doctors, another suggestion was to shorten medical education for some doctors – to introduce a category of health providers with a lower level of medical education. None of these measures were implemented (Seip, 1984: 223–24). However, there was a fourth suggestion, which was instigated. In 1918 a grant system was introduced for medical students who committed themselves to work in a district for three years after qualification (Box 1).

During the 1920s, the situation for doctors changed. Student capacity was increased, and at the same time the Ministry of Health and Social Affairs – due to the difficult economic situation – amalgamated districts, withdrew vacant posts, and reduced the salary of some doctors. During the period 1924–1935, 34 posts were withdrawn, 21 district physicians were given a reduction in salary, while five were given an increase in salary, but only because they were given responsibility for a larger area as a result of the amalgamation of districts.

As a result of an improvement in the national economy, health districts were again divided up after 1935. In 1939, there were 377 public physician posts, that is to say, 27 less than the recommended number in the plan from 1914. In 1930, the Director General of the Health Services, Kars Wilhelm Wefring (1867–1938), ascertained that the time of the doctor shortage was over. By the beginning of the Second World War, there was a danger of high unemployment among doctors (Box 151).

15.3 Being Employed – Conditions of Employment

The Public Medical Services Act of 26 July 1912 added to and reinforced the regulations in the Health Act of 1860. Regulations about the duties of public physicians with regard to prevention, control, and administration were to be found in this Act. In addition, the Act confirmed that physicians had a duty to provide medical care to the population in their district, in return for an appropriate fee, and to such a degree as attention to their public duties allowed. The duty to provide medical care was secondary to the physicians' public duties. In practice, the situation turned out to be the reverse.

The preparatory documents and the actual implementation of the Act evoked debate, both in the Parliament and in doctors' circles. In particular, there was strong debate about the point referring to changes in the status of district physicians and city physicians. These were no longer to be senior government officials, appointed by the Government, but were to be employed as junior civil servants appointed by the Minister of Health and Social Affairs. In 1918 they came under the new Civil Servants Act. Chief county physicians and chief city physicians continued to be senior government officials.

However, the debates had an effect: the new civil servants were given strong protection against being dismissed – much stronger than that which was laid down in the Act. The letter of appointment continued to be drawn up by the Royal Council, and it was decided that the regulations in the Civil Servants Act about dismissal of civil servants should be "presumed not to apply to city physicians and district physicians, who are covered by the Public Medical Services Act of 1912" (circular from the Ministry of Health and Social Affairs, 17 Jan 1920).

Despite these steps, it took many years before the doctors came to terms with "the new arrangement." The fear of losing status was strong. A communication from Dr. Fredrik Emil Adolf Roscher (1891–1962) from Arendal to the District Physician Committee of the Medical Association asked them to deal with the matter. In his opinion, the situation with regard to the large number of vacant posts would be improved if one could again: "reinstate public physicians to their earlier dignity and give back to them the authority and security which this entails . . . (and) that public physicians should, as previously, be appointed as senior government officials" (Tidsskrift for Den norske Lægeforening (TDNLF), 1918:125).

The District Physician Committee acted on this communication, and requested that the Ministry of Health and Social Affairs should alter paragraphs 3 and 5 of the Public Medical Services Act, so that city and district physicians again should be appointed as senior government officials (TDNLF, 1918:190). The Ministry was, however, unshakable.

15.4. Changes in the Law and Regulations

The Public Medical Services Act was under continuous "surveillance," and as early as June 1920, a Public Medical Services Act Committee was appointed to consider an eventual revision. In addition, the Committee was to prepare a general act on the rights and duties of doctors. The work resulted in two acts: the Revised Public Medical Services Act and the Act on the Rights and Duties of Doctors and Dentists. Both of these Acts were dated 29 April 1927. One of the changes in the first Act was a more precise definition of authorization given in §8 on who could be employed as a public physician. This concerned candidates who had been educated abroad. They could now be employed in public posts after having passed a special examination.

In addition, the change in the Act permitted the simplification, abolition, or rearrangement of health districts. Five years later, a regulation was added that specified that allowances for meals and heating of the doctor's office should be paid by the municipalities, while travel allowances should be paid by the State (the Act of 27 May 1932). Further changes to the Act in 1934 permitted the transfer of public duties to private practitioners, and allowed re-location of district physicicans and city physicians as required (Act of 15 June).

A change in the organization of public medical services in the years between the wars deserves to be specially mentioned. This concerned the establishment of chief county physician posts in every county. As early as 1920, an important addition to §7 of the Public Medical Services Act (Act of 16 July) was made. This stated that:

> "For every county, except for the towns of Kristiania (Oslo) and Bergen, a chief county physician post shall be established. The chief county physician shall also hold an office of district physicians within the county. In counties where it is regarded necessary because of the workload, the chief county physician can still be employed without also taking over the position of district physician, with the necessary allocation of salary."

Even before this addition to the Act was made, eleven counties had appointed a chief county physician. His duties were to carry out overall surveillance of the county's medical and health services. The cities that had a chief city physician were exempted. "In addition, throughout the county, in all doubtful cases, they shall examine whether poor mentally-ill people need special treatment or care ..." (Box 147).

The authorities worked continuously to improve, adapt, and impose new duties on the public physicians. New regulations, based on the Health Act of 1860, the Public Medical Services Act of 1912, and later acts on social services, were drawn up and published three times in the years between the wars: Regulations for doctors. On the special notifications and reports which are laid down in the law and monthly or yearly reports concerning their services. A separate chapter – comprehensive and detailed – dealt with the special duties of public physicians. New editions of the regulations which came out in 1922, 1928, and 1939 reflected the important role played by the various reports. According to §20 of the Doctors Act, failure to report, or else inaccuracies in filling out or sending in reports, could lead to fines, and, in the worst cases, to dismissal.

15.5 Fixed Salary and Pension

Why did some doctors apply to work in the district, and what tempted them to be employed by the State? There were certainly many reasons, but Tryggve Hauan (1909–), who took his medical exams in 1936, gave some reasons which, in his time, were undoubtedly important motivating factors for many doctors:

> "It provided a fairly high status in society. In addition, it was, at that time, the only medical position which provided a fixed salary and a pension. In my opinion, these two factors, and particularly the pension, were important for many doctors when deciding to become public physicians" (Personal communication, 1994).

After a decade with great fluctuations in the economy, it was understandable that these factors were of importance.

The proportion of total income which the fixed salary for public duties accounted for varied greatly. Certain districts were "lucrative," that is to say, the size of the population meant that income from treatment services was significant. Such income was correspondingly low in other districts, for example in most districts in Northern Norway. Through the Public Medical Services Act of 1912, the authorities tried to compensate for these inequalities by introducing different classes of salary, determined according to income possibilities in the different districts (Berg, 1986: 252). In the same way, the location of the district in relation to central areas was taken into account. As an example, the so-called "Hålogalandstillegget" is mentioned, which was a supplement, introduced by Royal Resolution in 1921 – a supplement of up to 700 kroner for all civil servants (in full-time employment) in the diocese of Hålogaland in the northern part of Norway. Some other remote districts in other parts of the country also received this special advantage, such as Røldal district, which had only 800 inhabitants. This supplement was gradually withdrawn during the 1920s and was ended completely in 1927 (Box 202).

In March 1917, because of high prices and the shortage of doctors, the authorities decided to appoint a committee to propose new salary regulations and regulations for enrolling public physicians into the new State Pension Scheme (Box 202). However, the Committee did not confine itself to these two matters. They also reported their opinions about calculation of seniority, moving expenses, traveling expenses, housing conditions, holidays, and clinic expenses. These were matters about which the public physicians' professional bodies were concerned throughout all years. (The District Physicians Committee was established as a subcommittee of the Norwegian Medical Association in 1913, and later the District and City Physicians Association was established in 1934 and was the forerunner of the Public Physicians Association that began in 1945).

15.6 Further Education and Leave of Absence

As early as 1893, the Norwegian Medical Association had demanded that a specialist qualification should be established for the work of public physicians. Nearly 40 years passed before a privately funded course was established. The course continued for three years, but when the State was scheduled to take over responsibility for funding in 1934, the course was disbanded for financial reasons (TDNLF, 1935: 1381). However, it stopped for only a year, and then continued until 1940. Eight years later it was re-established, under the Director General of the Health Services, Karl Evang (Nordby, 1989: 161). On the other hand, the State had funded courses for a number of years, from the health services budget, in forensic medicine, public health, psychiatry, and tuberculosis, for chairmen of the board of health, and had given grants to public physicians who applied for these courses. For economic reasons, funding was withdrawn in 1922–23 during the first economic crisis.

There were several factors which motivated district physicians to apply for further education. One factor was the ever-increasing competition for public posts. Another factor was that new developments in medicine and changing patterns of disease highlighted the need for new knowledge. Last, but not least, district physicians were faced with new challenges in the field of prevention. In other words, a high level of knowledge was required from them. Apart from having to meet the regulations of the Health Act about "monitoring public health," high level skills related to controlling epidemics and tuberculosis were necessary, and they had to organize conditions for the mentally ill. The authorities stressed the fact that tuberculosis, epidemic diseases, and mental illnesses were important topics of which district physicians should have a good command. They could extend their knowledge about more traditional medical topics as junior doctors in hospitals and other institutions. Hygiene and public health, however, had to be learned by private studies and by attending courses. It was not until the end of the 1920s that public health was given more comprehensive coverage during actual medical training. During times of demand for public medical posts, great importance was placed on different specialist qualifications when evaluating applicants. Thus, many of the district physicians with permanent posts had a broad training background, particularly regarding psychiatry and lung diseases. The specialties reflect those areas where it was felt that the need for skills was greatest. It is interesting to note that examination marks were regarded as very important, since a first-class honors degree gave three years more seniority than a second-class honors degree. In evaluating applicants, previous practice in hard and difficult districts was taken into account (TDNLF, 1928).

Applications to take further education were a headache for the authorities. On the one hand, they encouraged doctors to take further education, but at the same time they had a tough job dealing with so much study-leave, because they had to employ temporary staff and finance them. Not only that, one result of further education was that some doctors disappeared from the service. The Director General of the Health Services was one of the people who complained about the problem:

> "It is, of course, a big advantage that public physicians apply to take further medical education, but on the other hand, I find it bad that they take advantage of the study-leave which they are granted as public physicians, in order to gain further specialist education, and then to leave the services."

He therefore recommended that before study-leave was granted, it should be clarified whether the physician intended to come back to the public medical services after his leave (Sos.dep 1934, Box 202).

The chief county physicians in Troms and Vest-Agder pointed out the difficult situation which study-leave created. In 1930, as many as two-thirds of the health districts in Troms were manned by temporary staff, while some years later, at the end of 1938, six out of 13 district physician posts in Vest-Agder were filled by interim appointments. It was therefore proposed that no more than one-third of physicians should be granted study-leave at any one time (Box 202).

During the 1930s, the possibilities for getting study-leave were good, though the formal conditions were relatively stringent. In 1935, new rules were introduced, with the condition that the applicant must have had at least three years practice in a permanent post. The applicant himself had to arrange for an approved replacement who had "experience as a doctor and who will be resident in the district." The district had to be managed without incurring extra public expenditure. Finally, if leave was granted, the doctor had to return to his post and work for as long a time as he had been on leave (from foredrag til kgl res nr 37. Avgjort av Kongen 13. mars 1935) (Box 202).

The utilization of temporary district physicians – for which there was a great demand – was an excellent way of giving employment to young unemployed doctors. They gained valuable experience and useful knowledge. For the district physicians themselves, being able to apply for leave in order to take further education was a valuable perk. They worked in isolation and the amount of work was always large. They had minimal time and opportunity to read medical literature. Therefore, both courses and house officer posts were of great importance, socially and professionally.

15.7 The Time of Persecution

By 1923, the plan for expanding public medical services had more or less been carried through. There were 400 public physicians in the country. The population's access to medical help had improved considerably, and preventive public health work was showing good results, even though there was still much to be done. But the good times came to a sudden end. The public economy deteriorated. Savings had to be made, and the State found it necessary to make a series of cuts in the years to come. Doctors received the first signals in the form of a circular dated 20 April 1923. The Ministry of Health and Social Affairs pointed out that traveling expenses for journeys in the call of duty "have greatly increased during the last few years, so that they now make up a sizable sum in the National budget." Doctors were asked to take economic considerations into account when choosing routes and modes of transport, and to combine different errands (Box 148).

In June 1923, the government-appointed State Rationalization and Saving Committee presented its report. One of the matters which concerned the public medical services was a proposal that the Director General of the Health Services and his staff should move into the Ministry of Health and Social Affairs, and that the Department of Health should be dissolved. The proposal was not followed up (Seip, 91–92).

More interesting proposals from the Committee were to abolish the post of district physician, to build more modest doctors' residences, and to provide that the municipalities should take over responsibility for a large part of the salary of midwives. After consideration by the Ministry of Health and Social Affairs and the Parilamentary Committee (Stortingets næringskomitè nr. 2), the head of the division, Olaf Lundamo, stated in a memo that:

> "As stated, the proposition of the Saving Committee is unlikely to result in so large saving as was thought. In particular we note that the proposed dissolution of health districts meets with strong opposition from the municipalities" (Note of 18 May 1924, Box 148).

The Parliament was not convinced by the comments from the Ministry of Health and Social Affairs, and in 1925 the Government was asked to simplify the medical services. The Government responded, as noted above, by withdrawing posts and making the districts bigger (Seip, 94). Several doctors were given a reduction in salary. However, it seemed as though doctors in general, with regard to salary, maintained their position as top income earners. In 1929, the statistics on income show that country doctors had an average salary of about 11,550 kroner and doctors in towns had 16,800 kroner. In the country, only lawyers and directors earned more, while doctors in towns were right at the top (Larsen, 1986: 384).

Protests against the reorganization of the medical services surfaced up quickly. The Director General of the Health Services warned against weakening the preventive work which the district physicians took care of

> "... by making changes in the Public Medical Services Act which have redressed a strongly felt deficiency, and if irreparable damage is not to occur, then the basis, given in our Health Act and Public Medical Services Act of 1912, must be fully maintained" (referred to in St meld nr 18, 1926, Innst. nr 2, pp. 191–192).

The Norwegian Association of Public Health followed this up with a statement in 1927, and protests came from the chief county physicians and the county governors, and of course from the district physicians themselves. The district physician in Otta, R. Müller (1869–1935), who was an exponent of the latter group, was blunt in his statements:

> "I believe that district physicians throughout the country should be aware of the fact that the authorities seem to be after us, and will make it as difficult and awkward for us to carry out our duties as possible, so we can just as well say: the authorities would gladly get rid of us in order to put all medical services in the mold. They allow us to drift towards a situation where we shall be inundated with doctors, so that competition and the fight to earn a living shall crush doctors' demands."

Müller encouraged the Norwegian Medical Association to gather district physicians together to discuss methods and means of defending their interests.

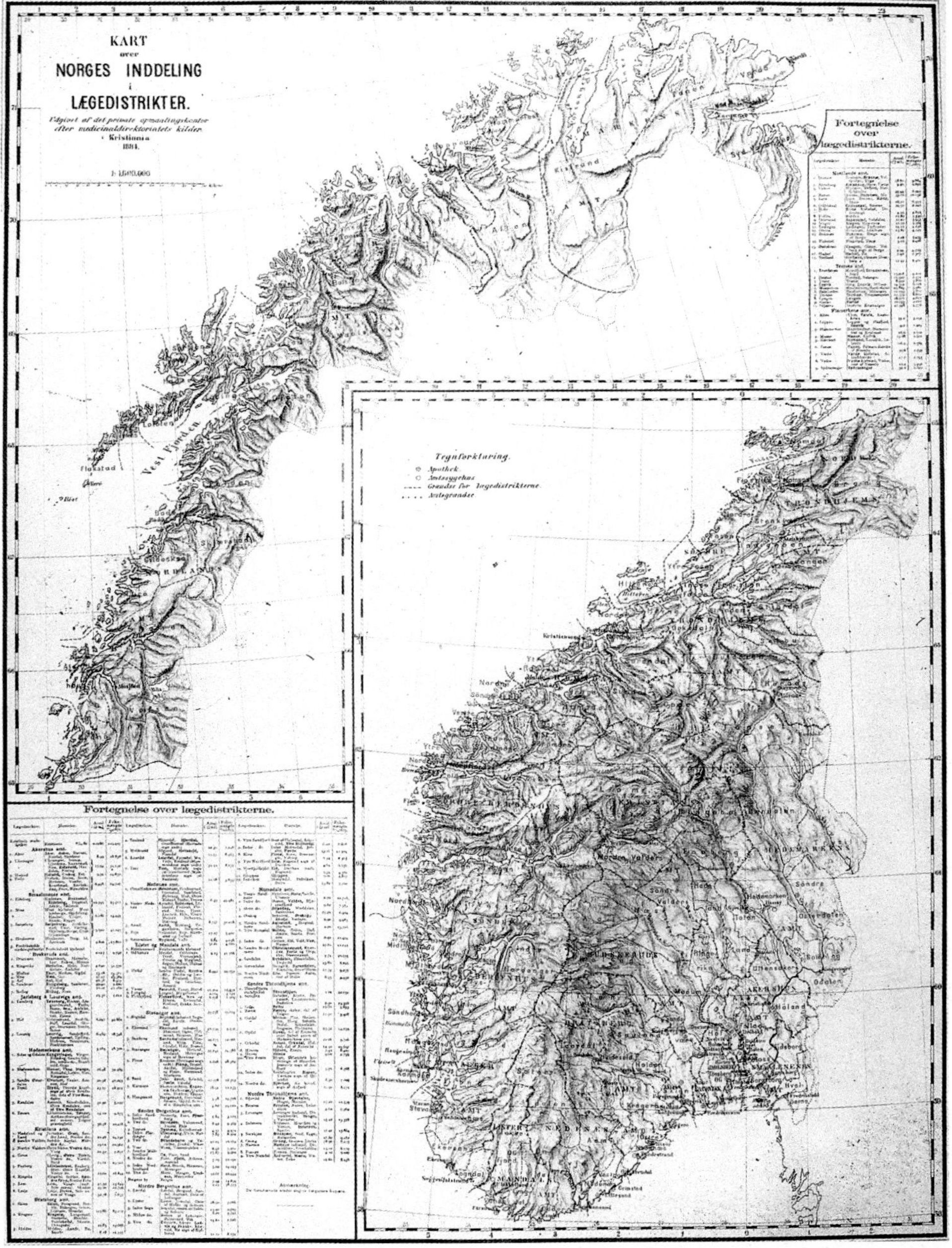

Figure 46: Map of Norway showing the districts served by the physicians (Courtesy University Library, Oslo).

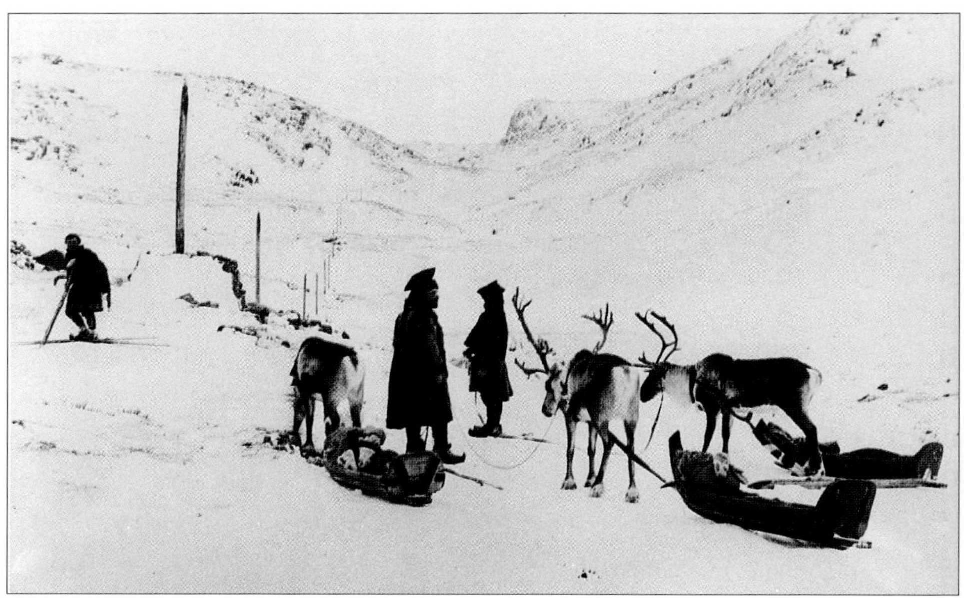

Figure 47: Dr. Anders Bredal Wessel (1858-1940) on house call travel near Bugøynes in Finnmark around the turn of the century.

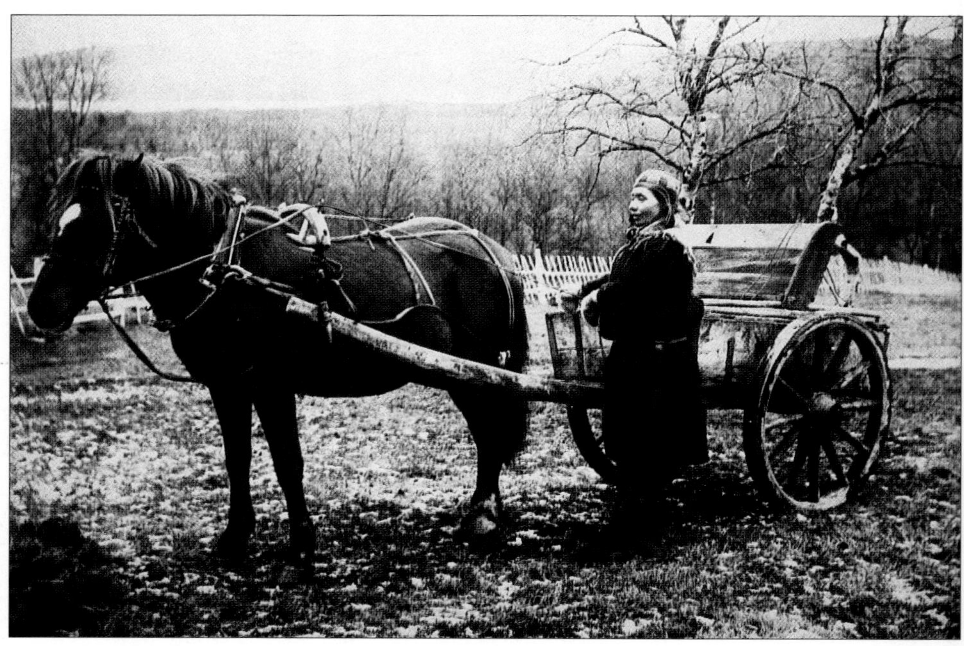

Figure 48: When there was no snow, horse and carriage had to do, but roads were often scarce in rural Norway. Both photos (figs. 47 & 48) were taken by the wife of Dr. Wessel, Ellisif Rannveig Müller Wessel (1866-1949), who produced a remarkable photographic documentation from Eastern Finnmark for the period 1895-1915. However, most of her material was lost during the World War II bombing of Kirkenes. She was also well-known as a revolutionary politician and as an author.

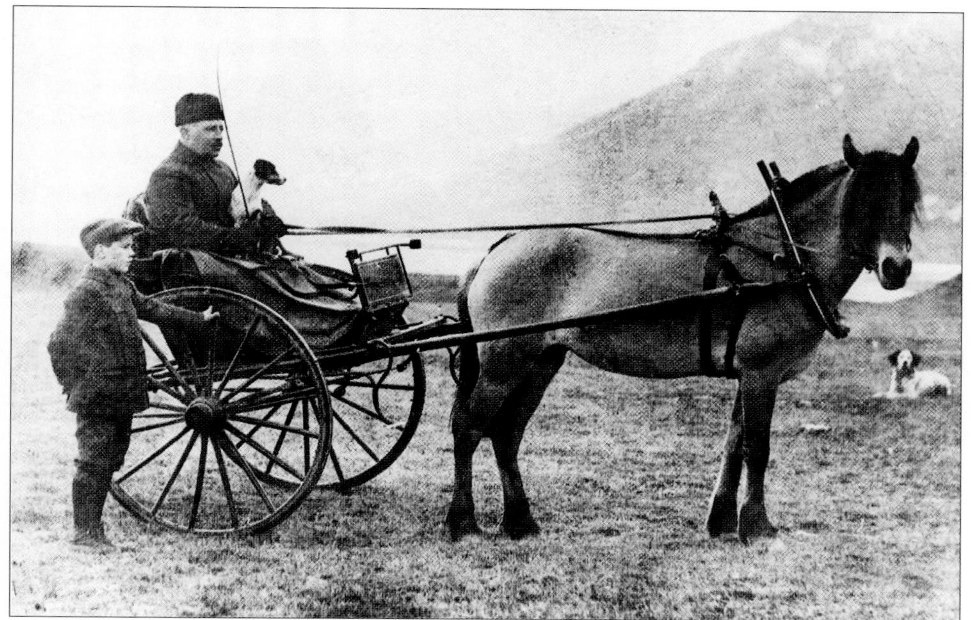

Figure 49: Better transportation was of paramount importance to increase the amount of medical work which could be accomplished in one working day by a rural doctor. Dr. Birger Lærum (1872-1953) is seen here in his horsecart at Voss in Western Norway around 1912. (The boy is his son Ole Didrik Lærum (1901-1972), later professor of transportation at the technical university in Trondheim (Courtesy Ole Didrik Lærum, Bergen).

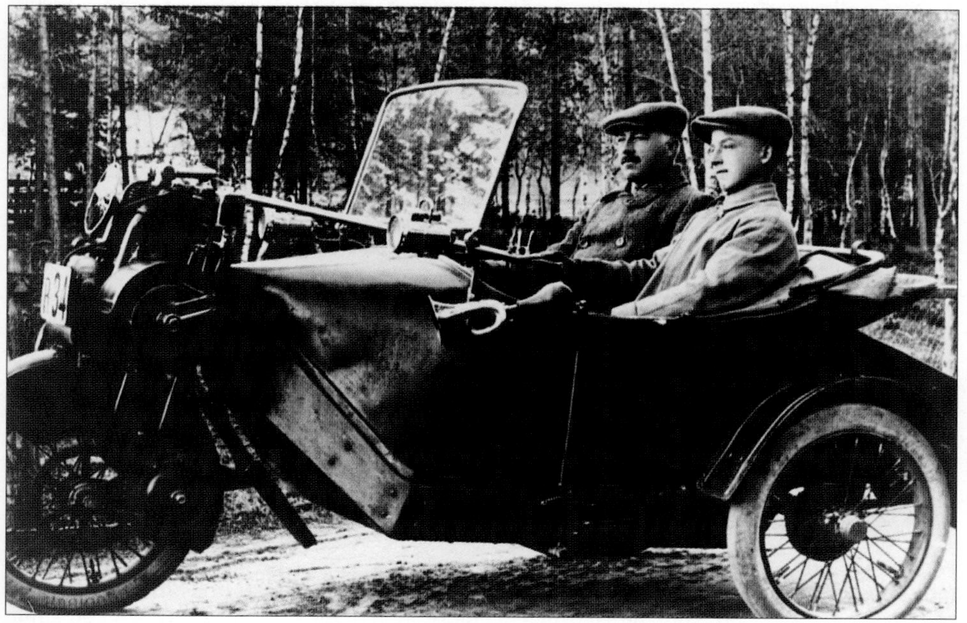

Figure 50: This photograph from 1922 shows Dr. Lærum in his Phaenomobile 9 Hp, 1913, together with his driver John Turvold (Courtesy Ole Didrik Lærum, Bergen).

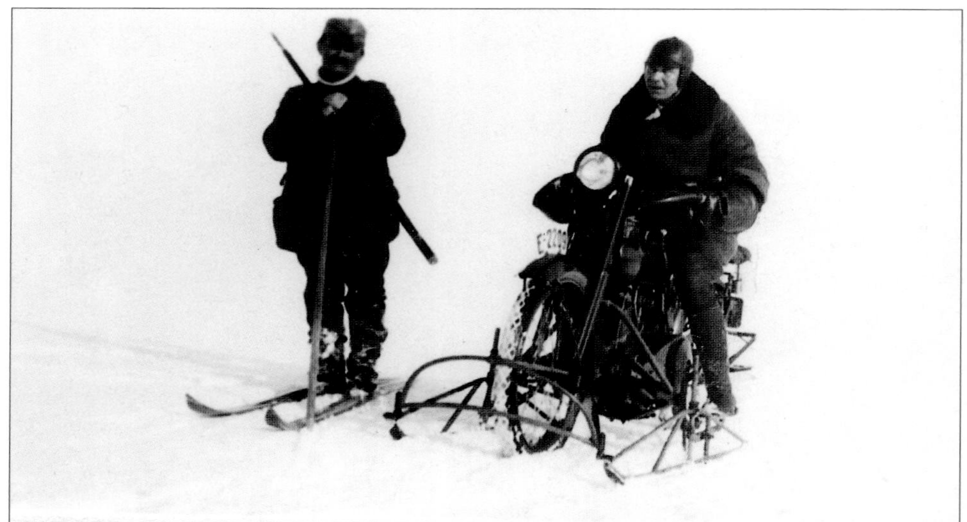

Figure 51: In the municipality of Østre Slidre district physician Carl Einar Isachsen (1892-1970) equipped his Harley Davidson motor bike as a sledge in winter. Photo from 1922 (Courtesy Department of Medical History, Univertsity of Oslo).

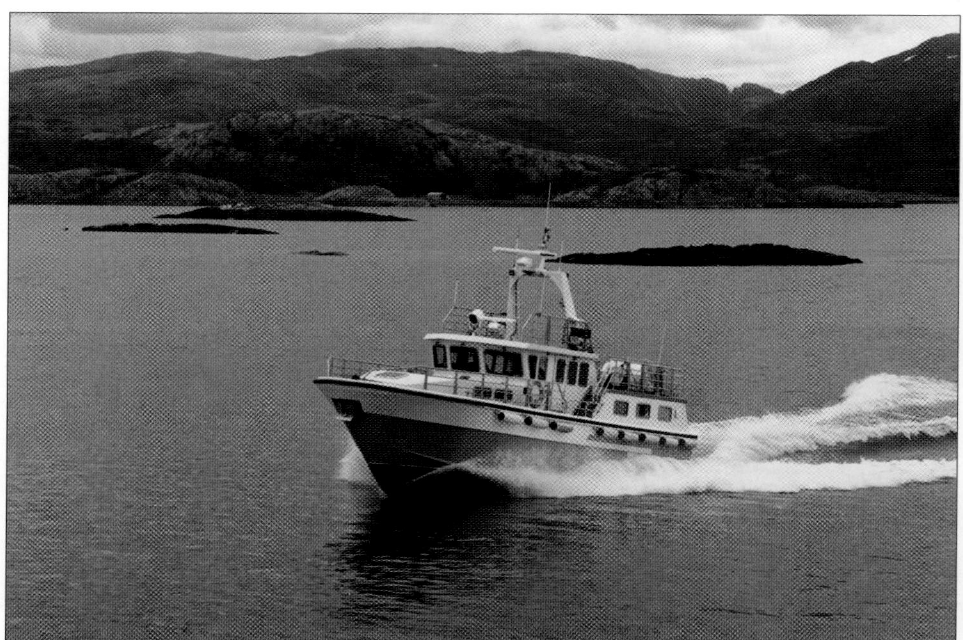

Figure 52: Still, even in the age of helicopters and ambulance aircrafts, the boat is indispensable for the health services in Norwegian coastal districts. Here is the doctor's and ambulance vessel "Tjøttagutt" cruising near Sandnessjøen in the county of Nordland on a rare quiet day (Photo: Øivind Larsen 1996).

"When it comes to the crunch, we just might have a few cards in our hand, which the Government and Parliament have not reckoned with. At least we have some sort of a monopoly over the sick" (TDNLF 1928: 75–76).

15.8. New Dangers

The protests did not help. Posts were continuously withdrawn, and new threats lurked round the corner. In 1932, the Government appointed a new committee, this time called the Saving and Rationalization Commission. Norway was now experiencing its last and worst depression. During the winter months of 1932–34, 40 percent of trade union workers were unemployed. The Agrar Party (Bondepartiet), which was in power at the time (May 1931–March 1933), proposed a brutal policy of cut-backs, which other governments would also perhaps have been forced to do. In 1932, the Ministry of Justice sent a circular to the municipalities, giving them notice that

> "the municipality has a duty to provide help only in emergency situations – when a person is completely stripped of the means of existence and when all other options are closed. The municipality's duty according to the law goes no further than ensuring that the person involved does not starve..." (Seip, 1987: 276 ff, Bull, 1979: 103).

The Saving and Rationalization Commission concentrated on recommending areas which could be delegated from central administration to the counties, on cutting expenditure and on re-allocating expenditure between the different administrative levels (Seip, 1994: 92).

With regard to public physicians, the Commission proposed a range of recommendations for saving money, particularly with regard to limiting traveling expenses.

The recommendations of the Commission for Saving and Rationalization, which applied to public physicians were:

- Co-operation between district physicians and health insurance doctors.
- Simplification of doctors' salary system.
- Proportional allocation of traveling expenses, when district physicians carried out public and private duties on the same journey.
- Cutting out special journeys for controlling cleanliness in schools.
- Further restriction of district physicians' journeys to the administrative office.

In addition, the Committee recommended considering further abolition of posts and amalgamation of districts with vacant posts with neighboring districts (Box 148). However, the most sensational recommendation was the statement that

> "the income of district physicians should be based mainly on medical practice, and, for most posts, public duties should be a secondary occupation" (Ot.prp. nr 29, 1934, p. 1).

This could not be interpreted in any other way than as a downgrading of public health work, or even as an attempt to undermine the whole public medical services. This statement stood in clear contrast to the signals which had been given earlier, such as in the Public Medical Services Act of 1912.

In the spring of 1933, the Government presented the matter to the Parliament. A proposal was put forward to withdraw 143 district physician posts and to establish 105 new chief municipal physician posts, the latter with a subsidy from the state to the municipality of 1,000 kroner per doctor. In this way, the State could save large amounts of money, since there was a big difference between this and the basic salary which the district physicians received – at that time between 3,100 kroner and 6,600 kroner, not including age subsidy. The Government did not oppose the statement of the Commission that public medical duties should be regarded as a secondary occupation.

Before the case came up for debate, the Health Committee had been given the opportunity to comment (Report of the Health Committee on Public Medical Services. Budget-innst. s. nr. 53). A majority of the Committee were strongly opposed to the Government's proposals. The chairman, Signe Swensson (1888–1974), stated that if one should accept these proposals, then one would abandon the principle of district physicians. He pointed out that one matter which

> "has been discussed regularly in the Parliament, and has always been adopted – is that one has never wanted to use the principle of municipal physicians with state subsidy..." (p. 942).

Signe Swensson was a former teacher, who had qualified as a doctor in middle age. She had also worked as district physician and physician to fishermen on the coast of Trøndelag for a few months.

The debate in Parliament was long and intense. A small minority of members of the Parliament, such as Nils Christian Nilsen Mjaavatn (1883–1951) and Jens Hunseid (1883–1965) – the latter had resigned as Prime Minister for the previous Agrar Party just a few weeks earlier – supported the proposed changes to the law and the withdrawal of posts which these changes entailed. Hunseid defended the proposition by stating that the development of communication and the large number of doctors had created a completely new situation. Even though that was true, the members, not surprisingly, set down the condition that their own remote districts should not be hit. In their opinion, the withdrawal of posts in central areas should not lead to great problems. In those areas, there were enough private doctors who could take on different tasks. Also, the gentlemen did not seem to be opposed to the proposal to establish chief municipal physician posts with state subsidy, to partly replace the district physicians.

The minority members were given a direct reply. Signe Swensson stated that:

> "Such a recommendation that the plan should be adopted, such as given by Mr. Mjaavatn, can also be given by me. I can well say that savings must be made, but do not save on this and that district" (p. 947).

The member Anton Olai Normann Ingebrigtsen Djupvik (1881–1951) also commented on Mjaavatn's statement: "I was also most surprised after listening to Mr. Mjaavatn. The first part of his speech was, in reality, a defense of this plan. As long as he moved around down there, the plan was excellent, but when, in the last part of his speech, he had come up to Bindalseidet and Helgelandsflesa, it was not good enough" (p. 962).

The plan to establish 105 new chief municipal physician posts, to replace the district physician posts, was controversial for several reasons. First, it was completely unrealistic to think that the municipalities could manage such an expenditure. They struggled with poor economy just as much as the State did. It involved transferring an expenditure to the municipalities that they did not have the means to meet. Second, it was completely unthinkable that the municipalities could appoint their own doctors. Cornelius Enge, a member of parliament, from Helgeland – one of the many who expressed horror over the proposal of the new medical plan – asked:

> "If it is such that we shall also go in that direction, that incompetent, ignorant people out in the districts and villages shall be the ones to appoint men who shall care for the sick and lead public health work in our country, then I think that we have gone so far in attacking our culture, that we have come so far into the much discussed culture pause, that the situation begins to be critical" (p. 951).

The proposal for the new Health Plan was not adopted. Most of the people involved in the debate defended the district physician system "with a full understanding of its importance for health work," as the Journal of the Norwegian Medical Association could confirm with satisfaction. The Parliament agreed that the public medical services could be rationalized by readjusting and abolishing health districts from time to time as found defensible by the Ministry. This only involved continuing the practice of earlier years.

Agreement did not last for long. The finances of the State continued to be at rock bottom, and in the spring of 1934, the government under Mowinckel (repr. liberal party "Venstre") had no alternative but to present new proposals for saving (Ot. prp. nr 29, 1934, on the Act on changes and additions to the Public Medical Services Act). Before this – in April 1933 – the Central Board of the Norwegian Medical Association had adopted a proposal in which they clearly rejected "that which can only be regarded as an unbounded lack of concern towards public physicians" (TDNLF, 1934: 439).

The Government's new proposals again gave rise to protests. One of the new proposals involved giving the Government the authority, if necessary, to move district physicians or city physicians to another public physician post. This could be done without giving compensation – perhaps from a central, rich district to any remote post. Another proposal made it the possible to transfer "public duties," such as the work of chairman of the board of health, to private doctors. The Director General of the Health Services tried to protest, but the Ministry had nothing to add other than that they had to stick to the proposal for financial reasons (Box 166).

The chief county physician in Buskerud, Sverre Kjølstad (1887–1957), put forward many of the same views as the Director General of the Health Services (Kjølstad was president of the Norwegian Medical Association from 1923–1938). He expressed strong views in the newspaper Aftenposten, under the headline: "Shall our public medical services be undermined?" In this article, Kjølstad talks about a complete destruction of the plan for public medical services, and a complete break with the arrangements for doctors of 1912 and the thoughts that lay behind this. The most hair-raising element of the Ministry's proposal was that public duties should be transferred to private practitioners. It was exactly this that one would get rid of, when the Royal Commission for Doctors of 1898 was appointed.

> "A private practitioner will, and must be, always so dependent on his clientele, from which he gains his livelihood, that preventive public health work would easily go off the rails."

He wrote further that district physicians are the backbone of the public medical services, and particularly among young doctors, there is a continually increasing understanding of the huge socio-medical tasks which have been entrusted to them (Aftenposten, Wednesday afternoon, 11 April 1934).

The elderly district physician in Trysil, Otto Mejlænder (1865–1944), expressed himself in less polite terms. He spoke of

> "the continuing period of persecution over the last few years against public physicians' economy and salary for their responsible work in prophylaxis and public medical services. ... And what kind of competence does the Ministry of Health and Social Affairs represent, with its ever-changing bosses and its old paper-pushers?"

Mejlænder's concern was to arouse attention for

> "the trend which for many years has been pushing the Norwegian medical profession in the direction of simplifying and proletarianizing them, particularly with regard to public physicians" (TDNLF 1934: 439, 440).

The Norwegian Medical Association, which had supported the Director General of the Health Services, had carried out its own persistent lobbying, this time without success. Both proposals were adopted and incorporated into the Public Medical Services Act as the new §16. However, the Health Committee did get in an addition:

> "A person who is moved against his will shall not receive a lower fixed salary in the new district than that which he had earned before moving, calculated from the currently applicable salary scale."

It seems natural to ask: Did the medical profession have no understanding of the country's huge economic problems? Why did doctors, as a socially privileged group, not show solidarity with the authorities who were trying to make ends meet, and with the many people who lived on the poverty line? Many of the statements made by doctors during the time between the wars were interpreted as biased contributions as they battled to maintain their security, power, and position. The work of the Norwegian Medical Association which made the greatest impression on the general public was advocacy in the areas of doctors' economy, salary, tariffs, and residences (see T. Skoglund in TDNLF 1986, 1221). Seen from the outside, it seemed as though the medical profession stood united in the battle to at least maintain the status quo, and that they were not interested in giving an inch, even in these times of extreme crisis.

However, many of the doctors' statements can also be looked upon as a stage in their endeavors to build up a comprehensive health service, and by this means to give a better life to the many people who were suffering, both in the short and the long term. One of the ways these sentiments were expressed was through medical reports and personal communications. Public physicians, and particularly district physicians, had a unique vantage point from which to view society. More than any others, they obtained in-depth knowledge of the living conditions of the local population, and through their patients they came into close contact with the many ways in which suffering was expressed. This gave them a form of insight which they passed on with great authority, and which was difficult for the authorities to ignore. Therefore, when doctors warned against running down public medical services, there were many who listened. In the debates in the Parliament which followed the authorities' proposals for cuts in the years of crisis in the 1920s and 1930s, there were many signs that a number of politicians had sympathy for this side of the story, and that they understood that health services as such were of great value to the population, particularly in times of crisis. In the light of this background, it is therefore not surprising that the proposals for saving and rationalization of the different governments were rejected so often.

In other words, the debates about doctors and medical services in the years between the wars illustrate the dual nature of the value orientation of doctors. On the one side they fought for their own self-interest. Public physicians, the Norwegian Medical Association, and the Director General of the Health Services stood united in this battle. On the other side, the same parties adopted the role of persistent advocates for the interests of others, for building up a healthy and well-functioning society for the common good.

15.9. District Physicians – Identity, Role, and Practical Work

What did it involve, being a district physician? Health commissions were established in each municipality, according to the Health Act of 1860. The public physician in the municipality was chairman. The commission was given wide authority, and had the right and duty to initiate measures which could prevent disease amongst the municipality's inhabitants. The office of chairman gave the public physician a very special position in the local community. It gave

> "the administrative basis for significantly raising the status and standing of the doctor in society. The welfare of the whole local community was, in a manner of speaking, his area of interest and responsibility" (Larsen, 349).

Thus, much of the foundation for the future powerful role of the district physician was already laid – a role associated with authority and status. The fact that he was a senior government official, associated with the rich traditions of the century-long bureaucracy, meant that he was already placed in a central position.

According to the historian Jens Arup Seip, the profession based much of its professional identity on the concept of its distinctive education from erudite schools and universities. By virtue of medical education, the profession represented "knowledge and information." Physicians regarded themselves as representatives of the aristocracy of refinement, of intelligence, and of the spirit. Their training gave them access to an elite status and upheld the identity of the profession. It gave legitimacy to the right of senior government officials to be the "ruling elements in the society of the state." Before 1884, but also to a large extent before the huge political upheavals which took place at that time, the chief government officials held decisive positions in politics and in the State Administration. At the same time, it was they who set the norms in politics and culture by virtue of their prestige (Seip 1994: 203–220).

The role of the doctor is also portrayed in novels and dramatic works. In the second half of the nineteenth century, we see a profession whose ethics were built on a strongly rational foundation that claimed that life and health should be preserved using all reasonable means. The picture which is painted of the doctor is of the authoritarian, strict, conscientious, and society-minded professional, such as Doctor Stockmann in "En Folkefiende" (An Enemy of the People) by Henrik Ibsen (1828–1906) and district physician Baarvig in Jonas Lie's (1833–1908) "Niobe." Coldness and sobriety are also characteristics which are associated with the role. As a reflection of the new ideological trends at around the turn of the century, a new type of doctor began to emerge. The role of doctor obtained a softer profile. The doctor took on the additional role of spiritual advisor, and the good doctor was portrayed as the one who treated his patients with emotional attachment and intellectual alertness. The "art of medicine" is practiced and praised, and the doctor also manages in conditions where his purely scientifically based knowledge is inadequate, such as the doctor in Knut Hamsun's (1859–1952) "Pan." See also E. Rasmussen, "Legen i norsk litteratur," TDNLF 1961, 701–05).

Through medical studies, professional practice, and often also through family connections (quite a few district physicians were sons or daughters of senior government officials), doctors had developed a common identity and common norms and values – cultural, social, and professional. These norms and values often contrasted markedly with those they encountered among people who lived in the district, and there was no doubt about which norms prevailed.

The cultural and social background of doctors, as well as their professional competence and authority, almost automatically commanded respect and deference, and placed them, right from the day they arrived at a new place, in a unique position in the local community. Thus, right from the start, there were many advantages associated with their position.

However, they had to keep within strict norms in order to maintain their position, because it was primarily through patient treatment that they won trust (see Berg 1: 79). After a few years in the same place, the district physician was in possession of a wealth of knowledge about the internal dynamics of the local community, about the villages and the welfare of the village people. Possession of this type of knowledge generated power. Knowledge was primarily important in order for the doctor to develop his diagnostic and therapeutic skills, but, in addition, it provided the conditions for the development of a relationship based on loyalty and dependence between the doctor and the local people, a relationship in which the doctor played the strong part.

15.10. Did Public Physicians Manage to Maintain their Position in the Years Between the Wars?

The fact that district physicians and city physicians lost the status of senior government official when the Public Medical Services Act came into force in 1912 probably contributed to weakening their position – at least within the medical profession. The shortage of doctors and the low pay of public employees during and in the first few years after the First World War undoubtedly reinforced this trend.

However, it is uncertain how much effect these factors had at the local level – whether or not the local people had a lower opinion of the authority and status of the doctors. There are many signs which indicate the opposite. There is no doubt that the relationship between district physicians and the local people became closer during the 1920s and 1930s. There are several reasons for this. There were many more doctors, and development of the health insurance scheme meant that more people with limited means could visit the doctor.

The new systems of communication also played a role. The telephone, improved roads, cars, and motorboats connected the doctor and the village people. And through this, the doctor's position as a person of authority was strengthened in the eyes of people. Other factors that also seem to have contributed to strengthening the role and position of the doctor in the eyes of people are that medical science made advances in these years and that district physicians obtained a broad and comprehensive education.

To what extent their role and identity was further consolidated through collegial bonds or contact with superiors (the chief county physician, the Director General of the Health Services, and the Ministry of Health and Social Affairs) is uncertain. Personal reports from the years between the wars indicate that it was local things – patients, working conditions, family, and nature – which meant the most for the doctor. Contact with colleagues was rare, as was professional and more informal contact with superiors. The latter was mainly in the form of circulars and regulations. Both lack of time and long distances restricted or prevented contact. The subsequent strong bond between the Directorate of Health and the public physicians was formed after 1945, at the time when Karl Evang was Director General of the Health Services. In other words, the class consciousness and collegial bonds which they had formed when they were students were neglected while they worked in the district. These contacts were re-formed to a certain extent during periods of further education.

What about unions? Did the District Physicians Committee and the later District and City Physicians Union contribute to unity within the service – solidarity, confidence and belief in their own importance? This is not likely. The doctors themselves do not seem to have been particularly conscious of this. As the district physician in Lillestrøm expressed it "... one sees very little of what these gentlemen do" (TDNLF 1933, 155).

15.11. Public Medical Services

According to the historian Anne-Lise Seip, the road to the welfare state was paved in the years between the wars. At this time, a gradual transition from the "social help state" to the welfare state began – from a society where social policy was established according to the premises of the liberal society with narrow scope for the collective element and wide scope for private measures, to a society where some of the principles of the social help state were further developed, but in which new measures were also implemented. Such new measures were universal benefits, adjustment of laws and relief measures to different groups, centralization along with greater public responsibility, professionalization and "corporatization" in the form of negotiation with professional and industrial bodies. The development of the welfare state moved forward particularly rapidly during the 1930s (Seip 1994: 15–16). The social democrats and the left wing of the Liberal Party (Venstre) became more and more vociferous in their demands for finding state solutions in the form of welfare guarantees such as social security, wage guarantees and a definite nutrition policy (Nordby: 80). The new ideas were clearly expressed through a range of laws and revisions of the law within the health and social sector. The social security system was definitely in the mold.

More and more attention was focused on socio-medical themes within the health care field. Public health, nutrition, and mental health were areas that were given priority. Seip writes that attempts were made to organize work in these areas as broad popular movements, with doctors at the forefront (Seip, p. 123). In 1920, the Norwegian Association of Public Health (Den norske hygieniske forening) was formed, and from the beginning of the 1930s several voices demanded that the university teach social medicine as such. Public health work ranged from sanitary and environmental strategies to individual measures, from prophylaxis of infections to prophylaxis of disposing factors, from preventive measures to constructive measures, and from sick and infectious adults to healthy but weak children (Alsvik, 255–56). In 1934, the Director General of the Health Services could confirm that

> "work directed against disease and towards better community health in our country... moves more and more in a preventive direction, and during the time since the new arrangements for doctors came into effect, we have acquired a range of important new laws and regulations with the same aim" (TDNLF, 1934: 437).

In many ways, public physicians, and in particular district physicians, played a central role in this process of modernization. They acted both in implementing matters, and in setting the premises. In practice, this involved new tasks, great pressure to acquire new skills, and the capacity to adapt. The district physician had an extensive field of work, as chairman of the board of health, member of the committees for child care, building and surveying, sobriety, and health and safety at work, school physician, physician at the center for the diagnosis of tuberculosis and physician responsible for supervision of the mentally ill and the poor, and so on. He gained great insight, which he, among other things, disseminated through medical reports. For health planners and politicians, this knowledge was of great importance. Within most of these areas, great ideological and professional changes, and changes in the organization of services, were taking place.

Many district physicians complained over the increasing amount of administrative work, and particularly that the "public duties" were too demanding and took up too much time. Time early in the morning and late at night were often used to prepare board of health meetings, to fill in forms, to send applications, and to answer official notifications. Just collecting information for the yearly medical reports on the health status of the district came to be a huge job, according to the various amendments to the Regulations for doctors. The consequences were severe if they were careless about sending in reports. They could be given fines, and in a few cases they could even be dismissed. District physician Johan Fredrik Øvrevik (1883–1968) in Nordmøre was sent to court, because, in 1938 he had not sent in his report to the Directorate of Health in time (Vatten, 1978: 34). Usually such cases resulted in fines of 300–500 kroner. The money was paid into a Public Physicians' Fines Fund, which was administered by the Norwegian Medical Association. This fund was used for colleagues and their dependents (Box 168). The verdict on Doctor Øvrevik seems to be meaningless. According to himself and others, he had never refused when asked for help and had never accepted payment from poor people. He asked: "what is most important, to write reports or to help people?" (Vatten, 1978: 34).

However, most doctors did their duty, but complained over the growing amount of administration. The district physician in Lebesby, K.A. Schrøder, was one of those who complained about "these retched reports." He stated that there was a mass of correspondence: private, municipal, county, departmental, etc. There were numerous applications about contributions... There were people who were mentally ill, who had tuberculosis, who were crippled, there were children under probation. There were boards of health complaints about rubbish, bird excrements, boat houses, drinking water, and schools. There were circulars from the ministries, which began to diminish, if anyone at all should get to know anything, reports from the county governor and chief county physician and the National Insurance Administration, mostly about the new social security benefit (manntallstrygden), and so on. (Schrøder, 1936).

"Manntallstrygden" was a part of the health insurance scheme. Health insurance for special groups was adopted in 1909. Neither the very rich nor the very poor were included at this time. In 1920–21 there was pressure to extend the insurance scheme to cover other groups, but because of the savings policy, the authorities withdrew several of the proposals. However, a new period of expansion began from 1933, and by a change in the law, health insurance was extended to cover new groups. "Fiskertrygden" or "manntallstrygden" was introduced in 1922, and it became a sought-after benefit (Seip, 198–201).

There were also other forms to be filled in which were time-consuming. In these times of crisis, the Ministry of Health and Social Affairs tried continually to reduce doctors' traveling expenses, and the Ministry carried out thorough control of claims for traveling expenses. Inaccuracies and attempts at cheating were called to attention. Before the claim came to the Ministry, it had to be approved by the chief county physician. To get a few kroner refunded could take a long time. Doctors had to give a detailed description of clinic days and journeys. How many patients had they seen, what type of patient and how many public duties had been carried out at the clinic and during journeys back and forth? (Box 168).

15.12. Curative Work – Trials and Rewards

As a district physician, one had a two-fold task. Public duties had to be attended to, and as we saw in the Public Medical Services Act of 1912, these should be given priority over other duties. In addition, patients had to be taken care of. In the Act on the Rights and Duties of Doctors and Dentists, it was clearly stated that doctors had to be prepared to provide help at all times. For many, this was an impossible combination. Usually, it was public duties that suffered, and curative work that dominated daily life, for most of them.

Set working hours was an unknown phenomenon. The law laid down that doctors had to be on duty 24 hours a day. According to § 7 in the Act: "Every doctor has a duty, when requested, to give such immediate medical help which either he personally or his deputy is able to provide." To be off duty – even if only for a few hours – was not possible, unless he had made arrangements with a deputy, or else had given clear instructions about where he could be reached. Being off duty for more than one day had to be approved by the chief county physician.

The overall impression from personal reports from the years between the wars is that the work of a doctor was constant toil – always on duty, always on call. In some periods they worked day and night. The days were divided up into some hours for patients in the clinic, then home-visits to the sick, often with long and tiring journeys. Days in the administrative office in other parts of the district or in the neighboring district – if the post there was vacant – were also usual. In some districts, and particularly in the north, this could involve an expedition of several days in order to get there and back. In 1939, the district physician in Vardø wrote about his days in the administrative office. He had to take the express boat to and from Båtsfjord, the local boat to Havningberg, a fishing boat to Syltefjord and then return from there to Vardø with the local boat (Box 168). By looking at the map, we can see that this was not exactly a Sunday trip. Trude Johnsen (1872–1954, cand. med. 1903), who was one of the first female district physicians, obtained permission from her father, director of the local Works, and authorization from the Director General of the Health Services, to go to Finnmark in 1913. She practiced in Northern Norway for 10 years. She managed to serve the districts of Alta, Kautokeino, and Talvik together, and she tells about journeys of up to 13 days at a time and round trips in and out of the fjords of 330 kilometers with the means of travel available at the time (Kvinnelige studenter 1932: 154, 155).

Knut A. Schrøder tells about traveling 170–180 kilometers to visit the sick in Laksefjordbotn, and journeys to the administrative office of 130–150 kilometers.

Even though these examples were extreme, journeys in most districts were long and tiring. District physician Øvrevik managed to get a little sleep on the boat on the way to visiting the sick, or else on a kitchen stool while he waited for a child to be born. His children relate:

> "We just do not understand how he managed his workload. When he came back from Tustna, he washed, changed his shirt, shaved, drank coffee, and then went straight to the clinic where the waiting room was full of patients. The same pattern was repeated day after day. He slept a short while on the boat, and it was this that kept him going" (Vatten: 13).

Øvrevik was district physician from 1918 until 1955 in a coastal district in Nordmøre.

The most moving stories are about contact with patients. The doctors often give the impression of having an almost paternal relationship with them. There are numerous reports about the satisfaction of having solved a medical problem, and about having been able to help, or else about being powerless in the face of sickness and wretchedness. At times, the many epidemics and tuberculosis wrought havoc, and the fight against disease could often feel like a struggle against all odds.

The most gripping stories are accounts of childbirth. Managing a complicated birth and saving the mother and the child gave life meaning. If things went wrong, it was never forgotten. Karoline Mathisen (1898–1981, cand. med. 1925) was substitute for the district physician in Lyngen, and she gives us an insight into how it was:

> "It was often not very pleasant to come home to the doctor's residence, completely exhausted after a long tiring journey into one fjord or another, with your head thumping from the noise of the engine, your stomach empty after the usual serving of coffee and bread – and so to see the horse carriages, perhaps one, perhaps several, waiting in the court-yard. One was not always in the mood to drive for a couple of hours in biting snow, perhaps to have to sit and watch over a difficult birth until the early hours of the morning. But the feeling of being a reasonably useful member of society, of having a task, always worked as a tremendous stimulus in such cases" (Kvinnelige studenter 1932:160).

Rewards were also to be found on other "levels." Many regarded having worked in the district as extremely useful experience. At the time when there was a shortage of doctors, there was talk about ordering doctors to remote districts. Member of the Parliament and later Director General of the Health Services, Karl Wilhelm Wefring (1867–1938), complained in a debate in the Parliament in 1917 that doctors congregated in central areas, and argued that the experience they could gain in remote districts would be to their own enrichment,

> "... because I believe, especially for younger doctors, that being a country district physician is extremely stimulating. It is extremely stimulating, because one learns to rely on oneself. In practice, one is faced with tasks where one has to deal with the matter oneself, without being able to rely on others. In addition, one comes into contact with people from the highest to the lowest, indeed all levels of society, and in this way one gains experience which is useful for the rest of one's life" (St. forhandl. no. 90, 1917, 30 mars, s 713).

The rewards were, in other words, connected with the joy of being able to master things, of being independent, of learning to rely on one's own strength and getting to know people and the country.

Life in the open and experiences of nature also meant a lot. We can again quote Karoline Mathisen:

> "The life of a district physician seems to be – despite all the toil – like a refreshing holiday, when one comes from the fatigue of the indoor life of the infirmaries. The long journeys in sunshine and starlight, over a calm, glittering sea or in storm and seaspray, give plenty of time for dreaming and meditation, something which one had almost forgotten... And exactly because it is rare for work to be so personal, when one can gain insight into strange fates and living conditions, that the work is also rewarding, and gives much pleasure. I believe that most doctors, who have spent time in the country, will be glad of the wealth of experience, knowledge of people and common sense which it has given them" (Kvinnelige studenter, 1932: 158, 161).

Another type of reward, but perhaps a less noble one, was being able to earn a reasonable salary. A doctor's income gave access to material goods – goods which could contribute to distancing the district physician from the village people. District physician Emil Moe tells about a visit to his brother, Knut (1892–1972), in 1929.

> "He was district physician in Tysnes, and had had a car for three years. He looked very good when he sat in his three-seater Citroën with a 12 horse-power engine and open top. He sat there in his fur coat, with a fur hat, long leather gloves and an expression on his face which said that he was lord of all he surveyed" (Moe, 1994:19).

15.13. Complaints Against Doctors

Not all district physicians tackled all their tasks according to the rules. In the years between the wars, as always, there were "rotten apples" who threatened the reputation of the profession. The complaints which reached the top – the Ministry of Health and Social Affairs – were few, but serious.

Complaints from patients were very rare. There was no tradition for such. As the father of a patient expressed it:

> "Even though, in the year of the Lord 1924, it seems as though, in the Kingdom of Norway, it takes about ten lay persons to one royal government official in order for one to be believed, I shall still, as briefly as possible, recount the event."

The man accused the doctor of drunkenness and "improper conduct in his work." The complaint was not supported by the executive committee of the local council in the municipality, so the case was therefore dismissed (Box 158). Other complaints were about sexual abuse of servants, about improper conduct towards female patients, about inappropriate medical treatment, about having refused to visit dying patients, about having constantly told patients off, and so on. Last but not least, there were many complaints about lack of attention to public duties.

Doctors were able to defend themselves, but not all of them were equally professional in their defense. In 1924, a district physician received complaints that he was difficult to get hold of during working hours, because when he was absent he did not notify the local sickness insurance fund or the local council, and that he did not hold board of health meetings. The doctor replied that the complaint had to be seen in the light of the communist propaganda "which manifests itself everywhere." In addition, the people who complained were

> "... spokesmen for loose, untrue, evil gossip, while they failed to take into account my enormous contribution to the health district of..., since I am primarily an eminent, clever doctor with a unique education... and I have personally sacrificed large sums of money in order to improve the doctor's residence (Box 154).

There are only a few cases in which the sources give information about doctors being suspended. In a couple of cases the matter was dealt with by giving early retirement or invalid pension (Box 154, 156, 158).

15.14. *Helpers*

Stories of toil, vivid experiences, and rewards are recurring themes in doctors' accounts from the 1920s and 1930s. But we can also read in these accounts a tribute to the helpers who assisted them in their work, both to the men who drove them both on the land and on the sea, and to the nurses or the new health visitors in areas where they were to be found.

In 1925, the Nurses Association established a post-graduate school in nursing and social health work. This school was closed down after the war, and the National School for Health Visitors was established in 1947 (Berg, 1987: 48).

The work of spouses was taken more for granted. Doctors' wives, for most of them had a wife, stood by in good times and in bad, and were essential in order to run the "business." They did everything from serving food to long-distance travelers, answering the telephone, washing the clinic, sterilizing instruments, assisting with simple operations – to carrying out some of the tasks themselves. Very many of them were qualified nurses and they made constant use of their vocation, without being remunerated.

15.15. *Conclusions*

For public physicians, the years between the wars was a time of upheaval, but also a time of construction and consolidation. Despite a strong external pressure, primarily caused by the great upheavals in society, the doctors managed to strengthen their position. Their professional management was carried forward, doctors kept their professional independence and control over their own business, and public medical services were strengthened both quantitatively and qualitatively.

It seems natural to ask how and why doctors managed to stand up against the pressure. The strong attachment to the service was consolidated through the central, state-financed professional management. The threats directed at the professional management were always rejected by the doctors' allies – the majority of the democratically elected members of the Parliament. The cultural and social bonds which, in particular, had been formed during their medical studies, were solid enough to withstand professional isolation. External threats about changes in terms of employment, reduction in salary, cut-backs in the number of posts and the number of districts served to unite the profession more closely. With their "monopoly over the sick," their solidarity, and their strong allies in political circles, public physicians were, in the long run, unassailable.

Accounts about district physicians from the years between the wars also provide the opportunity to reflect over repetitions, over the lines through history, over how a shortage of doctors or a surplus of doctors can provoke the same reactions and the same recommendations for measures to meet the problems. In times of crisis we hear about remote municipalities which are hard hit, about demands to increase the number of medical students, about importing foreign doctors, about special advantages in the form of extra salary and subsidies, and last but not least about compulsory service.

When solidarity is threatened in times when there is a surplus of doctors and competition for jobs, we register fear for loss of status and position, and demands for better education. Demands for lower salary and for better services and additional services come from the employing authorities and from consumers.

Threads can also be traced on other levels. In times of public "poverty" we see the continuous fight over which level of bureaucracy shall pay for public services: the state, the county, or the municipality. In the history of district physicians, we can clearly see the status which is attached to the different levels. The government initiative in the 1930s to replace a large number of district physicians with community physicians, who would be employed by local, democratically elected bodies instead of the central professional management, was one of the most threatening proposals that was forwarded during this period.

At the individual level, over and over again we find the powerful, eternal conflict between public duties and curative work – between meeting immediate and obvious needs, against using time on preventive work and work orientated to the future. Which tasks should come first, and what should be given priority? Public tasks were the tasks which were put aside first.

Building up the modern welfare state began in the years between the wars. For doctors, this meant new tasks, new groups of patients, and demands for a stronger focus on preventive work – partly from a changed perspective. We also experienced changes in patterns of disease and developments in medical science. Public physicians met these challenges by gaining further qualifications, by taking further courses and by specializing: not to disappear from the services, but in order to be better able to meet the challenges they came across in the districts.

Specialization and further education also had side-effects. Through greater professional weight, the doctors achieved greater trust from the local population: their social status was strengthened. In meetings with colleagues and superiors, the collegial bond, their role, and their professional identity were strengthened. Thus, by the beginning of the Second World War, public physicians were a strong group, but also a group that would come to meet new and different challenges.

References

Alsvik, O. *"Friskere, sterkere, større, renere." Om Carl Schiøtz og helsearbeidet for norske skolebarn.* Thesis in history, University of Oslo 1991.

Bain, M. H. *"I hine haarde dage." Legeberetninger fra Lurøy legedistrikt.* Lurøy 1979.

Berg, O. "Verdier og interesser – Den norske lægeforenings fremvekst og utvikling." In *Legene og samfunnet.* eds. Larsen, Ø., O. Berg and F. Hodne Oslo: Seksjon for medisinsk historie, Universitetet i Oslo og Den norske lægeforening, 1986.

Berg, O. *"Medisinens logikk."* Oslo: Seksjon for medisinsk historie, Universitetet i Oslo, og Den norske lægeforening, 1987.

Bjørnsson, B. "Legesituasjonen i Norge." *Sosialt arbeid* 39(1965),: 34–44.

Bull, E. *Klassekamp og fellesskap 1920-1945. Norges Historie, vol. 13*, Oslo: Cappelens forlag, 1979.

Forsdahl, A. "Utdrag av medisinalberetninger fra Finnmark 1863-1929." *Fylkeslegens skriftserie nr 5-1991*, Fylkeslegen i Finnmark 1991.

Forsdahl, A. *Sunnhetstilstanden, hygieniske og sosiale forhold i Sør-Varanger 1869–1975 belyst ved medisinalberetningene. ISM skriftserie nr 2.* Tromsø: University of Tromsø, Institute for Social Medicine, 1992.

Forsdahl, A. *Utdrag av medisinalberetninger fra Sulitjelma 1891–1990. ISM skriftserie nr 27*, University of Tromsø, Institute for Social Medicine, Tromsø 1993.

Furre, B. *Norsk historie 1905–1940.* Oslo: Det Norske Samlaget, Oslo 1972.

Gogstad, A.C. *Helse og hakekors.* Bergen: Alma Mater, 1991.

Johnsen, T. "Fra mine distriktslægeår." In *Kvinnelig studenter 1882–1932*, Oslo: Gyldendal, 1932.

Hodne, F. "Økonomisk vekst og helse." In Larsen, Berg, Hodne, *Legene og samfunnet.* Oslo: Seksjon for medisinsk historie, Universitetet i Oslo, og Den norske lægeforening, 1986.

Larsen, Ø. Parts 4 and 5 in Larsen, Ø., O. Berg, and F. Hodne, *Legene og samfunnet*, Oslo: Seksjon for medisinsk historie, Universitetet i Oslo, og Den norske lægeforening, 1986.

Lund, O. *Som lege bak Lofotveggen*, Oslo: Gyldendal, 1975.

Løken, K. *Karjoldokt'ern*, Oslo: Cappelen, 1974.

Mathisen, K "Inntrykk fra distriktslægedager nordenfor polarcirkelen." In *Kvinnelige studenter 1882–1932*, Oslo: Gyldendal, 1932.

Mellbye, F. *Slit med helsa. Bilder fra medisinske samtid.* Oslo: Gyldendal, 1989.

Moe, E. *Den siste distriktslege.* Published by the author, Stord 1994.

Nordby, T. Karl Evang. En biografi. Oslo: Aschehoug, 1989.

Nordby, T. "Statsutviklingen under Arbeiderpartiet" and "Det offentlige helsevesenet – en fagstyrets høyborg." In T. Nordby ed., *Arbeiderpartiet og planstyret 1945–1965.* Oslo: Universtitetsforlaget, 1994.

Rasmussen, E. "Legen i norsk litteratur." *Tidsskrift for Den norske lægeforening*, (1961):701–705.

Reichborn-Kjennerud et al. *Medisinens historie i Norge.* Oslo: Grøndahl & Søns forlag, 1936.

Seip, A. L. "Helse som samfunnssak," in *Sosialhjelpstaten blir til. Norsk sosialpolitikk 1740–1920.* Oslo: Gyldendal, 1984.

Seip, A. L. "Fattiglov og fattigvesen i mellomkrigstiden – et forsørgelsessystem under krise," *Historisk tidsskrift*,3 (1987):276–300.

Seip, A. L. "Veien til velferdsstaten," in *Norsk sosialpolitikk 1920-75.* Oslo: Gyldendal, 1974.

Seip, J. A. *Utsikt over Norges historie. Første del.* Oslo: Gyldendal, 1974.

Seip, J. A. "Flerpartistaten i perspektiv," *Nytt Norsk Tidsskrift*, 3–4(1994): 203–220.

Skoglund, E. "Legers videre- og etterutdannelse," *Tidsskrift for Den norske lægeforening*,14(1986):106;1220–1226.

Vatten, I. Å. *Doktor`n vår*. Trondheim: Rune Forlag, 1978.

Official documents

Stortingsforhandlinger nr 90, 1917, 30. mars.

St.meld. nr 18 – 1926, Innst. nr 2.

St.meld. nr 85 (1970-71). Om helsetjeneste utenfor sykehus.

Innstilling om Legetjenesten og tannlegetjenesten. Innstilling I fra komiteen til utredning av spørsmålet om tilstrekkelig tilgang på og spredning av helsepersonell (Helsepersonellkomiteen) oppnevnt ved kongelig resolusjon av 22. november 1963. Avgitt i juni 1967. St. prp. nr 108 (1937).

Ot. prp. nr 29 (1934).

Ot. prp. nr 46 (1938).

From the National Archives (Riksarkivet):

Sosialdepartementet, Medisinaldirektoratet, Legekontoret. (Ministry of Health and Social Affairs, Directorate of Medicine, Doctor`s Office) The boxes 1, 147, 148, 151, 154, 156, 158, 168, 197, 202.

From Tidsskrift for Den norske lægeforening: (Journal of the Norwegian Medical Association)

1918: 125, 190.

1928: 75-77.

1933: 155.

1934: 437, 437.

1935: 1381.

1942: 336.

1961: 701-705.

1986: 1221.

Other references

Eriksen, S., Article in Morgenbladet 12. april 1934.

Gedde-Dahl, Tobias M. "På helsa løs. En leges opplevelser i det tyvende århundre." Oslo: Manuscript owned by the family, 1991.

Hauan, T. (M.S., born 1909, cand. med. 1936) in interviews with A. Schiøtz, 27. July, 14. September, and 3. December 1994, and 3. August 1995.

Kjølstad, S., Article in Aftenposten, Wednesday afternoon 11th of April 1934.

Schrøder, Knut A. Letter to his friend Dr. Hans Krag Sandberg, Kjøllefjord 1936. Owned by the Schrøder family.

CHAPTER 16

Norwegian Doctors in Times of War

ANDERS C. GOGSTAD

16.1 Norway During the Second World War

When the Second World War suddenly came to Norway on April 9th 1940, neither the armed forces, the political authorities, nor the population were prepared for the events that, in the following days, months and years, would deeply affect the daily lives of every Norwegian and cause profound changes in society. The medical profession was no exception.

In spite of the overwhelming strength of the German attackers, the Norwegian Government decided to fight, and the sparsely equipped armed forces kept fighting the Germans for two months, assisted by a limited number of British, French, and Polish troops. In May 1940, the bleak outlook for the allied forces in France made a withdrawal from Norway necessary. The small Norwegian armed forces could not resist the Germans alone, and an armistice was made on June 10th. This day was the beginning of the five years of total German occupation under the Nazi system.

The Norwegian people, who were considered to be "pure Germanic," were generally treated in a milder way than the people in other German-occupied territories, at least during the first years. As the war changed to the disadvantage of the Germans, and as a growing resistance movement came into existence, an ever-increasing number of Norwegians were detained, tortured, executed, or sent to concentration camps. A total of around 40,000 Norwegians spent varying lengths of time in German prisons or camps in Norway or Germany. During the first two years, the pro-German Norwegian nationalist collaboration party, "Nasjonal Samling" (NS), had a proportionally high number of members – 43,000 at its height in 1942. Most of the members were recruited during the years 1940–41, when depression and pessimism were widespread in the population after the defeat of the allied forces.

The NS party, supported by the German administration, tried to influence the population with Nazi propaganda, with the aim of gaining sympathy for its ideas and changing society according to national-socialistic principles.

The Germans had stated that the NS party would only be allowed to take over complete control of the administration if that the party succeeded in gaining widespread support in the population. From the beginning, there was widespread reluctance and resistance within the population to the attempts of the collaboration party to instigate Nazi ideals, and the resistance movement increased strongly during the latter years of the war. Antagonism increased, and severe confrontation became more frequent.

16.2 German Civil Administration and Policy in Norway

As early as April 20th 1940, Adolf Hitler nominated Gauleiter Josef Terboven as Reichskommissar in Norway, directly responsible only to him. Terboven became the real leader and dictator in Norway during the five years of occupation, until he committed suicide on May 8th 1945.

A few months after the German military occupation of Norway, April-May 1940, the German civil occupational administration system, the Reichskommissariat, was established. In September 1940, Reichskommissar Terboven appointed a puppet assembly of cabinet ministers as heads of each of the ministries. Most of them were members of the NS party. The health services also came under the rule of the Kommissariat under the new Minsitry of Internal Affairs. The Reichskommissariat had its own "Abteilung Gesundheitswesen," whose leader, Dr. Fritz Paris, discretely influenced health policy.

The aim of German politics in Norway was a gradual introduction of a national-socialist administration system, based on the ideology and experiences of the German system. According to Adolf Hitler, Nasjonal Samling was to be the instrument. The leader of NS, Vidkun Quisling, was given the executive position.

With the consent of the Reichskommissar, part of the strategy of NS was to gain political control over the professional bodies, such as doctors, lawyers, dentists, teachers, and trade unions. This control was gained by appointing authoritarian leaders, so-called commissarian leaders, for each professional association. These leaders were usually members of NS who were loyal to the "new time." They were approved by the Reichkommissar and were responsible to him.

These measures were met with great resistance from those professional associations which were initially selected for the strategy. In June 1941, 41 associations sent a collective protest to the Reichskommissar. The Norwegian Medical Association was one of the leading associations in the action against the Reichskommissar.

16.3 The Norwegian Medical Association under German Control

The Germans and the NS considered it of special importance to gain control over the medical profession as soon as possible, since the medical profession had great influence and a wide range of contacts.

On June 15th 1941, representatives of the 41 associations were called to "eine Besprechung" with the Reichskommissar in Oslo. The decree about rule of the professional bodies by the Kommissariat was announced here. Some of the leaders present were immediately arrested, among them the Secretary General of the Medical Association, Dr. Jørgen Berner (1883–1964). One of his colleagues, the surgeon Axel Christensen (1879–1943), who had been a member of the NS party since before the war, was appointed as the new leader of the Medical Association. He left the "Besprechung" and marched directly to the offices of the Medical Association and tried to get in contact with the Central Committee. The Committee refused any form of cooperation. Within a short time the Medical Association was paralyzed, and was boycotted by the members during the rest of the war. Most of the members withdrew their membership immediately.

The much curtailed NS-controlled Medical Association attained no political influence during the war, and was finally reduced to a mere subsidary of the Ministry of Internal Affairs.

This NS strategy for gaining public support failed. They did not gain sufficient control of the professional associations, and could therefore not use these to influence and control the population. The Germans therefore had to give up their original political plans, and during the latter years of the war, it was military considerations that mainly determined the occupation policy in Norway.

From time to time the former members of the Medical Association were threatened and told either to re-enter the Association or to pay a license fee in order to practice. In most cases these threats were rejected without any serious consequences, as the German authorities wanted as peaceful a co-existence with the medical profession as possible. It was in their own interest to keep the health services intact and to maintain the health conditions of the population.

In 1942, out of 2,700 doctors, there were only 133 who were registered as members of the NS party. In addition, between two and three hundred had given in to pressure from the authorities and had paid their fees. They were thus considered to be disloyal to the illegal leadership.

16.4 The Illegal Leadership: the "Doctors' Front"

As early as in the autumn of 1941, a number of young physicians organized a specific medical resistance organization, "the doctors' front," under the leadership of Dr. Hans Jacob Ustvedt (1903–1982) and Dr. Ole Jacob Malm (b. 1910). The key persons lived in Oslo, but some of them were allowed to travel around the country with a German permit, on the pretext of a fictitious scientific project (OJM).

A secret network for distribution and secret contacts between reliable patriotic colleagues and other persons was established all over the country. This network was never disclosed at any time during the war.

Thus, most Norwegian medical practitioners had to continue their practice, isolated from any association, and with only occasional secret contact with the usually unknown illegal leaders. The former legal council of the Medical Association did not play any specific role in the illegal organization. Members of the doctors' illegal committee also played a prominent role in the leadership of the coordinated civilian resistance committee, the so called KK, later part of the central management of the "Home front."

A special situation had arisen, because the General Director of the Health Service, Dr. Karl Evang (1902–1981), had gone into exile in London in June 1940, together with the King and the Government. However, the majority of civil servants in public departments in Oslo and in local administration elsewhere in the country stayed at their posts during the rest of the war, in spite of the new political system, as did most of the doctors serving in hospitals and public health services. Only a small number of radical doctors in the central administration were dismissed on political grounds. In general, it was not considered unlawful or disloyal to the legal Government in exile to work in public services during the occupation, according to international war laws. None of these officials were charged with collaboration during the later purging processes, unless they had been members of the NS party or had committed other crimes of treachery.

An important part of the illegal activities of the members was secretly to re-establish the reduced military medical services, which had become disorganized since the war operations in Norway in 1940. The purpose was to serve the civilian population and Norwegian partisans, in case a later allied military invasion of Norway should take place. A comprehensive clandestine organization was built up, based in hospitals, with private and public doctors and nurses. Medical equipment and material was hidden, smuggled from Sweden or stolen from the Germans, and finally stored in secret places in selected hospitals, schools, and other buildings all over the country. With a few exceptions, these stores were never discovered by the Germans during the war.

Fortunately, it never became necessary to use the equipment during the war, but the equipment was very useful after the war for civilian purposes such as in the reconstruction of the hospital services.

Participation in the resistance movement was dangerous, and the risk of being exposed was great. A number of doctors were either arrested or had to flee to Sweden or Great Britain under dangerous circumstances. Many of the doctors who worked near the Swedish border rendered vital assistance to refugees during their long marches through the forests to the border. Many of the doctors who worked in the Western fjord districts gave important assistance to people embarking on the dangerous voyage over the North Sea to Great Britain.

Many doctors ended up in Norwegian or German prisons or concentration camps, where some of them were executed, died from other causes, or became seriously ill.

16.5 The Working Conditions of the Practicing Doctors in Norway During the War

A stream of laws and decrees covering most sections of the health and medical services came every year from the Ministry of Internal Affairs. They were comprised of such things as an order to close the pre-war open clinics for sexual information, a decree on establishing expanded mother and child health centers, hygienic instructions, rules and regulations concerning special food distribution to patients with specific diseases, re-organization of the municipal Boards of Health according to the "leader-principle," and new restrictive acts on tuberculosis prevention. There were issued strict decrees on compulsory vaccination, as well as comprehensive regulations on protection against veneral diseases. A comprehensive new legislation was, however, not passed until after the war. A national mass-radiography service to detect tuberculosis was also established in accordance with pre-war planning that had been done for such a service. New restrictions on the sale and extended control of narcotic drugs were imposed.

It must be admitted that certain parts of this set of regulations were not unfavorable from the point of view of preventive medicine. Thus, some of them continued to be valid after the war – usually after a certain revision of texts or headlines.

The Reichskommissariat did not issue separate decrees for the health services, with one exception: a decree about special care for children with German fathers and their mothers, according to the so-called concept of "Lebensborn."

A decree on posting doctors for medical duty, particularly in remote districts, was passed and remained valid until 1951.

Norwegian doctors who served in German medical institutions were very few. Both the German military and civilian administration in Norway had their own German medical service and staff. When necessary, co-operation between Norwegian and German doctors could take place locally, for example, in order to combat epidemics. It also happened that Norwegian civilians consulted German military doctors in remote districts with limited access to ordinary medical services. Some Germans occasionally also consulted Norwegian specialists.

The revision of the Norwegian Act of 1934 on sterilization of human beings was more serious. The law was in reality suspended during the occupation, and a new "law" that agreed better with Nazi ideology became valid, fortunately not before 1943.

The Norwegian system of pre-paid medical care in accordance with the National Sickness Insurance was not changed by the Germans, probably because its main principles were similar to those already existing in Germany at that time.

As was the case previously, the responsibility for primary health and medical care was carried out by the private practitioners and doctors working as district physicians. In order to protect the health of the working population, an increasing number of doctors were engaged as part-time factory doctors and industrial health officers at many enterprises. This took place with the silent consent of the German authorities, but for totally different reasons: It was in their interest to have a healthy number of workers available so that the Germans could maintain their production schedules.

The daily life of the general practitioner could often be dull and gray, but the relations between doctor and patient were generally not overtly influenced by the war conditions. The clinical practice had to be carried out in the shadow of numerous decrees, rules, and regulations. The doctors had also been deprived of the support and advice from their own association, since in reality it was as good as dissolved. Questions and practical demands were handed over to the NS or the German authorities. In contrast, they also met with the medical authorities of the clandestine resistance movement with their frequently reverse orders.

The lonely doctor thus had to proceed in the face of contrasting ethical demands and do his work in the "battle-field" between the "legal" and "illegal" authorities, both demanding loyalty. They frequently had no choice out of consideration for their patients, even if nearly everyone personally took a strong patriotic stand. It is not erroneous to describe their situation as difficult, stressful, and often frustrating.

Their colleagues in hospitals and other health institutions were in fact in more favorable positions. They worked within a social and loyal professional network and had access to personal advice and social support when critical decisions had to be made.

16.6 The Health Condition of the Norwegian Population During the War

There exist several studies on different aspects of the health status of the Norwegian population during World War II. Here we can summarize only the most important traits: The failure of the food supply led to various symptoms caused by deficient diet, which reduced resistance to infections, particularly in the cities. Hygienic problems increased, access to medical services deteriorated, and resources in terms of hospital beds, economic appropriations, and the number of health personnel were reduced, particularly during the final years. An increasing danger of infections arose from the hundreds of thousands of foreign soldiers and prisoners of war. Serious epidemics broke out, among others of diphtheria, poliomyelitis, streptococcus, and gastrointestinal diseases. The number of serious accidents increased considerably.

The crude death rate of the population had gradually decreased before the war from early 1930s until 1940. During the German occupation, the total death rate increased moderately, but markedly, particularly among males and in the age groups below 45 years. Children too had a high death rate, due to an extremely high occurrence of infectious diseases. Infant mortality, however, declined moderately, especially in the cities, probably due to increased resources in mother and child health care.

In all age groups, mortality was generally dominated by injuries and violent causes of death, in addition to infectious diseases. The concept that cardiovascular diseases became less frequent due to favorable changes in diet and lifestyle is doubtful. The statistical decline in mortality from these diseases actually started before the quality and quantity of the diet was reduced to any extent, and the rise began before the diet and nourishment really improved after the war. Furthermore, the routines for reporting death, and the nomenclature was changed already in 1941, making comparisons between the pre-war and war period difficult. Thus, the figures may be misleading. In addition, the high frequency of violent and unknown causes of death may mask the possible effects of chronic and lethal diseases.

After the occupation, the health status improved very quickly, evidently due to rapid access to medical resources, organized by the Norwegian public authorities in exile and also because of considerable support from American relief organizations.

16.7 Norwegian Doctors as Refugees in Sweden

More than one hundred Norwegian doctors and around two hundred medical students were compelled to flee to Sweden during the years 1941–45. A small number made their way to Great Britain to enroll in the Norwegian or other allied forces.

The number of Norwegian refugees in Sweden gradually increased to over 45,000. The majority were young men who were eligible for military service. It was considered necessary to register these persons with the aim of giving them basic military training, in case the political situation in Sweden should allow implementation of full military training. As the war developed to the disadvantage of the Germans, the Swedish government gradually liberalized its neutrality policy and permitted the training of Norwegian troops under the camouflage of being police-forces. Around 12,000 men joined the "police" forces in Sweden.

A leading Norwegian surgeon, Dr. Carl Semb (1871–1971) from Ullevål Hospital in Oslo, played an important role in planning and implementing the registration and military training of Norwegians in Sweden during the war. He was promoted to colonel, and in May 1945, he was appointed as chief of the combined Military Medical Services for all the Norwegian military forces (Forsvarets Sanitet).

At the Norwegian Legation in Stockholm, the Director General of the Health Services had established a Norwegian Public Health Service section. This was a branch of the London office, placed directly under the Director General of the Health Services and the Norwegian Government in exile. From 1943, the chief of the Stockholm Section was Dr. Hans Jacob Ustvedt, the former leader of the illegal "doctors' front" in Norway. During the following years, the section acted as the clandestine contact chain between the doctors' resistance movement in Norway and the health authorities in exile in London.

The majority of Norwegian doctors and medical students who fled to Sweden after 1943 were mobilized as "police" troops, most of them in the forces' Medical Corps, after proper military and supplementary medical training courses. Some of them worked in the Swedish Health Services.

Some of the police troops were transferred to Finnmark after it was liberated by the Red Army in the winter of 1944–45, and the rest of the troops were transferred to Norway immediately after the armistice to assist the allied troops in demobilizing the German forces in the country.

16.8 Norwegian Doctors in the United Kingdom

In London, Dr. Karl Evang immediately started to reconstruct the civil health administration as a section of the exiled Norwegian Ministry of Social Affairs. A group of Dr. Evang's earlier medical colleagues in Oslo were secretly called to London, some of them having to be transported across the North Sea under very risky conditions. Together with other medically qualified refugees in the UK – doctors, nurses, and medical students – the civilian and military health authorities had enough qualified medical staff at their disposal for manning both military health services and civil public health services, at least during the first few years. The Norwegian military services in the UK consisted of an Army group of about 3,000 men, a Navy group of about 7,000 men, and an Air Force group, partly based in Canada and Iceland, of altogether about 2,000 men. The Norwegian merchant navy was also very important for allied warfare. About 30,000 Norwegians sailed on fixed convoy routes over all the oceans and they were considered to be an invaluable aid to allied transport needs. More than 3,000 men lost their lives.

The merchant sailors were not considered to be military service men, so they could not benefit from the medical services of the Navy. Thus the Government had to establish a "Norwegian Public Health Service" for civilian Norwegians in the UK and overseas, mainly for the civilian sailors. They had considerable health problems. Diseases such as tuberculosis, venereal diseases, mental problems and general medical conditions needed to be cured rapidly and effectively in order to keep the crews able to sail. Thus a network of Norwegian hospitals and convalescent homes were founded in the UK, the United States, and Canada.

The large number of civilian medical institutions in the UK, in addition to the military medical services in the UK, Canada, and Iceland, required more and more qualified medical staff. Inevitably, as time went on, there existed an increasing shortage of qualified medical officers and specialists in all fields. In the UK, Norwegian medical students in exile solved many problems, and they were able to satisfy many urgent needs after taking short special courses.

As early as the summer of 1940, Dr. Evang started a campaign in the United States for relief to Norway. He had great success, and he spent long periods there. Much of the medical equipment, food, and medicines from his fund-raising campaigns was of great use to the Norwegian health services in the reconstruction period immediately after the war. Dr. Evang and other Norwegians made contact with a number of influential American colleagues and established many close personal contacts. This made it possible for young Norwegian doctors to gain access to several American postgraduate schools after the war, where they could obtain additional professional qualifications.

16.9 The Purging process and the End of the War

The process of purging Norway of collaborators after the war was given high priority by the Norwegian Health authorities in London. As early as 1943, the Director General of the Health Services decided to appoint an investigation committee to carry out this process. In the spring of 1944, the management of the doctors' illegal organization in Oslo was asked by the Director General of the Health Services to nominate its own local investigation committees in Norway. However, it was emphasized that these professional investigation committees should not substitute for the legal prosecuting committee, only supplement it. No one should be sentenced for treachery unless he had been given the opportunity to defend himself and account for extenuating circumstances. The professional committees in London and Oslo coordinated their work in the months after liberation.

Approximately 7,000 Norwegians had served as volunteers in the Waffen SS at the Eastern Front, and of these approximately 5,000 saw active duty. About 20 doctors and medical students took part in the military medical services on the German side. Five lost their lives, the rest were put on trial after the war, accused of treachery, and sentenced to many years of inprisonment.

Public sentences for the NS doctors were generally no harder than those for other categories of NS members. Those who were imprisoned were usually released after they had served half their sentence and they were immediately allowed to resume their work. The Medical Association, however, continued its own internal evaluation process of members who had a questionable past. The process concentrated on those members who were not put on trial, but had either paid their fees to the NS top management or else had paid license duty to the Ministry. In addition to the 133 NS members who were given a public trial, another 37 members were excluded from the Medical Association, 20 members were reprimanded, and 152 were acquitted. At that time, being excluded from the Medical Association had some serious consequences. No longer did the physicians have the right to practice for the National Sickness Assurance and to qualify for a medical specialty, and in addition he was subject to the general personal stigmatization. However, the wounds seemed to heal rapidly. In the course of 8 to 10 years, nearly all sentenced and excluded members were accepted as ordinary members again.

During the war, contact between the clandestine medical organization in Norway and the legal health authorities in London was continually maintained through the Stockholm legation, partly by the aid of couriers and refugee reports, partly by radio-link messages and cipher-code letters. Under such circumstances, it was unavoidable that misinterpretation of directives and instructions and other misunderstandings arose. But, as soon as peaceful conditions were reestablished, all misunderstandings were cleared up, and the legal management of the Norwegian Medical Association was reinstated.

As soon as the war ended, in agreement and in cooperation with the political health and social authorities, the members of the Medical Association started enthusiastically to re-construct the health services of the country and to restore the health of the people, which had suffered considerably during the war.

Altogether, 22 doctors and 29 medical students lost their lives on the allied side in the battles, concentration camps, or prisons, or as a result of military accidents or by execution.

References

Andresen, R. *Fra norsk sanitets historie*. Oslo: NKS forlaget, 1986.

Blindheim, S. *Nordmenn under Hitlers fane*. Oslo: Noregs boklag, 1977.

Dahl, H.F. *Vidkun Quisling – En fører for fall. Vol II*. Oslo: Aschehoug, 1992.

Dedichen, H.G. "Norsk helsetjeneste i Storbritannia under krigen 1940–45," in *Nordisk medicinhistorisk årbok,* København:1945, 189–198.

Ekman, S. and Grimnes, O.K. *Broderfolk i ufredstid*. Oslo: Universitetsforlaget, 1991.

Fabritius, H.F. "Sanitetsarbeidet i Sverige under krigen," *Nordisk Medicin*, 37(1948): 545.

Farnes, O. *Lege på mange fronter*. Oslo: Dreyer, 1982.

Florelius, S. "Sanitetsoppsetningene ved de norske 'polititroppenes' feltavdelinger i

Sverige," *Sanitetsnytt*, 11(1965).

Gogstad, A.C. *Helse og Hakekors*. Bergen: Alma Mater forlag, 1991.

Gogstad, A.C. *Slange og Sverd*. Bergen: Alma Mater forlag, 1995.

Grimnes, O.K. *Et flyktningesamfunn vokser frem*. Oslo: Aschehoug, 1969.

Grimnes, O.K. *Hjemmefrontens ledelse*. Oslo: Universitetsforlaget, 1977.

Howarth, D. *The Shetland Bus (new edition)*. Glasgow: The Grafton Books, 1991.

Høidal, O. *Quisling – a study in treason*. Oslo: Universitetsforlaget, 1988.

Kjelstadli, S. *Hjemmestyrkene Bd.I. Hovedtrekk av den militære motstanden under okkupasjonen*. Oslo: Aschehoug, 1959.

Klaveness, S.T. *Oslo kommunale sykehus i krigens tegn*. Oslo: Cammermeyer, 1947.

Kreyberg, L. *Etter ordre eller uten*. Oslo: Gyldendal, 1976.

Kreyberg, L. *Kast ikke kortene*. Oslo: Gyldendal, 1978.

Kvittingen, J. "Norsk helsetjeneste i London mai 1940 til mai 1941," *Norsk Bedriftshelsetjeneste*, (b. 1984) 62-78.

Kvittingen, J. "Fra den kongelege norske marines sanitetsteneste i Storbritannia under krigen. 1940–1945," *Tidsskrift for Den norske lægeforening*, 107 (1987): 1688–89.

Loock, H.D. *Quisling, Rosenberg und Terboven. Zor Vorgeschichte und Geschichte der nationalsozialistischen Revolution in Norwegen*. Stuttgart: Deutsche Verlags Anstalt, 1970.

Lønnum, A. *Helsesvikt – en senfølge av krig og katastrofe*. Oslo: Gyldendal, 1969.

Malm, O.J. "Polititroppene og sanitet i Sverige," in *Forsvarets sanitet: 50 år under felles ledelse 1941–1991*, ed. O.J. Malm. Oslo: Forsvarets Overkommando, (1991):29–33.

Nordby, T. *Karl Evang. En biografi*. Oslo: Aschehoug, 1989.

Rasmussen, S. *Barmhjertighetsfronten. Norges Røde Kors 1940–45*. Oslo: Halvorsen og Larsen forl., 1950.

Riste, O. *Londonregjeringa Vol II*. Oslo: Det norske samlaget, 1979.

Semb, C. "Den militære sanitets organisasjon," *Sanitetsnytt*, 11 (1965):3–25.

Skre, R.K. *Bjørn West i aktiv innsats*. Oslo: Gyldendal, 1946.

Strøm, A. "Lægeforeningen under okkupasjonen," *Tidsskrift for Den norske lægeforening*, 81(1961): 674–7.

Thiis-Evensen, E. *Sånn var livet*. Skien: Arne Kunstforlag, 1992.

Tranøy, K.E., and Sars, M. *Tysklandsstudentene*. Oslo: Cappelen, 1946.

Wyller, T. *Nyordning og motstand*. Oslo: Universitetsforlaget, 1958.

Øyen, O. *Milorg D13 i kamp*. Oslo: Norsk kunstforlag, 1961.

CHAPTER 17

Post-war Health and Post-war Medicine: Some Personal Impressions on Prospects and Realities from the 1940s into the 1960s

ØIVIND LARSEN

17.1. Health, Disease, and the Image of the Doctor

Dear readers,

Following a series of chapters pretending to cope with standards of objectivity and historical balance, some personal accounts could be appropriate. The personal perception of health, disease, and of the health services, as experienced by ordinary Norwegians, might be useful as an illustration of the historical facts. However, systematic information of this type is rather scarce when one looks over the shoulder, back into decades that have faded into the past.

When looking for sources, I found that my own experiences were nearest at hand. I suppose that readers of my generation, at least partly, will be able to tune into my reflections.

I was born in the capital of Oslo in 1938. Because of the demographic pattern described in another chapter, almost all children in Oslo of my age had relatives, and especially grandparents, in the countryside. And so had I. When the 1940–45 war was going on, I was sent on long visits to my grandparents' farm in a rural district south of Oslo. I suppose that my parents considered the situation to be better and safer there.

When the war ended, it was still some time before the living conditions could be regarded as normalized, especially in the city, so vacations were still spent on the farm. My basic impressions of health, medicine, and doctors took form during these years.

When I look back on what I observed as a boy in the post-war years, with my present medical and historical eyes, it strikes me among other things that there must have been quite a lot of disease around. People lived with their diseases and were afraid of them, but in a strange way they accepted them.

Among the elderly people who were our relatives and neighbors, chronic disease of some sort had an appalling prevalence. I have no statistics at hand; probably nobody has, because many of these complaints never became cases for the health services, at least not to the same extent as in later periods. Of these ailments, arthritis and other diseases of bones and joints, for which no real treatment could be offered, threw shadows over daily life for somebody in most of the houses I knew of.

Tuberculosis had hit hard when the grown-ups of the time were young. Histories of earlier pleurisy were heard of, and there were always lurking fears that the slumbering disease would reappear. But tuberculosis was also a matter that affected the children. From my Oslo days, it must have been in my first year at school in 1944, I recall the rather intensive screening activity and the class being summoned for tuberculin tests. And some of the pupils, probably those who had a positive family history, had to appear before the lung specialist of the Health Board for further examinations.

Hygiene also was a matter that the school had to deal with. Snappish and militant school nurses checked our heads for lice, and meticulously recorded our height and body weight.

Contemporary principles of nutrition were implemented in the schools of Oslo. Cod liver oil was served with or without a spoon, whether you could stand it or not. The school meal supplied basic calories and vitamins, and contributed to the maintenance of brown cheese as part of Norwegian culture.

However, what I primarily remember of medical matters from those remote years were the infections, and not least the fear of such diseases. The grown-up generation still had fresh memories of the ravages of the Spanish flu at the end of World War I. A late complication which hit some of the survivors was the so-called lethargic encephalitis, where scaring Parkinsonistic symptoms could be the dominating trait.

The outcome of infection treatment was still dubious, or at least regarded so by nervous relatives, and I remember the anxiousness in the house when my younger cousin got pneumonia. But anxiety was indeed appropriate: One of my playmates died from what must have been meningitis, at the age of eleven.

Thoughts were swarming in the heads of children when death and disease came up. However, it was not always so easy to know when to be afraid, and when not, because some sorts of disease were perceived as quite normal. As far as I can recall, vomiting and diarrhea were simply part of life during summer.

Of course, I now know the reason for the gastrointestinal problems. The reason was probably also well known in the 1940s. But it made little difference, one kept to the traditional lifestyle. The culprit obviously must have been our well, where the water buckets for the household were filled up, as we had no tap in the house. To this very day I can recall on my tongue the spicy taste of our drinking water. The taste was probably not from esoteric and health-promoting minerals. It was the taste of heavy pollution.

The drinking water hygiene was especially endangered when the ever-recurring drought made the wells almost dry. And these problems were quite widespread. When I worked as an assistant to a district physician in another part of the country in the early 1960s, inspection and hygienic approval of drinking water wells were frequent tasks.

In Oslo, milk was pasteurized, but in the countryside fresh milk still could be bought from open pails in the grocery stores, or directly from the cowshed. We had a refrigerator, but that was uncommon; the neighbors had to make do with the coolness of the cellar, or by hanging the bucket on a rope in the well.

But I do not think that anyone in that particular district, or in other rural districts, regarded the lack of water pipes and showers, or the privies used even in more densely populated areas, as a nuisance or especially detrimental to the standards of life.

Although hygiene and sanitary thinking had been prime issues in medicine between the wars, the general implementation of it had to be completed after the war in large parts of the country. The silent hygienic revolution in the first decades after the war should not be forgotten.

Stomach problems prevailed in the neighborhood of my grandparents' farm. The most feared of all diseases, at least among the children, was poliomyelitis. Around 1950, cases were heard of nearly every day. And most of the patients were children and youngsters of our own age. There is a novel, written by the Norwegian author Gerd Brantenberg (1941–), called Sangen om St. Croix (The Song about St. Croix, a primary school in the city of Fredrikstad). The novelist has quite precisely caught the anxiety and the doomsday feeling that arose when rumors spread about there being poliomyelitis in nearby dwellings.

There is a phenomenon that has struck me in recent years. When I look back now on newspapers from those earlier years, the recurring cases of poliomyelitis or other epidemic diseases were only mentioned quite briefly, if at all. In the 1990s, only a suspected case of a possible epidemic covers front pages of newspapers. Of course press practices have changed, but perhaps there has been a change in attitudes toward disease too.

The initial symptoms and signs of poliomyelitis are those of a gastrointestinal disease. That very fact produced some difficult dilemmas: When was the ailment one of the usual infections or of food poisonings, and when was it the initial phase of a poliomyelitis? When should the doctor be called?

One time, when it was my turn to be in bed, sick and shivering from fear, the doctor was called. The nearby township had two private general practitioners. Both of them were highly respected and admired. They were overworked, but in spite of that they were said to make housecalls anytime. Some people were most in favor of one of them, but others gave their vote to his colleague. Let me call him the one who came to see me Dr. X. I remember how he examined my belly, and then reassured me and my grandparents that this was nothing to bother about and that in few days I would be running around again, which was what I actually did.

The paternalistic utterings of the beloved doctor were just what the situation required. Again, when reconsidering what happened from my medical background, I am quite sure that his diagnosis was based only on probability: aching stomachs from other reasons were by far more common than poliomyelitis. And in addition, if it had been poliomyelitis, it would not have been terribly dangerous because the non-paralytic cases were the most common.

I feel that the image of the doctor as I experienced it as a boy in this coastal district of rural Norway was a rather general one. Knowledge, skills, helpfulness, and authority were virtues assigned to the doctor, and in return he or she gained a central place in the local community. I must admit that a vague image of this kind was of some importance when I later chose to enter medicine myself.

However, I cannot remember that the local hospitals and other health institutions in the district had a comparable reputation. Hospital beds were few and they were, as a rule, only considered when an operation was necessary, in cases of epidemic disease requiring isolation, or in other complicated cases. To be sick at home, and to be nursed at home when old and frail, were still the traditional ways of thinking.

Back in Oslo, there was no single and outstanding, well- known and well-informed doctor who knew us all as the doctor in the country did. Some called for one general practitioner, others for another. When my right arm broke because of violent play in the school-yard, hours of waiting and subsequent and similar controls at the hundred-years-old municipality emergency station were required to restore it.

But the city of Oslo had large hospitals:

Ullevål Hospital, the National Hospital, and some others, and just outside the old city borders, the Aker Hospital. Hospitals still had high fences, gates, and guardsmen watching them. For us who had no other ties to hospitals than as patients or relatives to patients, the hospital world was a strange world, an alien world with frightening overtones. I think that the old fear of the general hospital as a place that gave one a dubious chance of returning home, or the image of asylums and sanatoriums as dreadful places was still a reality among many people even as late as the post-war years.

Things changed rather rapidly. When I started to consider to study medicine in the mid 1950s, signs of modernization of the health care system were apparent to everybody. In the town near my grandparents' farm, a brand new hospital of an unheard of size was opened in 1955; and something similar happened at almost the same time in other places, even in nearby neighboring towns. And a new health insurance scheme was a main political issue.

Was there a philosophy behind all this? What was the longterm policy that was meant to change the situation in the entire country?

17.2. The Evang Impact

When I later, as a young doctor, started to work in the office of a district physician, I found a grey cabinet with large drawers in the corner. The never-ending stream of circulars from the central health authorities were filed here, and old circular letters were replaced by new ones. Thus the grey cabinet contained an updated set of papers telling what to do in matters of public health. The cabinet was the implement for executing a health policy. But what was this policy like?

The so-called Heath Clark Lectures at the University of London for the year 1958 were given by a Norwegian physician, the Norwegian Director General of the Health Services, Dr. Karl Evang (1902-1981).

The series of lectures was delivered at The London School of Hygiene and Tropical Medicine and covered five topics: the main types of existing health services, the role of the hospital, the role of the general practitioner, the role of drugs, and the public health service. If time had permitted, Evang noted, he would have covered three additional subjects too: medical education in relation to health services, types of medical and auxiliary personnel, and specific health service problems in technically underdeveloped countries (Evang 1960).

Fifteen years later, in 1973, after having retired from his position as Director General of the Health Services at the age of 70 in 1972, Evang gave lectures at the medical school of the new University of Tromsø in northern Norway. The next year, in 1974, a book was published, based on these lectures. The title was Helse og samfunn – sosialmedisinsk almenkunnskap. Health and Society – general knowledge on social medicine (Evang 1974). Here, his thoughts were updated and further developed.

In 1957, a book in English entitled Health Services in Norway appeared, and the fourth edition of it was published in 1976. Later on, other authors reviewed the situation, (Strøm 1980) (Siem 1986), but I cannot remember that the overall picture was that clear, at least for me and others outside the political and public health circles, when the process of transformation was at its height in the post-war period.

Why mention this in connection with the development of the medical profession? Karl Evang was Director General of the Health Services for 34 years, being appointed in 1938 to assume office by January 1, 1939. His biographer, the historian Trond Nordby, vividly portrays his strong personality (Nordby 1989). Political commitment and professional work went hand in hand.

Throughout his entire period of duty, Evang maintained a clear policy for the development of a nationwide, uniform, and centripetally orientated health system, managed by medical professionals, and based on a wide definition of health and medical responsibility.

Social and psychological conditions were regarded as of prime importance, and in his thinking the philosophy of the German sociohygienists of the twenties was replaced by the corresponding extended notion of health which was settled in the health definition of the World Health Organization in the forties.

The coverage by the health services should be universal, and to maintain the health of the population should be a public responsibility.

The objectives were to be reached through central planning, in which the quality of the services was the factor of importance. The writings by Evang through the years are crucial for the historical assessment and understanding of the development of the medical profession during his years of strong and paternalistic rule. They give a documentation of a consistent philosophy behind the long-term planning, and behind the day-to-day decisions as well.

Politically, Evang was controversial. In the pre-war years he belonged to the influential intellectual leftist movement Mot Dag (Towards Dawn). Social and economic problems in the 1930s made the importance of a social approach in health matters obvious. It goes without saying that this general attitude sparked political resistance when he was appointed Director General of the Health Services by the labour government, but he also attracted enemies through his overt and pragmatic policy on taboo matters, such as contraception and sexual life counselling.

Evang was controversial among many of the members of the medical profession, mostly because of his strong belief in central planning and steering. However, his respect for medical knowledge and proficiency as the one and sole basis for health planning and management turned out, paradoxically, to be a most important line of defense against the agressors among lawyers, economists, and politicians for the same medical profession throughout the entire Evang period.

Evang's high position as a civil servant and the rather independent placement of the post of Director General of Health Services in the political system, allowed him to put his ideas into practice. When World War II broke out and the German occupation changed life in Norway for five years, his efforts to build up a health system in Norway in one way was hampered, but in other ways was enhanced.

Evang himself spent the years of war in exile in Great Britain and in the United States. In these countries he acquired extensive professional contacts on all levels and became one of the founders of the World Health Organization (WHO). At the end of the war, Evang had to make a choice between the international arena and Norway. He decided to return, but nevertheless he continued to work with the WHO during the rest of his professional career, and thus remained a central person in international health care work.

Back in Norway, the implementation of his plans for the health services was dependent on the general central planning policy maintained by the Norwegian labour party, which held the leadership in the years of restitution after the war. Evang's idea for the health services was a system lying somewhere in the middle between the American and the Soviet systems. He wanted to combine the high quality and efficiency he had observed in the United States with the universalism, the public responsibility, and the central planning he admired in the Soviet model. And the possibilities of implementation required that he was in the position to do so.

For the members of the medical profession, the Evang health policy had important bearings. On one hand, his deep concern for the district physician system as the local hub of a state-run health system made these jobs attractive, both in terms of personal economy and of public and professional esteem. There also was a career ladder available in this field: For a district physician, a junior job in the directorate could lead to being selected for study abroad on a grant to attend a School of Public Health, in order to acquire a degree as a Master of Public Health. Then the road might be open to a position as a county medical officer, an important, high-ranking link in the Evang health administration chain.

On the other hand, Evang promoted the erection of hospitals, and the specialized, central hospital was his favorite. The growing hospitals in the 1950s and 1960s required qualified staff. Hospital work became an attractive field for new doctors and recruited young M.D.s as never before.

Just like earlier brands of health policies from the times of Frank in the eighteenth century onwards, Evang's was also totally dependent on, and intermingled with its context. When the surroundings changed, health policy was at stake. The acceptance in society of central planning, and the acceptance of a certain professional paternalism, legitimated through a medical education, was a prerequisite. The same was true for the feeling of an obligation toward the health and well-being of population groups, not only of the individual person – and an accepted notion of health as a superior value. A national economy which allowed for an expansion of health expenditures, and politicians who were willing to accept them without too many objections, constituted additional necessary elements.

When the Evang period approached its end, these prerequisites started to fail. His own political position in the leadership weakened. Although still a member of the labour party, in his consistent political views on important matters for example on the Norwegian relationship to the North Atlantic defense system (NATO), on the plans for a European Union Evang all the time positioned himself on the left wing. This position became more and more visible as the labour party over the years gradually turned more toward right in its general attitudes.

At the end of the 1960s, general antiautoritarian waves also rolled over the health system. Both the paternalistic role of the physician and the strong leadership position of a Director General of Health were challenged. Despite the new prospects of future oil incomes, the national economy did not allow for an unquestioned expansion in health costs anymore. And the population no longer accepted the claim that excellent health was the only road to happiness. A trends toward the glorification of individualism, which was gradually replacing the former era of solidarity, seemed to have started.

If we assume that the training given at the universities heavily influences the shaping of the professional self-image, a glance at what happened at the Faculty in Oslo might be illustrative. In the 1930s hygiene and bacteriology were growing disciplines. The social hygienic activity of Carl Schiøtz was continued by his successor Axel Strøm (1901-1985), who took over the chair in hygiene in 1940. The professor in bacteriology, Theodor Thjøtta (1885-1955), had a reputation as a brilliant and enthusiastic head of his institute. Voluminous textbooks were published, that were read not only by medical students, but also served as handbooks for the general public.

The journal founded by Schiøtz in 1934,

Liv og Helse, was published because there was a strong belief in health education. Also, outside the University, sociomedical research was performed, for example, by Karl Evang.

In 1952, Haakon Natvig (1905-) was appointed professor in hygiene; social medicine was given the status of a separate institute under the leadership of the previous professor of hygiene, Axel Strøm. The academic disciplines of hygiene and social medicine gave the medical students a background for their future work, not only in general practice, but especially in the role as a district physician with all the comprehensive responsibility that adhered to that role in the Evang period.

To a district physician, having a broad overview of medicine was a virtue in itself, even in a period when the complexity of the science involved made firsthand knowledge of everything involved impossible to attain. To the doctor in the field, voluminous handbooks were still available, the textbook on hygiene by Natvig, published in 1958, being the best example. And the institute of hygiene at the University of Oslo was involved in a research and teaching activity that covered many different aspects of individual and environmental health factors: clothing, garbage collection, air pollution, and food-borne epidemics are only a few of the examples.

But something happened.

The broad-scale approach was overtaken by the general tendency of reductionism, the need for specialization, and the tendency to split up the disciplines. This reflected the situation elsewhere in the society. Community health in the municipalities was increasingly complicated and called for personnel with a more specialized background: engineers, veterinarians, administrators. Even if the district physician and the later municipality physicians carried a public responsibility, fields of medicine that previously had been near the center of interest for many physicians slid out to the periphery. For example at the University of Oslo, which had the largest national faculty, the approach toward medical teaching followed suit. Especially after the resignation by Natvig in 1975, the institute concentrated on certain parts of the former pallette of activities. Epidemiology, a field with obvious potential, became a core topic. Previous fields of interest were gradually taken over by others, partly by institutions outside the University for example regarding air pollution, food hygiene, nutrition, and occupational health. Of course this change has to be assessed in light of the development within the sciences involved. The growing complexity of each science precluded the possibility of maintaining top competence on a broad scale; concentration was a necessary strategy. What was lost, however was the overview and sense of comprehensiveness that had been taught to the students by the old hygienists as a preparation for work as a district physician.

A similar process also affected social medicine, as social politics was a growing field that also existed outside medicine. Social medicine became more and more focused on the problems of the weaker groups, and the handling of the complicated sick insurance system.

The exclusion of topics clearly related to the community-orientated physician, and the shift away from the general, social points of view, probably added to the weaker standing of the physicians in this matter and weakened this aspect of their professional role in the years to come.

The general belief in health education and prevention admittedly was hailed at festive occasions and at other times, but the discontinuation in 1972 of the journal Liv og Helse for reasons of interest and economy is a documentation of the prevailing realities. The climate for medicine had altered.

But new physicians entering the corps of district physicians as a rule attended a special course offered by the health authorities from 1948 onwards, brushing up their knowledge in public health and stimulating their enthusiasm. Karl Evang participated as a brilliant teacher and a persuasive orator. But still, clouds were gathering as the 1970s approached.

When Karl Evang resigned, a period was over, not only for him, but also in the history of the medical profession.

17.3. Doctors, Population, and Patients

The elderly lady seated herself in the chair beside my desk in the district physician's surgery.

Nothing happened. She was silent, and she remained silent. After a while I carefully tried to find out in what way she expected me to help her:

"What is the matter with you?"

Her hands were tightly folded around her purse on her lap. Her reluctant answer, uttered with submissiveness and respect, impressed me:

"I thought that the doctor was the one who was supposed to find out what was wrong with me."

The author of these lines served as an assistant to the district physician in Hemne, a coastal region of Trøndelag in 1963. The encounter described was with one of my very first patients, and it illustrated what proved to be some quite typical traits of the general practice there at that time: An astonishing esteem and confidence in the doctor, paired with a sort of culture collision. Disease was something private, you were not supposed to talk too much about it.

Another experience, some time later: It was a Sunday morning, the telephone was quiet, and my notebook for the day was still empty. A couple of days before I had made a home visit to an asthmatic child in a remote fjord. I instituted some treatment, but I did not feel comfortable with the situation, so I rang the farm and inquired about the condition of the child. To a stranger in the community, the information I received probably would have sounded rather reassuring. But by now I had attained a certain grip of the local way of talking and use of understatement. I drove some one hundred kilometers to the place where the fjord ended, and was picked up at the shore by the boat of the farmer. Upon arriving at the house shortly afterward, I found the child half-suffocated, bluish in the face, gasping for air, in a state far beyond the therapeutic possibilities available on the spot. Needless to say that my immediate transportation of the child and its parents to the nearest hospital took place at the highest speed my VW beetle could perform on curved dirt roads. The child survived. But I learned something again: Defeatism and a possible element of neglect in matters of health still had not yielded, and had to be taken into account.

A general practice in the countryside at this time could be very rewarding. To a rural population like my clientele in 1963, the doctor had something to offer, which was relatively new. He had possibilities which he did not have shortly earlier. Dangerous diseases like pneumonia or tuberculosis were not so threatening anymore, due to the syringes and the tablets of the physician. Less than twenty years before, no antibiotics were available. Arthritis, back ache and muscular pain, hitherto regarded as part of their destiny by a population engaged in hard, manual work on their farms and on board their fishing vessels, could now be relieved by means of new drugs. New tablets could also be prescribed for the nervous mind, and hormones could correct menopausal distress. However, although already heard of, oral contraceptives that

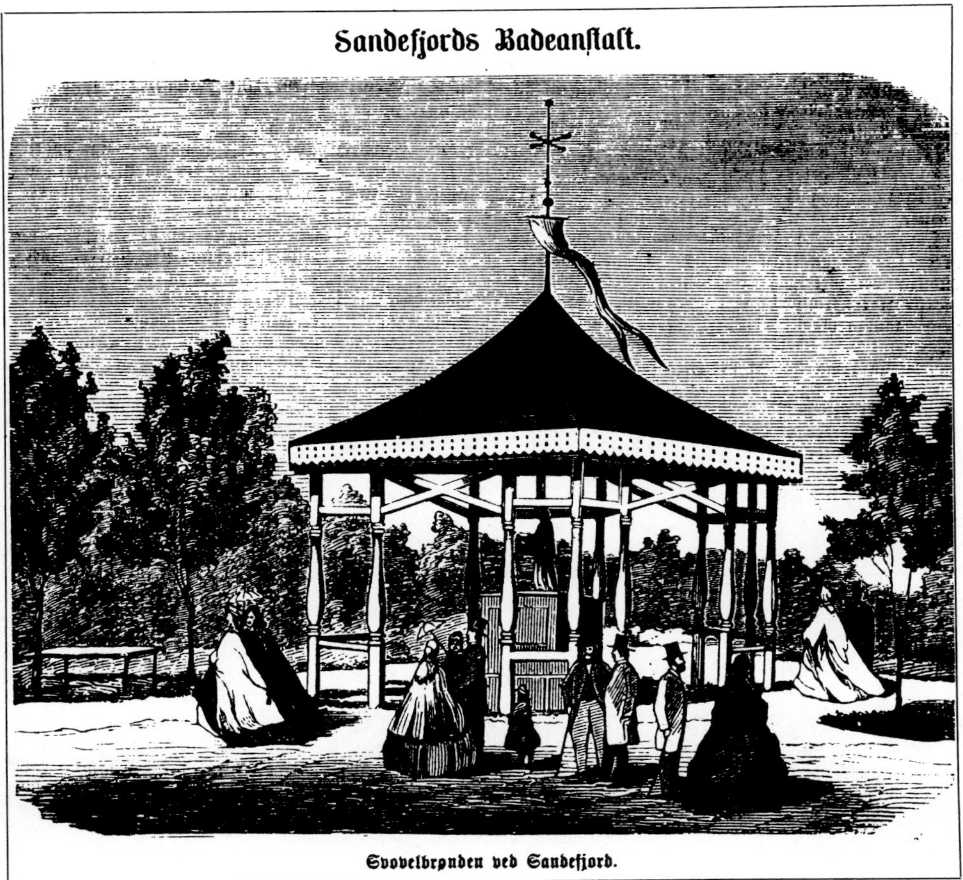

Figure 53: Balneology never became a major medical field of work in Norway. One of the enterprises was the Sandefjord spa, and this picture from the Skilling-Magazin of June 16, 1866 shows the sulphur well and the pump.

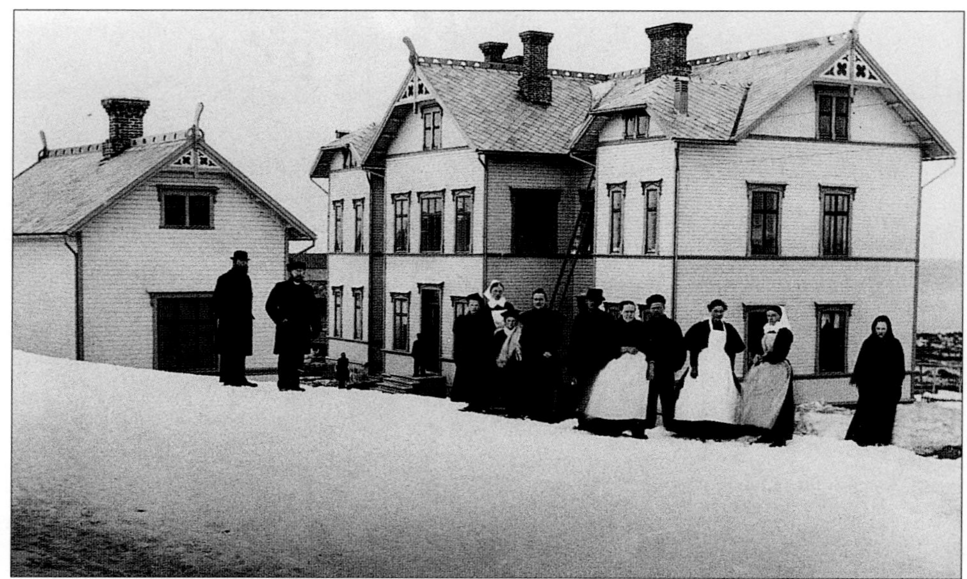

Figure 54: The hospital in Vadsø in the county of Finnmark at the turn of the century (Photo: Ellisif Wessel).

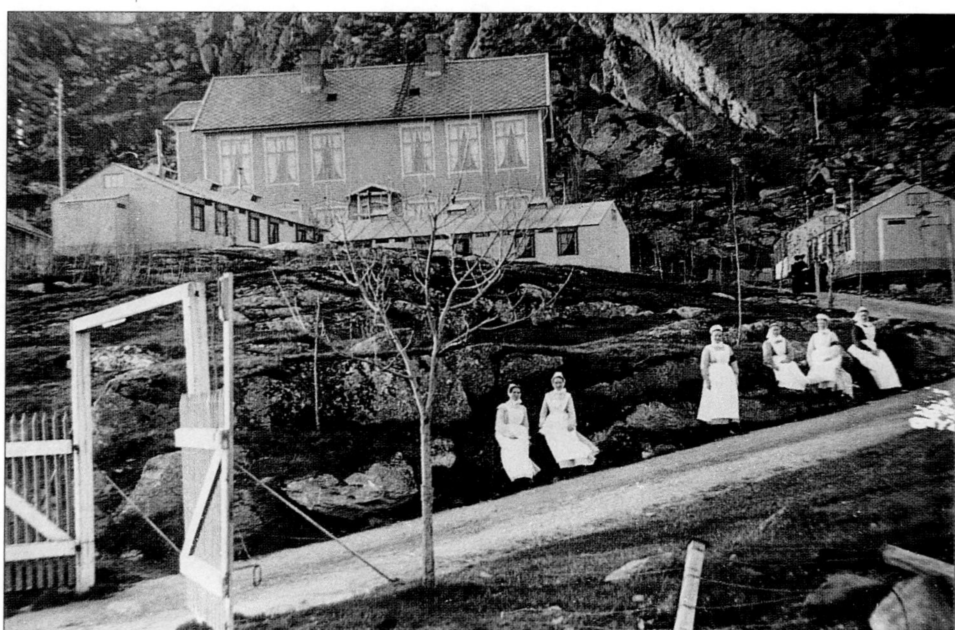

Figure 55: After the great city fire in Ålesund on the Western coast of Norway on January 23, 1904, substantial aid was provided by Germany, whose Emperor Wilhelm (1859-1941, Kaiser 1888-1918) was a true friend of the Norwegian fiords. The low buildings in front of the hospital are the so-called German barracks (Courtesy Aalesunds museum).

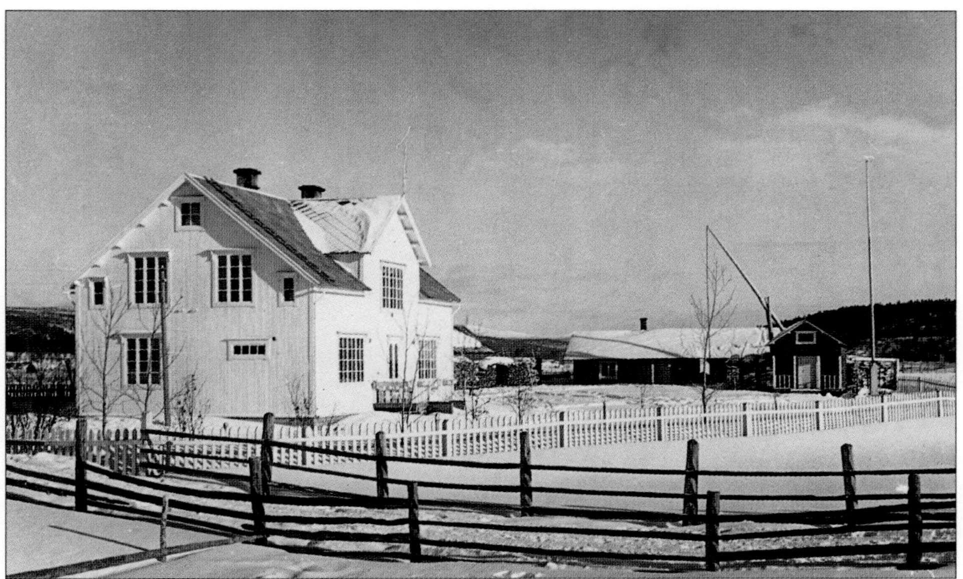

Figure 56: Dr. Tryggve Hauan (1909-) still has vivid memories of how terribly cold it could be in this pre-war house for the district physician in Karasjok in Finnmark (Schrøder photo-album, courtesy Aina Schiøtz).

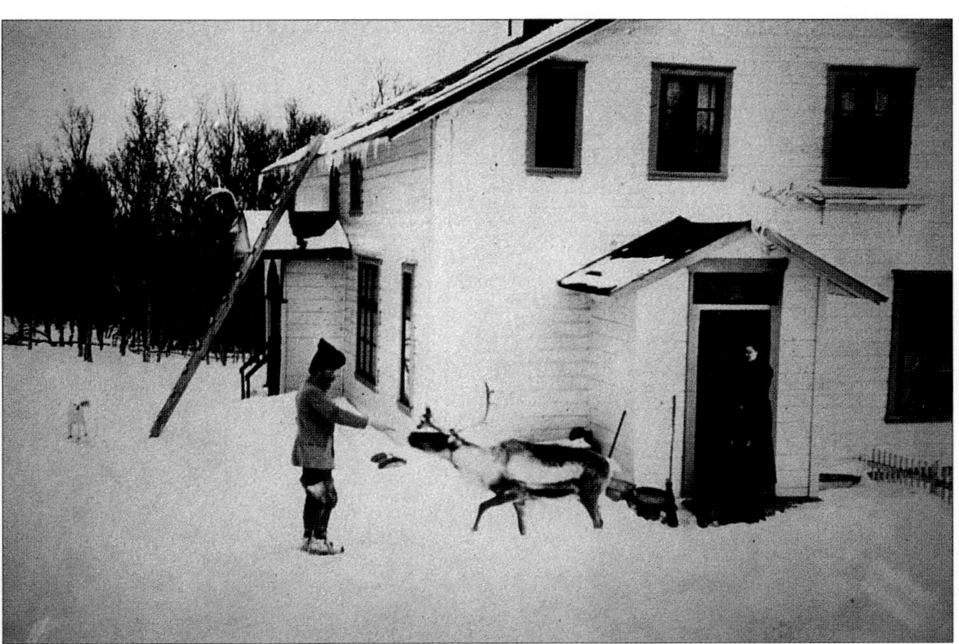

Figure 57: Outside the physician's home in the Finnmark municipality of Sør-Varanger at the turn of the century. Dr. Andreas Bredal Wessel (1858-1940) and his reindeer (Photo: Ellisif Wessel).

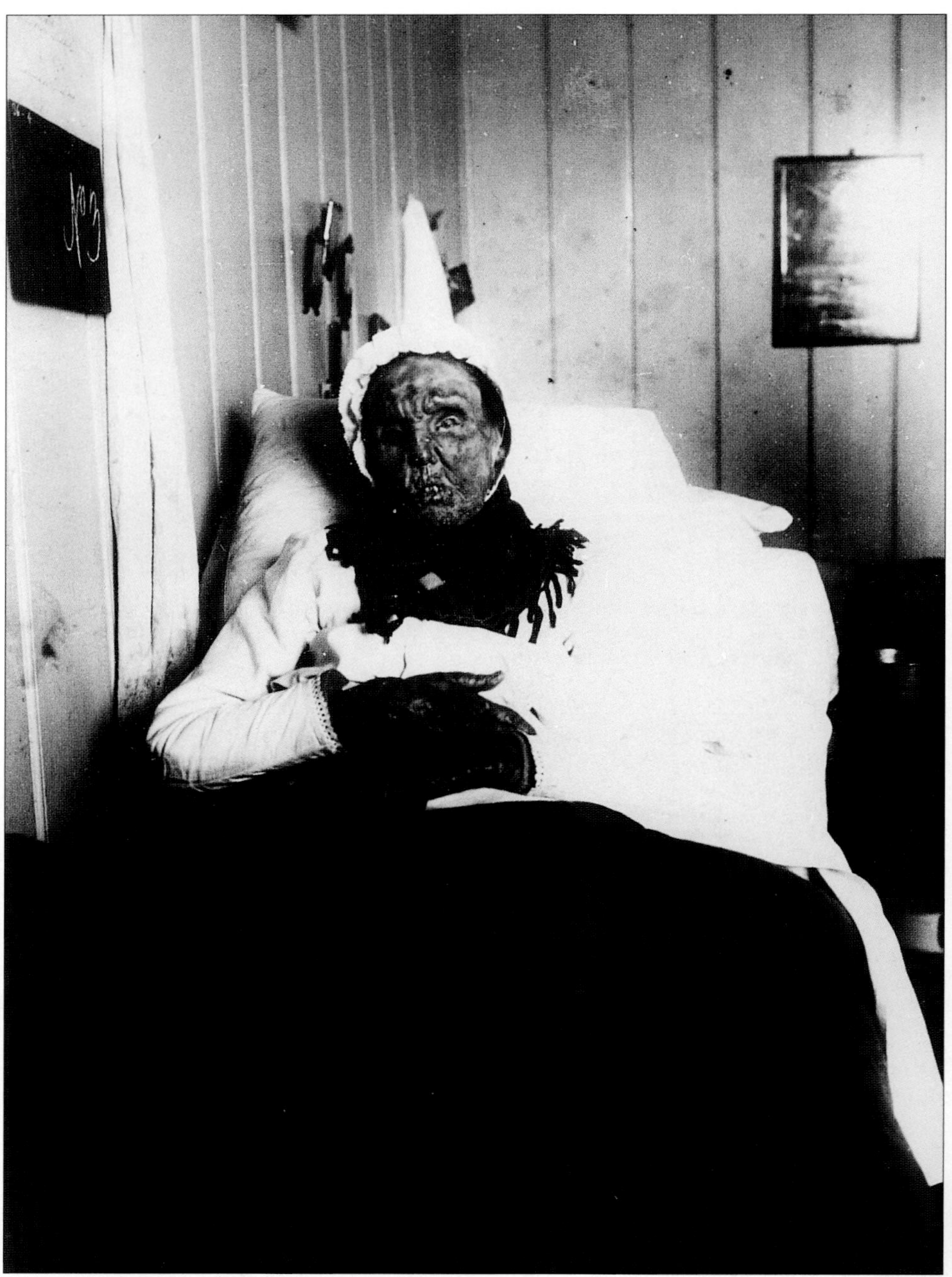

Figure 58: At the nursing home for leprous patients in Bergen around 1900 (Photo: Knud Knudsen. Courtesy University Library, Bergen).

might have given a new dimension to private life, were not marketed in Norway until 1967.

The services of the general practitioner were met by a growing demand. Obviously, the attitudes toward health had undergone changes: more and more of the everyday complaints, strains, and hazards were medicalized and turned into a task for the doctor. But the increasing demands also led to a lack of physicians in primary health care; in the countryside many positions for district physicians were vacant, and the working days became long for those physicians who were available in the neighborhood. Since they were being reimbursed from the sickness insurance without questioning, a greater part of the doctors of that time could work as much as they wanted and obtain a good income; a favorable personal economy became a hallmark of general practice.

However, the feeling of being constantly overworked and tied up, as was the situation for many a private general practitioner or district physician, could be a heavy burden for which there could be only partial be compensation, both for the physician and for his family.

An interesting change of another kind could be observed in these years: The medical activity of the practitioner involved more and more people, and more and more economy. A common setup had been that the physician, as a rule a male physician, had his wife as his combined secretary and nurse in the surgery. His practice in fact was a family business, a system with long traditions in other fields of the Norwegian society: farms and shops were run in the same way, and the wife of the minister was an indispensable part of church life, preparing meetings and gatherings and staying behind. In fact, a highly conservative family pattern, consisting of a stable marriage and a loyal and enthusiastic spouse, was a sort of prerequisite for the district physician system of Evang and his predecessors. But could that requirement be maintained in the years to come?

Within medicine, the demands for assistance increased. More laboratory work was expected to be done in the surgeries, and the paperwork increased in complexity. A need for hired assistance emerged, and the idea of establishing group practices and health centers was discussed.

Better communication, roads, reliable cars, boats, and so on increased the capacity of the doctor. It became easier to make house calls, but also easier for the patients to come to the doctor's office. The simultaneous development of hospitals made the possibility of referral to a policlinic or admittance to a hospital ward more readily available, a situation which in its turn made the general practitioner more efficient and therefore he could see more patients.

In addition to transforming the local health services, this process also did something to the local society. Just as the running of a hospital or another type of health institution could be an asset to the community in terms of economy, the activity by the general practitioner could also release an important redistribution of public money. A consultation or a home visit made wheels turn outside the practice: the taxi owner, the crew on the doctor's boat, the local ambulance might have been put into action; the pharmacist would have another customer, and so on. This side of the medical development should not be overlooked.

What were the prospects for general practice in this situation?

Medical students of the 1950s often listened to the complaints of doctors they met at the medical school. When they had finished their studies in, say, the thirties, settling on a corner as a private practitioner was often the sole option. And the knowledge acquired to pass the examinations did not automatically qualify them for that scenario.

The work in a solo practice was a lonely job with only few contacts with colleagues. There was still no systematic postgraduate training program for general practitioners, as will be treated in more detail elsewhere in this book.

The attitude that medical knowledge needed continuous updating, and was not to be left to the initiative of the individual physician only, was yet to be developed. The Norwegian Medical Association had admittedly had postgraduate training as a main concern since around 1910. Specialist training under the auspices of the Association had been introduced in 1918, and general updating courses had been offered from 1935. But it was not until the 1960s that the structuring of a comprehensive system took place, a system which gradually involved the medical faculties and the Medical Association more and more, and made the participation in courses not only a moral obligation or a collegial duty, but also a compulsory requirement for the obtainment and, in some disciplines, also the maintenance of approval in medical specialties. The general professional norm of upkeep of knowledge was institutionalized and settled.

From the 1960s onward the course system

TABLE 17.1
Diagnoses, the district of Hemne, Norway, July–Dec. 1963 (Larsen 1965)

Diagnoses	Number	Percent
Cardiovascular diseases	284	10.9
Respiratory diseases	268	10.3
Skin and venereal diseases	237	9.1
Skeletomuscular diseases	234	9.0
Injuries	214	8.2
Psychiatric diseases	143	5.5
Psychosomatic diseases	25	1.0
Gastrointestinal diseases	154	5.9
Pregnancy checkups	135	5.2
Vaccinations, dressing of wounds etc.	132	5.1
Eye diseases	97	3.7
Acute contagious diseases	95	3.7
Neurological diseases	90	3.5
Blood diseases	77	3.0
Urinary tract diseases	68	2.6
Ear diseases	63	2.4
Gynecological and obstetrical diseases, brest diseases	60	2.3
Observation cases	54	2.1
Various diseases	92	3.5
Attestations ect.	78	3.0
Total number of patient contacts	2,600	100.0

TABLE 17.2
Patient contacts, the district of Hemne, Norway, July–Dec. 1963 (Larsen 1965).

	Day	Night/ weekend	Total	Percent
Office consultations	1,711	41	1,752	67.4
Home calls	178	131	309	11.9
Vaccinations, prescriptions, telephone consultations	518	21	539	20.7
Total	2,407	193	2,600	100.0
Percent	92.9	7.4	100.0	

was gradually made universal. Both the enthusiastic participation and the large number of physicians who were engaged as teachers and instructors maintained the norm, assisted by funds administrated through the Medical Association, which made most of the courses free of charge for the profession's members. In addition, courses and meetings were also arranged by pharmaceutical firms, often through local doctors' clubs.

But around 1960, this system still was far from developed, at least not for the general practitioners. The attraction of learning more was mainly connected with entering the medical specialties and with hospital work. And the general practitioners were generalists by definition.

The introduction of a mandatory hospital and general practice service in 1954 in order to achieve the official and final authorization as a physician, had a twofold objective: to relieve the quest for practical training and to supply the periphery of Norway with doctors and health services. Although two-thirds of the "turnustjeneste," the mandatory service, took place in a hospital six months in a medical, and six months in a surgical department, the remaining six months of working as an assistant to a district physician usually provided important and necessary practical training for all new doctors, and taught the future general practitioners in more detail what it was all about.

A common complaint, even as late as in the 1960s, was that there was only a distant concordance between the skills and knowledge attained at the University and the problems encountered in general practice. The patients used as examples in the University hospitals did not reflect the diseases represented in the doctor's waiting room. Table 17.1. and table 17.2. (Larsen 1965) give only a personal glimpse of this situation, and show the author's experiences during six months in a rural general practice in 1963. Apart from the circulatory diseases, which had been duly focused on in the curriculum, coughing, sneezing, and other common complaints that had only scarcely been heard of at the University played a dominating part as compared to the more rare diseases which had been treated in detail by the teachers. And the distinction between the important and less important, between the frequent and the less frequent, when to react on a faint suspicion, and when to wait for developments and calm down the nervous family, had not been a prominent subject in any university lectures. Vacation

TABLE 17.3
Operative procedures and injections performed in general practice 1952 – 1955 (Bentsen 1970)

Nature of procedure	Number of procedures: Absolute figures	Per 1,000 persons yearly: Males	Per 1,000 persons yearly: Females	Per 1,000 consultations
Suture of larger wounds	67	4.5	1.3	1.7
Reduction of shoulder dislocation	7	0.5	0.1	0.2
Radical operation of nail	8	0.3	0.5	0.2
Obstetrical procedures	10	–	1.0	0.3
Removal of larger skin tumours, drainage of deep abscesses	17	0.9	0.7	0.5
Suture of small wounds, removal of small tumours, biopsies, etc.	465	26.1	15.0	11.9
Paracenteses of ear drum	83	3.3	4.3	2.1
Removal of wax from ear	199	12.0	5.5	5.1
Removal of foreign body from:				
Cornea or conjunctiva	75	6.3	–	1.9
Nostril or ear canal	13	1.1	–	0.4
Pharynx or oesophagus	3	0.1	0.2	0.1
Catheterisation	57	3.4	1.6	1.5
Gastric washout	4	0.2	0.2	0.1
Treatment of crural ulcer	101	1.6	8.1	2.6
Incision of abscesses, etc.	686	34.0	27.5	17.6
Anaesthesia for wounds, etc.	544	31.0	17.0	13.9
Local anaesthesia for myalgia, tendinitis, etc.	191	7.4	10.0	4.9
Intra-articular injections	38	1.8	1.7	1.0
Injections treatment of varices	112	1.7	9.0	2.9
Intravenous injections	167	6.2	9.1	4.3
Other injections	2,590	100.0	137.2	66.4

jobs, acquired on the students' own initiative, were the place to get an impression of such important topics.

The need for doing something to the medical curriculum became obvious; an earlier confrontation with live patients and with the general spectrum of diseases in the society became more and more necessary. In some lectures, practice-related problems were treated, but it was not until around

DIAGRAM 17.1

Consequences of disease (Bentsen 1970). Employment situation of the impaired and the impairing diseases at Dec 31, 1955. Age-group 18–69 years. Relative distribution.

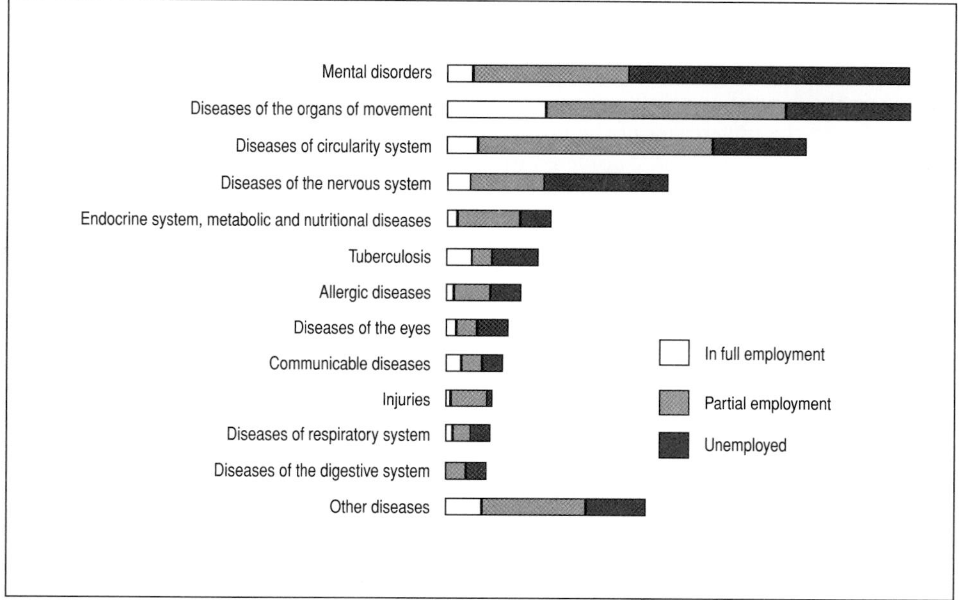

1980 that the outplacement of students in general practice during the curriculum became formalized.

One of the main causes for this alleged distance between theoretical training and the challenges of general practice might have been a lack of proper knowledge of what the work of the general practitioner really was like in quantitative terms. Some minor papers dealing with this topic had appeared, but in the years 1961 through 1966 a series of fourteen articles were published in the Journal of the Norwegian Medical Association. Bent Guttorm Bentsen (1926–), later professor of General Practice at the University of Trondheim from 1978 on, had carried out a survey of the workload in his practice in Nes in Eastern Norway in the years 1951 through 1955, later on published in English in 1970 (Bentsen 1970). For this probably rather typical rural district of the 1950s, Bentsen gave a thorough description of the population, of the medical care given, of the morbidity of the population, as experienced from the point of view of a general practitioner, and of the consequences in terms of mortality, impairment, disability, and economy.

The comprehensive overview presented by Bentsen documented the complexity and distinctive character of a general practice, the social impact of the diseases and the handling of them, and he discussed the research problems that arose when someone tried to figure out the peculiarities of first line medicine (Table 17.3. and Diagram 17.1.). At the time, much of this sort of systematic knowledge was new, and therefore of great practical importance.

But still the pursuit of a professional career first and foremost belonged in other parts of medicine, even if the importance of primary health care was fully recognized both by the profession and by the authorities.

Norway also had changed. The demographic transition represented the big issue in the transformation of the society, but in the post-war years important processes took place as well. A substantial centralization pulled a stream of migrants from the countryside to the central areas. Of course this trend affected the preferences of the physicians too. Urban Norway was considered to be attractive.

On the other hand, the established district physician system belonged to the old structure. People were now moving to urban areas, often to suburbs where one apartment house could contain the homes of a number of people exceeding that of a traditional township in rural Norway, only without a district physician. Why not set up a private practice in such a city?

I must say that, I experienced the patient encounters of the intern service in general practice in 1963, as described above, as very stimulating.

Sixty-five new medical doctors graduated from the University of Oslo in 1962, and I was one of them. As of 1996, 34 years later, six of them have died. Among the rest, only about five, or less than ten percent, are general practitioners. Three are in the public health services; one of them, Anne Alvik (1938–) succeeded Torbjørn Mork (1928–1992), who took over after Karl Evang as the Director General of the Health Services. The others are hospital doctors, specialists, work at universities, or have other kinds of medical work.

When we were rallying around on dirt roads or in shaky boats in the 1960s, earning both gratitude and money, and having a rewarding time in general practice, or working as assistants to district physicians in their often very interesting public health duties, why did so few plan a career in first line medicine? And why did the same phenomenon also apply to other classes from medical school in these years?

In my own case, I sometimes wonder about it because the image of the general practitioner had been so vividly present and so strong before I entered medical school. I still remember the fatherly doctor who calmed down the situation, and on obviously unclear grounds promised me a good prognosis when the epidemic was threatening during my boyhood. I still recall the respect we felt for him and for his colleagues.

Was there a crisis under way in 1963? A cultural crisis for general practice, with a complex set of intermingling elements?

I did not think so then, but I do think so now.

References

Bentsen, B.G. *Illness and general practice.* Oslo-Bergen-Tromsø: Universitetsforlaget, 1970.

Brantenberg, G. *Sangen om St. Croix.* Oslo: Aschehoug, 1979.

Evang, K. *Health Service, Society, and Medicine.* London: Oxford University Press, 1960.

Evang, K. *Helse og samfunn.* Oslo: Gyldendal, 1974.

Evang, K. *Health services in Norway.* Oslo: Universitetsforlaget, 1976.

Larsen, Ø. "Legesøkning i et distrikt i Trøndelag," *Tidsskrift for Den norske lægeforening,* 85(1965): 1770–2.

Nordby, T. *Karl Evang.* Oslo: Aschehoug, 1989.

Siem, H. *Choices for health.* Oslo: Universitetsforlaget, 1986.

Strøm, A. *Velferdssamfunn og helse.* Oslo: Gyldendal, 1980.

CHAPTER 18

The Development of Primary Care Medicine after the Second World War

EVEN LÆRUM AND PER HJORTDAHL

18.1. Modern General Practice

General practice is defined as the general diagnostic, therapeutic, and preventive part of medicine directed toward each single individual. It represents the front line service to the local society, and has also a foothold in the community, and the interaction between health, and environment. Consequently, the primary physician has to get involved with the people under his care, and with the local society.

The aim of this chapter is to look at the main characteristics of the professional development in primary care medicine from the Second World War up until today, and to describe some important events were related to education, research, and academic life. Further, there have been important changes in the running and the organization of the primary health care services, and changes in the population have required adjustment in the situation of the primary physicians.

18.2. The 1950s and 1960s

"The Hard 1950s and 1960s" is a title in a Norwegian book on the development of primary care medicine (Fugelli et. al. 1984). The chapter describes the first two decades after the Second World War. From the turn of the century up until the Second World War, biotechnology produced impressive results in medicine. New remedies were developed which radically changed the treatment of previously crippling and often deadly diseases. We got vaccines which could prevent epidemics, and new techniques made a much earlier and more precise and reliable diagnosis possible.

Both among the population and among the politicians a considerable belief was developed in the possibilities of specialized hospital medicine. At the same time, physicians were attracted by the professional status which the specialties gave. As a consequence, conditions for the general practitioner working outside the medical institutions were deteriorated.

Thus, the first decades after the Second World War became critical for general practice in Norway. The ideals of the profession were at a discount and so was the general practitioners' general status among the population and within the profession. General practioners felt that their work carried low prestige and they had difficulties attracting recruits. The general practitioner was not part of the progress within technological and specialized medicine, which first became evident in the hospitals. Similar conditions for general medicine also caused concern in many other European countries, and one can even say globally.

At the beginning of the fifties, a deliberate campaign was initiated in order to make visible the importance of the corps of general practitioners, and to show the necessity of having a well-developed primary health care service, based on a general practitioner firmly established in the local society. This view was also gradually realized by the authorities. In addition, expenses increased alarmingly in the hospital system and specialized medicine.

From 1955 to 1965 there was a decline in the number of primary physicians, and the average age increased from 45 to 55. In many places there were up to 8,000 people per physician, and the word "crisis" was often used. Many general practitioners worked under a severe pressure with continuous call duties, without stand-in arrangements, and without time for holidays. Equally, there was little time for family life, for keeping oneself professionally updated, let alone for writing publications.

An obvious sign that something had to be done came in 1967, when a committee, specially appointed for considering primary health care, delivered its recommendation. Several measures were proposed, including the suggestion to emphasize further and higher education, and to increase the weight placed on general medicine during the basic medical training.

But, although the committee pointed out the prevailing difficulties for the general practitioners and suggested a number of measures for improvement, it was opposed by both the Medical Association and the primary physicians, particulary because of the proposal of stricter rules for setting up a practice. This was contrary to the concept of general practice as a freely accessible type of medical work.

The General Practitioners' Association (Aplf) had been established in 1938 as an Oslo-based organization. The Association after World War II played an increasingly important role in the reformation of general medicine, and the reshaping of the working conditions for general practioners. Several small steps had to be taken; among other things, there was a breakthrough when the general practitioners succeded in having removed the restrictions on prescriptions for medicines free of charge in the case of life-threatening or chronic diseases, introduced in 1960, after a five-year-struggle. This right now was not reserved for the specialists only any longer; an important symbolic victory.

The national meetings of the Norwegian Medical Association became lively arenas for discussions concerning working conditions in general practice. Gradually, good contacts were established to the secretariat of the Norwegian Medical Association, and to the Journal of the Norwegian Medical Association. A special pension scheme for general practitioners was introduced in 1961, followed by the sickness benefit scheme in 1963.

A fund for the postgraduate training of physicians was established in 1967. By means of financial support from this fund, regular courses, study tours, and research could be set up. The General Practitioners' Association introduced a series of courses held in mountain resorts at regular intervals, and this initiative became particularly important. These courses were meeting places for general practitioners; experiences could be exchanged and unity and solidarity established a process of professionalization of the general practitioners. A stronger sense of identity for the general practitioner followed, which in turn awakened an interest in establishing general practice as a medical specialty. This required a systematic postgraduate education scheme, which even drew some international attention.

The Oslo group within the General Practioners' Association, which started in 1948, gradually gained strength during the 50s. A central issue in these years was to strive for the improvement of the standard fees.

In the 60s, the focus was first and foremost on the strengthening of the professionalization of the general practitioners through efforts to establish opportunities for the physicians to attend courses, and emphasizing the working conditions and the social security for the primary physicians. There was a drive to achieve just as good terms for doctors in primary health care service as were for the hospital specialists.

During the five-year period after 1965, a small group of enthusiastic primary physicians went on study tours to Denmark, Great-Britain, and The Netherlands, where general practice was beginning to be consolidated with, among other things, a system of permanent patient lists. They gained valuable experience and promoted the struggle for introducing general practice as a separate subject in the universities.

Gradually there was also a general acceptance of the importance of introducing general practice also into basic training for the students. The Norwegian Medical Association also gave priority to this goal, and in 1968, which became a memorable year for Norwegian general practice, the first institute for general practice was opened at the Red Cross Clinic in Oslo. In addition, a professorship was established as a gift from the Norwegian Medical Association to the University of Oslo. The first professor was Christian F. Borchgrevink (born 1924).

The foundation for establishing general practice as an academic discipline was thus settled, and general practice could aim at achieving the same status as the other established specialties.

18.3. The Promising 1970s and 1980s.

The important introduction to the 1970s was the establishment of the Institute of General Practice at the University of Oslo. Four years later a similar institute was established in Bergen. In 1973 and 1975 Institutes for Community Medicine and General Practice also were set up at the University of Tromsø and of Trondheim.

In 1971 the Government put forward its own parliamentary report about health care services outside the hospitals, in which it was pointed out that, in a European context, Norway was comparatively far ahead regarding the professional development of general practice.

However, in this report a lot of the attention was paid to the principle of fixed salaries for the primary physicians, a principle which was opposed in medical circles. The report mapped out a co-ordination of health care and social welfare services in the muncipalities. What was central to the whole public health system in the 1970s, however, was the legislation on hospitals, which involved a considerable upgrading of the specialized institutional health care services.

A basically new medical curriculum was launched at the University of Tromsø in 1971. General practice and social medicine received a prominent position in a study plan that was also radical in other ways. The experiences from this curriculum at the new university played an important role later in the further revision of the medical training at the other Norwegian universities.

At the beginning of the 1970s, several muncipalities also supported the establishment of private general practice, in the form of subsidizing physicians' and health care centers. In 1974 the first fixed-salary position was established at Stovner Health and Social Welfare Center in Oslo.

Everyday life for most of the primary

physicians still contained considerable work pressure, but many of them were encouraged by their belief in the possibilities for the further development of primary care medicine. Gradually there was also an increase in the number of recruits.

In 1972 a special journal for general practitioners called "Utposten" was founded. The name means "the outpost," and in the Norwegian language the word also has connotations to the pioneering state of primary care medicine. The journal has existed ever since and is doing very well as a grassroots' periodical.

During the 1970s, the population in general became increasingly suspicious to the health care system. One of the reasons was the fact that costs were mounting considerably within the hospital system. In addition, the population's expectations were increasing. Many, including politicians, realized the necessity of restraint and the need to develop further a decentralized and well-functioning primary health care service.

During the same period, research within family medicine was increasing, even though this had already been started in the mid 1950s by Bentsen (Bentsen 1970), with his basic work on the frequency of sickness and the use of the health care services in a general practice. An explanation for the increase in research this time was that Norway by now had established institutes for general practice in all the medical faculties. Another important step toward increasing research was taken by the establishment of a General Practice Research Committee, which brought together the repective institutes, the General Practitioners' Association, and the Public Health Officers' Association.

During the 1970s a lively discussion went on between the Norwegian Medical Association and the health authorities. The Medical Association struggled to maintain general practice as an independent and liberal occupation, while the authorities wanted to take over the running and responsibility for the primary health care service, and employ the doctor at a fixed salary.

In order to give a definition of general practice and state the objectives of primary health care service, a small but important pamphlet was published as a co-operation venture by the associations for general practioners and public health officers (Aplf Oll 1977).

Also internationally, the closing of the 1970s was an important period for primary health care service. In 1977 WHO defined its aim of health for all by the year 2000. This was followed up in 1978 during the conference at Alma Ata, where primary health care service was singled out as the most important mean for achieving this ambitious goal.

> "Herein primary health care is defined as essential health care based on practical, scientifically sound, and socially acceptable methods and technology made universally accessible to individuals and families in the community through their full participation and at the cost that the community and the country can afford. It forms an integral part of both the country's health system of which it is the central functionand main focus, and the overall social economic development of the community" (Bærheim 1994).

In 1979, the first Nordic Congress of General Practice was held in Copenhagen in Denmark, and was followed by an equally successful congress in Bergen in Norway two years later. The Nordic Congress now takes place every other year, and circulates among the five Nordic countries.

A new legislation on health services in the counties was introduced in 1984, under a much more austere economic situation than in the previous decade, but with the suggestion to develop further the decentralized health care service, in which each county would be the responsible unit.

The Norwegian College of General Practitioners (NSAM) was established in 1983. Contrary to the Association of General Practitioners, the new body was not to be politically active, but should stand for professional development, research, and international communication. The Scandinavian Journal of Primary Health Care, which has been of considerable importance to researchers in primary health care in Scandinavia, was established the same year.

During the last half of the 1980s, the primary physicians' working conditions began to improve considerably. There was a good coverage of physicians in many places and the many health centers were well-equipped and administratively well functioning units with plenty of facilities for diagnostics and treatment, such as x-rays, electrocardiographic equipment, good laboratories and, not least, staffed with well-educated supporting personnel. Professional activity was advanced, and many primary physicians saw it as a sign of quality to become as independent as possible from the specialists and the hospitals. Financial incentives contributed to this development.

This development was also evident in the fact that primary physicians became key figures within the steadily more extensive care for the elderly, with the expansion of old people's homes and nursing homes. The 1980s were experienced by many primary physicians as a promising decade, when their position was settled, and the standing of primary care medicine was felt to be clearly defined and appreciated in the eyes of the public and medical colleagues of other disciplines.

18.4 Research in General Practice

In general practice, as in other types of professional work, research is systematic collection of information and data, which is processed and passed on to others, usually by publishing. The aim is to obtain new knowledge. Some call research "organized curiosity". And the continuous acquisition of new knowledge is one of the characteristics of a profession. Without research of its own, also practical medicine would be in danger of dying out. However, research is not always just acquiring new knowledge. Just as often it can be about modifying, verifying or rejecting existing information and accepted truths.

From the earliest days of Norwegian medical journals in the first half of the nineteenth century and onwards, articles and casuistic reports document that professional curiosity has been well established among Norwegian physicians. Important clinical observations and also results of large-scale studies for example those by Carl Schiøtz (1877–1938), appeared from Norwegian primary health care at an early stage.

However, modern research in general practice in Norway can roughly be divided into three main phases: the first steps, the manifold phase, and the consolidation, and deepening phase.

At the beginning of the 1950s, research in primary medicine was at a low ebb, although with one important exception: the studies by Bent Guttorm Bentsen (1926–) of an inland population in south-eastern Norway in 1952–55. The results of his investigations were first published in the form of 14 articles in the Journal of the Norwegian Medical Association. His work received international recognition, and was a decisive first step in research on general practice. However, throughout the 1950s and 1960s, there were only a few other research projects and publications, except for some descriptions of practices, mostly simple mappings of health and morbidity in the population covered by the general practice in question.

Research activity increased throughout the 1970s and 1980s. But in the 1990s a new phase commenced marked by a succession of single projects, based on genuine general practice problems in the primary physician's daily life, under the motto: "Dig where you stand." Besides the registration of work and medical topics of interest in primary health care practices, the clinical side of general practice more and more came into focus. Grants for general practitioners, given by the Norwegian Medical Association, were an important precondition for primary care physicians to be able to complete small projects based on their own practice and clinical everyday life.

A penetrating and in-depth phase with more large projects on the doctorate level was begun in the 1980s. A decisive force behind this new phase was the establishment of a four year program for research in general practice in the Norwegian Research Council.

Then focus in this program was on: clinical primary medicine and the doctor/patient relationship. The following are typical research topics and examples of projects: Urinary infections as encountered by the primary care physician (Bærheim 1994); diagnosing of pneumonia in adults in general practice (Melbye 1992); studies on fever in general practice (Eskerud 1995); studies on urolithiasis in general practice (Lærum 1983); cancer in general practice (Nylenna 1986); and continuity of care in general practice (Hjortdahl 1992).

Research on general practice had a broad selection of subjects. It applied itself to almost every medical field and much of the activity was the result of one simple person's efforts, often her or his only larger research project.

However, in this phase there has also been an increasing and lasting tendency to consolidate professional areas, where groups have agreed on penetrating into special problems and research methods. One example is a group in Trondheim (Johannessen 1992), where general practitioners and gastroenterologists for 15 years have charted the problem of dyspepsia as related to symptomatology, the patient's personality, social conditions, method of examination, therapy and the development of methods of research.

The scope of research has also been demonstrated by others, for example the group performing investigations in Ullensaker, a municipality outside Oslo, where the main subject of study is muscle and skeletal problems, and diabetes.

Another group, consisting of general practitioners, an urologist, a nurse, and a physiotherapist, have studied the problem of incontinence, with its base at the department of general practice at the University of Bergen. At the department of general practice in Oslo, a group is working on the improvement in quality of the doctor/patient relationship in clinical practice.

The number of monographs and articles from general practice has gradually increased. The number of papers was small in the 1950s, but has increased considerably. From 1960 until 1996, a number of approximately 25 doctoral theses have been defended, dealing with a variety of problems from the field of general practice.

General practice has no specific research methods of its own. Approaches from several disciplines have been used, according to the research problems just as in other research. Methods from, among others, sociology, psychology, anthropology, epidemiology, statistics, and pharmacology are applied. The methods can be descriptive, analytical, observational, and experimental (APLF 1988).

A considerable part of the research on general practice has been initiated by the pharmaceutical industry, in the form of clinically controlled trials, for the purpose of testing new drugs. In this type of project, however, the general practitioner has, as a rule, performed the research in accordance with a protocol presented by the drug company.

Norway has some special advantages for doing epidemiological investigations. It is relatively simple and easy to use geographically well-defined population units to chart the spreading of definite health problems. Some municipalities also has the advantage of a low migration activity. The system of personal identification numbers for all Norwegians, by which every person can be identified by a 9-figure number consisting of birth date and a specified number, also is very advantageous.

There exists a basic field of problems within research in general practice: formulating a classification system that is agreed upon internationally. Such a system is indispensable for comparative work and studies over time.

Taxonomy, or classification development, has been important in Norway, as in other countries. This work has been going on an international level from 1985 on, as part of a co operative effort between WONCA (The World Organization of Family Doctors) and the World Health Organization. A collection of standardized implements for primary health care research has been built up. The most important is the primary health care central classification (ICPC-International Classification of Primary Care)(WONCA 1991). Norway has taken an active part in this work.

The four university institutes for general practice have played an important role in the initiation and guidance of general practice projects. General practitioners also often have contacted the institutes on their own initiative for advice and help with problems they wished to bring into focus. Research activities at the institutes have become rather extensive, despite a very limited scientific staff.

The grants available to general practitioners have been important for the development of research on general practice. Since 1977, the Norwegian Medical Association has provided the means for research grants that support one to six months of study. A total of 36 scholarship months are available each year for the time being, and more than 150 general practitioners have received such grants.

Within the framework of a special training program in connection with the abovementioned Norwegian Research Council Program of 1986, seminars and courses on qualitative methods, multivariate analyses, rating scales, classification, and publishing, etc. were offered. Thirty researchers took part in this program, which was an important start of the consolidating phase in the research. A majority of the participants aimed at completing a doctoral thesis. Thus the program has been very important for consolidating the status of primary care medicine as an academic discipline.

From the point of view of professionalization, an interesting point should be mentioned. In the beginning, many grassroot practitioners were resistant to research which aimed at a doctorate. However, this has changed. Some of those who were most reluctant and afraid of losing their footing in practice, have later become advanced theoreticians and full-time academics. Gradually the understanding that there exists an exciting world of research outside the universities, has taken hold.

18.5. Who was – and is – the Primary Physician?

After the turn of the century, two main types of primary physicians appeared in Norway: the district physicians and the general practitioners with a private practice. The district physicians were based in the Norwegian countryside, on the stormy coast, and in the narrow valleys all over the country, while the general practitioners mainly were located in larger towns and villages.

In an earlier chapter of this book the

reader will have learned how it was established by law that each district should have one or more district physicians. The system provided doctors even for the most remote areas of Norway.

The district physician in most cases was a combination physician; employed by the State as a public officer to take care of the socio-medical and preventive work in the local environment, and at the same time he worked as an independent private general practitioner, treating the local population. The County Medical Officer of Health was the professional superior of the district physician for the public medical work, whereas the district physician was his own boss in his general practice.

Many districts were large, often entailing long trips when home calls sick calls were required. Usually it was necessary to be on call for weeks in a row. The work of the district physician was physically demanding, and the majority of the doctors were males. And the wife of the doctor had a key role in the primary health care service. She acted as the switchboard operator, adviser and buffer, often both day and night when her husband was out on a sick call or occupied with some other work. Because of the husband's irregular working hours and frequent absences, she often had sole responsibility for the family as well.

This combination of public and private activities involved hard work. But it developed pride in the profession and respect in the local communities. As pointed out in several of the chapters in this book, the Norwegian district physicians had a strong and deeply rooted position among the population outside the large towns, and were respected by their colleagues, politicians, and public authorities.

In the big towns, the role of the primary physician developed differently. Here the situation was clearly dichotomised. A few public physicians in full-time positions as public health officers took care of the preventive and socio-medical tasks, while a larger group of privately practicing general practitioners were working in curative medicine. These general practitioners did a large and necessary job for the town's population, but they also were relatively vulnerable as a professional group. As private fee-for-service practitioners, they were dependent on access to patients and on running of their practice profitably.

They often ran their practice alone, and as sole practitioners who were confined by the work they did behind their consultation-room doors, they were easily isolated both professionally and geographically, even if they were situated in the larger towns.

There were more female doctors among the general practitioners in the cities than among the district physicians.

To be a general practitioner was in principle to be engaged in free trade well into the second half of the twentieth century, when restrictions of different kinds gradually appeared. Anyone with a medical education could set up a general practice wherever he or she wanted. Of course, this was regarded as an advantage, but it was also a professional and personal challenge.

As covered elsewhere in this book, after the Second World War, an increased weight was put on hospitals and specialized health care institutions. During these years, private general practice became almost invisible, was low in prestige, experienced worsened working conditions, and the recruitment was low.

This particularly affected the primary care doctors in the towns, but also many positions for district physicians were vacant. During the 1950s and 1960s, there were only about 800 private general practitioners and around 400 district physicians in Norway. A vicious cycle had been set in motion. Vacancies increased the work-load on the remaining doctors, which in turn could lead to new vacancies. As we already have discussed, the primary health care service was on the verge of a breakdown.

From the end of the 1960s and up to the 1990s, dramatic changes have taken place. Many of them are part of the general development of the Norwegian society. The wave of decentralization and the 1984 law on health services in the municipalities resulted in the discontinuation of the system of district physicians as a state-run arrangement. The responsibility for the primary health service of the local population was turned over to the municipalities. The district physician became a municipality doctor, and instead of being a state official in the part of work containig public duties, he or she was turned into a muncipality employed adviser.

The general process of change in the role of females in the society also affected primary medicine. The old system of general practice as a family business, with the doctor's wife as his assistant, no longer could be maintained. In modern Norwegian marriges the two spouses normally have occupations of their own; this is the case in the medical world as well. At the same time, female doctors in increasing members entered the profession as independent practitioners. This resulted in the requirement and demand for more organized working and family conditions, as they related to both female and male primary physicians.

During this period, there was also a general awakening of social awareness among the students. The newly qualified and socially conscious physicians found primary health care service to be a challenge. Prevalent anti-authoritarian attitudes dismissed the authoritarian model of the district physician system. Many young doctors also rejected the system of general practice as a free trade, and wanted to be able to commit themselves to social problems and to have fixed-salary positions. The muncipalities' responsibility for the primary health care service, combined with many young professionals' wish for more regulated working conditions, resulted in many communities, including in the larger towns, in the establishment of positions as muncipality physicians for general health care, with a fixed-salary and fixed working hours.

Different arrangements for remuneration were introduced, but the common denominator was a base of fixed salaries and fixed working hours.

In the years which have elapsed since 1970, the number of primary physicians in Norway has doubled. A quarter of the country's doctors are now general practitioners in the 1990's, and 30 percent of these are women. The average age for primary physicians is at present 43 years, the lowest among the different groups of the medical profession. In the countryside there is now an average of 1.300 inhabitants per primary physician, with a range between 890 and 1.600. About 2.000 of the primary physicians have been educated as specialists in primary care medicine, and another 500 are in the process of training for approval as specialists. There are 450 specialists in community medicine, of whom 8 percent are women.

The Norwegian general practitioner of the 1990s usually works with curative medicine four or five days a week, and devotes the rest to other activities, such as maternity care and preventive health work.

The primary care physician has an average of 20 to 25 consultations each curative day, and spend 17 to 20 minutes with each patient (Hjortdahl 1992). More than 80 percent of the Norwegian population are in contact with a primary physician one or more times during the year. The population seeks a primary physician an average of 2.6 times per year, and those who go to the doctor have an average of 3.3 visits yearly (Berg et al. 1994).

18.6. The Paradox: Specialized Generalist

The Norwegian debate on the requirements for a specialized education of doctors started at the end of the nineteenth century. At that time anyone who had completed medical studies could call him- or herself a specialist, and there were examples of people who did this immediately after graduation. Collegial rules for the first specialists were adopted by the Norwegian Medical Association in 1918 and approved by the authorities in 1925. More and more specialties appeared during the next decades, and there was a steadily increasing number of doctors who were becoming specialists.

For many years general practice was not part of this development. It was looked upon as the simple and ordinary part of doctoring that was left behind after the specialists had taken their share. Many general practitioners felt that they among the population and their colleagues usually were looked upon as medicine's jack of all trades and master of none. This was an unpleasant and unsatisfactory situation for the doctors involved.

Being a specialist was connected with a considerable prestige and, as a rule, also with better financial terms. So the delineation and definition of a specialty had social connotations, beyond signifying special scientific or medical competences.

And in addition to this, the rapid growth and increased emphasis on technology both in society at large and in medicine in general in the 1950s and 1960s contributed to the relative disparagement of general practice. In many ways, it is easy to understand why many young physicians in the 1950s and 1960s went in for a specialist training, and turned away from general practice. At the same time, however, some enthusiasts discovered specific qualities hitherto overlooked in being a generalist.

An international co-operation also was instigated about finding the identity of general practice. England was the leading country in this work, but physicians from Denmark, Holland and Norway were coworkers. An international group was established, in order to outline definitions and descriptions of aims in the general practitioners' roles and tasks (Leenwenhost Working Party 1974).

A basic element in this new assessment of general practice is that the patient and the patient's problems must be understood in a bio-psycho-social frame of reference. A general practitioner with knowledge of the patients, often obtained over a long period of time and under different conditions, and with specific knowledge of the local environment, can use this professional knowledge in a broad context.

Most of the diseases the primary care physician sees are minor and self-limiting. But now and then, and unexpectedly symptoms appear that can be signs of serious diseases. One of the general practitioner's most important tasks is to be able to invalidate the suspicion of a serious disease. To be on the alert toward serious diseases with low prevalence requires its own working methods and interpretations of diagnostic tests and reports.

This understanding of primary care medicine started to get a foothold in Norway toward the end of the 1960s. And the aim was to get general practice recognized as a medical specialty of its own. This goal was reached in 1985.

In 1962 a special fund for postgraduate training of doctors was established. This arrangement was based on an agreement between the State authorities and the Norwegian Medical Association. This fund became a useful tool for the committee working with postgraduate training for general practitioners (with a Norwegian abbreviation it was called the VEAP-committee) in their efforts to turn general practice into a full-fledged specialty. The demand for establishing a complete specialty, not only a minor approval arrangement, such as had been launched in 1973, was brought forward regularly, and a proposal was accepted, valid from January 1, 1985. A specialty committee for general practice then replaced the VEAP committee.

Two main principles were established with the introduction of this new specialty. The first was a recognition that basic medical training educate generalists, and that the discipline of general practice has a content lying considerably above that general level. General practice therefore justified its own postgraduate studies and specialty. Externship and practice were considered most important for achieving the sufficient level of knowledge, and the attitudes and skills necessary for the specialty of general practice. Emphasis was therefore put on clinical general practice during the postgraduate studies. The other main principle was the importance of a continuous follow-up training. It was not only the general practitioner's general knowledge, skills, and attitudes the first years after the basic education and externship that mattered. Just as important was how these qualities could be updated and maintained through a period of 20 to 30 years of professional life in a busy clinical, private practice. Continuous postgraduate studies were therefore emphasized, resulting in a mandatory recertification arrangement for the specialists in order to stay licensed as a specialist in general practice.

The specialty education in general practice presently consists of four elements, and it takes a total of five years to complete. The requirements are four years in general practice as the main part, with an additional year at a clinical hospital ward, or in an outpatient department. At the same time, the candidate has to participate in a longitudinally working collegial group consisting of five to eight persons. These groups are guided by an experienced general practitioner who has also been educated as an instructor. The group meets on an average of one day per month during a two-year period, in the candidate's local environment; in this way the training program can be completed without major breaks in clinical practice or continuity of care with their patients. The last element of the training consists of 400 teaching hours in courses during a five-year period. Some of these courses relate to preventive and environmental medicine, epidemiology, research, law, economics and management others to clinical subjects. A specific textbook is used for the training program.

The first requirement for the renewal of the approval every five years is that the candidate has maintained a minimum of one year of clinical practice during this five-year period. Another requisite is a minimum of 200 hours of specified refresher courses. The last requirement is a minimum of 3 months of hospital service, teaching, or research during the period.

There are no written examinations in the specialization procedures for general practioners. For the general practitioners, the standard fees make it financially advantageous to become a specialist, and to keep the specialty updated. Although continuing education and specialization is not obligatory in Norway, most practitioners consider it as very worthwhile.

Norway is different, in a positive way, from the system in many other countries with a similar specialist education, because emphasis is placed on the opportunity for the candidates to complete their training while running their own practices. In the training program, educational weight is placed upon general practice instead of on hospital-based medicine.

The educational scheme for specialization of general practitioners has been in effect for more a decade and is considered successful by the practitioners themselves. The specialization has contributed to an improvement of the professional quality of general practice, and it has increased its status for recruiting new colleagues. Of decisive importance has been the Norwegian Medical Association's strong support and management in connection with development, drawing up, and implementing the educational program.

During this period, an upgrading of general practice also has been put into effect in basic medical education. The Norwegian medical faculties now accept general practice as one of their major clinical disciplines, on an equal footing with internal medicine and surgery.

18.7. The Economics, Organization, and Running of the Primary Health Care Service

In the last decades of the nineteenth century, some sickness insurance arrangements of different kinds appeared, a legislation on this was introduced in 1911. However, it was not until 1956 that sickness insurance covered the entire population. Since the introduction of a complete social and sick relief system in 1967, replacing several older arrangements, the premiums have been levvied on the taxation bills of every Norwegian citizen. It has been a general principle for the doctor in Norwegian primary health care to be paid by fee-for-service. The services to be reimbursed and the amounts are negotiated between the state and the Norwegian Medical Association. A written bill is sent to every patient, but only a moderate amount of this is paid by the patient. The magnitude of the own-risk charge is varying between 10 and 20 percent of the expenses of a consultation. This system was introduced in 1925.

For a long time, direct settlement, an arrangement whereby the patient paid the whole amount which has been charged for the consultation directly to the primary physician, and later got the expenses reimbursed by national insurance office, was the standard procedure.

After the Second World War, however, most of the general practitioners entered into agreements directly with the local national insurance offices, so that the patients only had to pay the deductible amount; the balance of the total due was regulated directly between the doctor and the national insurance office. This system was considered to be very convenient by the patients, and also suited the doctor and the insurance office. But there is a psychological risk: both the patient and the doctor can easily lose sight of the real cost of the various services. The actual expenses are hidden from the patient, who only sees the deductible amounts. This can influence some patients' demands and expectations of the health care services and make them unrealistic. The public authorities also have had some difficulties in handling this arrangement with the doctors, and long-range economic health planning was difficult.

In the middle of the 1970s it was time to change the organization and payment methods in the primary health care service, for administrative reasons and because incentives were needed for doctors to take up posts in less favored regions. The system of fee-for-service reimbursement did not work well in remote areas with sparse populations, long travels, and a wide panorama of diseases. Fee-for-service rewarded fast consultations and technical examinations. Doctors who spent time discussing socio-medical problems lost income. There were signs of a budding structural crisis in the big cities as well. There were only private general practitioners in Oslo in 1970; they were few in number and the geographic distribution within the city was uneven. The new suburbs which appeared at that time had few or no general practitioners and little chance of recruiting any. For newly qualified doctors, it was viewed as an economic mishap to practice in Oslo; one had to look forward to a heavy work load, and little professional prestige.

Consequently, the chief public medical officer in Oslo, Fredrik Mellbye (1917–), introduced the first four fixed salary positions for primary physician in cities at the Stovner health care and social welfare service center in 1974. These doctors were called Community Medical Officers and had the same functions as the district physicians in the rural areas; they had some public preventive work, but the emphasis was placed on curative general practice. The difference between the district physician and the city-doctor was not so much the professional content as the organization and running of the services. The district physician in the countryside was running a private business in addition to his salaried public tasks, he or she received reimbursement per consultation for curative activities, had a heavy load of work, and had many on-call duties. The city medical officers on the other hand, had a fixed salary, fixed working hours, and in many cases no on-call duty.

The Norwegian Medical Association resisted the introduction of such fixed-salary positions, which was looked upon as a threat to general practice as a free, liberal profession. The arrangement, however, was considered successful by the political authorities, and also by many young physicians who for various reasons wanted more organized working conditions.

In the course of a few years, more than one hundred positions for "city doctors" were established, geographically distributed over the whole of Oslo. This arrangement was repeated in other cities as well, such as Tromsø, Bergen, Bodø and in the muncipality of Bærum. The system also spread to the rural areas of Northern Norway, where they were experiencing problems with recruitment. Twenty-five positions for district physicians in Northern Norway were converted to fixed-salary positions in 1978. These positions were considered attractive by many physicians, both because of the work and the salaries, and recruitment improved. This arrangement was later expanded to include some two hundred positions around the country.

A new law on primary health care was passed in 1984. This law was partly the result of a political desire to decentralize public services in general, and partly a wish to improve the planning and financial control of the health services. The formal, and partly the financial, responsibility for primary health care service was transferred to each muncipality by this law.

For many muncipality officials, it became a matter of principle that the local health care service should be run by muncipality-employed physicians. The result often was a bureaucratic and formal structure with strong political and administrative elements, which easily conflicted with the clinician's individualistic patient-oriented culture. This potential conflict between bureaucracy and individual doctoring diminished many physicians' enthusiasm for the fixed-salary system during the years to come.

The system of fixed salaries for general practitioners was at its peak in 1990, covering almost 40 percent of all general practitioners in Norway, that is, 1,200 doctors compared to 30 percent in 1984. Then the trend was fairly abruptly reversed. It started with a few fixed-salary positions being reverted to fee-for-service reimbursement, and the trend continued like a landslide. Within three years, the number of fixed-salary doctors was down to the 1984 level, and the number has decreased even further.

The reversal took place for several reasons. A general political de-ideologizing of social democractic ideas as guiding principle for health care has taken place; more liberal tendencies with general political pragmatism and result-orientated public management systems and health plannings have-taken over.

At the same time, the Norwegian Medical Association has also become more pragmatic. The standard fees have been adjusted to make it easier for the general practitioners to work in accordance with their professional standards, and to run a quality practice with reasonable profit.

Up untill the end of 1960, one-person practices dominated Norwegian primary care, but then the first private group practices came into existence. This became rapidly a popular form of health care service. Many interdisciplinary centers were started in Oslo and other places, where primary health care service, social welfare service, and sometimes the health insurance office as well were located under the same roof and administration. This produced certain advantages due to a more rational operation, but there were also many disadvantages, such as professional conflicts and problems of cooperation. Most of these interdisciplinary centers have now been dissolved, or are being run as separate units within the same building.

Primary care group practices are still popular, however, and can be found all over the country. About one-fourth of the primary physicians still run one-person practices, but most work in groups of two to four doctors and some in even larger units.

During recent years, there has been a revolution in the use of medical technical equipment, and many of the procedures that earlier were confined to the hospitals have now been transferred to primary care. Norwegian general practitioners to a larger extent carry out such procedures and laboratory analyses in their own offices. National structures for safeguarding the quality of the primary physicians' laboratories have been implemented and almost all country's general practitioners participate on a voluntarily basis in these quality assurance activities.

Most Norwegian patients of the 1990s today can see the primary care physician of their choice. They may change physicians as often as they wish, whenever this is practical and geographically possible. Similarly, doctors can refuse patients when their appointment books are full. During periods when there is low coverage by primary physicians, it can be difficult for some patients, particularly for the old and the chronically ill, to get in contact with the primary health care service. Moreover, the free choice of primary physicians has led to unfortunate disruptions in the doctor/patient relationship. This lack of continuity of care led to initiatives from patients, politicians, and many general practitioners to establish a list patient system, similar to those in England, Holland and Denmark. Under this scheme, the population in a particular area is listed with the general practitioners who are available, and every person has his or her regular doctor to apply to. The physician in turn has a group of the population for whom he or she is wholly responsible. This system is now under trial and has been evaluated in four Norwegian counties. Should this arrangement prove to be satisfactory in Norway also, and should it be introduced as a general system by political decision, it will require a drastically new organization and operation of the primary health care service in Norway.

References

APLF 1938–1988. *Tidsskrift for Den norske lægeforening,* (1988):108(29b).

Aplf Oll. *Tanker om morgendagens primærlegetjeneste.* Oslo: Den norske lægeforening, 1977.

Bentsen, B.G. *Illness and general practice.*Oslo-Bergen-Tromsø: Universitetsforlaget, 1970.

Berg, O. and P. Hjortdahl. *Medisinen som pedagogikk* (Medicine as pedagogics) Oslo: Universitetsforlaget, 1994.

Bærheim, A. *Lower urinary tract infections in women. Aspects of pathogenesis and diagnosis. Thesis.* Bergen: Division for General Practice, Department of Public Health and Primary Health Care, University of Bergen, 1994.

Eskerud, J.R. *Studies on fever: Clinical aspects in general practice, perception, self-care and information. Thesis.* Oslo: Department of General Practice and Department of Pharmacotherapuetics, University of Oslo, 1995.

Fugelli, P. and K. Johansen (eds). *Langsomt blir faget vårt eget. Festskrift til Christian F. Borchgrevinks 60 års dag og Sigurd Humerfelts 70 års dag.* Allmennpraktikerbiblioteket. Oslo-Bergen-Stavanger-Tromsø: Universitetsforlaget, 1984.

Hjortdahl, P. *Continuity of care in general practice. Thesis.* Oslo: Department of General Practice, University of Oslo, 1992.

ICPC – ICHPPC – Defined – IC – Process – PC. Klassifikasjoner og definisjoner for primærhelsetjenesten. WONCAs internasjonale klassifikasjoner og definisjoner tilrettelagt for Norge. Translated into Norwegian by Bentsen, B.G. Oslo: TANO, 1991.

Johannessen, T. *Controlled trials in single subjects: a comparison of the symptomatic effect of cimetidine versus placebo in single patients with dyspepsia.* Trondheim: Faculty of Medicine, University of Trondheim, 1992.

Leenwenhost Working Party. *The general practitioner in Europe.* The Netherlands: Leenwenhost Group, 1974.

Lærum, E. *Studies on urolithiasis in general practice. Thesis.* Oslo: Department of General Practice, University of Oslo, 1983.

Melbye, H. "Diagnosis of pneumonia in adults in general practice". Tromsø: *ISM skriftserie 24.* Institute of Community Medicine, University of Tromsø, 1992.

Nylenna, M. *Cancer – A challenge to the general practioner. Thesis.* Oslo: The Norwegian Cancer Society, Department of General Practice, University of Oslo, 1992.

CHAPTER 19

Home Visits or Hospital Beds?

GEIR STENE-LARSEN

19.1. Introduction

When the health authorities set to work on their part of the reconstruction after the Second World War, they faced not only a series of immediate problems caused by the effects of the war on the society, but also significant problems which were the result of the lack of national health planning before the war.

In many places, premises and equipment were in a poor condition, there was a lack of personnel, and the distribution of hospital beds throughout the country was unsatisfactory. Thus, the health authorities on the one hand had to work toward a general re-equipping and raising of standards in the hospitals, and on the other hand try to counteract the damaging effects of the structure of hospital services, which was out of line both with medical development and with availability of resources in society.

19.2. Structure of Hospital Services

When the Sickness Insurance Act (Syketrygdeloven) of 1911 introduced the principle of reimbursement of fees for hospital services (kurpengeordning), the hospitals obtained a secure economic position, because the hospital remuneration system based the funding of hospitals on their actual running costs. By this method, a proportion of the total hospital expenses was taken over by the state, making the system very advantageous for hospital owners. Local authorities saw, to an increasing degree, the benefits to be derived from investing in hospital services, both from a health-political and social point of view. But, they also saw that there were financial reasons for doing so. Increased tax-income and the increased demand for goods and services that the hospital brought about, made it, in many cases, profitable for a community to run a hospital.

As a result, the development and expansion of the hospital services took place at great speed. In the course of a few decades, more than one hundred hospitals were established, and the number of beds increased dramatically, from 3,407 in 1900 to 8,107 in 1920, and to as many as 19,172 in 1940 (Table 19.1). This expansion occurred at the initiative of local authorities and voluntary organizations, but was often based on local desires and needs. Usually, the hospitals were small general hospitals, that primarily provided surgical services.

In order to have better control over the development, the Directorate of Health established the National Hospital Council (Statens sykehusråd) in 1946. This council

TABLE 19.1
Treatment capacity at somatic hospitals in Norway from 1939 to 1992

Year	Number of treated patients	Number of beds
1939	189,089	6,594
1947	273,366	7,238
1950	287,043	8,071
1955	330,454	9,488
1960	381,285	12,398
1963	414,443	14,795
1970	–	–
1975	–	–
1980	600,538	20,696
1985	647,916	22,065
1990	645,027	20,268
1992	649,461	19,104

was to ensure that plans concerning the hospital coverage were made in each county, and that resources were utilized across county borders. The Director General of the Health Services at that time, Karl Evang, believed that a restructuring of the health institutions was imperative. He strongly believed in the benefits of centralization, and he advocated that one large central hospital, with the main responsibility for the county's health services, should be established in each county, and that many of the small hospitals should be closed down. However, this initiative met with great resistance, because local communities were opposed to changes in the position of local hospitals. Therefore, the attempted reduction of the number of hospitals did not succeed in the following decades.

DIAGRAM 19.1
Number of hospitals in Norway from 1939 to 1992.
Source: Statistics Norway. Statistical Yearbook. «General hospitals» include somatic hospitals, private clinics, and cottage hospitals. «Mental hospitals» include only psychiatric hospitals, and not psychiatric clinics.

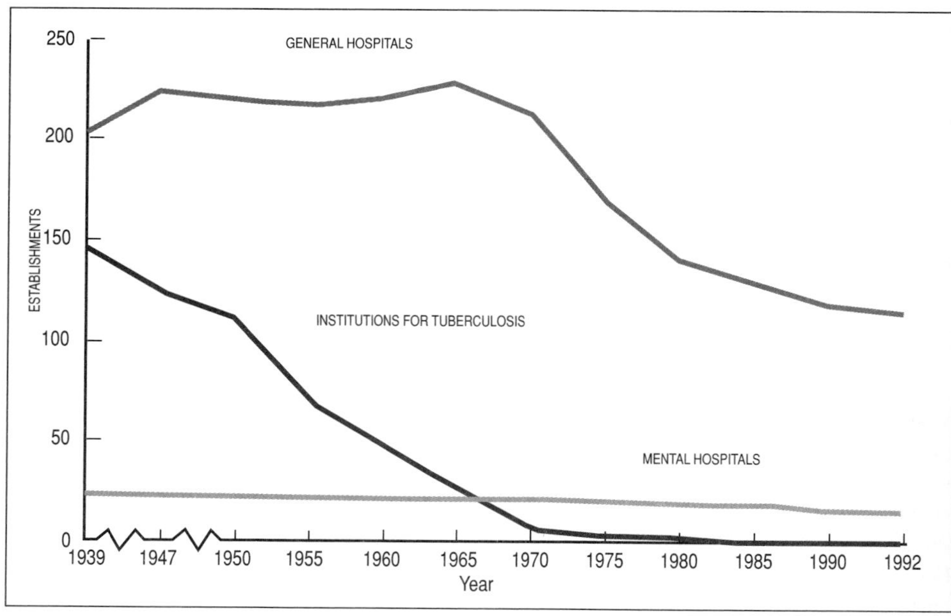

DIAGRAM 19.2
Number of hospitals in Norway from 1963 to 1992.
Source: Statistic Norway. Statistical Yearbook. «General hospitals» include only somatic hospitals. «Clinics» are private clinics run by individual doctors or organizations. «Cottage hospitals» include both ordinary cottage hospitals and small maternity homes. «Specialized hospitals» is a collective term for hospitals which offer specialized services for orthopedics, rheumatism, and epilepsy

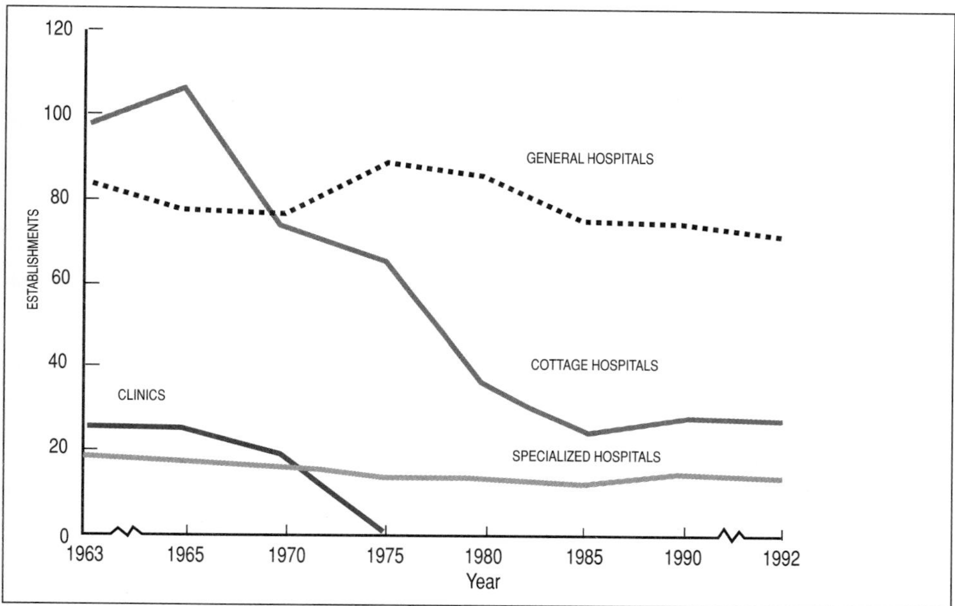

19.3. National Control

The great expansion in the number of hospitals that took place just after the turn of the century has had consequences for the structure of the hospital services right up to the 1990s. As shown in Diagrams 19.1 and 19.2, the number of somatic hospitals has remained largely unchanged since 1939. The large structure of existing hospitals has continuously been a barrier to innovative thinking.

One of the intentions of the Hospital Act (Sykehusloven) of 1969 was to remedy this situation. This law was intended to coordinate local plans for hospitals and priorities on the national level. As a consequence, private clinics and most cottage hospitals were closed down (Diagram 19.2).

However, the great turning-point first came with the Report to Parliament nr. 9, 1974–75. As a result of this report, real national control over the establishment of hospitals was achieved for the first time. At the same time, a system was established which in principle could ensure equal health services for the entire population, that is to say, equal access to hospital services, independent of geographical location and social position.

The principle of regionalization involved giving defined areas of responsibility to all hospitals in the country, as part of a coordinated nationwide plan. Hospitals were divided into four main categories: local hospitals, central hospitals, regional hospitals, and national hospitals.

Local hospitals were given responsibility for first line hospital treatment. These were small hospitals, which usually only had departments of internal medicine, surgery, and radiology. Central hospitals were given responsibility for conditions which went beyond the competence of local hospitals, either in terms of professional skills or in terms of the resources available. These hospitals were to offer a broad range of specialist services, have a relatively large catchment area, and have the main responsibility for the hospital services in the county. The regional hospitals were to have tasks which crossed county borders. They were to have medical responsibility for a region, and had to have an even higher grade of specialization than the central hospitals. The national hospital was to have a particularly broad range of specialist services and to work on a national level.

The country was divided into five health regions, each region being allocated a regional hospital. These regional hospitals were to have equal professional status, but one of them (Rikshospitalet, the National Hospital) was to function as the national hospital. In this way, all hospitals which belonged to the system were allocated a defined geographic catchment area, while at the same time every citizen belonged to a specific hospital at all levels of specialization, from the local general hospital level to the most advanced regional and national hospital level.

The most important arguments for introducing the principle of regionalization were that it made planning easier and that it made it possible to make the most rational use of both highly specialized personnel and of advanced and costly equipment. As it was impossible to provide specialists on all subjects and to provide all the latest technological developments in all hospitals, a hierarchical system according to specialty was chosen, which conveyed patients to the level of specialization required by their specific condition, while at the same time ensuring that care was provided at the lowest possible effective level.

The process of regionalization involved a radical rearrangement of the financing system. The distribution of professional medical responsibility was arranged within a defined financial framework, and the counties were given economic and administrative responsibility for running hospitals. The finances available for running hospitals therefore no longer automatically followed the accrued costs, but were given as block grants, according to the county's financial situation. The hospital budget was meant to cover all expenses for hospital services within the hospital's catchment area. A system of reimbursement was introduced in cases where it was necessary to cross county borders, the so-called guest patient arrangement, in order to correct for extra expenses associated with treating patients from other counties. On the whole, these arrangements involved a strong incentive for cut-backs and control of costs. However, there has still been a significant and steady increase in hospital running costs during the decades that have followed. (Diagram 19.3).

19.4. Technological Advances

As early as the end of World War II, the rapid development in medical technology had made it necessary to re-evaluate the organization of the hospital services. Improved surgical techniques, new methods for clinical examinations, and more effective medication made it not only possible to treat more patients and more seriously ill patients than before, but also made it necessary to demand more from the service providers.

In situations where non-specialized personnel and small local units had earlier been suficient, highly competent specialists were now needed, and large, specialized hospital departments were required, in order to fully

DIAGRAM 19.3
Total running costs of somatic hospitals in Norway from 1970 to 1992. The figures are not adjusted for inflation.

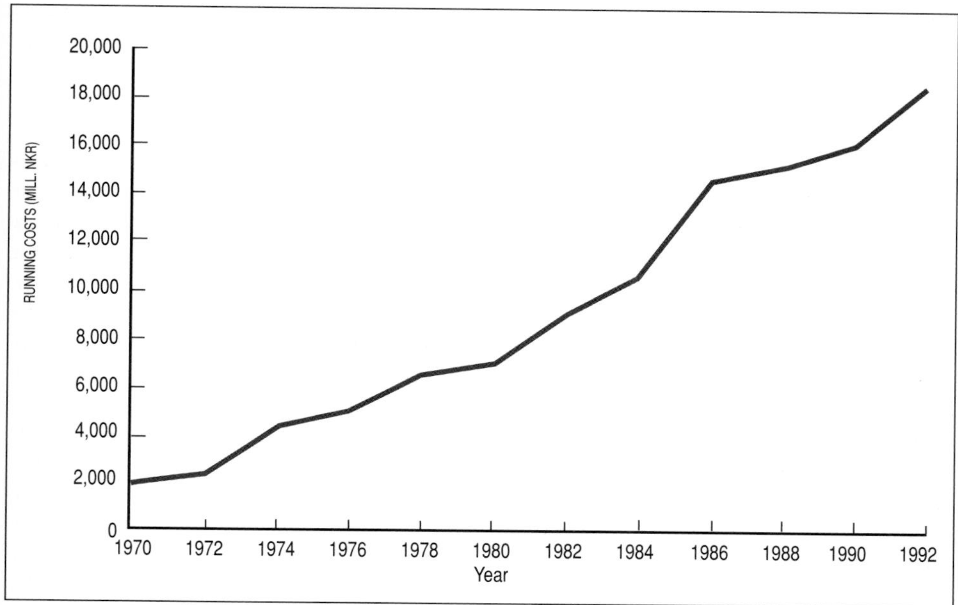

exploit the treatment possibilities available. This trend progressed, and there is little doubt that the technological advances have been one of the strongest driving forces in the expansion of the modern hospital services.

The growth in new methods of treatment made the old type of hospital that was not divided up into departments obsolete. Hospitals subdivided into three departments were established instead, with internal medicine, surgery, and radiology departments. Later on there were also the more differentiated hospitals, which in addition had special departments for other specialties, such as gynecology, pediatrics, ear, nose and throat diseases, and anesthetics. The establishment of such special departments led to an increased demand for their services, and to a steadily increasing need for medical specialists.

19.5. Increased Specialization

Doctors themselves have been driving forces behind the increasing specialization. They have ensured that the new technology has been adopted and, to a large extent, they have dictated the professional development within the hospitals. As they gained sufficient experience in using the new techniques, they developed routine procedures which they delegated to assistants, while they themselves moved on to new tasks.

Thus, increased knowledge has been one of the most important reasons for the marked specialization in hospitals during the post-World War II period. This expansion has brought about new medical specialties, for example, gastroenterology, cardiology, hematology, and endocrinology, thoracic and vein surgery, and orthopedics, and these in turn have led to a sectioning of the traditional internal medicine and surgical departments.

As a result, the level of education among the personnel has changed dramatically. For example, at the beginning of the 1990s, more than 90 percent of all Norwegian specialists in internal medicine were also specialists in one of the sub-categories of internal medicine. In the same way, hospitals right down to the local hospital level have acquired a very highly specialized medical staff.

Changes in the panorama of diseases have also influenced this development. The great increase in the number of elderly people and the number of people with cancer has formed the basis for new specialties, for new specialists, and for new special departments. During the last decade, geriatric departments have been established, both in the regional hospitals and in several of the county hospitals, and departments of oncology have been established in the regional hospitals. In contrast, the marked reduction in the number of cases of tuberculosis has led to a dramatic reduction in hospital services for this category of patients (Diagram 19.1). At the end of World War II, there were more than one hundred institutions for the treatment of tuberculosis, whereas in 1990 there were no units reserved solely for this purpose.

19.6. Effectiveness and Changes in Treatment Ideology

One of Karl Evang's great ideas was that the hospitals should be the health centers of the future. There all citizens were to have access to the best that medicine had to offer, and there most of the health personnel were to have their place of work. The aim was that the hospitals should provide both preventive and curative services, and should cater to medical needs at all levels, including the services provided by general practitioners. It was thought that physicians could not provide high-quality service without access to the equipment and laboratory services at disposal in the hospitals.

However, this policy had to be abandoned. The strain on the hospitals soon became so great that it was necessary to limit their area of responsibility. The idea of incorporating preventive work into the hospitals' responsibilities was one of the first ideas to be abandoned. Then it was realized that it was neither possible nor desirable that general practitioners should do their work in out-patient departments in hospitals, because their work was too dependent on close contacts with patients and knowledge of local conditions. Consequently, to an increasing degree the hospital became an arena for narrow, specialized medicine, where demands for efficiency steadily increased.

As possibilities for diagnosis and treatment of disease in hospitals improved, the scope of hospital activity also expanded. The number of admissions to hospitals greatly increased, from just under 300,000 admissions per year in the 1950s to about 650,000 per year in the 1980s and 1990s (Table 19.1). The number of deaths in hospitals also increased significantly, from about 7,000 per year in the 1940s to about 20,000 per year in the 1980s, perhaps reflecting a change in the view of the hospital's responsibilities toward dying people (Diagram 19.4).

At the same time, length of stay per hospital patient was dramatically reduced. Average length of stay went down from 22 days just after the Second World War to just over seven days in the 1990s. This reduction coincided with a gradual reduction in the number of hospital beds and a significant increase in out-patient facilities. One of the most important signals in the above-mentioned Report to Parliament concerning a regionalized health service was that hospitals should intensify the out-patient side of their activity, a recommendation that indeed was followed.

Altogether, this led to more intensified medical treatment and increased reliance on

Diagram 19.4
Number of patients who have died in hospitals in Norway from 1939 to 1992.
Source: Statistics Norway. Statistical Yearbook. Includes only numbers from somatic hospitals.

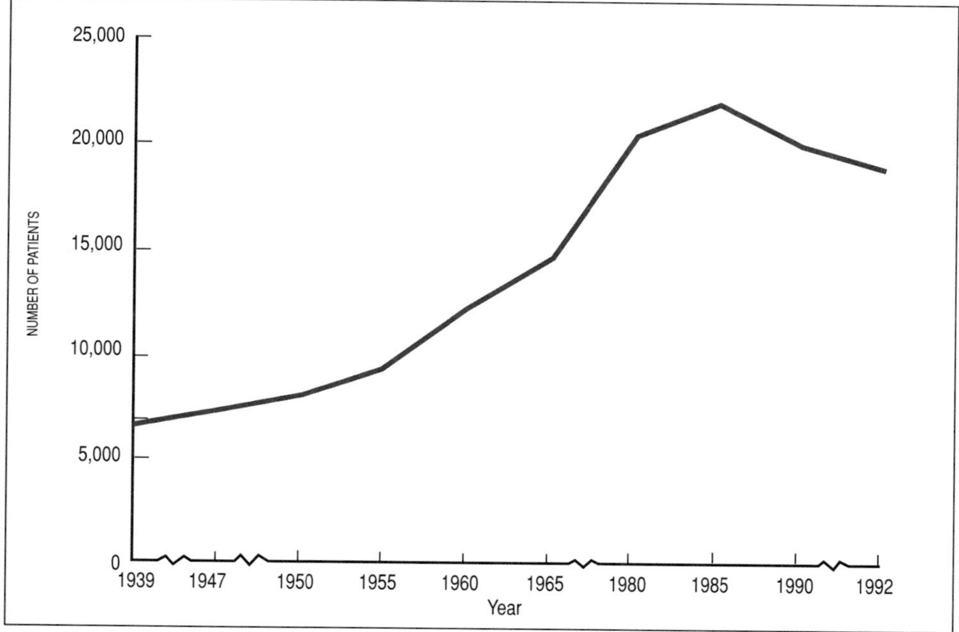

technology-based procedures. Time was no longer valued as a resource but seen as an expense. Whereas long stays in hospital, with rest and peace, previously were recommended, early dismissal and self-help were now advocated. A more careful treatment ideology was replaced by a new and aggressive approach. Conditions such as cardiac infarction and stomach ulcer were no longer treated with rest and long curative stays in hospitals, but with medication, surgery, and active training.

During the 1970s and the 1980s, technological advances made it possible to handle even complicated conditions by means of out-patient procedures, or with very short admissions for examination and treatment. New, gentle procedures based on the use of fiber optics and micro-invasive surgical techniques considerably reduced convalescence time for many patients. Therefore, hospital beds were increasingly replaced by out-patient clinics and day surgery wards.

At the same time, a larger share of responsibility for follow-up and rehabilitation was transferred to the patients themselves and to the primary health care services. Thus, the main trend has been that responsibilities and focus, to an increasing degree, have shifted from health services to self-care, from the institutions to the primary health care services, and from the health services to the home of the patient.

These trends have been particularly noticeable within psychiatry. While there has been a 30 percent reduction in the number of beds in somatic hospitals during the period from 1975 to 1992, 80 percent of beds in psychiatric hospitals were cut during the same period (Diagram 19.5). New medication and new approaches have made year-long stays in institutions unnecessary.

But, capacity in residential departments has also been reduced on the grounds of treatment philosophy. Particularly in the 1980s, leading psychiatrists strongly advocated that patients under psychiatric treatment should live in their own homes, and should stay in their own environment in order to prevent problems associated with institutionalization and withdrawal from society. Today, in the 1990s, there is a steadily increasing number of professionals who maintain that this ideology has led to a too great reduction in residential care, and that there now is a need to increase residential capacity again.

19.7. Decentralized Responsibility

While the period from 1945 to 1975 was devoted to hospitals, one might say that the

DIAGRAM 19.5

Number of hospital beds in Norway from 1939 to 1992.

Source: Statistics Norway. Statistical Yearbook. «General hospitals» include somatic hospitals, private clinics, and cottage hospitals. «Mental hospitals» include only psychiatric hospitals, and not psychiatric clinics

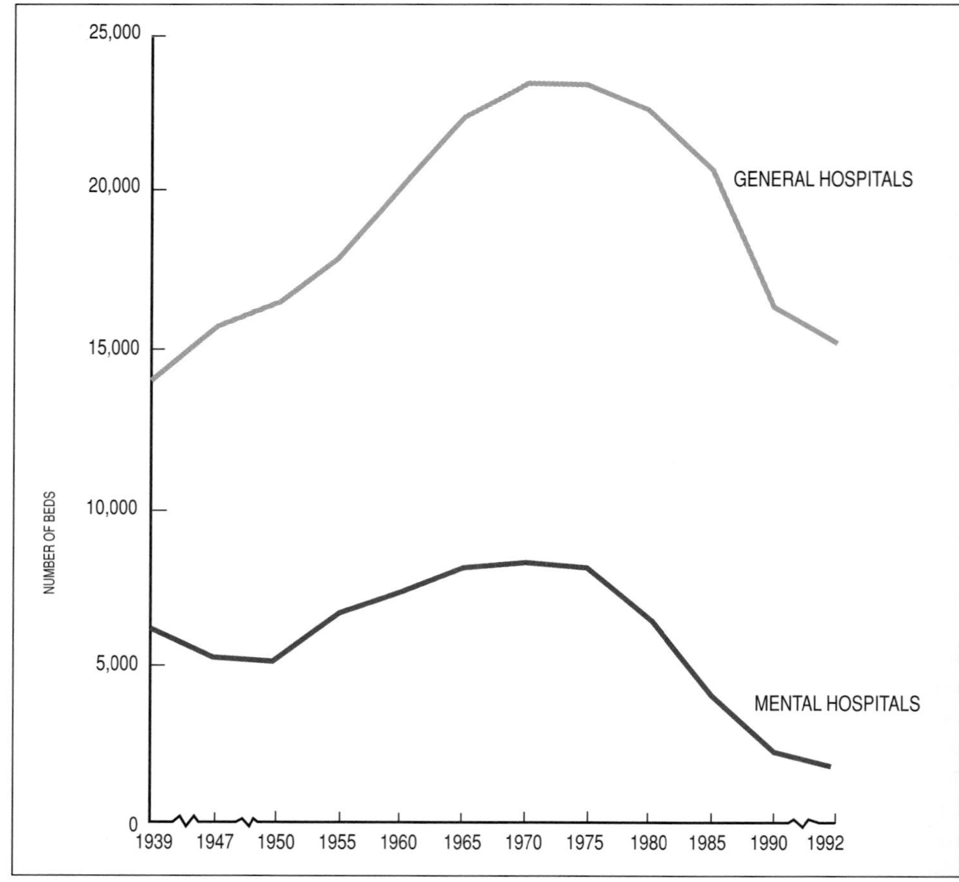

period from 1975 to 1995 has been devoted to the primary health care services. During this period there has been a massive build-up of home-based services and general practitioner services. Today, the Norwegian health services emerge as a decentralized system based on the local communities. Hospitals still provide professional impetus, but have not attained the dominating position which the health authorities in the period of reconstruction after the Second World War hoped that they would attain.

The greatest challenge faced by the health services today probably lies in the interface between the hospital and the primary health care services. The increased specialization and technological development in the hospitals have created an increasing need for systems which can ensure that the patients' needs are put into a general perspective. There are a lot of indications that this coordinating role will be allocated to the general practitioners and the primary health care services.

However, whether or not this role can be fulfilled depends upon good co-operation between first and second line services. It is probably here that the greatest potential for increased efficiency and improvement lies.

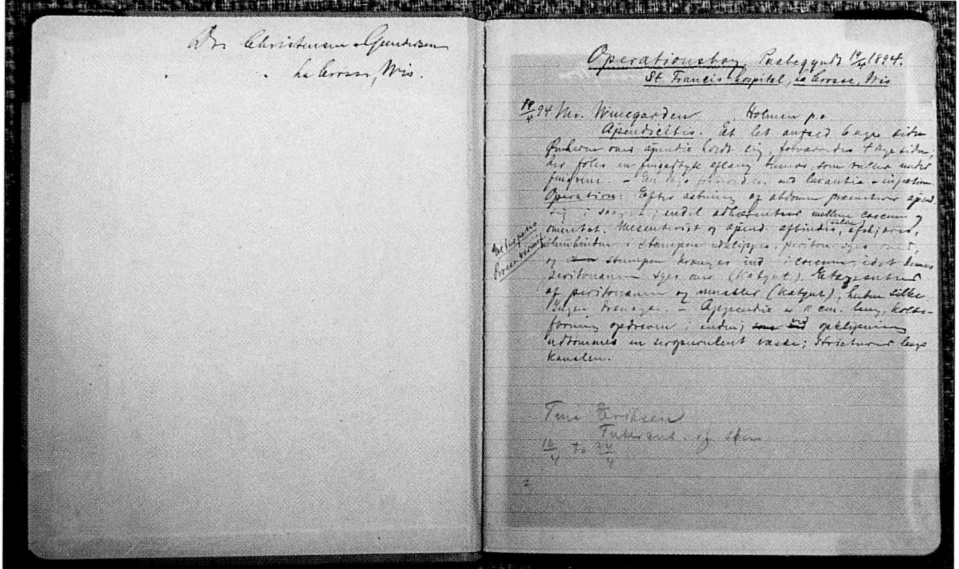

Dr. Christensen & Gundersen
La Crosse, Wis.

Operationsbog. Paabegyndt 10/4 1894.
St. Francis Hospital, La Crosse, Wis.

Figure 59: Patient record in Norwegian 1894 by Dr. Christian Christensen (1852-1919) and Dr. Adolf Gundersen (1865-1938) at St. Francis Hospital, La Crosse, Wis. U.S.A. (Photo: Øivind Larsen 1996).

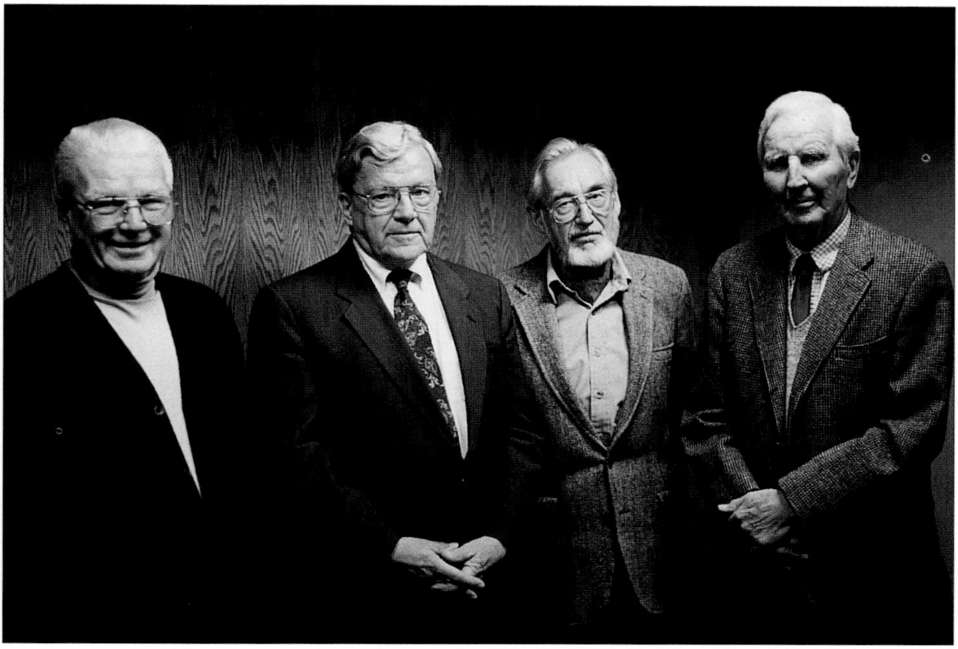

Figure 60: Medicine with a Norwegian heritage is practiced at the Gundersen Clinic, La Crosse, Wis., U.S.A. in 1996: From the left Dr. Sigurd B. Gundersen Jr. (1924-), Dr. Adolf L. Gundersen (1925-), Dr. Rolv Slungaard (1922-), and Dr. Thorolf Gundersen (1911-) (Photo: Øivind Larsen 1996).

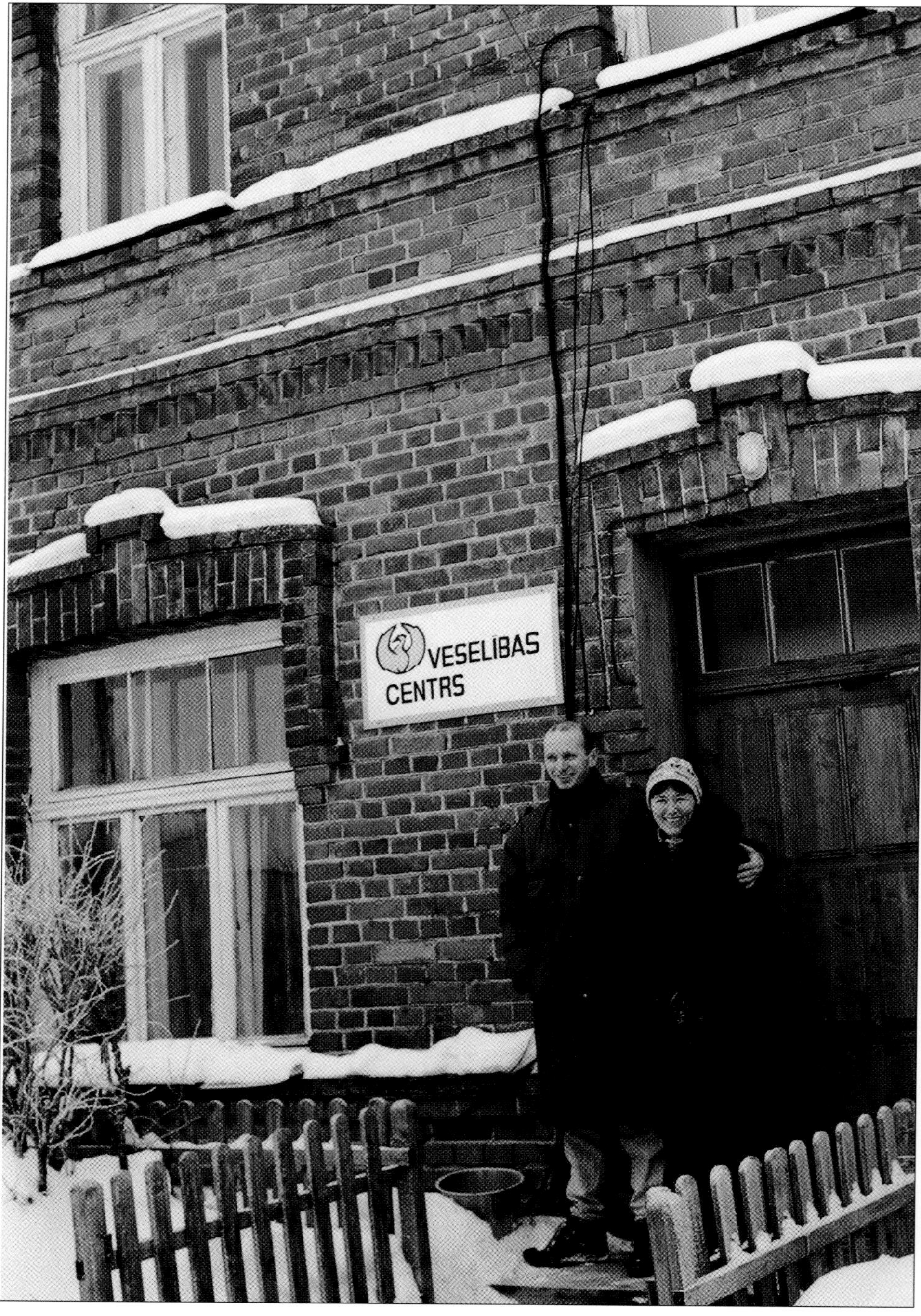

Figure 61: Norwegian physicians have often been found abroad. Here is one example from 1996: Dr. Øivind Juris Kanavin (1955-) who runs a Norwegian-style health station in the Latvian village of Madliena together with the midwife Annemette E. Riisgaard (Photo: Øivind Larsen, January 1996).

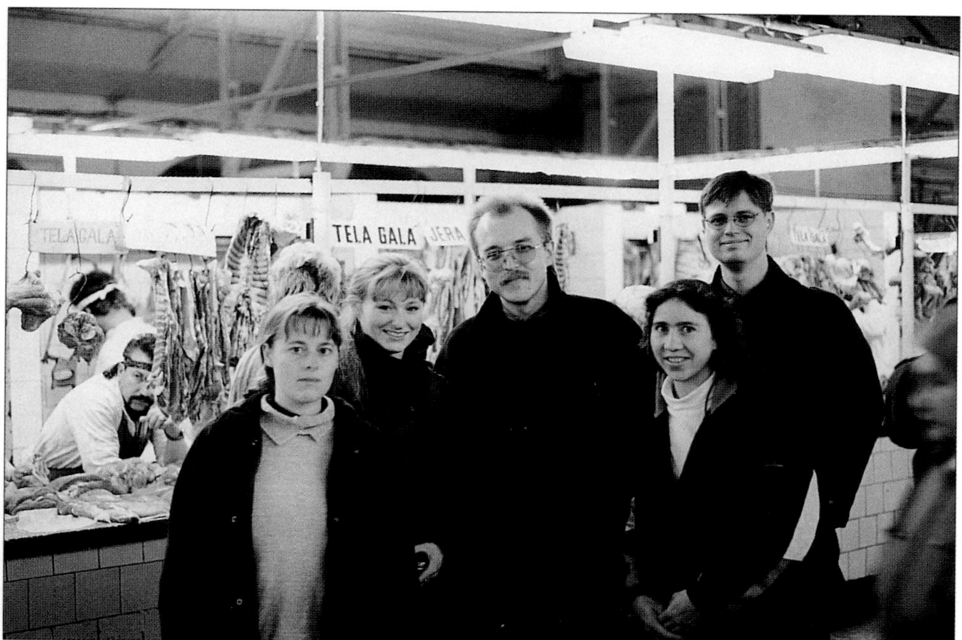

Figure 62: Going abroad as a medical student may bring perspective and insight applicable to medical knowledge intended for later use in the Norwegian health services. The teaching program in family medicine and community medicine at the University of Oslo gives interested students the possibility of going abroad to various countries where arrangements for training have been set up, for some weeks of their curriculum. This example is also from the Baltic country of Latvia: Norwegian students are comparing the principles and practice of food hygiene on the Riga food market with Norwegian conditions. From the left: Hilde Lunde, Christina Voss, their Latvian medical teacher, Dr. Guntis Kilkuts, Ellen Ann Antal, and Erling Tjora (Photo: Øivind Larsen, October 1996).

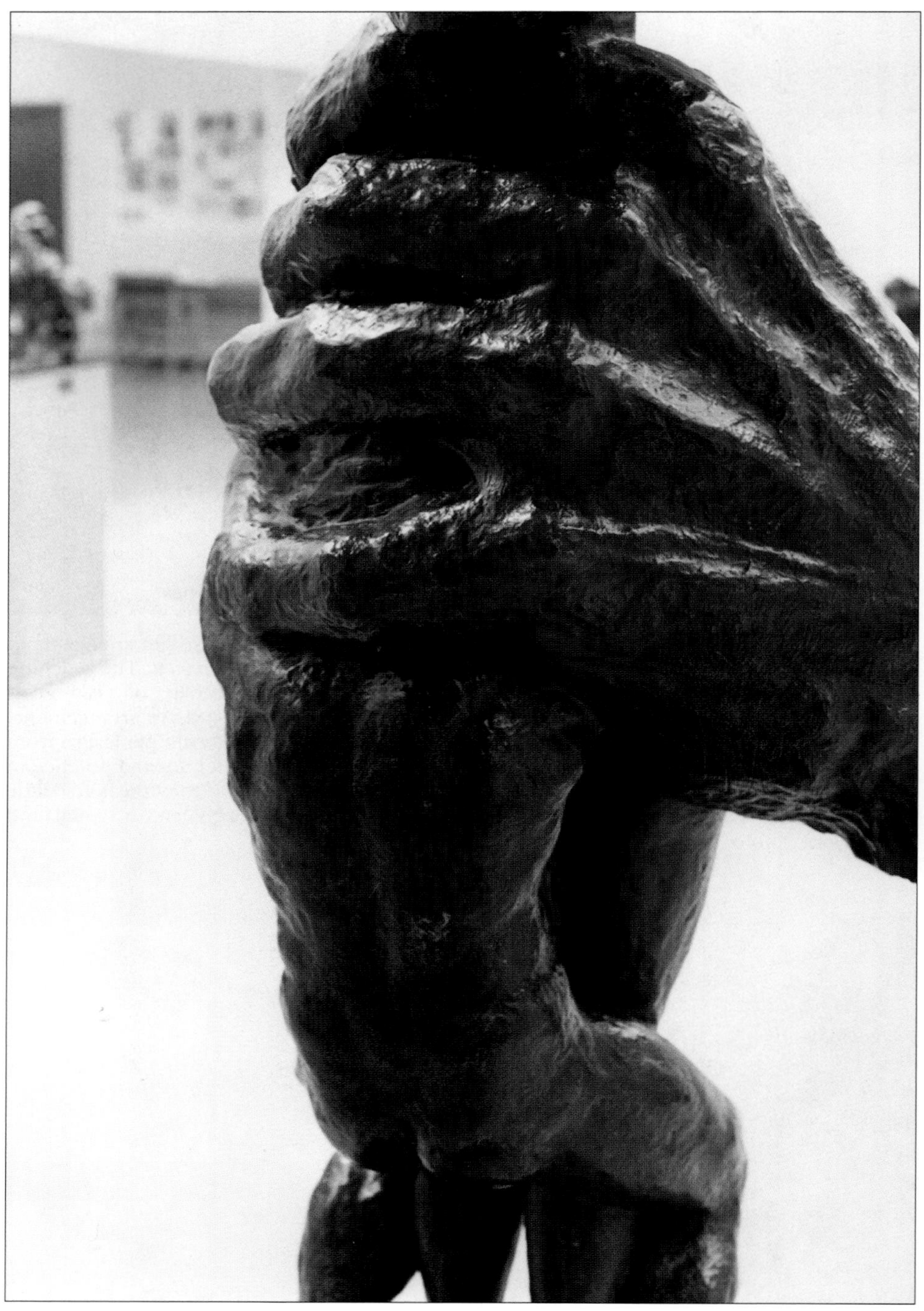

Figure 63: Cancer. Detail of a sculpture by the Norwegian physician Kaare Kristian Nygaard (1903-1989). Dr. Nygaard lived and worked as a surgeon in the United States most of his life, but was appointed professor of sculpture at the New York University 1981-1983. The sculpture was photographed at an exhibition in Lillehammer in Norway in 1987 (Photo: Øivind Larsen).

CHAPTER 20

Medical Students Abroad

TORSTEIN BERTELSEN

20.1. The Medical Degree from Foreign Universities: The Situation up to 1945

Before the Second World War, with a few, rare exceptions, there were no Norwegians who went abroad to take their medical education. In the years right before and right after the war, the number of physicians with foreign degrees who applied for a Norwegian medical license increased: refugees from Central Europe, a few Norwegians who had studied in allied and neutral countries during the war, female physicians who had married Norwegians, and a few foreigners who wished to work in Norway. But there were only a handful applicants a year.

The "Law on physicians rights and obligations" (Legeloven) of 1927 regulated medical practice and licensing in Norway. In the preliminary work that was done before this law was passed, attention was paid to whether the medical faculty in Oslo, still the only medical faculty in Norway, should decide on who should get a license to practice, as it had done before, or not (Indstilling fra Den kongelige lægelovkommission 1908, Odelstingsproposisjon No 28, 1924). Both The Norwegian Medical Association (DNLF) and the majority of the medical faculty were of the opinion that the faculty should still have this authority. But the Ministry was more foresighted, and did not rule out the possibility that another medical faculty could be established and that the two faculties could have different opinions on who should be allowed to practice. They therefore thought that the Ministry of Social Affairs should have the last word, and this was the way it turned out.

The law of 1927 determined two possible ways of attaining a license to practice:

1. The physicians with a Norwegian medical degree automatically received an authorization. According to several older laws, only the physicians with an authorization, that is, a Norwegian degree, could be appointed public health officers.
2. Those with a foreign degree could attain a license to practice (Licentia Practicandi) by way of a royal decree, after a declaration concerning the person's abilities was obtained by the medical faculty. Some physicians were given a general license without time limitations, while others got a license within a specified field or position, and sometimes also for only a limited time-span. The faculty usually demanded that the applicants for a Licen-

tia Practicandi should take exams in all the clinical disciplines of the Norwegian Study and also that they should have two years of deputyship in Norway. Other demands depended on which country and university the applicant came from.

This was practiced strictly before "Legeloven" (The law on physicians' rights and obligations) became law. The commission working on this law from 1908 refers to several earlier applications. Also, applications from Norwegians with degrees from North-American universities were mentioned. These were probably emigrants who, after completing their medical training, wanted to return to their "old-country." However, almost all of the applications were refused. The medical faculty considered it dubious that a study that could be finished in three to four years abroad should give the same rights as a Norwegian education.

The demands from the law of 1927 were not much different from those of other countries. Physicians with a foreign degree who wanted the right to practice faced new exams and obligatory deputyship everywhere, even in their home countries.

From the end of the 1920s, the medical faculty in Oslo had educated about 100 physicians annually. The pre-clinical part of the study was open, and the number of applicants increased steadily. The clinical part of the study, however, did not have room for any more than approximately 100 students annually.

Thus, toward the end of the thirties, some students had to wait for several years after completing the pre-clinical part of the studies before they could start the clinical part. After a while, the increasing number of students waiting to continue their studies made conditions at the faculty unbearable. The average length of training had increased from 7.3 years in 1930 to 9.5 years in 1939 (Universitetet i Oslo 1911–1961, 1961, Vol II). As a result, parliament was compelled to limit the admission to the pre-clinical part of the studies to 100 students per year as well. It was agreed that this number was high enough to sufficiently cover the need for physicians.

In 1940 there was one physician per 1,270 inhabitants in Norway (SSB 1978), while one physician per 800 inhabitants was considered desirable. But, as a result of the favorable demographics of the profession, it was thought that this goal would be reached within an acceptable period of time. It was not a question of a lack of physicians. On the contrary, the harmful effects on society that would be caused by an overproduction of physicians were regularly discussed (Universitetet i Oslo 1911–1961, 1961).

But then came the war and the years of occupation. Many students, including medical students, fled across the North Sea to take part in the Norwegian military forces being established in Great Britain, Canada, and The United States. Others fled by way of Sweden. An attempt was made to continue running the University in Oslo, but the Nazi governments pressure to Nazify the university gradually became unbearable. Professors were to be appointed by the Ministry, without consent or advice from the university. In the fall of 1941, the university's rector, Didrik Arup Seip (1884–1963), was removed from his position and later sent to Germany for internment. New rules and regulations for the university made it possible for the Ministry to give priority to students with Nazi sympathies in selecting students for the closed studies, among them medicine.

The confrontation between the university and the new rulers led to the closure of the university on the 30th of November 1943, with an arson fire in the university's great hall being given as the triggering cause. Between 600 and 700 students, many of them medical students, were deported for the rest of the war. One group was sent to an SS training camp in Alsace (SS Ausbildungslager Sennheim), another group to the Buchenwald concentration camp. The persistent German attempts to re-educate the students to the Nazi ideology failed completely.

When the war ended in the spring of 1945, Norway was 200 to 300 physicians short, compared to normal conditions. At the same time, all medical students had had their education delayed three or four terms. It was also predicted that a number of physicians would be deprived their right to practice because of disgraceful conduct during the war. The university in Oslo, still the only university in the country, had problems finding space, both for the delayed students who now came back to their studies, as well as for the two to three generations of students that had not yet started their education.

20.2 The Privileged Students Abroad – It Began in Denmark and Sweden

Just a couple of weeks after Germany's surrender, the rector of the University of Copenhagen, Jens Nørregaard (1887–1953), came to Oslo. Seip, the Norwegian rector, who had just returned from Germany, requested that the universities of Aarhus and Copenhagen educate a number of Norwegian medical students. The Norwegians wished that 70 to 80 freshman students, as well as 25 students who had finished the first part of their studies, could be admitted to Danish universities as early as the fall semester of 1945. They also wished that 25 studens who were to finish the first part of their studies in January 1946 could continue their studies in Denmark.

Both of the Danish universities agreed to comply with the Norwegian request, because, as it is written in a note dated 4 October 1945 from the dean of the Medical Science Faculty in Copenhagen: "In this unique situation in Scandinavian history, one could not say no to the Norwegian request for help in a time of hardship."

The two medical faculties had taken on an enormous responsibility. However, the good-will toward Norway and Norwegians that was felt throughout the Danish population was important. At the same time, negotiations took place with the consequence that 20 students of pharmacy and 18 students of odontology could undertake their studies in Denmark. This attitude was to a large extent the result of irritation and disappointment with the Danish government's policy of co-operation with the Germans during the first years of the occupation. Many had hoped for what they called "Norwegian conditions."

The medical faculties of Aarhus and Copenhagen went one step further. In a proclamation to the Danish medical profession, it was called an "undeniable duty to welcome and educate Norwegian students" (Møller 1945). They managed to find accomodation for all of the Norwegian students, many times for free. The issue was treated at the highest level, and all of the authorities were just as helpful. An extra fuel ration of 500 kilos of turf was granted for each room made available. In a letter to the rector of the University of Copenhagen, dated 8 August 1945, the minister of Trade, Industry, and Shipping stated: "I hope that we, through this, can contribute to not scaring anyone from taking on this beautiful assignment because of worries about fuel." And the minister of Social Affairs provided the necessary funds. The higher authorities wanted to be part of projects that definitely were popular with the Danish people.

20.3 New Admission Requirements

While these preparations were made in Copenhagen and Aarhus, the University of Oslo was deciding on the entrance requirements for both students who were to study in Oslo as well as those who were going to Denmark. A group of professors was assigned to investigate the possibilities for opening the medical study for students who, because of their efforts during the war, were hindered from attaining sufficiently good grades on their examen artium (the University qualifying examinations).

The first draft of the admission requirements was ready on the 2nd of July, and started like this:

> "The examen artium results alone are, especially this year, not sufficient to, on an objective basis, judge the qualities of a student that will make him or her a good physician. The examen artium results do not measure the idealism, the courage, the generosity, and the independence that are characteristic for the group of our youth that was in the frontline of the battle for our country's independence. – The group of our youth that we would prefer to have among our physicians to be."

The faculty was aware of the difficulties connected with this task. The fact that the university two years earlier had "strongly opposed" the priorities concerning closed studies given to those with political sympathies toward the Nazis made it difficult to make rules that favored those who had their loyalties on the opposite side. Admittance to the medical study was not to become a reward for fighting on the right side during the war. The final rules, therefore, emphasized that they only applied to those who had their grades spoiled by their war efforts. The Ministry of Education and Church affairs, which had to sanction the rules, stressed this point.

How good the grades of the applicants would have been without their cited efforts during the war was, of course, impossible to document. Therefore, the rules that not only decided the requirment of a main grade that was "very satisfying," but also the need for documentation of war efforts, resistance activities, imprisonment, and so on, were in reality a reward for national attitudes during the war.

Originally, these modified rules were intended to cover everyone who had applied for admission to medical studies in 1945. However, when it was clear that a large number of students could study in Denmark, it was decided that the modified rules should only apply to them, and only for the year 1945. The normal rules, those based on the grades at the examen artium alone, were to apply to the students who had to study in Oslo.

At the same time, Sweden offered to accept a number of Norwegian students as well. Seven freshmen were admitted to the old universities. In addition, medical education was started in Gothenburg, something that had been discussed for some time, but was now realized rapidly, with the Norwegians among the first students. Pre-clinic studies could not start as quickly, but the large Sahlgrenska hospital could, on short notice, establish clinical education for 39 students, divided into one class in the fall of 1945 and one in January of 1946.

Based on this, the medical faculty in Oslo decided to transfer to Sweden all the advanced students who were supposed to go to Denmark. Instead, the faculty decided on its own to increase the number of beginner students in Copenhagen and Aarhus from 70–80 to 120. Notice of this was sent by telegram to Denmark on 31 August 1945, only two days before the students were to arrive. This irritated the medical faculty in Copenhagen, but did not stop the project.

20.4 How Was this Possible?

Three months after the negotiations had started, 120 Norwegian students had already arrived in Denmark, 35 in Aarhus and 85 in Copenhagen. The number of admitted students was increased by more than one third to make room for them. First and foremost, it was good-will both among the authorities and the staff and students at the universities that made this possible. It was considered an imperative duty. The Norwegians were not considered strangers, and they quickly became a natural part of the student body. The fact that the universities' request for extra funds for the project were modest also helped the project. What was to happen later on was not a concern to begin with.

The medical curriculum, both in Aarhus and in Copenhagen, was another condition that made the project possible. The medical study was open, as it had been in Norway up until 1940. Both faculties were therefore used to large freshman classes, which were reduced by 50–60 percent after the following exams.

However, the high percentage of failure did not apply to the Norwegian students. They had lost time during the war, and were one or two years older than their Danish fellow students. Perhaps the special entrance requirements for the "Danish" students also contributed to the selection of a more mature and goal-oriented student group, something that led to good results in all of their examinations.

All the large hospitals in the Copenhagen area, to some degree, were part of the clinical part of the studies. This made the planning of the studies flexible, both for the students as well as for the administration, and provided widespread opportunities for practical training and experience in hospital wards and polyclinics.

The medical faculties in Sweden could not accept more than seven Norwegian medical freshmen. They probably did not feel that the admittance of Norwegian students was their "imperative duty" to the same extent as the Danes did. In neutral Sweden, people did not feel the same relief over Germanys fall as people in Denmark and Norway did. And Sweden had already introduced school teaching and educational plans that did not easily allow room for sudden or large increases in the student numbers.

The same year that the two Danish faculties increased their beginner classes by including 120 Norwegians, and 7 students were admitted in Sweden, the University of Oslo raised its intake number from 100 to 150. More students than that was not considered necessary. The placement of Norwegian students in Denmark and Sweden, along with the high number of new students in Oslo, was thought once and for all to solve the problem of delay in medical studies that the war had created. Later, there was to be a return to normal conditions with the education of 100 new physicians per year. The fact that this was the plan was confirmed the following year, when the medical faculty turned down an offer from Aarhus to receive more Norwegian students.

20.5 A Special Law for Medical Students Abroad

From the very beginning, it was planned that the students who were sent to Denmark and Sweden by the faculty should receive the same authorization as those with a Norwegian degree (Odelstingsproposisjon No. 76 1949). To make this possible, a law had to be passed that gave the foreign degrees a status equal to the Norwegian degree.

In the fall of 1948, about ten of those who started their studies in Denmark could move to the new medical faculty in Bergen, and a few others transferred later on.

The law passed on the 8th of July 1949 emphasized that it only applied to candidates who in advance had been chosen for this study by a Norwegian university or a postgraduate college. This applied to the medical students sent to Sweden and Denmark, as well as to a number of pharmacy and odontology students, but not to anyone who had gone out on their own initiative.

According to the law, the University of Oslo should certify that the candidates had been chosen in advance for medical studies abroad and thus made sure that the medical education did not get out of control. Even applicants who, on their own, had managed to get a place at the same universities and had passed the same exams, could receive an authorization.

According to the law, authorization could only be given to candidates who returned to Norway within six months after finishing their education. Since Norwegian authorities had made it possible for the students to study abroad, they were of the opinion that they also had the right to call the newly educated candidates back home to fill the empty spaces in the health care service as soon as possible. The students did not find this demand unreasonable either, but the law was never carried out. Some students started a specialist education in Denmark or Sweden before they returned, and a few settled abroad permanently. The law never applied to any of the later students who went abroad, and it was abolished in 1970.

We can estimate that this planned and organized education of physicians abroad produced an extra 150 new physicians in the years between 1949 and 1954, a welcomed addition at a time when a shortage of physicians was becoming a problem in many places in the country. However, this was also a group that, with its particular backgound, education, experiences and professional connections abroad, was to make itself felt within the Norwegian medical profession, both politically and professionally.

20.6 Students Abroad "of Their Own Initiative" – The Breakaway Faction

When the medical faculty at the University of Oslo in the summer of 1945 negotiated with the universities in Denmark and Sweden about the admittance of Norwegian students, the assumption was that this should be an isolated event to help recover from the problems caused by the war. Later on, Norway would educate the physicians it needed itself, as had been the rule since the University of Oslo was established in 1811. It was, however, predicted that some students would apply to foreign universities without having been admitted to the University of Oslo first. This possibility also had to be under control. In the entrance requirements to the medical study in Oslo, the faculty therefore added a new item that said that:

> *"Norwegian students who are not admitted to the medical faculty in accordance with the prevailing terms, but who have studied medicine abroad of their own initiative and taken a medical exam there, cannot count on getting a licentia practicandi in Norway."*

In spite of the fact that this regulation clearly was in conflict with the physicians statute of 1927, which said that a license was to be given after an individual assessment of the candidate's qualities, it was silently accepted both by the Senate of the University of Oslo and by the Ministry of Education and Church affairs. The ruling was not only limited to 1945, but became a regular part of the entrance requirements. The following years the ruling was referred to in all letters to the many applicants who were not accepted into the medical study in Oslo.

The medical faculty in Oslo went one step further when it notified the applicants that the University could not recommend a currency-license for medical studies abroad. A currency-license was at that time necessary for all stays in foreign countries.

The Ministry of Education and Church affairs followed suit. A newly established "Office for studies abroad," later renamed "Office for cultural relations with countries abroad," were to give practical advice to students who wished to study abroad. However, this did not apply to medical students. In a circular letter sent to potential students abroad, it was stated that physicians educated abroad could not count on receiving a license to practice in Norway, and that it would not be recommended to give a currency-license for such studies.

20.7 A Good Proposition from Aarhus

In spite of this, there were many students who, after receiving a refusal from Oslo, wanted to go abroad to study medicine.

Germany and Austria, which had accepted a large number of foreign students before the war, had been our enemies through five years of war. The first five or six years after the war ended, it was out of the question to go to these countries to study. This would almost have been considered treason. A small number of Norwegian medical students were admitted to studies in allied or neutral countries, mainly in Great Britian, the Netherlands, and Switzerland, but also a few in the United States and Canada. A large majority, however, tried to apply for studies in Denmark and Sweden. Aarhus received so many applications from Norwegian students that the Medical Faculty there, in 1946, expressed their willingness to the University of Oslo to find room for more than the 35 students they had agreed to admit the previous year.

The faculty board in Oslo discussed the matter a couple of weeks later, and came to the conclusion that they would not accept the offer. In a letter to Aarhus, dated 12 September 1946, the dean, Torleif Dale, expressed their gratitude for the generous offer, but stated that the University of Oslo from now on was capable of educating the number of physicians the country needed. In addition, the faculty found it difficult to come to fair terms in a competition for the study places made available in Aarhus.

Before the letter with the answer was sent to Aarhus, neither the countrys highest health authorities, The Directorate of Health/The Ministry of Social Affairs, nor The Ministry of Education and Church affairs were allowed a say in the affair. The faculty obviously felt that it could decide on its own the number and the placement of the medical study positions, as well as how many physicians the country needed. Both the faculty and The Norwegian Medical Association were firmly convinced that 100 new physicians per year would cover the country's needs. This corresponded with the yearly admittance of new medical students to the faculty in Oslo, and consequently there was no reason for admitting more people to the study.

The Norwegian Medical Association did not attach any importance to the analysis of the need for physicians, recently made by the Director General of Health Services, Karl Evang (1902–1981), who had concluded that 150 new physicians should be educated per year for the first few years and that after that, a stable number of 125 new students per year would be required.

20.8 "Evasion of Our Rules"

Moreover, the faculty in Oslo went to great lengths to prevent individuals with possibilities to study abroad from realizing their plans. In 1947, a physician who contacted the faculty in Aarhus about a position of study for his son had his request refused after the faculty in Aarhus had checked with the faculty in Oslo. The dean of the Oslo faculty referred to the principled stand it had taken because competition was very fierce, and an evasion of the rules would seem unfair to the many who did not have sufficient financial possibilities and connections to get admitted to foreign universities. He therefore suggested that they should write to doctor Christophersen and tell him that it was not possible to get his son admitted to the University of Aarhus.

As early as 1945, when the threat of denied license to practice was added to the entrance requirements, a majority of the Oslo faculty had already developed a strong dislike for Norwegians who went abroad to study medicine "on their own initiative."

To begin with, the official justification for this standpoint was the principle of fairness, the consideration for all of the students who, for various reasons, could not go abroad to study, and the alleged problems involved with selecting the students who were to be permitted to go. Later came the worries concerning the cost of having students abroad, and finally, when the conflict intensified toward the end of the 1950s, questions were asked about the professional qualities and moral standards among the students abroad. The real reason for the opposition, however, was probably simpler: worries that with so many physicians the source of income would decrease.

Such worries were not unusual among Norwegian physicians in the years before and after the war. This can be seen from several cases in which doctors protested against colleagues establishing a practice on their turf, or against the establishment of specialist wards in neighboring towns.

It was Axel Strøm (1901–1985), professor of Hygiene from 1940 and Social Medicine from 1952, and dean of the Medical Faculty from 1956, who for decades was to lead the campaign against students abroad. And for obvious reasons. Apart from being the first among equals at the faculty, he was also the President of the Medical Association from 1948 to 1952. He did not try to conceal the fact that he defended the economic interests of the medical profession.

In an article in The Journal of the Norwegian Medical Association (Strøm 1952), Strøm claimed that 100 new physicians annually was enough to cover the demand. The "optimal demand for physicians," meaning the number of physicians the country needed so that "all citizens would have just as easy access to medical help and to full medical services under all circumstances," was probably somewhat larger. This aim, however, was unrealistic. The authorities have "after the war pursued a hard-lined policy of cutbacks towards the physicians' incomes, so that these now have reached a level where many doctors cannot manage financially without a work effort and working hours that go beyond the reasonable and in many cases beyond the responsible."

"The real demand for physicians, that is the number of physicians the country has financial ability and will to support," was therefore of much greater interest. As early as in 1950, the faculty in Oslo suggested a prohibition against the admittance of physicians with degrees from foreign universities, both Norwegians and foreigners. Exceptions to this were only to be made in special cases, for example, for persons with "exceptional qualifications."

The faculty in Oslo's dislike of medical studies abroad was well known at the other Nordic faculties, and they followed Oslo's wishes loyally. Between ten and fifteen years were to pass before the universities in Denmark and Sweden once again admitted Norwegian medical students.

20.9 New Countries of Study

It was more difficult for the faculty in Oslo to influence the universities further south. After some time, Germany and Austria had become more politicaly acceptable, and they also welcomed foreign students. These were inexpensive countries to study in. An increasing "emigration" of Norwegian medical students to universities in South and Middle Europe started around 1950. They left of their own accord. Through the letters of refusal from the University of Oslo, they were familiar with the threat that they would be denied a license to practice after they had completed their studies.

This, along with the announcement that the University could not recommend them for a currency-license, contributed to making these students look somewhat like dissidents who did not want to follow the laws. Nevertheless, an increasing number of people started doubting that this threat could be carried out in the long run. Their battle for the right to practice would not be fought before they had passed their examinations, in six or seven years time. A lot might have happened before that time. In 1952–53 there were a little more than 100 Norwegian medical students at foreign universities, not counting the privileged ones in Denmark and Sweden (Diagram 20.1). Approximately two thirds of these were in Germany and Austria.

The majority of these pioneers were supported by resourceful parents, people who could demand a reasonable explanation for why a young physician, educated at a highly respected foreign university, could not receive a license to practice in Norway. As many as 17.5 percent of them were children of physicians, compared to 14 percent of the medical students in Norway (Bruusgaard and Gjestland 1976). It is impossible to assess how many students were deterred from a medical study abroad by the threats of being denied a license after graduation.

20.10 *The Truth is Revealed*

The threat to deny licenses to physicians educated abroad "on their own initiative"

DIAGRAM 20.1

The State Educational Loan Fund's registration of medical students abroad «of their own initiative» 1952–1995

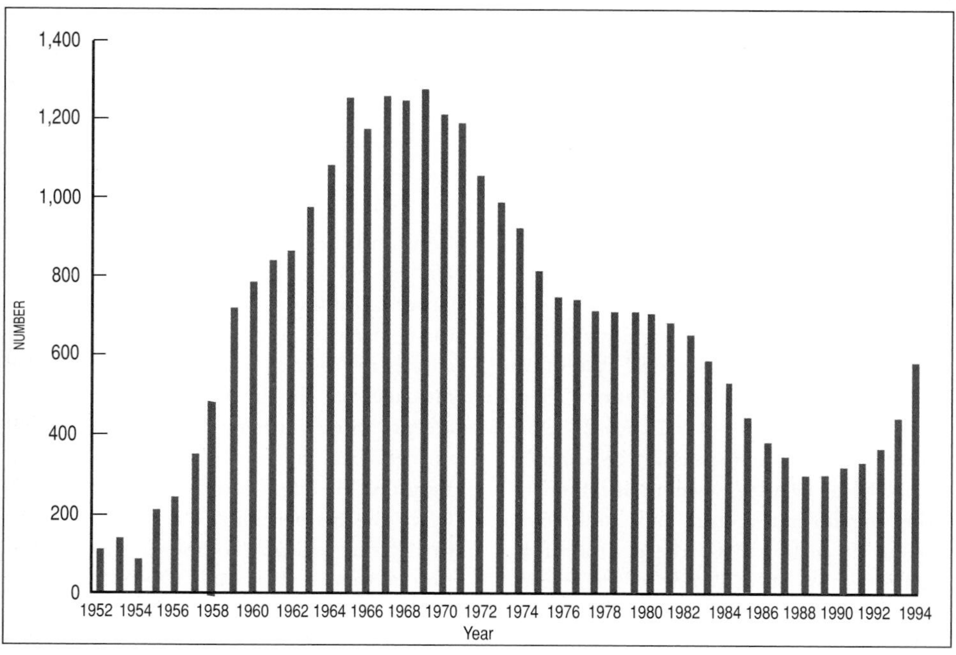

was widely distributed and was well known to everybody interested in the matter. Nevertheless, it created quite a stir when a student, in the fall of 1953, went to see the dean of the Medical Faculty in Oslo and told him that he, in a conversation with the rector at the University of Aarhus, had been shown a letter in which the University of Oslo had requested the University of Aarhus not to admit any Norwegian medical students, except for those who had been selected by the faculty in Oslo in advance. The new rector of the University of Oslo, Dr. Juris. Frede Castberg (1893–1977), immediately wrote a letter to his colleague in Aarhus. The medical faculty did not know of such a letter, but he had been informed from different sources that such letters had been written to Danish and Swedish universities. He assured his colleague that the Senate "now at least" no longer wished that Norwegian students be refused on such a basis.

The answer from the rector in Aarhus, dated 26. September 1953, made it quite clear that the faculty in Oslo twice had expressed that, on the grounds of their principles, they were opposed to Norwegian students being accepted in Denmark. It was the letter of refusal from Oslo of Aarhus' offer to accept more Norwegian students, dated 12 September 1946, that was so conveniently referred to, along with the long-forgotten letter about the chief physician's son.

For Castberg, a lawyer with administrative law as one of his fields of speciality, and who had claimed that our legal system was one where "all coincidence is banned" (Universitetet i Oslo 1911–1961, Vol. I, 1961), it must have been embarrassing to learn that the Medical Faculty, without intervention from the former rector, had gone so far beyond its authority. Castberg wrote in his memoires that the attitude of the Medical Faculty after the war was very hostile towards Norwegian medical candidates from foreign universities (Castberg 1971). We shall come back to this later.

The student John Berglund (b.1934), who had started the commotion, was not content with oral assurances of the University's new attitudes toward studies abroad. He demanded a written statement, which he received. In this statement, the dean of the Medical Faculty, professor Georg Waaler (1895–1983), declared void any previous agreement or request for the refusal of Norwegian students.

20.11 *"Declaration"*

> The student John Berglund has been to see me as dean of the Medical Faculty at the University of Oslo, because he intends to apply for medical studies in Sweden. As the existence of an agreement or a request from the Medical Faculty in Oslo that the other medical faculties in Scandinavia refuse to admit Norwegian students to the medical study might be used as reason for refusal, I would like to state that the University's and the Faculty's stand is no longer in accordance with any such agreement. If it exists, it will therefore from our point of view be regarded as terminated, so that we no longer will contribute to hindering Norwegian students from studying in Sweden.
>
> G. Waaler
> Dean of the Medical Faculty

Berglund did not benefit from his efforts. He was not admitted to the medical study either in Aarhus or in Stockholm, in spite of the declaration. He had to start his medical studies in Austria (Graz). But then came the message that the faculty in Oslo would not accept exams from any German or Austrian universities, as we shall see later on. Berglund therefore had to apply for a transfer to the Netherlands (Utrecht), where he finally succeeded in completing the education he wanted (Berglund 1995).

20.12 How Great Was the Demand for Physicians?

In the years around 1950, a certain concern about the low number of new physicians was spreading, both among the authorities and the public. The faculty in Oslo still admitted only 100 students annually. The authorities had become more skeptical and refused a proposal from the faculty for a collective ban on all physicians educated abroad. The Ministry was now of the opinion that the "law on physicians rights and obligations" (Legeloven) gave each individual applicant the right to have his or her "abilities" assessed for a Norwegian license. This, however, should have been apparent as early as 1945. The real reason for the refusal of the suggestion was probably that the authorities now had discovered that the Medical Faculty had a pursued union policies little too enthusiastically, instead of educating a sufficiently large number of physicians. In a Report to Parliament the Ministry concluded that, in a transitional period, 175 physicians should be educated annually, and after that 150 per year (Stortingsmelding No. 45 1950).

The main reason for Castberg's letter and Waaler's declaration was probably to distance themselves and the Senate from the somewhat dubious dealings of the Medical Faculty. Nothing was done to relieve the pressure on the students abroad. The letter and the declaration were not made known among other students who planned to try their luck abroad. And, as far as we know, none of the other medical faculties in the Nordic countries were informed. Anyway, the number of Norwegian students admitted to the medical faculties in our neighboring countries did not increase until many years later.

There was no change of attitude in the Medical Faculty. Only six months after the John Berglund incident, Axel Strøm made clear the faculty's restrictive attitude toward studies abroad in two articles in the Journal of the Norwegian Medical Association (Strøm 1954a and 1954b). The old arguments were used again:

> "It would be unreasonable and undemocratic if Norwegian students who, because of financial benefits and connections abroad, could be admitted to studies abroad, were to become Norwegian physicians... while their less fortunate friends who perhaps were as good or better physician material, were cut off from the medical career."

But, these noble arguments did not have the same persuasive force as they had had right after the war, when the sense of togetherness and equality between high and low, rich and poor had been an important factor in the struggle against the common enemy. Now the authorities also claimed that the faculty's attitude was in contradiction with the trends in other countries toward mutual recognition of university exams.

At least the faculty no longer claimed that its own education of new physicians was sufficient to meet the demand. It had become too obvious that this was not the case. Silently, the higher numbers from the Report to Parliament had to be accepted. However, in reply to a question from the Ministry, the faculties in both Oslo and Bergen claimed that the Director General of Health Services' estimate of 125 physicians annually was sufficient, and would also cover future needs within education and research.

20.13 Within the Framework of the Law

A new proposal from the faculty to the effect that all students with a foreign medical degree applying for a Norwegian license must pass Norwegian examinations in all subjects in the clinical part of the study was also rejected. The Ministry was of the opinion that the rules had to stay within the confines of the law and that an individual evaluation should be made. Then one could formulate certain basic requirements that had to be fulfilled, as proof of sufficient proficiency. And this was the way it was to be. The following requirements had to be fulfilled, according to professor Strøm (1954a and 1954b):

1. The first condition for being evaluated at all was that the foreign examination had been passed at a university that was recognized by the faculty as "giving an education of similar character as the Norwegian one."

Such an approval or refusal had to be based on a professional evaluation of the educational standards of the university. Without approval of the university, no applicant could be considered "proficient." One saw the difficulties in such an evaluation of the different universities, but was of the opinion that one could consult a report made by the American Council on Medical Education and Hospitals, where also the percentage of failure of physicians from different countries was given. The universities in Denmark and Sweden were the first to be approved, as were the universities in the Netherlands, Great Britain, Paris, Strasbourg, Albany, and Zürich.

2. Examinations had to be passed in those subjects the faculty decided in each individual case.

This would usually mean full Norwegian examination of the clinical part of the study. In other words, the foreign medical degree was regarded as equal to the Norwegian preclinical part of the study, while knowledge of the clinical subjects had to be documented again by passing full Norwegian examinations.

3. The applicant had to go through practical duty similar to the Norwegian internship arrangements.

Since mandatory internship service had been introduced in 1954 for Norwegian candidates, this was a reasonable demand. But, for the candidates who took their education abroad, the duration and the character of the practical duty was to be assessed by the faculty in each individual case. In addition, the applicant had to find the position on his or her own. Only by coincidence would it be possible for an applicant from a foreign university to enter the regular internship system, stated Professor Strøm.

When all of the above requirements were fulfilled, the Director General of Health Services would give a statement in which he would also take the moral standards of the applicant into consideration. The rules were made public by the Ministry of Social Affairs/The Directorate of Health in the summer of 1953 (Sosialdepartement 1953). Almost all of the students abroad found the rules unnecessarily strict, but were pleased with the fact that the students abroad "on their own initiative" for the first time were accepted as a new group of students that both the medical faculty and the Ministry had to take into consideration.

20.14 No German or Austrian Universities Were Accepted

The faculty quickly decided that German and Austrian universities could not be approved as "giving an education of similar character as the Norwegian one." The professional standards in these countries were supposed to be too low. Axel Strøm reminded his readers that "the deterioration of German and Austrian medicine had started long before the war, namely from the time the Nazis came into power" (Strøm 1954c). In addition, these countries had been through five years of war. He was probably right. But, nine years had now passed since the end of the war. The fact that it was still easier and more acceptable to discriminate against our old enemies than against others is not mentioned. But those who remember the mood from those days will know that, to a great degree, this was the case.

Probably the most important reason for making Germany and Austria particularly negative cases was not mentioned, either. At that time (1954), it was known that of the 86 Norwegian citizens studying abroad, 67 were studying in Germany and Austria. By refusing to recognize medical examinations from these countries, one could, in one stroke, remove 80 percent of the Norwegian students abroad who could apply for a Norwegian license. This would be a substantial blow to what Strøm had called "the problem with physicians educated outside Norway" (Strøm 1954a).

20.15 The Legation Was Notified

The Medical Faculty at the University of Oslo issued a report on medical studies abroad (Det medisinske fakultet 1954). This was passed on to the legation in Bonn on 6 November 1954. The report and the letter stated:

> "According to the information that is gathered about the medical education in Germany and Austria, the Medical Faculty finds that it cannot be regarded as equal to the one that is given in Norway. The study at these universities do therefore not meet the requirements made by the faculty. The faculty can therefore for the time being not approve education at German and Austrian universities as basis for taking tests at the Medical Faculty in Oslo.

From the legation, the message was passed on in a letter to known students, amongst others, in Heidelberg on 16 November 1954. Here it is stated that the Ministry of Education and Church Affairs had recommended that the students apply for a transfer to the following universities that were recognized by the medical faculty: Zürich, London, Cambridge, Oxford, Sheffield, Durham, Leeds, Manchester, Liverpool, Bristol, Wales, St. Andrews, Edinburgh, Glasgow, Aberdeen, Strasbourg, Paris, Toulouse, Utrecht, Groningen, Amsterdam, Leiden, Toronto, The Albany Medical College, U.S.A, and the universities in Denmark and Sweden. But, this list of "recognized" universities was almost fictitious, because at the same time, in the letter to the legation in Bonn, it was stated that:

> "students cannot for the time being count on being admitted at the universities in Denmark and Sweden. It is also very difficult to get admitted to British universities."

With this declaration, almost all universities of most interest to Norwegian applicants had again been removed from the lists. Left were a couple of universities in the United States and Canada, which could only be of interest to the wealthiest; three French universities where the language was a serious obstacle for most Norwegians; and four Dutch universities that everybody knew had room for only a very limited number of foreign students.

We have earlier mentioned a student, John Berglund, who had been affected by this decision. He had courage and backing enough to immediately manage to be admitted to a recognized university. We do not know how many others did the same. Neither do we know how many students felt forced to give up their medical studies after Germany and Austria were ruled out.

It was a consolation that Statens Lånekasse (The State Educational Loan Fund), in the letter to the legation in Bonn, had stated that it would not categorically deny students (in Austria and Germany) continued loans. Professor Axel Strøm thought that this was regrettable and found "reason to point out that the granting of such loans does not mean that the person will get a Norwegian license. Those considering going abroad this year to study medicine should bear this in mind" (Strøm 1954a).

Still, many regarded this as a sign that the authorities were changing their mind and that the faculty in Oslo could not ban physicians from German or Austrian universities forever. They continued their studies.

20.16 *"Attack on the Faculty"*

In the middle of the 1950s, more and more people voiced critical opinions about the restrictive policies toward the medical students abroad. The chief physician at the Eye Clinic in Bodø, Anton Johnson (1893-1967), immediately wrote an answer to the two articles by Strøm in the Journal of the Norwegian Medical Association.

Johnson was critical of Strøm's statements, particularly because of "the many Norwegians who study medicine in Germany and Austria, and also because of common courtesy toward the medical research and universities in these countries" (Johnson 1954).

In relation to these two countries, politeness was not common, but Johnson could more easily do this, because he had been a prominent member of the resistance during the war. Chief physician Johnson also felt that there was a certain amount of bad feelings toward those who studied abroad. The Medical Faculty's use of the expression "unreasonable and undemocratic" to describe these studies pointed in that direction. In Johnson's opinion, the faculty had in this matter exceeded its competence and infringed on social aspects that should have been the Ministry's field. He also stated that it is often energetic and especially interested students who take upon themselves the task of studying medicine in a foreign country.

In his reply in the same number of The Journal of the Medical Association (Strøm 1954c) Axel Strøm would not rule out the possibility that there might be a change in the faculty's decision about the German and Austrian universities. "It is a fact that among the students who study abroad there are many sons of colleagues," he states in his answer, and continues: "Since I wrote my report in The Journal, I have been contacted regularly by both colleagues and others. These have all been on behalf of a student abroad and have all – apart from some neutral inquiries – represented an attack on the faculty."

As mentioned before, many of the medical students abroad were children of physicians. Thus, it is understandable that many of them wrote to Strøm. He was not only a member of the Medical Faculty, where he was soon to become dean, but also the newly retired President of The Norwegian Medical Association.

These "attacks on the faculty" were now also being made by some of the faculty's own members. Professor Carl Semb (1895-1971), a well-known surgeon at the Ullevål Hospital, had a son who studied medicine in England. When it was revealed that the Medical Faculty had asked the Bank of Norway to deny medical students abroad a currency-license, there were strong confrontations between him and the strongest proponents of a restrictive policy (Semb 1995).

The complete disqualification of the universities in Austria and Germany could not last for long. In 1955, only two years later, the faculty in Oslo had to recognize the University of Graz, and a few months later also the University of Vienna and a number of German universities as providing an education similar to the Norwegian universities. But, the catch was that the study had to be followed by three years (Austria) or two years (Germany) of internship duty.

20.17 *Discord over the Process of Validation*

In accordance with the law of 1927, which states that the Medical Faculty in Oslo (the only medical faculty in Norway at that time) was to provide a statement on the candidate's proficiency, it was assumed that the exams mentioned in item two above were to be taken there. But now the situation that the Ministry had predicted when making the law had become reality. A new medical faculty had been established in Bergen, with the same professional functions as the one in Oslo, but seemingly without the possibility to evaluate the proficiency of physicians with a foreign degree. This was a privilege that the faculty in Oslo wanted to keep for itself, but that was taken away in a somewhat surprising manner.

During the treatment of the first application to the faculty in Bergen for approval as a Norwegian physician from a physician educated abroad, it was concluded that §22 in the university law gave them the possibility to recognize the exams he had passed in Switzerland as parts of a Norwegian Medical Education. In that way, the Oslo Faculty's monopoly of recognizing foreign educations was broken. With knowledge of the place of study abroad, the individual teacher could decide whether the foreign exam corresponded with the Norwegian one in duration and contents. If this was the case and the applicant then took additional exams in the national subjects, forensic medicine, hygiene, and social medicine, he or she could be given a Norwegian degree from the University of Bergen. This meant automatic authorization on the same terms as the faculty's own candidates.

The faculty in Oslo did not accept this interpretation of the law. Axel Strøm, who became dean in 1956, did not want to put up with the new Bergen faculty's infringement on what had so far been Oslo's territory. On the other hand, dean Jørgen Løvset (1896–1981) in Bergen, would not accept being directed from Oslo. In a new case, there was quite a nalsh correspondence between the two deans. It went so far that Løvset, in a letter to Strøm on 10 December 1956, hinted that the applicant might seek legal advice to have his case tried. The faculty in Bergen got support from two of the professors in Oslo, the newly retired dean of the faculty, Georg Waaler, and Carl Semb, whose son had now finished his medical exams in England. They had contacted the Director General of the Health Services and the Ministry of Education and Church Affairs and had received confirmation that the University Law for Bergen made it possible to recognize foreign exams as part of the Norwegian education. This was a view that could easily be supported by the dean in Bergen, professor Erik Waaler (b. 1903), who at that time (1956) also had a son who considered studying medicine abroad.

The law pertaining to the University of Oslo did not have a similar rule, and the majority of the faculty did not want it, either. Only after having passed the examination according to the requirements mentioned above could the foreign examination be evaluated as equal to the Norwegian exam and had to make do with a license to practice (licentia practicandi) after application to the Ministry of Social Affairs. This was important to the medical students abroad, partly because of the prestige of having a Norwegian degree, which was considered superior, and partly due to financial and practical reasons, since a Norwegian exam was necessary to get appointed to posts such as District Physician.

20.18 Common Guidelines. The Rector Had to Interfere

Even though the approval of foreign medical exams led to different results at the two universities, the Ministry demanded that the procedure and requirements for exams and so on must be the same. A committee from the two faculties started to work on this.

The composition of the committee reflected the attitudes at the two faculties.

Bergen appointed Professor Erik Waaler, who, like his brother Georg Waaler in Oslo, had a liberal attitude toward students abroad. This also applied to the other member from Bergen, dean Jørgen Løvset, who as we have seen, had vigorously fought in the first acceptance cause for a student abroad.

The representatives from Oslo were totaly different. The fact that Axel Strøm, who now was the dean of the Oslo faculty had a very restrictive attitude, was well known. And Frederik Leegaard (1891–1970), professor in physiology, had been the chairman of the committee that earlier had proposed that all candidates with foreign examinations had to pass all Norwegian examinations, also those from the pre-clinical part of the studies.

The committee could quickly agree that all candidates with foreign exams had to pass exams in all the national subjects, mentioned above. But here agreement ended, both within the committee and also between the two faculties. After engaging in a long tug of war trying to reach a common agreement, the two faculties issued separate proposals for the Senates in Bergen and Oslo, respectively.

Both proposals stated that, as a rule, all candidates with foreign exams, except those taken in Denmark and Sweden, had to pass Norwegian tests in all clinical subjects. But, only the proposals from Bergen added that the demand for a Norwegian test did not apply if the exam at the foreign university could be regarded as equal to the Norwegian exam.

This would give the faculty in Bergen the possibility to carry on with its practice of giving foreign students Norwegian degrees. This arrangement could not be accepted by the faculty in Oslo, where full Norwegian exams in the clinical subjects were demanded.

Again, the Senate in Oslo, under Frede Castberg, had to intervene. Castberg writes about this incident in his memoirs:

> ...but also the "guidelines" that the Medical Faculty proposed in response to the new University law of December 1956 were in my opinion far too strict... According to the faculty's proposal, there would in no case be any possibility to accept any exam in these subjects from a single university in the entire world, apart from the Nordic countries. This was in my opinion unreasonable. . . . I therefore had to propose to the Senate that they, in this important matter repudiate the Medical Faculty. The discussion in the Senate proceeded in a calm and friendly manner. The members of the Senate, apart from Strøm, accepted my proposal, which therefore became the University's point of view (Castberg 1971).

In an accompanying letter to the Ministry of Education and Church Affairs dated 20 December 1956, the Senate strongly supported the position that foreign clinical examinations should be recognized, even if they were from universities outside Denmark and Sweden. The ministry agreed to this liberal attitude. In the summer of 1957, equal guidelines were made for both the universities. Each applicant was to be evaluated on an individual basis by a committee that was to give a statement to the Faculty Council with a recommendation on whether the applicant should be accepted without any further examination, or had to be tried in one or several subjects where his or her examination could not be approved. In this evaluation, the place of study, the duration of the studies, if the study plan had been followed, examination grades, and practical work as a physician, if any, was to be considered.

In the last field, most of the candidates had extensive experience. The lack of physicians had become more noticeable, and medical students received good deputyships, even early in their studies, either in Norway or in Sweden, where the lack of physicians was even greater and salaries considerably higher.

The individual evaluation of the applicants was so complex and demanding that the process could take up to a year. It was therefore necessary to work for more schematic regulations, without a too great reduction of the individual assessment laid down by the law. The work in the interfacultary committee went on, always with Strøm and Waaler as guardians of the view of the two faculties.

20.19 Travels to Foreign Universities

When the medical faculties in Bergen and Oslo were to assess candidates from several different universities, it was necessary that there be at hand sufficient knowledge of the curriculum, tuition, and professional demands at the different universities. Erik Waaler in Bergen recognized this need, and was supported by the Ministry of Education so that he could travel to the places of study those that were of most interest in this case. Two specialists in internal medicine traveled with him, docent Sigurd Humerfelt (b. 1914) from Bergen and docent Knut Aas (1910–1992) from Oslo.

The three undertook a visit to several universities in Germany, Austria, the Netherlands, Switzerland, and France in January and February of 1958. Waaler and Humerfelt also visited several universities in Great Britain in October and November of the same year.

The travels had been well prepared, due to the fact that Waaler had sent a thorough account of the background for the visits to his colleagues at the different foreign universities. They did not think it strange that one wanted to obtain a closer knowledge of the education of students who later were to become physicians in Norway. The fact that Waaler was a known scientist among many colleagues outside of Norway probably contributed to the warm welcome the delegation received in most places.

By attending lectures, demonstrations and exams, as well as having thorough discussions with both teachers and students during the four or five days that each visit lasted, they attained useful knowledge of the subjects. This was the basis for their recommendations as to whether further education or tests were needed or not.

It would be too extensive to give the results from the individual universities. They can be read in the two reports given to the two faculties at the end of their journeys (Waaler, Humerfelt and Aas 1958, Waaler and Humerfelt 1958). Both positive and negative aspects are mentioned. The main conclusions, however, are given in the following:

> It is obvious to us that the education at the universities we visited can give the active and skillful student very good opportunities to learn a great deal, as well as a good opportunity for self realization. The possibility of not meeting standards is, however, at hand.
>
> Our main impression is that the tuition at the places we visited is good and that their professional requirements are no less than ours.

The emphasis on the good possibilities and also the possibilities of not meeting the standards were due to the less stringent curriculums that were usual in several countries, as opposed to the more school-like teaching that, already then, had become the ideal in Norway. The freer curriculum, with a higher emphasis on a thorough theoretical education and examinations where the clinical practice, to a larger degree, has to wait until the internship duties after finished studies, gives the intelligent and highly motivated students the possibility to determine their own progress toward a possibly brilliant result. There is, however, also the risk that the not-so-gifted and less motivated students will not be able to keep up.

Something that the delegation did not

consider, or at least forgot to mention in their reports, was that it was these free study plans that made it possible for many universities in southern Europe to accept so many foreign students. If they had had a school-like study with mandatory tuition in small groups, like the faculties in Oslo and Bergen had, they would also have had to limit their number of students to a great degree.

A lot of criticism has been directed toward these journeys, both at that time and afterward, in particular from the students abroad themselves. The students were positive that their own university gave the best education. They were unfamiliar with the reason for the travels, with whom the delegation was in contact with, as well as what they were interested in and what was reported. As a result, it was easy to say that it was unseemly that teachers from two small universities in a small country went to inspect universities that had accepted hundreds of its country's medical students. This view was of course also shared by some of the members of the faculties in Norway.

Upon further study, the question appears not quite so simple. The knowledge required of physicians was, and to a large extent, still is, based on cultural factors, the pattern of settlements, as well as social conditions. Especially in those days, the emphasis put on the different subjects could be very different from country to country, depending on the problems a young physician was likely to face. There is a difference between London and a fishing village in Northern Norway, also medically, but not everybody was willing to understand this.

In addition, there was the question of mutuality. There were hardly any examples of countries that mutually acknowledged other countries' medical degrees without demands for further education or practice. Between many states within the United States this is still the case, and even within the European Union there are still certain requirements. Should Norway alone, without any further ado recognize any exam from a foreign university without any agreement of reciprocity? Of course not.

The delegation, of course, could not refrain from commenting on the overproduction of physicians. At this time, in the beginning of 1958, the number of medical students abroad had reached 450 (Diagram 20.1). The delegation regarded this number as very high, and all the members of the delegation agreed that, if possible, there should be some regulation of the number of Norwegian medical students abroad. The delegation, however, wisely did not put forward any proposals of restrictions in any way.

The contact between the delegation and the students was arranged through the university administration, and by the network of student representatives that had been set up at universities all over Europe, the United States, and Canada, by the Association of Norwegian Students Abroad (ANSA), since the establishment of this organization in 1956.

The medical students' reactions to the visit from their own country varied significantly. For some, this was a sought-after opportunity to vent their aggression toward the Norwegian universities and authorities. In their opinion, Norwegian universities and authorities, who had not created enough positions of study, where now, on top of everything, coming to inspect the oldest and most distinguished universities in all of Europe. The delegation was referred to by these students as the "commissars" (Siem 1990).

Many others, however, remember the meetings with the delegation as much more positive (Humerfelt 1996). The delegation was always warmly welcomed by the students, and most of the students understood that the visits were an important sign that the Norwegian authorities realized that the country soon would need the students abroad and therefore wanted to arrange for their return to Norway.

Reading the reports from the delegation's travels today, one gets the impression that the criticism, both then and later, has been unjustified. The reports leave a sober, thoughtful, and mainly positive description of the conditions at most of the universities where there were Norwegian students. This contributed, to a large extent, to deflate the arguments of the greatest adversaries of the students abroad, and also created a professional basis for the new rules of acceptance of foreign medical degrees.

The faculty in Bergen found the experiences gained through these travels so important that they suggested and received funding for the establishment of a post as guardian for the students abroad. Trygve Gjestland (b. 1911), professor in hygiene in Bergen, was appointed and started the position in 1961. He established a secretariat for the students abroad at the University of Oslo, but it never reached the same importance as the delegation had had, when it came to establishing contacts with the foreign universities.

20.20 The Guidelines Become Common Rules and Common Law

The new rules were determined by a Royal Resolution the 30th of January 1959. In addition to examinations in the national subjects, the opponents had managed to push through that all candidates had to pass a clinical test in either surgery, internal medicine, or pediatrics. But new detailed rules concerning additional tests and practical duties for applicants from the different universities were more important. With this, the individual evaluation of the individual applicant was reduced, but it ensured that candidates with examinations from the same university were treated equally. From now on, the students who went abroad knew what would be demanded of them. But still, the applicants in Bergen had their foreign education recognized as part of a Norwegian education and received authorization as Norwegian physicians, while the applicants in Oslo could only get their education recognized as similar to the Norwegian one and had to make do with a Licentia Practicandi.

20.21 Could They "Be Let Loose on the Population"?

The introduction of the new rules did not take place without resistance from the opponents of studies abroad. Only two weeks before the Royal Resolution was laid on the table, Dr. Martin Seip (b. 1921) wrote a feature article that appeared in a Norwegian newspaper under the title "University Politics Fallen Short" (Seip 1959). A large part of the article was written in the form of an attempt to throw suspicion on the students abroad, regarding both their professional knowledge and their moral attitudes:

> In all countries of culture, great emphasis is put on ensuring the best possible control of the physicians that are to be let loose in the population. This applies both to their level of knowledge and especially to their ethical attitude to the medical work... The sparse experiences we have made with the additional exams for Norwegian physicians educated abroad indicate that their level of knowledge, on an average is noticeably lower than that of our own students, in some cases questionably low...
>
> Our medical faculties can, through additional exams etc., have some amount, although unsatisfactory as it might be, of control of the students abroad's knowledge of medicine. But, these students' ethical attitudes towards the medical profession can not be controlled... it is hard to avoid elements that are unwanted from a moral point of view.

As an university teacher, Seip should have understood that "sparse experiences" with additional exams was an insufficient basis for a general evaluation of the professional qualities of the medical students abroad. The attempt to throw suspicion on the students' moral standard was particularly vicious. There was no reason to believe that there were more unwanted elements among them than there were among students in Norway. Also, Martin Seip had to know that the students in Norway were not subjected to any kind of moral evaluation or control either, as he had tried to give the impression of.

The danger was particularly great because so many studied in Austria and Germany:

> This is especially unfortunate. It was in these countries that Hitler had a hard grip on almost all scientific life. And the repercussions from this are far from conquered. It is still seldom one reads a good medical, scientifical report from these countries.

Seip wanted to stop the *"uncontrolled mass production of physicians at German and Austrian universities"* and the *"misuse of five to six million kroner in foreign currency."* The money should instead be spent on expanding the medical education in Norway. In his opinion, the country's need for physicians would be covered when the 600 who already had gone abroad came home. Loans and currency should be granted only to 30 or 40 new medical students abroad per year, chosen by our own medical faculties.

The same day that Martin Seip's article was printed in Dagbladet, the front page of the same newspaper stated that there was not one single practicing physician in the town of Svolvær in spite of the fact that 10,000 men were expected to be at the Lofoten fisheries that year.

Others disagreed with Seip, as can also be seen from the response he got. The General Secretary of ANSA, mag. art Johan R. Ringdal (Ringdal 1959), reminded Seip of the positive reports from the delegation about the universities in Germany and Austria. Seip answered that the most important point in their reports was that there was a need to restrict the number of medical students abroad. Anything else the delegation had stated was of less importance.

20.22 *"Considering this Serious Situation"*

Seip's article in Dagbladet was followed up on by Dean Axel Strøm only a couple of months after the new rules were put into force. He gained the approval of the Faculty Council for a letter (dated 15 April 1959) to the Ministry of Education and Church Affairs in which they expressed their concern. The liberal rules and all the publicity around them had left the impression that "the authorities would like people to study medicine abroad." The number of medical students abroad was not 550 as ANSA had reported, a number that up until now had been used in all prognoses, but could be as many as 690 (Diagram 20.1). It was claimed that such a high number made all prognoses on the supply of new physicians obsolete, and that it would make it impossible to go through with the extra exams and the internship duty for all the medical students abroad, especially since the faculties in Bergen and Oslo the same year had increased the number of new students to 130 per year.

"Considering this serious situation," the Faculty Council recommended that new prognoses be made on the supply of new physicians, and that the completion of the practical duty be discussed with the Ministry of Social Affairs and the physicians organizations at once. Information campaigns directed toward potential students should also be initiated, with the aim of reducing the number of students who wanted to go abroad to study medicine. They should be warned that the rules for approval of foreign exams (which were only two months old) could be changed and made stricter. The Ministry should also consider other ways of reducing the number of students going abroad to study medicine.

Both Martin Seip's feature article and Axel Strøm's letter to the Ministry bear signs of despair. It was probably a coordinated effort from the two union-companions. They had not managed to prevent the new, more liberal rules from being approved. Now they made a last, desperate attempt to stop the flow of medical students going abroad and to keep the faculty in control of the medical education.

But it turned out to be too late. They did not manage to persuade Dean Alfred Sundal (1900–1991) and the faculty in Bergen to affiliate themselves with the letter to the Ministry. Even worse, the letter did not lead to any reaction from the Ministry. Almost every day, the newspapers told stories about the serious lack of physicians in many districts, especially in Western and Northern Norway. In political circles there was talk of a legislation ordering physicians to the areas that were most affected. ANSA had also become a force that had to be reckoned with. A Member of Parliament asked if the Government planned to make the situation easier for the students abroad. The Minister, Birger Bergersen (1891–1977), who himself was a Professor at the Faculty of Odontology, answered that most of the staff at universities, both in Norway and abroad, considered it "an advantage to the academic life if approximately 20 percent of the students at universities and colleges were foreign students." He also stated that the work on Nordic exam validity was developing in a satisfactory manner (Stortingstidende 1958). A European agreement on approval of university exams was to be signed in December 1959, and the report from a ministerial committee (Kleppekomiteen), which recommended large increases in the number of positions of study, including medical, was on its way. Under such circumstances, the Government could not listen to advice that recommended limiting the number of students abroad. The Ministry was of the opinion that there would be need for both the medical students abroad as well as for an increased number of physicians educated in Norway.

With its opposition toward the medical students abroad and its reluctance to increase the number of students at home, the medical faculty in Oslo was about to lose the confidence of the Ministry, both concerning medical students abroad and the medical education as such. The Ministry gave the faculty in Bergen the task of starting pre-clinic education as soon as possible. And a couple of years later, when committees regarding possible universities in Trondheim and Tromsø were appointed, the faculty in Oslo was set aside. In both committees, the medical expertise came from the Medical Faculty in Bergen. In the end, the Brodal committee, which had been established as a counter-weight, was not taken into consideration (Bertelsen 1991).

20.23 The Opposition Fades

The effort from Martin Seip and Axel Strøm was to be a last, desperate attempt before they had to accept the fact that it was not possible to stop the flow of medical students going abroad. The new rules had come to stay.

At first, the differences in the legislation concerning the universities in Oslo and Bergen were an advantage for the Ministries. By keeping to the more liberal legislation at the University in Bergen, the authorities could act more freely, and had also been able to liberate themselves from the complete control of the supply of new physicians that the Medical Faculty at the University of Oslo had had earlier.

For the faculty in Bergen, the fact that

they had been able to break the Oslo faculty's monopoly on the approving of medical exams from foreign universities felt like a victory. It was a small step toward liberation from and equality with the faculty in Oslo.

After a while, however, it became a problem that an unproportionately large part of the candidates from abroad preferred to apply to Bergen, in order to get a Norwegian degree and authorization, rather than just a licentia practicandi from Oslo. Thus, in 1959, 21 students applied for approval of their exams in Bergen, while only one applied in Oslo. Bergen had to limit the number of applications it could consider. In turn, the faculty in Bergen suggested to the Senate that they should ask for a change in the law concerning the University of Oslo, so that it would be possible for the faculty in Oslo to recognize foreign exams as part of a Norwegian degree as well. Another argument for this was that the two different laws could leave the false impression that medical degrees from the two faculties had a different professional status.

But the Senate in Bergen did not share this view. It preferred the view held by the University of Oslo, that it would be more appropriate to change the law concerning the University in Bergen to bring it into line with the law concerning Oslo. Particularly, it was pointed out that there were practical difficulties concerned with translating the foreign grades to Norwegian ones.

The Parliamentary Committee of Education and Church Affairs stressed the equal status of the physicians educated abroad and the ones educated in Norway (Forhandlinger i Odelstinget 1959–60). The fact that so many applied to Bergen instead of Oslo showed that it was considered "more prestigious having a Norwegian degree than a foreign degree with an attestation of having the additional Norwegian education," the spokesman stated when the matter was discussed in Parliament. The committee wanted to state that this was an inferiority complex that the physicians educated abroad did not need to have. The changes in the Bergen law was not a degrading of the physicians educated abroad.

> *"An education at a foreign university will in many cases have provided knowledge and skills that we cannot expect that the students also would have acquired here at home" ... "The stay in a foreign student environment and a foreign professional environment is in itself an asset."*

The law concerning the University in Bergen was changed so that it had the same contents as that concerning Oslo, in this matter (Lov av 1. april 1960). The candidates from abroad, however, did not think this adequate. They were of the opinion that the changes in the legislation had deprived them of the possibility of attaining a Norwegian authorization that they had had in Bergen. A change in the legislation concerning the physicians' rights and duties had to be made before the foreign candidates could acquire full authorization after having finished the additional Norwegian exams and practical duties. This came in the summer of 1960 (Lov av 2. juni 1960).

20.24 Why Did They Go?

It has been a common view that the stream of students going abroad to study medicine was due to the lack of physicians, as well as the Norwegian authorities' failure to create enough positions for studying medicine. Much indicates that this is not the whole explanation.

When the students started going abroad, around 1950, there was no recognized lack of physicians in Norway. Indeed, medical education had started in Bergen in the fall of 1946, according to a plan that originated around the turn of the century, but the aim had never been to educate more physicians. It was more a question of giving the rich medical and scientific environment in the second largest town in the country the superstructure and prestige that a medical faculty would represent. When it finally opened, the reason given was the need of relief for the faculty in Oslo concerning the teaching of the approximately 100 physicians annually that the faculty had educated since the end of the 1920s.

A comparison with our neighboring countries shows that the coverage of physicians, measured in physicians per 100,000 inhabitants, was lower both in Finland and in Sweden than in Norway up until the 1970s. Both these countries had strong limitations on the admittance to the medical study (numerus clausus). The financial terms for physicians and their social status in these countries was, and is, not noticeably different from those in Norway. This has not, however, led to an emigration of medical students going to foreign universities on the same level as in Norway. And the few who have gone abroad have never been considered to be a professional political problem, as in Norway. They have been given their medical licenses in accordance with the rules at the time, without problems.

As early as the 1930s the number of applicants to the medical study increased in Norway. The long wait for being admitted to the clinical part of the study has been mentioned. After admission to the study was limited in 1940, and the grades at examen artium were to create the basis for the admission of new students, an aura of prestige and exclusiveness quickly developed around the medical study, an aura that never developed around any other studies, and attracted a disproportionate number of applicants to the medical study.

A survey made by the Associations of Medical Schools of Europe showed that Norway was the one among the 28 countries in the survey that had the most applicants to the medical study. Also, the number of applicants was independent of both the coverage of physicians and the amount of positions of study (Curtoni et al. 1994). The survey states:

> Denmark, Norway and Sweden are three Scandinavian countries with a certain cultural homogeneity. They have similar density of doctors and they admit to the medical studies a number of candidates that is not much different as a proportion of the population. But the trend of the populations shows remarkable differences in terms of the number of candidates: for every position available there are 2 candidates in Denmark, 7 in Sweden and 19 in Norway. What is the explanation of this difference? Economy, image of the medical profession, or other?

While the students in our neighboring countries who are not admitted to the medical study apply to other studies, the motivation among the Norwegian students for studying medicine is so strong that large groups take on the strain involved with studying abroad.

The first few years, the motivation was perhaps strengthened by the many youths who had been abroad during the war and who could contribute with their contacts, and later on by knowledge of and connections with the priviledged students who were chosen for studies in Denmark and Sweden.

There can hardly be any doubt that the opposition felt from the medical faculty in Oslo as early as in 1945 toward medical studies abroad kept many from going the first few years. But, when the two fronts in this matter became more visible and it was shown that the threat of being denied a license could not be carried out in the long run, this attitude became more of an incentive for the more determined students and their resourceful parents.

The position taken by the State Educational Loan Fund and the Bank of Norway of not denying the students abroad loans or currency-licenses was a considerable support in this matter. Many saw this as a signal that the higher authorities did not support the faculty's restrictive policy. If these institutions had followed the faculty's example, most of the students would not have been able to study abroad.

20.25 How Many Were They?

The State Educational Loan Fund figures on loan takers is the closest we can come to a registration of medical students abroad at any given time (Diagram 20.1). These are minimum figures, since we must assume that a number of students, for various reasons, did not apply for student loans.

The diagram shows that the number of medical students abroad increased strongly from the middle of the 1950s and reached a peak in 1969, when 1,289 medical students reported that they were studying abroad. In the first years after the war, the universities in Switzerland, the Netherlands and Great Britain received the most Norwegian medical students. But from the beginning of the 1950s, Germany has been the country that has accepted most students every year. In the 1960s, there were also many Norwegian students at the universities in Austria, and in the period 1970–1985, Denmark received a large number of Norwegians. As the countries in question started requiring their positions of study for their own students, the number of medical students abroad declined to about 300 around 1990. In the later years, however, the number has again increased, after medical schools with English tuition and aimed at foreign students were established in Hungary and Poland.

The records of examinations in Bergen as

DIAGRAM 20.2

Norwegian physicians graduated from Norwegian and foreign universities in the period 1952–1991

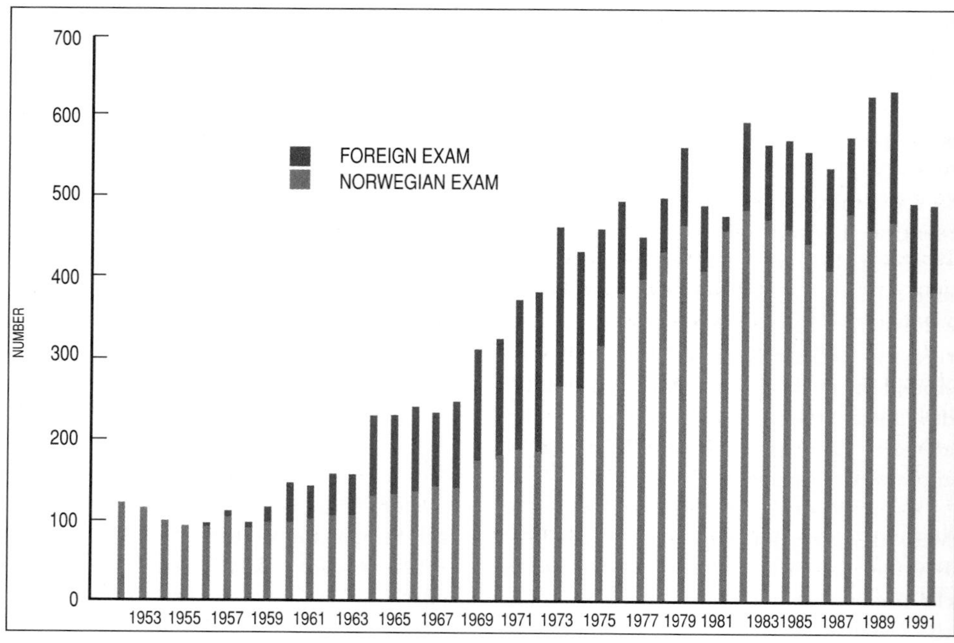

TABLE 20.1
Medical students abroad "of their own initiative" who got a Norwegian license during the years 1956–1991.

Country of study	Number of physicians educated	Percentage of total
Germany	ca 1,607	45
Denmark	" 393	11
Austria	" 357	10
Great Britain	" 286	8
Switzerland	" 214	6
the Netherlands	" 179	5
Belgium	" 143	4
Ireland	" 143	4
France	" 107	3
Sweden	" 71	2
Iceland +others	" 71	2
Total	ca 3,571	100

well as the numbers from Oslo, taken from The Journal of the Norwegian Medical Association, show that the two faculties together approved of 3,571 physicians with foreign degrees in the years from 1956 to 1991, 586 in Bergen and 2,985 in Oslo. These are minimum figures, since there seems to be some underreporting in the Journal. Diagram 20.2 shows the number of Norwegian physicians graduated from Norwegian and foreign universities in the period 1952 to 1991, and Table 20.1 shows an approximate distribution of the foreign graduates in the different countries where they had studied.

In addition, there were also about 800 physicians who, after having completed their pre-clinical education at foreign universities, continued their studies in Norway.

We may conclude that altogether about 4,500 Norwegian physicians have received ther entire or a fundamental part of their medical education at foreign universities (Table 20.2).

The integration of the physicians educated abroad into the Norwegian medical environment has taken place with only minor problems. They have entered positions in all divisions of the health services, medical teaching and research, and have in many cases been elected to high positions within the medical organizations. In other words, they have put all of the dismal predictions about their future to shame.

The Norwegian medical profession has, in the last 50 years, changed from being a homogenous group, educated at the same faculty in Oslo, by the same teachers or their pupils, to being a complex group, where two-thirds have been educated at one of Norway's four medical faculties, and one-third at more than 20 different faculties in 10 to 15 countries. There is hardly any doubt that this has contributed to a strengthening and differentiation of the country's medical environment, both professionally and in health politics.

Could we have managed without the physicians educated abroad? If the oppo-

TABLE 20.2
A general survey over all Norwegian physicians who completed parts of, or their entire education at foreign universities in the period 1945–1991

«Privileged» medical students who studied in Denmark and Sweden in 1945–1954:	about 150 physicians
Medical students studying abroad "of their own initiative" with a complete foreign degree, approved by the medical faculties in Bergen and Oslo in 1956–1991:	about 3,571 physicians
Medical students studying abroad "of their own initiative" who took over spare clinical study places in Bergen and Oslo in 1956–1991:	about 197 physicians
Medical students studying abroad "of their own initiative" who were accepted to the clinical study according to the Aker-Lørenskog plan of 1969–1986:	about 600 physicians
Total	about 4,518 physicians

nents had managed to stop the education of physicians abroad, Norway would – assuming that the Norwegian educational capacity remained unchanged – have had about 9,000 physicians instead of the 13,000 we have today. The large expansion of the social and medical services that have taken place in the last 50 years would have been very difficult to carry out. A substitution of the foreign candidates with an increase in the educational capacity in Norway would not have been possible. From the end of the 1950s, when it was accepted that the country would need a much higher number of physicians than previously thought, the number of medical study positions has increased as rapidly as the national economy and the supply of teachers would allow. First, the faculty in Bergen started admitting students to a full medical education, then two new medical faculties were established in Tromsø and Trondheim. But these new faculties, as well as the faculty in Oslo, could not have expanded fast enough to keep up with the need for physicians. Only by having physicians educated abroad, has Norway been able to meet its medical requirements.

References

Bertelsen, T. *Kampen for et medisinsk fakultet i Tromsø*. Bergen: 1991.

Bruusgaard, D., and T. Gjestland. *Medisinske kandidater fra norske og utenlandske universitet 1959–1966*. Oslo: Universitetet i Oslo, Institutt for almenmedisin og Sekretariatet for utenlandsmedisinere, 1976.

Castberg, F. *Minner om politikk og vitenskap fra årene 1900–1970*. Oslo: Universitetsforlaget, 1971.

Curtoni, S., et. al. *European investigation on the number of medical doctors and of students admitted in the faculties of medicine*, AMSE Newsletter, April 1994.

Det medisinske fakultet, Universitet i Oslo. *Orientering vedrørende spørsmål om medisinsk studium i utlandet med henblikk på å oppnå tillatelse til å utøve legevirksomhet i Norge*, 1 October 1954.

Forhandlinger i Odelstinget for 1959–60, 331–332.

Indstilling fra Den kongelige lægelovkommission. Kristiania: 1908.

Johnson, A. "Medisinsk studium i utlandet og Licentia practicandi i Norge for Læger med medisinsk eksamen fra utenlandsk universitet," *Tidsskrift for Den norske lægeforening*, 74 (1954):661-662.

Lov av 1.april 1960 om endring av paragraf 22. 3. ledd, i lov om Universitet i Bergen av 9.juli 1948.

Lov av 2. juni 1960.

Møller, K.O. "Udkast til Opraab til danske Læger om økonomisk Støtte til norske Medisinerstudenter," 1945.

Odelstingsproposisjon nr 28, 1924.

Odelstingsproposisjon nr 76, 1949.

Ringdal, J.R. "Borte bra – men hjemme best," *Dagbladet*, 27. January 1959.

Seip, M. Article in *Dagbladet*, 10. January 1959.

Seip, M. Article in Dagbladet 12. February 1959.

Sosialdepartementet, Helsedirektoratet: "Redegjørelse for studenter, som akter å studere medisin i utlandet", 23 July 1953.

SSB, *Historisk Statistikk*, Oslo, 1978.

Stortingsmelding nr 45, 1950. *Om behovet for akademisk arbeidskraft.*

Stortingstidende. Spørretime, 26 March 1958.

Strøm, A. "Lægebehovet i Norge," *Tidsskrift for Den norske lægeforening*, 72 (1952) 325–328.

Strøm, A. "Medisinsk studium i utlandet," *Tidsskrift for Den norske lægeforening*, 74(1954a):476.

Strøm, A. "Licentia practicandi i Norge for læger med medisinsk eksamen fra utenlandske universitet," *Tidsskrift for Den norske lægeforening*, 74(1954b):503–505.

Strøm, A. "Tilsvar til Anton Johnson," *Tidsskrift for den norske lægeforening*, 74(1954c):662–663.

Universitetet i Oslo 1911–1961. Bd I. Oslo: Universitetsforlaget, 1961.

Universitetet i Oslo 1911-1961. Bd II. Oslo: Universitetsforlaget, 1961.

Waaler, E., S. Humerfelt, and K. Aas "Kontakt-reise til medisinske fakulteter i Tyskland, Holland, Østerrike, Schweiz og Frankrike". *Report, 130 pages, Bergen: University of Bergen, Medical Faculty archive* 1958.

Waaler, E., and S. Humerfelt "Den medisinske utdannelse i England og Skottland." *Report, 45 pages, Bergen: University of Bergen, Medical Faculty archive* 1958.

Interviews:

Berglund, J. In interview with Bertelsen, T., 23 October 1995.

Humerfelt, S. In interview with Bertelsen, T., March 1996.

Semb, G. In interview with Bertelsen,T., 16 November 1995.

C H A P T E R 2 1

Preparing for the Inevitable Crisis? Medical Students After the 1970s

GUNHILD NYBORG

21.1. With Open Eyes into a Crisis?

In this period, many arguments have been raised against the medical profession being an attractive occupation. Some of the arguments that have met medical students and applicants to medical school are:

- An increasingly strained economy within the health sector has increased the pressure on the employees. This resulting effectiveness is experienced as a threat towards the quality of work (Tidsskrift for Den norske lægeforening 1995).
- Many argue that the status of the medical profession is devalued.
- To many physicians development has been unsatisfactory.
- The health sector has become the arena of a growing number of professional battles.
- Advances in medical technology have lead to a range of ethical conflicts connected to medical practice.
- More and more often, conflicts appear between the physicians' priorities and the expectations of the general public. Album (1991) argues that there is a certain ranking both of diseases and specialties according to prestige within the culture of the health care system. The "dramatic" diseases, and specialties which involve technologically advanced diagnostics and treatment, are the most prestigious ones. This may hamper work with the more common diseases.
- The media regularly publish stories of dissatisfied patients. More than half of the 1991 interns experienced the media's focus on physicians' mistakes as an extra burden to their work (Akre et al. 1991, Skaare et al. 1996).
- The legal system is considered a threat; Akre and Vikanes found that 36 percent of the interns experienced the fear of making mistakes dampening much of the joy of working as a physician (Akre et al. 1991).
- The growth of alternative treatment is felt as a challenge: Many patients, after innumerable visits to physicians, allege that they have been helped by chiropractors, acupuncture specialists, healers, homeopaths, and other groups who offer treatment not traditionally considered effective by university medicine.

Many studies of physician's living standards and working conditions in the Nordic countries, conducted during the end of the 1980s and the beginning of the 1990s, have disclosed a high degree of dissatisfaction, especially among the younger and the female physicians (Strandberg et al. 1989, Nordisk medicin 1991, Aasland et al. 1992). Studies have shown that the suicide rate among female physicians is markedly higher than in the average female population (Buxrud 1993). There seems to be a growing problem of physician burnout (Roness 1995). Those attending medical school during this period have heard about these studies during the course of their training. They have also observed that their medical lecturers have been in a stressed work situation.

In what way have these signals of a crisis influenced the students? Has the recruitment started to be affected? And what steps have the faculties taken to meet the challenges?

21.2. Recruitment to Medical Studies

The capacity for training new physicians in Norway has been adjusted according to the health authorities' and the university authorities' calculated demand for physicians. This national policy has also influenced the opportunities for Norwegian students to study abroad.

Medical studies have traditionally been very attractive in Norway. The number of applicants has been high. Since numerus clausus was introduced in 1940, the marks needed in order to be admitted to Norwegian medical schools have been high.

Beginning in the late 1980s, the number of applicants to the medical faculties has risen dramatically (Statistics for the Medical Faculty, University of Tromsø 1976–1996), and the requirements have increased correspondingly. Many young students have taken high school exams over again, in an attempt to improve their scores. This trend, however, is shared by many other fields of higher education, and can partly be explained by large cohorts in the 1960s and 1970, an increasing general interest in higher education, and growing unemployment.

In 1993 a study of all first-year medical students was conducted in order to explore the implications of the high admission requirements on the recruitment to medical school (Wiers-Jenssen 1994, Wiers-Jenssen et al. 1995). According to this study, 76 percent of the students had spent time improving their grades after leaving high school. Four out of ten students had spent one year, one out of four had spent two years, and one out of ten had spent three or more years doing this. Many students also took advantage of the possibility of getting extra credit for up to two years of other forms of education or for work experience. Hence, it was shown that the majority of these students had invested much effort in being admitted to the study, both during and after the completion of their high school years.

The studying abroad opportunities have been regulated through the student support system. In 1994, the Norwegian State Loan Fund for Education resumed giving extra grants for medical studies abroad. The result has been a new increase in the number of Norwegian medical students abroad; in 1995/96, the total had risen to nearly 600, in contrast to a low of 300 students in 1989/90. Many Norwegians now study in Hungary and Poland. In the academic year 1993/94, there were 19 Norwegian students who received their medical training in Hungary, and three in Poland. The following year, this figure had risen to 77 and 29, respectively. In the fall of 1995, there were 150 Norwegian students in Hungary, and 57 in Poland (the Norwegian State Loan Fund for Education 1995).

This enormous interest in pursuing medical studies becomes rather paradoxical when viewed in the context of the grim warnings which have appeared in relation to the occupation. What can explain this? Might it be that the profession is so isolated that its negative sides are unrecognized by "the outside"? In the rest of society, the discontent among physicians has not been acknowledged; physicians are still regarded as privileged, and the feeling of being privileged still characterizes the newest students (Haas et al. 1987). In a study of Norwegian interns in 1991, 26 percent answered that they at least once, during their time as interns, had regretted their choice of occupation (Akre et al. 1991, Vikanes et al. 1992, Akre et al. 1992). This may be a signal that some students have met obstacles that they were not prepared for during their training. On the other hand, maybe the interns have expressed a frustration that is natural as they make the transition from being a student to being a practicing doctor.

Does modern society, which is so influenced by the great power of the media and by the overflow of information, demand to have crises? Has the debate about the development in the profession perhaps been marked by a tendency to reinforce of the negative aspects in accordance with this?

21.3. Motives for the Choice of Medicine

What are the motives that lead one to choose this course of study in the existing climate? Studies at hand are not conclusive as to whether or not those entering medical school toward the end of this period have had different motivations than those who entered earlier on. Wiers-Jenssen (1994) explored the motivations for studying medicine among students commencing their studies in Oslo in 1993. Prospects for future work with human beings, and the opportunities for making a humanitarian and social contribution, were reported as being most important, especially to the female students. This may seem to have become more important to the new students during this period compared to earlier cohorts (Wiers-Jensen 1994, Larsen 1986). A possible explanation is that the outlook for working with human beings is becoming increasingly attractive in a modern society marked by alienation. If this is a trend, it has implications that raise questions about the fact that physicians who best avoid the burnout syndrome are those who chose their profession for reasons other than the wish to take on the role of a helper (Roness 1995).

Financial prospects and high status have not been motives of vital importance in respect to the students' choice of study in these surveys, but many students attached some importance to the matters. However, the data may to some extent be biased toward an idealistic motivation.

The strong focus on health in modern society may also explain some of the interest in the subject. Interest in the medical science as such seems to be important to many students (Wiers-Jenssen 1994, Larsen 1986). Medical school also qualifies as a higher theoretical education, which in itself is regarded as a necessity by many.

People with a university degree in any subject are in general no longer guaranteed work to their satisfaction after they finish their education. As a new feature, the prospect of a safe labor market was an important aspect to many in the 1993 study. Physicians in Norway have never experienced unemployment, as opposed to colleagues in many other countries.

21.4. Demographic Development Among the Students

The share of female medical students has increased throughout this period. In the mid-1990s, approximately half of the students are women. This development is also seen in most other academic courses of study.

The percentage of medical students getting married during medical school has increased (Larsen 1986). In addition to this, cohabitation has become more usual than before. 42 percent of the 1991 interns had children (Akre et al. 1991).

Thus, medical students of the last decades have to a greater extent had family commitments during their training than before. No studies from other fields of education are at hand, but the amount of time used by applicants to improve their grades before entering medical school has led to a higher average age among the students. Beginning in the fall of 1996, admission to all the four universities in Norway is to be coordinated. A new feature is to be introduced: nearly two-thirds of the new medical students will be admitted on the basis of their original high school certificates, and the admission of half of these again will be offered to applicants based solely on their certificate, with no extra points. This may contribute to lowering the students' average age.

An increasing number of medical students and physicians, both male and female, must also take into consideration their partners' career choices (Larsen 1986). This trend is shared by other occupations and results from the changing pattern of sex roles. The number of marriages in which both parties are physicians is increasing. In 1984, 15 percent of the physicians had a spouse who was a physician. Among those who were interns in 1991, approximately 35 percent had a spouse who was a physician with the share being larger for female than for male physicians (Akre et al. 1991).

The changing demographic structures have led to a new set of problems for the medical profession. However, the strain on young families seems to be an increasing and general problem in the modern Norwegian society.

21.5. Strain, Information Challenge, and Great Demands

Several studies confirm that at the beginning of their studies, the students have an idealistic approach (Wiers-Jenssen 1994, Haas et al. 1987, Becker et al. 1961). As they are confronted with the great amount of requirements, their attitude becomes more cynical, and they end up learning to prioritize what is needed to pass their exams. It seems that a few decades ago, the students gradually developed a greater confidence in their knowledge, and hence became more confident in themselves (Fox 1957). The amount of information becomes increasingly overwhelming, even to physicians who have finished their training (Nylenna 1995).

Bramness, Fixdal, and Vaglum found, in a study carried out at the medical faculty in Oslo in 1990 (Bramnes et al. 1991), that medical students' self-esteem was lower than that of the rest of the population. This somewhat surprising result may also reflect the stressful situation of information overload combined with the high demands on physicians' skills. Among the students in the early stage of clinical study, male and female medical students had an equal level of self-esteem. Among those in the late stages of medical study, however, the self-esteem of the men was higher than that of the women. This may be interpreted as a better adjustment to the strain factor of the student-physician role among men than among women. In 1991, Akre and Vikanes discovered that a third of the women interns, but only 13 percent of the men, felt a greater responsibility than they thought they could handle (Akre et al. 1991). There may be many reasons for these differences between the two sexes, but it is important to bear in mind their differences in communication patterns.

Is the medical training in step with society as a whole? This was the question posed

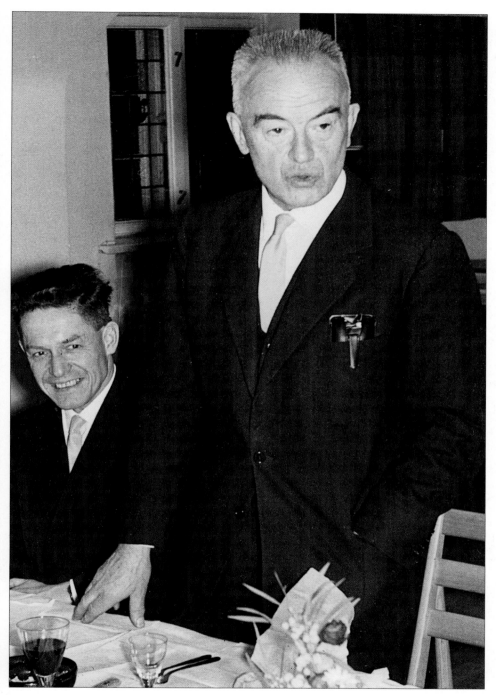

Figure 64: Director General of the Health Services 1938-1972, Karl Evang (1902-1981), a brilliant orator, giving a speech at a dinner concluding a course in public health. Such courses have been given annually since 1948, and have been an important element in the professionalization of district physicians. At Evang's right hand side: Dr. Knut Rein (1919-), then district physician in Vik in Sogn (Photo: Øivind Larsen 1964).

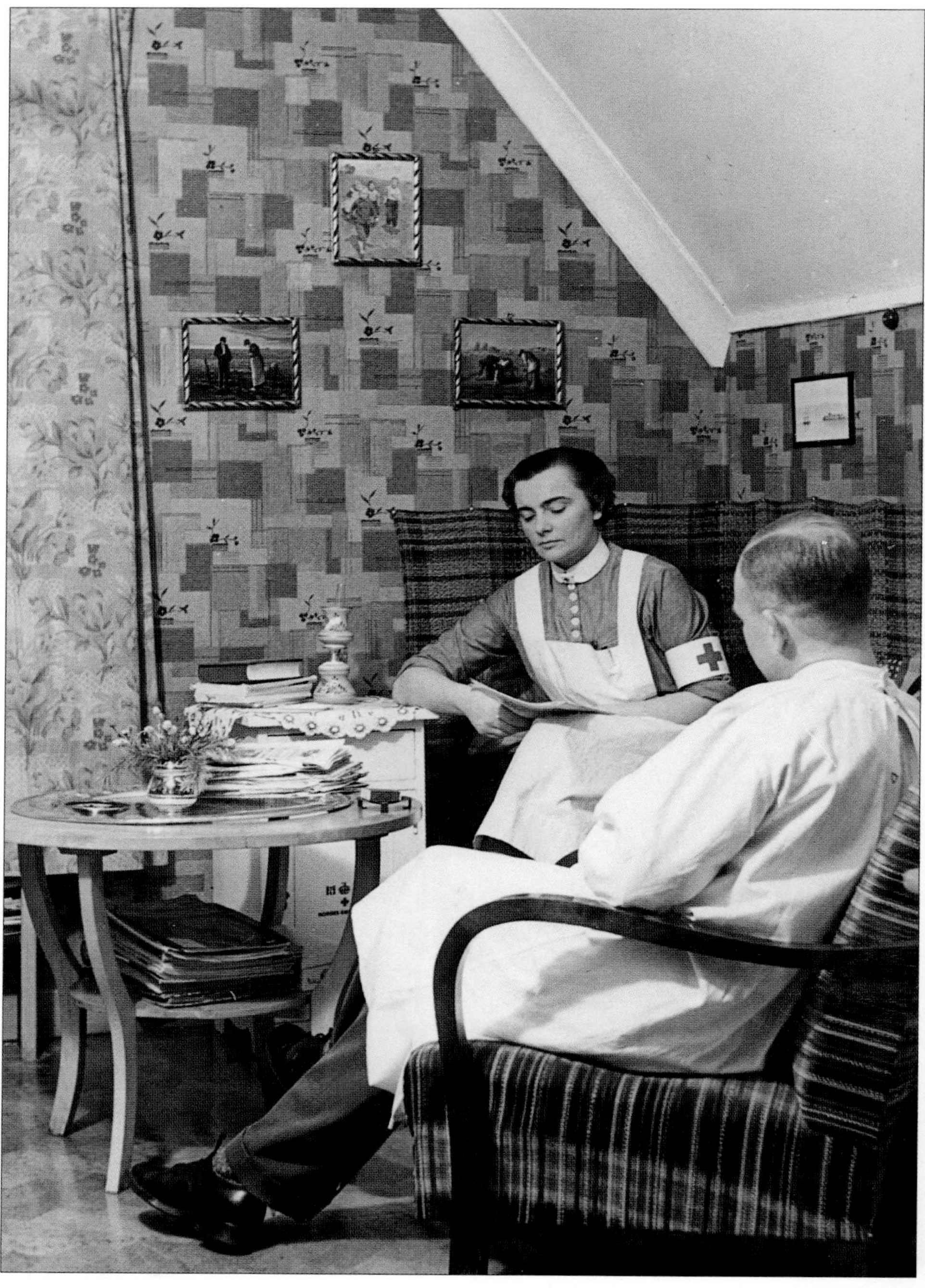

Figure 65: District physician and nurse having a break. (Dr. Knut A. Schrøder [1905-1988]; Kjøllefjord, Finnmark, 1930s. Courtesy Aina Schiøtz).

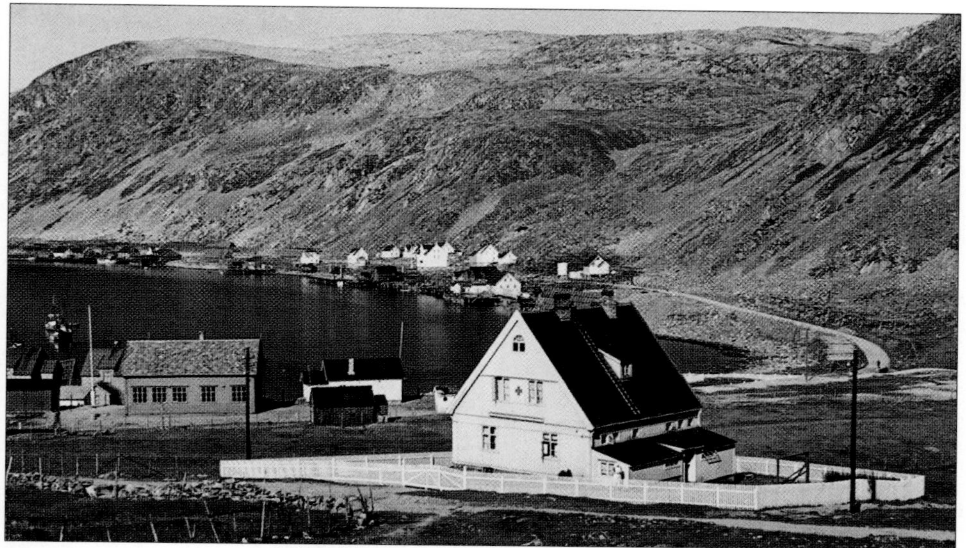

Figure 66: The Red Cross Cottage Hospital, Kjøllefjord, Finnmark, late 1930s. It was burned down during the German withdrawal in 1944 (Photo: Dr. Knut A. Schrøder, courtesy Aina Schiøtz).

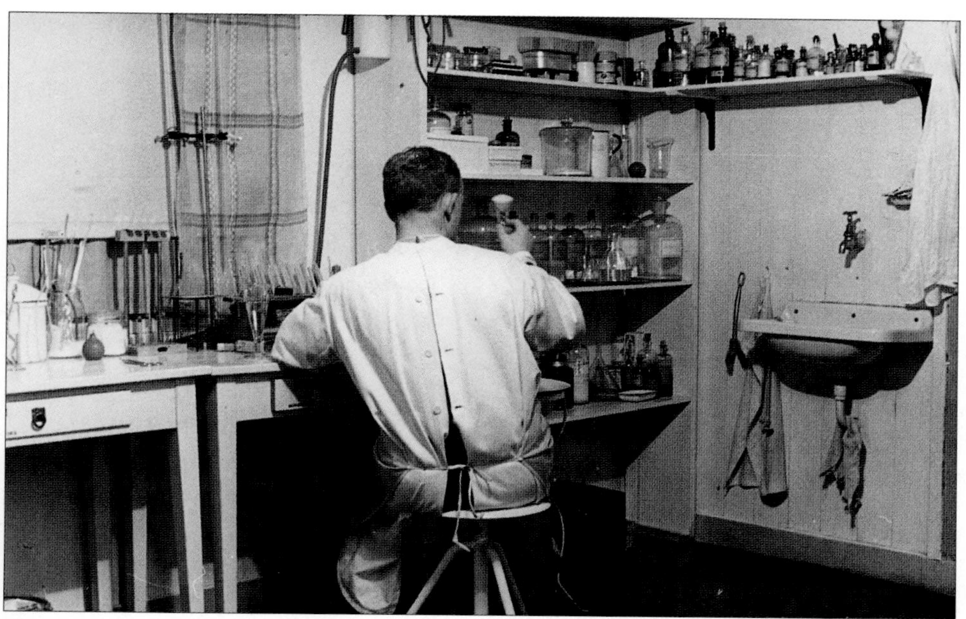

Figure 67: Laboratory work in the Red Cross Cottage Hospital, Kjøllefjord, Finnmark 1938-1939. (Dr. Knut A. Schrøder [1905- 1988], courtesy Aina Schiøtz).

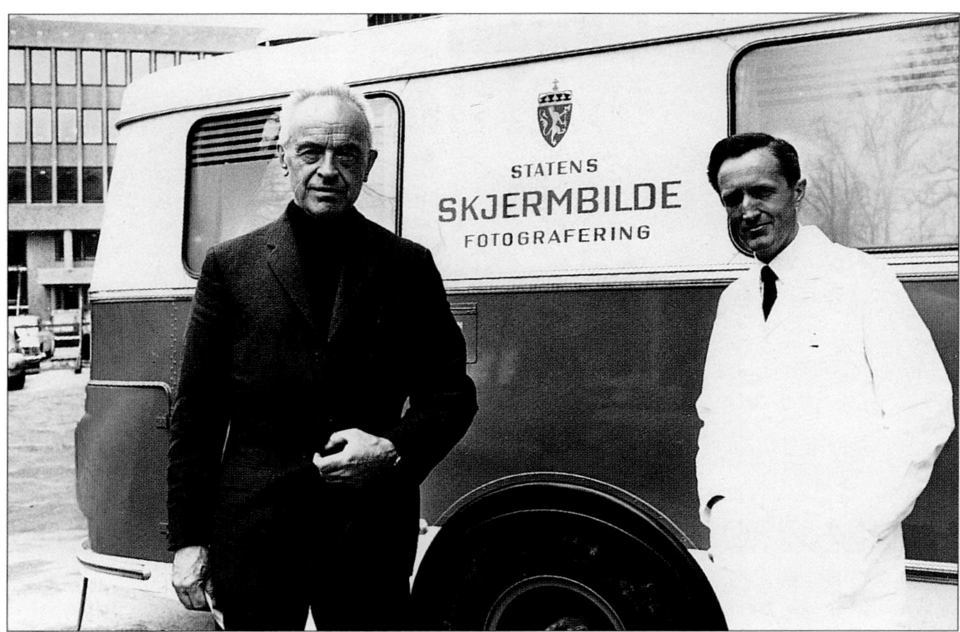

Figure 68: An ambulatory x-ray service was introduced in 1969 in order to perform selective lung screening. Karl Evang (left) and chief physician Kjell Bjartveit (1927-) (Photo: NTB).

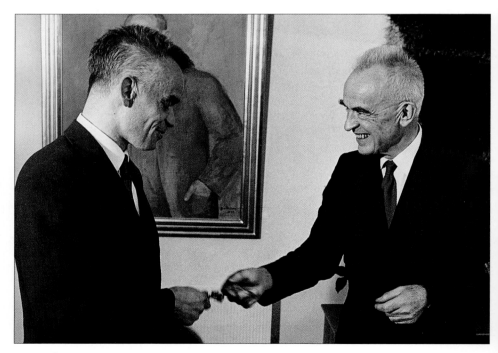

Figure 69: November 1, 1972: Thorbjørn Mork (1928-1992) takes over as Director General of the Health Services after Karl Evang (1902-1981) (Photo: NTB).

by the former Director General of Health Service, Karl Evang, in 1976 (Evang 1976). He thought that the system lacked a mechanism that ensured students would be able to meet a society where the role and tasks of the physician had become substantially different from what the university lecturers themselves experienced when they had finished their training. On the other hand, tacit knowledge cannot be learned from books, and the students need role models, in close relations, over a substantial period of time (Hjort 1991). Personal supervision of the students is expensive training, and in the late 1980s and early 1990s, for several reasons, the financial distribution to the education of medical students had been cut (Vaglum 1994). This, combined with the more stressed work situation that the educational staff is experiencing, has led to a situation where the students receive little personal follow-up. In a situation that places great demands on the physicians' skills, it may seem as though it has become more difficult to get the experience necessary to become confident in the role.

On the other hand, the interpersonal climate at the medical faculties has changed over the years, with a more relaxed relationship between students and teachers. The increasing number of female students may have contributed to this. This may have had a positive effect both on the students' socialization into the role as a physician, and on the faculty staff's ability to understand the students' frustrations. It may also have played a role in the recent adjustments of the curriculum.

21.6. *Reform of the Curriculum*

The medical training in Norway has largely been based on the same framework since 1844: first there is one unit of preclinical subjects, and then two units of clinical subjects. The students' achievements are given marks on a scale from 1 to 12.

In almost the entire period after 1844, many students and lecturers at the University of Oslo have argued in favor of a more practical approach in the curriculum, and a reduction of the excessive amount of theory. The curriculum has gradually been changed according to the society's needs, but the faculty has a long tradition of being reluctant to change (Larsen 1990).

Medical training has been taken up in Bergen, Tromsø, and Trondheim in the last 30 years. The University of Tromsø chose a new policy for medical training when medical education started in 1973. They offered a model with early patient contact and integrated training. In addition, the Tromsø students get extensive training in local hospitals and with general practitioners. Students trained in Tromsø have reportedly been more content with their schooling than those trained in other faculties (Kaisen et al. 1984, Akre et al. 1991). In a questionnaire conducted by Bramnes et al., 255 students early or late in their clinical studies in Oslo in 1990 gave an estimate of their clinical skills (Bramnes et al. 1992). The results showed that many students felt that they lacked sufficient practical experience.

In recent years, in-service training has also been introduced at the other universities, along with other reforms to the curriculum, such as an increased emphasis in communication skills. In 1996, the University of Oslo introduced a new curriculum, with problem-based learning and more practical training. There seems to be an increasing willingness to take radical steps to meet the demands of a society in rapid change.

The general impression in the debate created by the development of the medical profession is that there is an inevitably approaching crisis. But there are also positive signals. In some instances, improvements have followed in the wake of problems being uncovered. The students and the young physicians may have the capacity to cope with the demand of the profession if they are properly trained and prepared for the modern society. The change is inevitable; perhaps not the crisis.

References

Aasland, O. G. and, E. Falkum, "Hvordan har vi det i dag? Om legers helse, velvære og arbeidsglede." *Tidsskrift for Den norske lægeforening,* 112(1992):3818–23.

Akre, V. and Vikanes, Å. *Turnuskandidaten, menneskets beste venn? En kartlegging av turnustjenesten.* Oslo: Den norske lægeforening, 1991.

Akre, V., Å. Vikanes, and P. Hjortdahl, "Profesjonalisering uten styring? En undersøkelse om det faglige innholdet i turnustjenesten." *Tidsskrift for Den norske lægeforening*, 112(1992):2546–51.

Album, D. "Sykdommers og medisinske spesialiteters prestisje." *Tidsskrift for Den norske lægeforening*, 111(1991):2127–33.

Becker, H., B. Geer, E. Hughes, A. Strauss, *Boys in white. Student culture in medical school.* Chicago: University of Chicago Press, 1961.

Bramness, J. G., T. Fixdal, and P. Vaglum, "Effect of medical school stress on the mental health of medical students in early and late clinical curriculum." *Acta Psychiatrica Scandinavica*, 84(1991):340–5.

Bramness, J. G., T. C. Fixdal, and P. Vaglum, "Sosialisering til legerollen i studiets kliniske del. Del I: Studentenes vurdering av egne ferdigheter." *Tidsskrift for Den norske lægeforening*, 112(1992): 2207–10.

Buxrud, E. G. "Er helsetjenesten en god arbeidsplass for kvinner?" *Tidsskrift for Den norske lægeforening*, 133(1993):1869–72.

Evang K. "Følger medisinutdannelsen med i samfunnsutviklingen?" *Nordisk Medicin*, 91(1976):137–139.

Foreningen av yngre lægers socialpolitiske arbeidsgruppe. "Danske underordnede lægers arbejds- og livsvilkår." *Nordisk Medisin*, 106(1991):279–280.

Fox, R. C.: *Training for uncertainty. The student-physician. Introductory studies in the sociology of medical education.* Merton, Reader and Kendall (eds). Harvard University Press, 1957.

Haas, J. and W. Shaffir, *Becoming doctors: The adoption of a cloak of competence.* Department of Sociology, McMaster University, Greenwich, Connecticut, 1987.

Hjort, P. F. "Gode leger – hvordan blir studentene det?" *Tidsskrift for Den norske lægeforening*, 114(1994):3171–2.

Kaisen, A., G. A. Kjetså, R. K. Lie, R. Hjetland, P. T. Haaland, P. Møller, H. E. Oulie, T. Tveit, and J.G. Mæland: "Interns' evaluation of their preparation for general practice: A comparison between the University of Tromsø and the University of Bergen." *Medical Education*, 18(1984):349–354.

Larsen, Ø. (red). *Legene og samfunnet.* Seksjon for medisinsk historie, Universitetet i Oslo, and Den norske lægeforening, 1986.

Larsen, Ø., *Mangfoldig Medisin.* Det medisinske fakultet, Universitetet i Oslo, 1990.

Norske elever og studenter i utlandet. Oslo: Statens Lånekasse for Utdanning, 1995.

Nylenna, M. "Så mye å lese, så liten tid å gjøre det på." *Tidsskrift for Den norske lægeforening*, 115(1995):2043.

"Opptaksstatistikker." *Det medisinske fakultet, Universitetet i Tromsø, 1976-96.*

Roness, A. *Utbrent? Arbeidspress og psykiske lidelser hos mennesker i utsatte yrker.* Oslo: Universitetsforlaget, 1995.

Skaare, D. and G. Jacobsen: "Leger i gapestokk? Om legetabber og tabbeleger i norsk tabloidpresse." *Tidsskrift for Den norske lægeforening*, 116(1996): 265—9.

Strandberg, M. and B. Arnetz, "Kvinnliga

läkara mår sämre än sina manliga kolleger." *Läkartidningen*, 86(1989):4402–5.

Sunnanå, Lars Sigurd. "Orker vi å være sykehusleger lenger?" *Tidsskrift for Den norske lægerforening*, 155(1995):3315.

Vaglum, P.: "Legestudiet – fortsatt et menneskebehandlende studium?" *Tidsskrift for Den norske lægeforening*, 114(1994):3171–2.

Vikanes, Å., V. Akre, and P. Hjortdahl, "Medisinsk grunnutdanning i utakt." *Tidsskrift for Den norske lægeforening*, 112 (1992):2541–5.

Wiers-Jenssen, J. *Rekruttering til medisinstudiet. En studie av et årskull medisinerstudenter, med vekt på sosial bakgrunn, poengsamling, studiemotiver og ambisjonsnivå.* Thesis in sociology. Institutt for sosiologi, Universitetet i Oslo, 1994.

Wiers-Jenssen, J., P. Vaglum, and Ø. Ekeberg, "Repetisjon og privatisteksamener – veien til det medisinske studium." *Tidsskrift for Den norske lægeforening*, 115(1995):2659–62.

C H A P T E R 2 2

Organization and Professionalization of Medical Students – The Norwegian Medical Student's Association

JAN CHRISTIAN FRICH

22.1 Introduction

Norwegian medical students have organized parts of their social life in different sorts of societies from the early beginnings of the faculty in the nineteenth century. The oldest society for medical students (Medicinerforeningen) was founded at the University of Oslo in 1829. This society's main concern has traditionally been debates, celebrations, and festive occasions. The Norwegian medical students' periodical, Æsculap, bearing an appropriate classical name, has been published more or less continuously since 1920, presenting both political and medical articles. Also today the student life flourishes in the many societies at the four medical schools in Norway. Participation in this activity may be an important factor for each individual's own socialization into the medical profession. However, these societies are not dealt with in further detail in this chapter, as their objectives mainly are focused on spare time and leisure – albeit as important as this may be for the well-being of the students.

The aim of this paper is to focus on the medical students' endeavor to establish their own trade union, and how this led to a new organizational relationship between Norwegian medical students and the Norwegian Medical Association (Den norske lægeforening). In 1987 medical students were offered membership in the Norwegian Medical Association, through a newly established body, Norwegian Medical Students' Association – NorMSA (Norsk medisinstudentforening). Today the Norwegian Medical Students' Association organizes 95 percent of medical students in Norway. The history of the Association and its predecessors, the Organization for Norwegian Medical Students (Organisasjon for norske medisinske studenter) and the Medical Students' Interest Organization (Medisinstudentenes interesseorganisasjon), shows that there have been different opinions concerning student's membership in the Norwegian Medical Association, among both students and established professionals.

22.2. The First Initiative

Organized trade union activity among medical students in Norway was started in the mid 1960s. In 1965 an article appeared in the journal of the association of Norwegian Students Abroad (ANSA), taking up the medical students' desire for appointments in

Norwegian hospitals during holidays. At that time there was no organization that could assume the responsibility of promoting their cause. Such engagements were usually arranged on a private basis. This was especially problematic for Norwegians studying medicine abroad, due to the geographic distances and due to fewer personal contacts at hospitals in Norway. A debate followed among Norwegian medical students around the issue of medical students' participation in the labor market. Later in the year, on the 19th of December 1965, the Organization for Norwegian Medical Students (Organisasjon for norske medisinske studenter) was founded, mainly to improve the possibilities for students to get work during the holidays for a respectable professional and financial benefit.

However, these objectives were criticized by some medical students: "You give the other students the impression that medical students are avaricious and only interested in feathering their own nest" (Holm 1966). This can be seen as reluctance to perceive oneself as different from other students and as resistance against the professionalization of medical students.

The supporters of the organization opposed this assertion by insisting that medical students were in a special position, because, owing to their medical education, they are periodically active in the labor market practicing medicine.

During the next ten years the organization was instrumental in the procurement of summer jobs. It also managed to get the time-limited provisional license to practice as a doctor extended to cover the whole year. In spite of this, in 1980 the management of the organization went through a self-searching crisis. In an article in Æsculap in 1980, the author describes the union as being "without the legal right to negotiate or enter into contracts, and without any particular influence. This is the paradox which makes the situation so difficult." The organizational structure was questioned and thoroughly discussed: Which structure should be chosen, and which collaborations should one concentrate on? Other important areas of concern were how to secure the continuity of the work and how to gain more influence.

22.3 Questioning the Organizational Structure

Three alternative organizational models were suggested. The first alternative was to maintain the organization as an independent body. The management thought that this was the best solution. The second alternative was to establish a formal connection to the faculty bodies through the students' councils. One faction of students claimed that this could not work because the organization's main interest lay in the student's working and salary conditions, which was outside the councils' jurisdiction. The third alternative was to co-operate with the Norwegian Medical Association, including the Norwegian Junior Hospital Doctor's Association (Yngre legers forening). Some objected to this alternative, because the organization might eventually become totally dependent through the co-operation. On the other hand, it was claimed that this was the easiest way to gain influence. These considerations are interesting because they show how medical students conceived their own position as different from that of the established professionals.

At that time, however, the idea of co-operation with the students' organization was not endorsed by the Norwegian Medical Association. Students had never before been considered to be eligible for membership in the professional organization.

The Organization for Norwegian Medical Students discussed their future with the Co-operation Committee for Medical Students

(Samarbeidsutvalget for medisinstudenter). This discussion resulted in the formation of the nation-wide Medical Students' Interest Organization (Medisinstudentenes interesseorganisasjon), established in Tromsø on May 2, 1981.

The students emphasized that the new organization should primarily work on salary and working conditions, but in addition it was admitted that this necessarily implied a certain involvement in health politics. The students were particularly interested in the primary health service, because at the time it was most likely that a great percentage of young doctors would get their future work in this part of the health care system: "As a student it is important to be able to influence your own future" (Sandvik 1981). One also stressed the importance of working with matters concerning medical education.

In spite of the new enthusiasm, the Medical Students' Interest Organization still faced opposition in their efforts to gain influence. In 1983, at the National Council meeting of the Norwegian Junior Hospital Doctors' Association, the suggestion was rejected that the Medical Students' Interest Organization should be represented in the National Council; neither was the Medical Students' Interest Organization accepted as a negotiating partner in dealings with the Norwegian Association of Local and Regional Authorities (Kommunenes Sentralforbund).

22.4 Application for Membership in the Norwegian Medical Association

In 1985 the Medical Students' Interest Organization approached the Norwegian Medical Association with a request for membership for medical students. The application for membership was presented in a report, which the annual meeting of the Norwegian Medical Association accepted. This resulted in the formation of the Norwegian Medical Students' Association, established on January 1, 1987.

The Norwegian Medical Students' Association announced a broader program than its predecessors had. In addition to working on salary and working conditions, the Association intended to work on the professional content in practical and theoretical medical education, engage in health politics, participate in the debate about new requirements for doctors and the medical profession, and arrange courses for medical students. The Association later became a member of the International Federation of Medical Students Associations (IFMSA). In 1994 the Association became responsible for the publishing of the medical students periodical, Æsculap. The journal of the Norwegian Medical Association is also sent to members of the Association, which probably is an important factor in the socialization of medical student into the medical profession.

22.5 Organization and Professionalization

Although a lot of trade union work for medical students was completed during the twenty years that elapsed between the mid 60s and the time when the Norwegian Medical Students' Association was established in 1987, earlier attempts to establish a trade union for students were not successful for any length of time. The work failed due to the Association's lack of recognition as a negotiating agent, lack of support among the students, and lack of adequate finances. The agreement concerning student's membership in the Norwegian Medical Association was an important milestone.

The driving forces that led to the establishment of the Norwegian Medical Students' Association, can, at least partly, be described as the medical students' endeavor to become professionalized, in order to gain power so that they might influence their own working conditions, salary scales, and future as professional doctors.

The history of the Norwegian Medical Students' Association – NorMSA (Norsk medisinstudentforening) illustrates at least two points concerning the relationship between medical students and the medical profession: first, medical students may be ambivalent about their own status as members of a profession and second, established professionals may be reluctant to include a new segment, such as students, as members of the profession.

References

Aamodt, Arild. "Medorg – et Oslofenomen," *Æsculap*, 2(1980): 13–14.

Holm, A. "Løst og fast fra Medorg," *Æsculap*, 3 (1966): 14–15.

Sandvik,E. "Medisinstudentene får landsomfattende organisasjon," *Æsculap*, 2 (1981): 6, 12.

CHAPTER 23

The Changing Conditions for the Hospital Physician

STEIN A. EVENSEN

23.1. Introduction

My impressions, gained through twenty-five years as a physician of internal medicine at a university hospital, constitute just a small part of the real work that is experienced by Norwegian hospital physicians. In addition, I have made a personal selection of what I believe are the most important topics. Therefore, physicians in psychiatry and laboratory disciplines, for example, will certainly feel that some important matters are lacking.

The chapter deals with four areas regarding the situation of hospital physicians:

1. The altered role of the physician
2. The development within medicine
3. Focus set by the media
4. Organizational and administrative challenges

But first, a description of the recent past and some often quoted assertions about the health services:

In the first half of the twenty-five year period 1970–1995, everything seemed to increase: salaries, number of posts, and available resources. But the economic situation changed. The brakes were engaged, a better control of expenses was demanded, work input was intensified, and there was a growing quest for efficiency. Since then most things are more slow moving, waiting lists for hospital admission have expanded and frustration has increased. In the media there are complaints about increasingly difficult conditions in the hospital service, decay and failing quality. In the last few years there has been talk of a physicians' migration away from hospital medicine, a development which allegedly started within the disciplines of eye diseases, skin diseases and gynaecology. From laboratories and service departments in hospitals there have been particularly vociferous complaints.

Is this a correct picture of the situation?

A distinction must be made between the situation for those who work in hospitals and for those who are treated there. In the media, it is alleged that the quality of hospital services is gradually deteriorating and that hospital patients experience miserable conditions. This is hardly true. Quite a lot indicates that diagnostics and therapeutics have steadily progressed, and that the services provided to patients are good and have never been better. More and more auxiliary personnel with better education are available. Contact with the primary health services is better than it used to be in most places. Probably, expectations play tricks with us. The serious feature in the development is lack of capacity, which has led to long waiting lists for a range of diagnostic groups. This is a serious weakness in Norwegian hospitals, and a weakness which politicians must assume the main responsibility for.

With regard to conditions for hospital physicians, macro data from the previous period of ten years does not support the general impression of deterioration. The number of man-labor years for physicians in somatic hospitals increased by 13% from 1986 to 1993, while the number of vacancies fell by 6% (Table 23.1.). However, there are many indications that staff turnover in certain hospital posts has increased, particularly in the disciplines mentioned above.

There are several reasons for this. The fact that work in hospitals is experienced as more stressful, despite the establishment of several new posts, is among other things owing to increased demands and more complicated treatment procedures. Table 23.2 shows that while the number of beds in the period from 1977 to 1991 fell by 32%, the numbers of patients admitted increased by 11%. This is in line with the significant fall in length of stay during these years, which undoubtedly was a desirable development. But there are certain groups of patients whose length of stay may have fallen below a professionally acceptable level. This refers in particular to elderly patients. In addition, there has been a significant growth in the number of patients who have been examined and treated on an out-patient basis.

23.2. The Altered Role of the Physician

Changes in the role of the physician are perhaps more important than stress and strain at work. Key factors are the devaluation of the patriarchal image of the physician and a strenghtened patient influence. Some physicians certainly have struggled in adjusting to a situation with greater equality between physicians and other health professionals. And perhaps it is even more important to adjust to a situation which implies self-conscious patients, well informed about their own illness and willing to make clear demands on the physician. Or, to quote professor Ole Berg of the Center for Health Administration: "Patients are not so patient any more!" Here lie new challenges which physicians must learn to meet. The physicians' skill in communicating with patients is more important than before. This is an area which is given greater priority in the teaching of medical students in Norwegian universities.

Criticism can be justified or unjustified.

TABLE 23.1
Number of man-labor years for physicians working in institutional health services. Source: The Norwegian Medical Association.

Year	1986	1993	% change
Man-labor years	4,410	4,969	+13
Number of vacancies	236	221	–6

TABLE 23.2
Key figures from somatic hospitals.

Year	1977	1991	% change
Number of beds	22,652	15,318	–32
Number of patients treated	572,276	635,385	+11

Source: Official Statistics of Norway. Health Statistics.

Many hospital physicians believe that most of the modern criticism is unjustified, because it often is based on factors which are political issues and consequences of political decisions. Examples are the financial confinements under which hospitals must work, and the patient waiting lists. It is, however, a fact that too much unjustified criticism contributes to creating a poorer working environment.

Complaints about the treatment given is also a burden to the physicians. In the first half of 1995, 758 patients claimed compensation in Norway. This is much more than a few years ago, and as many as 698 were complaints about treatment received in somatic hospitals. Some people assert that the whole climate for physicians and patients has changed. It is perhaps a slight exaggeration, but it is said that it is no longer unusual for physicians to adjust their behavior (which perhaps is necessary!), and their examination programs and documentation routines in order to guard themselves against litigation from lawyers or patient organizations. This may lead to more patients undergoing unnecessary examinations. Up to now, this development has not become widespread, but the problem should be dealt with before conditions in the Norwegian health services become similar to those in the USA, for example.

Physicians' demands for working conditions more equal to those of other employees also have changed the role of the physician. When physicians, in the course of the last decades, began to be paid for over-time and inconvenient working hours, they at the same time had to accept more extensive supervision from their employers. In some places, hospitals refused to pay for over-time, which led certain physicians to chose to work for nothing, rather than face a moral dilemma. When this was combined with the hospitals gaining control of extra income, by removing the possibilities for the physicians to run private out-patient clinics, many hospital physicians felt severely degraded.

Previously, junior physicians experienced a relatively Spartan existence, but this could be endured, because they knew that when they were promoted to chief physicians, conditions would improve. This is a career development which still exists in several countries in Western Europe. In Norway, many colleagues have the title of chief physician, but in their daily work they also carry the workload and duties of a resident until they are approaching pensionable age. Furthermore, those who are promoted to chief physicians without the on-call duties of their subordinates, often experienced a cut in salary! It is reasonable to ask whether the central health authorities realized the adverse long-term effects of such contracts.

Some people assert that physicians have moved from a doctor's role in which the art of medicine was the ideal, to a working role where effectiveness and organization are given priority. Can the classical physicians's role be combined with a well-organized health service? It should be possible, but it is difficult. A good organization demands standards for documentation, reports and control. When time is limited, the consequence is that patient contact is reduced. In connection with my preparation of this chapter, I interviewed several older and younger colleagues. One of the grand old men in Norwegian internal medicine was clear in his utterances: "My experience of being a physician is that time shall be used to treat sick patients. Many physicians seem to use their time on other things."

23.3. The Development of Medicine

23.3.1. Information Technology Revolutionizes Access to Knowledge.

Today, physicians, like other professionals,

with the aid of a keyboard and a telephone line can gain access to large data banks within seconds. The latest treatment results for a disease can be found. References to articles which have been published on a subject can easily be collected and printed out. Data from projects with several co-workers can be put together and analyzed in just a few minutes. Up to now, we have seen only the beginning of a development with fantastic but also frightening aspects. Among them: How can we prevent personal medical data from coming into the wrong hands?

But there already is one consequence of the data revolution, about which, at the moment, neither most physicians nor the patients (and their lawyers) seem to fully realize the implications. There is no longer any excuse for not knowing! Previously, a physician could maintain that it was impossible to keep up with medical developments, at least for rare diseases or special forms of treatment. This is no longer acceptable. Practicing evidence-based medicine has been possible and also required because databases give access to available knowledge in a much more effective way than previously. The so-called Cochrane Collaboration can be an example of the way in which the development is moving. The results of controlled studies which fulfill certain basic quality criteria are registered in a computer, according to a system which claims to reflect accumulated knowledge in a representative way. It will certainly not be long before going against Cochrane recommendations will be associated with a significant responsibility. These recommendations will be available to patients, the press and lawyers, and in a few years a physician probably will take on a heavy burden of responsibility if she or he treats a patient in a way which is not in accordance with the recommendations.

23.3.2. Further Education

There is no doubt that Norwegian physicians have a good system of further education, thanks to a good professional effort and foresighted work by The Norwegian Medical Association. For many years, hospital physicians had a large part of their expenses for attending courses covered by funds accumulated and administrated through the Norwegian Medical Association. It has become important that physicians behave in such a way so as not to lose this arrangement. The warning signs are clear. Starting in 1995, contributions have been reduced due to failing accumulation of the funds.

23.3.3. Quality Assurance with Ethical Problems.

Quality assurance has been focused on since the second half of the 1980s. Many believe that there has been much empty talk and more questions about formalizing procedures and documenting activities, than documenting quality or lack of quality.

Certainly, there is a long way to go before the largest and most difficult tasks are solved in securing a permanent and reliable quality on the right level in all parts of the hospital work. It is first necessary to agree upon which end points of clinical treatment should be achieved to reflect good quality, and then to establish a way to monitor whether these aims have been reached in daily work. Outsiders will experience it as surprising and perhaps frightening that few departments have such an overview of their own activities. Only the most courageous patients will ask the surgeon the decisive question: "How many operations of this type have you done in the last year, and what were the results?" In the years to come, physicians must be prepared for a situation where aware and well-informed patients will demand such questions answered. There are several reasons why such answers may not be readily available. A more extensive documentation and revising is time-consuming, and neither hospital owners nor any other central medical authority requests such information. It is even more thought-provoking that some physicians do not seem to be interested in providing such statistics, either.

With regards to health services, Norway is divided into a patchwork of 19 mainly small counties, which only co-operate with each other to a limited degree. If adequate expertise and quality is to be built up and maintained among the health personnel, then the level of experience with the different diseases and their treatment must exceed a certain threshold. It is a fact that the total national experience with a range of complicated procedures has been too thinly distributed throughout the country to achieve highly competent and well-trained teams to meet the national demands. It is also a fact that many physicians are opposed to changing this situation, often supported by the county administration. Table 23.3 presents an overview of how many operations of different types are carried out in large, medium, and small hospitals each year and reveals that far too many operations are carried out in small hospitals, instead of patients being referred to centers where greater experience is available. The figures look even worse if they are further subdivided according to the number of operating surgeons in each type of hospital. The conclusion is that much work needs to be done to ensure the quality of clinical procedures. Norwegian physicians should take the initiative to carry out such work. To refrain from doing so is comparable to ignoring a timebomb!

Probably, the solution would be to designate centers of competence for relatively rare diseases and for diseases with complicated treatment, and to direct all such patients to these centers.

It is strange that hospital physicians have not been more conscious about exploiting the demands of society for better quality hospital services as a means to gain the necessary improvement of their own working situation.

23.3.4. The Complications of Branch Specialization

The steadily increasing branch specialization, and the more recent sub-branch special-

TABLE 23.3
Mean number of operations carried out in hospitals of different size in 1991. Source: The Directorate of Health, report series. Relationship between patient volume and quality of treatment, 4–93 (slightly revised.)

Procedure	Regional hospital	Large county hospital	Medium county hospital	Medium/small county hospital	Small county hospital
Aortic aneurysm	49	42	8	2.2	0.1
Resection of the oesophagus	6.8	1.2	0.2	0.9	0
Total colectomy	23	7	0.9	1	0.1
Resection of the rectum	42	34	9	9	2.5
Resection of the pancreas	11.2	3.7	0.6	0.7	0

ization, increases the risk that patients encounter physicians who know more about a very narrow sector of medicine, but perhaps little about the rest of medicine. Therefore, if the patient is misplaced during the diagnostic phase, this can, at the least, delay the onset of an effective treatment. This problem still is only associated with large hospitals and to the main specialties, but is nevertheless something that one should be aware of. Perhaps all large hospitals should ensure that there also exist posts and career ladders for the broadly orientated hospital physicians?

23.3.5. Hospital Medicine and Female Physicians

The number of women employed as physicians in the hospital service is increasing, particularly in junior posts (Table 23.4). But among chief physicians and surgeons and in research posts the proportion of women does not reflect the proportion of women physicians as a whole. More women are needed in hospital medicine. More women voicing their opinion could mean a lot in many ways, such as for the many unsolved problems within ethics and communication. There is no evidence that more women in hospital medicine should have negative consequences for salary development.

TABLE 23.4
The proportion of women among employed physicians.

Year	1991 %	1994 %
Senior physicians/ surgeons	14	16
Junior physicians	34	40
Research/scientific posts	23	29

Source: A. Taraldset, Tidsskrift for Den norske lægeforening 114(1994):2182-84

23.3.6. Focus by the Media

The focus on medicine by the media, on the fate of individual patients and on the role of the physician has increased substantially during the last few decades. There are several reasons for this.

First, disease and suffering attract media coverage, particularly when a dramatic story can be associated with an individual. Physicians must learn to live with this phenomenon, whether they like it or not. Physicians find themselves in a difficult situation if they are criticized in such a way that they feel is unjust, without having the opportunity to reply. Often, such controversy can be traced back to poor communication between physician and patient.

Second, society is much more open than it used to be. The media make use of their right to gain insight into medical matters.

Third, it is more usual than it was before to claim compensation if treatment does not give the expected result. Many patients believe, and not without reason, that media coverage increases the chances for their demands being met.

Certainly, the need for knowledge about the media, and the need for experience in dealing with them, came as a surprise to many physicians. The result is that many physicians, either rightly or wrongly, feel victimized by the media. But many incidents are self-inflicted, either because physicians are unwilling to co-operate with the press, or else because they do not make use of their right to read through and check articles or interviews to which they have contributed. Failure to acknowledge the fact that certain patients are extremely well informed about their diseases, sometimes better informed than the physician, can also lead to unfortunate episodes.

The physicians themselves must take a large part of responsibility for the unrealistic expectations which many laypeople have about what medicine can accomplish. For example, information is often presented to the media in such a way that the physician knows, or should know, that it will be misunderstood by laypeople. Physicians are perhaps no worse than others when it comes to promoting their own interests, but the side-effects can easily become substantial.

23.4. Organizational and Administrative Challenges

We only need to go back a couple of decades to find many examples of physicians who gave administrative tasks such a low priority that it was noticed and had repercussions. It was not until lawyers and economists took over director posts and other leading posts in many hospitals that physicians woke up. The situation has improved, but it will take time for the physicians to persuade others that they give administration full attention. In hospitals, it is still not unusual for physicians who apply for the chief physician post that is in charge of the whole hospital (sjefslege) to demand that they be allowed to practice their specialty while at the same time carrying top-level administrative responsibility. This is a clear sign that they regard administration as a second-rate business, in contrast to the nurses who have cultivated the discipline of administration for many years.

23.4.1. The Out-patient Department

The demands of hospital owners that out-patient services should be part of the department's ordinary services contributed to the significant increase in efficiency that occurred in hospitals in the 1980s. Instead of automatically admitting referred patients, patients were first assessed as out-patients, and then examined and given appropriate treatment. For the patient, this reorganization has meant that he or she meets the specialist at an earlier stage than was the case before. Decisions are taken more rapidly and unnecessary admissions are avoided. Also, patients are referred back to their own physicians more readily than previously. The out-patient department was allocated appropriate premises and an adequate number of health personnel.

An important consequence was that hospital owners at the same time acquired control of the private and economically attractive out-patient practices of chief physicians. Until 1979, chief physicians were allowed to work up to six hours a week with private patients, usually in their own clinic, and not uncommonly with the assistance of personnel who were on the hospital payroll. Thus, hospital owners had good reason to intervene. In many departments, the chief physician disappeared early in the day, went to his out-patient clinic and stayed there. The result was that the everyday work of the department often was carried out by relatively inexperienced colleagues, who not uncommonly delayed decisions until the chief physician turned up. It was at the out-patient clinic that the chief physician made the real money. A private business existed within the hospital, run by practitioners who payed little or nothing for the premises which they used. Of course, the nurses saw through this. Maybe this is why out-patient clinics even nowadays are regarded with scepticism by many older nurses.

There is still room for improvement. Hospital physicians who wish to work longer than normal working hours for adequate remuneration should be given the opportunity to do so when the workload in the department is greater than can be managed within the normal timeframes. Instead, the physicians often work other places in their spare time.

23.4.2. Can the Role of the Physician and the Role of a Financial Gate-keeper Be Combined?

The traditional role of a physician was straightforward and safe. The physician should do his best for his patients. He should always try to heal, and if that was not possible, he should relieve suffering and give comfort.

These aims are as good today as they have always been. But we must realize that the enormous technological possibilities that medicine has to offer have presented hospital physicians, in particular, with completely new problems. These relate simply to when, and according to which principles, procedures which are especially demanding of resources should be applied. This is particularly problematic if the chances for successful treatment are small, even if no resources being spared. It is even more difficult if the treatment is risky and the side-effects are mumerous. In large hospitals, the senior physicians in responsible and decision-making positions often are faced with the problem as to whether expensive treatment should be initiated or not. The choice is difficult, especially when the physician knows that such treatment for one single patient may demand resources equivalent to what is required for running the department's out-patient clinic for several months, or are equivalent to the resources required to carry out scores of hip-replacement operations or operations for cataract. Norway has a publicy financed health service which allocates block grants to hospitals, and the basic philosophy is one of solidarity. Saying yes to new, expensive treatment for desperately ill patients, for whom the chance of a successful treatment is small, means saying no to a large number of other patients, for whom the chance of a successful outcome of the treatment is fairly good.

A disturbing additional problem arises when the principle of solidarity is challenged by patients who demand expensive treatment. The typical situation is a patient in a higher social class, who with the help of the press, lawyers and personal contacts, demands that the State pay for treatment that has not yet been proved to be effective, as measured by the standards accepted by Norwegian medicine. Until recently, politicians have capitulated much too often, and have allocated large amounts to cover treatment for some patients, without ensuring that others in the same situation are offered the same alleged chances.

As treatment possibilities based on advances in medical technology increase and as patients gain greater insight into what medicine may offer specifically for their disease, problems associated with ethics and resource allocation arise. Common sense and logic indicate that only setting priorities based on consent, and a general attitude that the priority principles which have been agreed upon should be followed, can solve the huge problems. However, there still are many physicians who are opposed to allocation of resources according to such priorities.

It is not by chance that conflicts over priorities first became apparent in welfare states with publicly financed healthcare systems. It is also in such countries that systematic work on defining priorities has been carried through to the largest extent. In Norway, the report of a committee headed by the professor of theology Inge Lønning (born 1938), published in 1987, provided the framework. But work proceeds slowly. Eight years later, compulsory, nationally accepted programs exist for only a handful of diseases. Systematic experience with priorities is available only for the bone-marrow transplantation program.

The challenge for hospital physicians in the years to come will be to draw guidelines for the way in which national priorities shall be implemented on the local level in each hospital department. Politicians must decide on the overall framework, and the leadership in each hospital may give a general outline for the services which will be offered. But it is in the hospital wards that the daily decisions have to be made, by the physicians in co-operation with the nurses.

Some will say that this is how it has always been. The big difference is that the medicine of the future will demand that these highly complex decisions be made according to an accepted set of guidelines.

In 1994, the Norwegian Medical Association adopted the following addition to §12 of its ethical rules: "The physician must contribute to ensuring that medical resources are allocated according to general ethical standards. A physician must not in any way seek to obtain an unwarranted advantage, in terms of economy, priority or any type of advantage, for individual patients or groups of patients. In the case of lack of resources within his field of responsibility, the physician must report this to the superior authority."

23.4.3. Leadership in a Hospital Department

Demands from hospital owners for better documentation of medical services and transferral of budget responsibility to the departments seemingly have given the chief physician or surgeon in each department more scope and authority. But other factors modify this picture. If transferring of administrative responsibility is not also accompanied by an allocation of sufficient additional administrative personnel, the chief physician or surgeon in the department can be reduced to a mere administrative clerk.

Other challenges to the authority of the chief physician or surgeon who is in charge of the department, at least in large hospitals, are the consequences of subdivision of departments into specialized sections with their own struggle for authority and autonomy. In addition, the distinction between specialties has been blurred. Key words in the process to cope with these problems are the establishment of the so-called organ clinics and the introduction of intervention medicine, where tasks are transferred from surgery and medicine to radiologists and anaesthetists.

However, a main issue in the 1990s has been the nurses' demands to share responsibility for leadership of departments. But to claim leadership in a hospital department is to take over a far more comprehensive job than to administrate the department. That such a conflict could arise says something about the way in which the physicians have neglected administration. The situation has developed to the point that several hospital directors, with the support of the Norwegian Union of Municipalities (Norske Kommuners Sentralforbund), have formulated the phrase "det enhetlige, todelte lederskap" (the uniform two-part leadership), without even blushing at the phrase's obvious lack of logic and rationality. Is there any business similar in size to a hospital department that would fail to give one person the leadership responsibility? This battle culminated at the National Hospital during the autumn of 1995, when an attempt was made to introduce this administrative malformation as part of an administrative reform at the new National Hospital, then under construction. The physicians refused to accept the proposal, and in November 1995 the Norwegian Parliament confirmed that the responsibility of leadership should be traced to one person at all levels in the medical services.

23.5. Hospital Physicians under Pressure

In the 1990s Norwegian hospital physicians in a way have been forced into a corner. This seems surprising, because huge steps forward have been taken in diagnostics and treatment in hospitals during the last years.

But both the role of a physician and the external conditions have changed. Many hospital physicians feel that while demands for knowledge and performance steadily increase, their status has decreased. And as a confirmation of this fact, salary developments have been miserable for many years.

Unrealistic expectations on the part of the population, the politicians, the authorities, and the hospital owners contribute to the strain experienced in a hectic working day, and so do certain aspects of the increased influence by the patients on the decisions which are to be made.

Owners demands for better control of costs and for better documentation mean that a larger share of the physicians' working hours has to be devoted to administrative work. In addition, when physicians in private practice are, to a larger extent, their own master, earn more money, and have more spare time, it is not surprising that experienced physicians are leaving hospitals. It is also frustrating to administer scarce resources in an everyday situation where the gap between what is possible and what can be financed becomes steadily wider.

Hospital physicians should probably be more conscious about profiling and limiting their professional role, so that more time is devoted to patient work. A continous comparison of their own treatment results with established standards, and implementation of resource allocation at the ward level according to given priorities, will provide huge challenges in the near future. These challenges have to be met in a way which is generally agreed upon among the members of the medical profession.

Finally, an active effort to open up, thoroughly discuss, and resolve the issue of leadership in hospitals is necessary.

C H A P T E R 2 4

Doctors in Research – a World of Conflicting Objectives

OLE DIDRIK LÆRUM

24.1. Introduction

The shaping of the medical profession in any country has been and is dependent on both education and research. Without a continuous flow of new knowledge from science, practical medicine would die out. The aim of research is not only to provide entirely new procedures and approaches, but just as much to question and modify existing knowledge.

Although the era of modern medicine is short, development of the medical profession and its research activities has a long history. In this chapter, the development of medical sciences in Norway will therefore be reviewed, and some pioneering work of the nineteenth and early twentieth century will be highlighted. Thereafter, a survey of investigations in different areas will be given, with the main emphasis on the last thirty years.

24.2. The Development of Institutions

Medical research in Norway has mainly been done in hospitals and university institutes. Therefore, the development of the different hospitals and institutes had a great impact on the scattered research activities in the nineteenth century, as well as the more systematic development of medical sciences in the twentieth century.

The first university in Norway, the University of Oslo, was founded in 1811 under the name Universitas regia Fredericiana (Larsen 1989, Hopstock 1915). A medical faculty with three professors was established. In addition to those who graduated with the medical degree, candidatus medicinae, in the years 1815–1844, four academic theses were defended in the field of medicine. Thirty years then passed before there were any additional doctoral dissertations.

However, the university was not the first scientific institution in Norway. As early as 1767, the Royal Norwegian Society for Sciences was established in Trondheim, an institution which laid part of the foundation for the later University of Trondheim.

The main university clinic in Oslo, Rikshospitalet (the National Hospital), was founded in 1826, and is the one institution in our country which has had the greatest importance for medical research. Later, other municipal hospitals in Oslo, such as Aker Hospital (founded in 1871) and Ullevål Hospital (founded in 1887), were included as university clinics (Larsen 1989, Elster

1990, Reichborn Kjennerud, Grøn and Kobro 1936, Kristiansen and Larsen 1987).

In Western Norway, Bergen Museum was founded in 1825, and from the last third of the nineteenth century, active research took place both at the museum and in different hospitals in Bergen, as will be mentioned later. In 1912 the municipal hospital in Bergen moved to a new location outside the city, named Haukeland Hospital, and at the same time the Gade Institute for Pathological Anatomy was erected as a private foundation. Both the hospital and the Gade Institute were important pillars when the medical faculty at the newly established University of Bergen was formally opened in 1946 (Brunchorst 1900, Tschudi Madsen and Sollied 1931).

In 1968, Norway established two more universities, one in Trondheim and one in Tromsø. In both places, a medical faculty was connected to the local hospitals (Fulsås 1993).

In addition to the four medical faculties in Norway, medical research has been carried out in several other research institutes, both state owned and private. The universities have, however, still been the dominating research institutions. For cancer research, the Norwegian Radium Hospital, founded in 1932 outside Oslo, has been, and still is, of particular importance.

24.3. Medical Research in the Nineteenth Century

In this period most physicians in Norway worked as general practitioners in rural districts. Although there was a growing awareness of research possibilities, such efforts were scattered, and mainly carried out by single physicians. Moreover, most of the medical activities were connected to the only existing medical faculty, as well as to some of the hospitals. Very little research was done in general practice, although there were exceptions. Chorea hereditaria had been recognized earlier, but the first complete description of this condition as a defined, hereditary disease was given by Johan Christian Lund (1830–1906) in the valley of Setesdal in 1859. In 1872, the American physician Huntington (1850–1916) described the same disease under the name chorea major (Huntington's disease), but without knowing about Lund's earlier description. Lund made a thorough study of the symptoms and of the way the disease was inherited, based on registration of families in a local district (Ørbeck and Quelprud 1951).

Leprosy, or what later was called Hansen's disease, has been recognized as a disease in Norway since the Middle Ages. From the beginning of the nineteenth century, the incidence in this disease increased, reaching a peak in the 1850s. Hansen's disease mainly occurred in the coastal areas of Western Norway. Hospitals for the care of these patients had been established in Bergen, and active research took place there in the 1840s. A thorough description of the disease, based on direct clinical observations and autopsies, was given in an atlas which was published in 1847 by D.C. Danielsen (1815–1894) and C.W. Boeck (1808–1875). Danielsen was the head of the Leprosy Hospital in Bergen, and Boeck was a dermatologist who later became a professor at the University in Kristiania (Oslo).

From the middle of the century, Bergen was an internationally recognized center for leprosy research, where several famous clinicians, pathologists, and microbiologists came from Central Europe in order to study the disease, including such notables as Rudolph Virchow (1821–1902) and Albert Neisser (1855–1916). In 1873, Gerhard Armauer Hansen (1841–1912) described the leprosy bacillus, mycobacterium leprae. Because of his work, in some countries the leprosy bacillus has been called Hansen's bacillus. This was the first known case where a chronic human disease was attributed to bacillar infection, and it was done nine years before Robert Koch (1843–1910) described the tuberculosis bacillus.

A register of Hansen's disease was established for patients from all over the country, and these data are still important for the understanding of the epidemiology of the disease. Epidemiological studies on Hansen's disease also formed the basis for the hypothesis by Armauer Hansen that leprosy was a communicable and not an hereditary disease.

In 1899 Caesar Boeck (1845–1917), a nephew of C.W. Boeck, also a professor of dermatology in Oslo, described sarcoidosis as a chronic granulomatous skin disease.

24.4. Some Medical Discoveries in the First Half of the Twentieth Century

The founder of experimental cancer research in Norway was Magnus Haaland (1876–1935), who spent seven years altogether in different European laboratories studying transplantable tumors in mice. In 1904 he was a co-worker of Amadé Borrel and Elie Metchnikov (1845–1916) at the Pasteur Institute in Paris. Later he worked with Paul Ehrlich (1854–1915) in Frankfurt. From 1906 to 1911, he was at the Imperial Cancer Research Campaign in London working in Erwin Bashford's laboratory. He was the first to describe reticulosis, a virus-inducted lymphoid tumor disease in mice, and he demonstrated experimentally how transplanted tumor cells metastasize through the blood vessels in mice.

In 1911 he took over the position as the first head of the Gade Institute in Bergen, where he initiated important research in the field of clinically oriented microbiology, with the main emphasis on typhoid fever. Haaland's efforts through many years were a main factor in eradicating this disease in Norway in the 1920s.

Familial hypercholesterolemia as a cause of angina pectoris and cardiac infarction was first described in 1925 by the pathologist Francis Harbitz (1867–1950). The clinical condition was first described as an inheritable disorder by Carl Müller (1886–1983) in 1938. Soon after the discovery of the BCG vaccine at the Pasteur Institute in Paris, Norwegian clinicians started mass vaccination. In the 1930s, Olaf Scheel (1875–1942) and Johannes Heimbeck (1892–1976), as well as Konrad Birkhaug (1892–1980), a former co-worker of Albert Calmette (1863–1933) at the Pasteur Institute, made important contributions to documentation of the efficacy and mode of action of the BCG vaccine.

Phenylketonuria, or Følling's disease, was first described in 1934 by Asbjørn Følling (1888–1973). Later, Norwegian physicians made important contributions to the understanding of the metabolic defect underlying this disease (Lie 1984).

Paul Owren (1905–1990), professor of internal medicine in Oslo, founded a Norwegian school of thrombosis research at the National Hospital, which emanated from his discovery of coagulation factor V in 1947.

A general picture emerges of the first half of the twentieth century: Norwegian medical research was related to clinical work and direct discoveries on patients, though a growing amount of laboratory and experimental investigation was also carried out. Researchers worked on their theses alone, partly on the clinical wards, partly in laboratories and also in clinical practice. Finally, research by the medical profession was connected to university institutes and large hospitals.

24.5. Organizational Developments After the Second World War

The need for more systematic research in

Norway not only necessitated the development of laboratories and provision of technical equipment and other facilities, but also granting boards which could support both research fellows doing their medical theses as well as research in general. From the end of the 1940s and onwards, five different research councils were established by the Government. One of them, the Norwegian Research Council for Natural Sciences and the Humanities, had a division for medical research. This was the main granting body for medical research until the five state research-councils were merged into one single organization in 1992 under the name of the Research Council of Norway. Since then, medical research has been included as one of six divisions, covering all types of health research, ranging from psychology and dentistry to general medical research.

In addition, several private organizations were founded in order to support medical research such as cancer research and research on tuberculosis and other infectious diseases as well as arteriosclerosis. Traditionally, the yearly cancer campaign, when money is collected by the Norwegian Cancer Society, has contributed substantially to the funding of medical research in general, in which basic research related to cancer has been strongly supported.

24.6. From the 1960s to the 1990s

This has been a period of rapid expansion in Norwegian medical research, along with the development of regional hospitals and the different specialties in medicine, as well as with the rapid expansion in the education of doctors and recruitment programs for doctoral theses. Although it would not be appropriate to mention some contributions at the expense of many others, some areas of particular strength in the international Norwegian medical research will be indicated.

As already mentioned, cardiovascular and hypertension studies, as well as kidney physiology research, have had a strong position, not only at the University of Oslo, but also in other medical faculties. Apart from thrombosis research, extensive epidemiological and intervention studies on the relationship between fatty acids in the diet and risk of cardiac infarction have been carried out. Lipid and other nutritional research has also had an important position.

Norwegian biochemical research has made important contributions to the field of inborn metabolic defects, and several new syndromes have been described and characterized on a biochemical and genetic basis. Furthermore, Norwegian epidemiology has been regarded as being high class. In particular, the Norwegian Cancer Registry holds an important international position.

Since the 1960s, immunology has expanded rapidly, both in experimental and clinical areas. Several important international contributions have been made, which have been widely cited in the literature. This has been connected both to cellular and humoral immune mechanisms, transplantation immunology and to secretory immunoglobulins (Brandtzæg 1990).

Norway has a strong tradition in neuroanatomy and neurophysiology, dating back to the pioneering studies in Bergen and Oslo by the Arctic explorer and zoologist Fridtjof Nansen (1861–1930) in the 1880s (Brunchorst 1900). Today, these fields hold an international reputation, mainly connected to the Department of Neurophysiology at the University of Oslo. Pain, stress and sleep research are among fields which have a strong research tradition at the University of Bergen.

In cancer research, all four universities, as well as the Norwegian Radium Hospital, have been active at an international level. Today, important studies on hyperthermia, immunotherapy, toxins, and biological response modifiers, including growth factors and growth inhibitors, are being done. Norwegian clinicians are actively participating in large international clinical trials in cancer treatment.

In the 1960s, new methods for separating white blood cells in human beings were developed at the Norwegian Defense Research Establishment at Kjeller, which later became a standard for blood cell separation all over the world. Arne Böyum (born 1928), who originally described the sedimentation and centrifugation methods, has become one of the most widely cited Norwegian physicians in international literature.

Experimental surgery has had a strong position at the medical faculties both in Oslo and in Bergen, and has generated a long list of academic theses. Research in general practice and community medicine, as well as in preventive medicine and health services, has also been gradually built up at the four medical faculties and state research institutes, and has gained an international reputation.

It should not be forgotten that the Norwegian pharmaceutical industry has made important contributions in the field of X-ray contrast dyes through pioneering research done by the Hafslund-Nycomed Company (Amdam and K Sogner 1994). Likewise, research in medical technology has led to the development of several new products for the international market, including an artificial cardiac valve, diagnostic ultrasound apparatuses, and simulators and practical equipment for resuscitation of patients.

24.7. 1985 to 1995: Features of a Decade

During these ten years, medical research has been relatively stable, although several changes have taken place. Medical research performed by the medical profession has become more and more intergrated into health research, where collaboration with other categories of health professionals, including psychologists, dentists and others, has become the rule rather than the exception. Basic sciences have become more and more dependent on an interdisciplinary approach, to which biologists, biochemists, technologists and other experts have been important contributors. This is also reflected in the funding policy of the Research Council and other agencies. The mean age of medical researchers has become higher, but at the same time recruitment to doctoral degrees has doubled. Some features will be mentioned here.

24.8. Recruitment

In 1994, altogether 550 doctoral degrees were given by Norwegian universities. One fifth of these were medical degrees, and one quarter of them were obtained by women. To give an indication of the expansion, in the period 1990–94, 2,300 academic degrees were given altogether in Norway, representing about one third of all dissertations which have taken place in this country since the first one in 1817. In addition to the MD thesis, an increasing number of academic theses, submitted by representatives of other health professions and the basic sciences, have been presented at the four medical faculties.

Among candidates who spend three years as research fellows at university institutions, about three-quarters complete their thesis. In contrast to academic thesis programs at the natural science faculties, the physicians take their doctoral degrees at a higher age. Throughout the whole decade, the mean age for doctoral dissertations by physicians has been around forty years, and this age is only exceeded by their colleagues in the humanities.

From about 1985 to 1994, the annual

number of doctoral degrees obtained by physicians increased by 50 percent. Today it is compulsory to have an academic thesis degree in order to obtain a permanent position at a university. Traditionally, medical research in Norway has resulted in many theses, and one third of all the academic degrees that have ever been given at the universities have been based on medical dissertations (Bruen Olsen 1994, Skodvin 1991, Bruen Olsen and Skoie 1991, FoU statistikk 1995).

24.9. Research Personnel

At present, there are about 4.35 million inhabitants in Norway, and altogether 2,300 people work in medical research, including those in universities and in independent institutes. This represents about 18 percent of all scientists in Norway. Two thirds of these work in university clinics, and one third in ordinary university institutes. Altogether, about 60 percent of all physicians who work in university clinics are involved in research work.

Investigators in clinical subjects account for nearly one half of all medical researchers. Researchers in basic sciences account for 26 percent and in paraclinical fields 21 percent, while researchers in general practice and community medicine account for 8 percent of all medical researchers. During this period, the yearly increase in personnel has been one to two percent. The number of women has doubled. They now account for 22 percent of all researchers.

24.10. Funding and Infrastructure

Expressed as a percentage of gross domestic product (GDP), funding of Norwegian research has gradually increased during the last ten years, from 1.4 percent of GDP in 1983, to nearly 2 percent in 1993. This is lower than the average in the OECD countries. Although the amount of research money provided by the government has been relatively high, private support of research is far lower than in other countries that are comparable to Norway.

Since the main funding of medical research is from the Division of Health Sciences at the Research Council, this budget gives an estimate of conditions for doctors doing research. This division receives approximately 6 percent of the total budget of the Research Council (141 million Norwegian kroner in 1995) of which about one-half is grant money for physicians. The rest goes to the funding of research done by other health professionals, mainly psychologists and dentists, and also biologists.

The main part of the budget comes from the ministry of Education, Research and Church Affairs, although other ministries also contribute, mainly the Ministry of Health and Social Affairs, which contributes 20 percent. Private industry also contributes, but to a lesser extent (FoU statistikk 1995, Norges Forskningsråd 1995).

In general, funding by the Research Council is low, compared to funding from private organizations, mainly within cancer research. This makes research particularly susceptible to changes in the general economy of the country from year to year, which may affect fundraising campaigns for research. In particular, funding of running costs for laboratories and funding of technical equipment has been low.

24.11. Areas of Research

An important objective in the policy of the Research Council has been to support health sciences in general, and not exclusively basic medical research. Therefore, on one hand classical medical disciplines have been supported, including research in general practice. On the other hand, research programs have been established where new or expanding areas at an international level are supported. Specific programs for psychiatry, general practice, and geriatrics have been established, a national virus research laboratory has been founded, and in addition a large program for research on health, environment, and living conditions (HEMIL: Helse-, miljø- og levekårsforskning) was launched in 1987. This latter included epidemiology, occupational research, health and environment, preventive medicine, health services research, and also health problems related to developing countries. The HEMIL program was established as an interdisciplinary approach and led to the formation of new research activities.

Altogether, in this decade, general health, social and clinical sciences have been promoted more than the basic sciences (Søgnen 1994, Evaluering av HEMIL 1991).

24.12. Medical Research at an International Level

To what extent do Norwegian physicians participate in international research communities? As a background, it should be mentioned that from the 1950s on, many Norwegians studied medicine abroad, mainly in Germany, but also in other European countries. Today, about 16 percent of Norwegian physicians have been educated abroad, and 8 percent have a doctoral degree from another country. It should also be noted that Norwegian medical research has always had strong ties to other countries, mainly the United States, Great Britain, and Germany, in addition to the other Nordic countries.

Of all scientific workers in Norway, about one-third have been abroad for more than a year. One half of all physicians in research have been at a research institution in another country for at least half a year.

Although it would be desirable to have a higher proportion of our medical profession engaged in research spend a longer period abroad, nevertheless three-quarters of them go abroad every year to attend conferences or in connection with scientific collaboration. In most cases, attending a conference includes presenting a paper. Altogether two-thirds of all medical scientists in Norway have participated in an international cooperative research project, mainly with the United States and Western Europe (Marheim Larsen 1992, Sivertsen 1991).

Another question is to what extent the results from Norwegian medical research are published in international fora, and if they have an impact on international science. Compared to the other Nordic countries, Sweden and Denmark, the activity and international impact from Norwegian science in general is relatively weak, and below the average level for OECD countries. Per capita, Sweden has 60 percent more scientific articles in print on a whole than Norway has, while Denmark has 30 percent, and Finland 5 percent more. The frequency of citations of these articles is also lower for Norway than for Sweden and Denmark. However, within the different research fields, there is great variation. Thus, in medicine, Norwegian international articles are cited more than in other fields, although the other Nordic countries are also ahead of us in this respect. Especially in clinical medicine, there are many Norwegian articles, and they are often cited. Gastroenterology and hematology rank high, but also dermatology, obstetrics and gynaecology as well as cancer research and partly internal medicine have high activity and good impact.

In biomedicine, Norwegian articles have a high citation index in cell biology and genetics, while microbiology and physiology also have high publication activity, but a lower citation index.

Such figures, taken as a whole, can be misleading, since large individual differences occur between scientists within the same research fields. As has been argued, the impact of the journal in which an article is published, and the number of citations, may in several cases be misleading.

As a general conclusion, Norwegian medical research has broad international contact, but reflects the problem of a small country: since the number of scientists is low, the impact as a whole will not be high. However, as a part of international networks and in limited areas, Norwegian medical research is of high quality by international standards.

24.13. Research as an Integral Part of Professional Activities

Medical education in our country is research based, and, in addition, continuous education is almost compulsory for all doctors. This implies that new research data will quickly have an impact on professional activities related to patient work, which is constantly upgraded by this professional exposure to new knowledge. The Norwegian Medical Association has strongly promoted this concept, both through its journal and by establishing new areas of teaching and research at the universities through donating professorial chairs, as in geriatrics, occupational and general medicine, as well as by supporting university personnel engaged in continuing education.

However, active research is mainly connected to hospitals, where 75 percent of it is done in the university clinics. Although many physicians also participate in research projects in other hospitals, the magnitude of this is relatively low, and there has been no change for the last fifteen years (Bruen Olsen 1991).

Medical research is generally considered to be of high priority, although the funding and number of persons involved can vary considerably from one area to another. The policy has been to distribute research money in order to cover the medical fields as broadly as possible, but at the same time to concentrate on some main lines within each field. There has also been a policy to achieve a balance between the different regions in Norway, so that research is not too strongly centralized. Programs for research in general practice have been aimed at making scientific thinking and approaches available that are relevant to all types of health problems and patient care in the general population.

A special problem is created by the limited number of patients available for different clinical trials. To overcome this, Norwegian clinicians have been active in participating in international, and mainly Scandinavian and European, trials and networks. In this way, better data become available for improvement of patient care in Norway.

There are also other limiting factors for Norwegian medical research. One is the low mobility of medical scientists between the four universities. This is a general feature of Norwegian research as a whole, where co-operation between the four medical faculties and different disciplines has been hampered, despite attempts to overcome this. Limitations on working time available for research in the clinical wards at university clinics has been another issue of controversy. Owing to the difficult financial situation at the regional hospitals which function as university clinics, the work load for the single physician has increased during the last ten years. This means less time for each patient, and also less time for doing research. In 1981, the amount of working time spent on research at universities in general amounted to 48 percent, while in the clinics this was only 26 percent for those in full-time university positions. Since then, working conditions have become even more difficult, and the available time for research has become less. For the same reason, the possibility for young physicians to participate in research projects has become more limited.

Therefore, recruitment to doctoral degrees is more dependent than before on research fellowship for three years, where they work full time on their research project.

24.14. Conflicting Objectives

Since a high proportion of Norwegian medical research is done part-time, and in parallel with many other tasks, including teaching, clinical work, administrative duties, and committee work, it is often difficult to get the necessary continuity in research. At present, the strongest conflict lies in the interplay between all the different duties, which all together make the work load for an average physician in a permanent university position almost unlimited. This is also a consequence of belonging to a small country, where the same experts have duties in many different fields. In contrast, for those working in university institutes, who do not have clinical or laboratory duties, almost one half of working time is considered to be available for research. The real world is somewhat different in this case as well, since having many different tasks tends to reduce the time spent on scientific activities.

In particular, when there are strong conflicting interests between patient work and research activities, ethical problems may arise. Which duty is the most important in the long run: the medicine of today or of tomorrow? How can a reasonable priority be determined?

The fact that the mean age for obtaining a doctoral degree is around forty years is also problematic. On one side, clinical experience can be of critical importance in influencing the choice of research topic. Therefore, recruitment should not be restricted to the age groups between 25 and 30 years, as is becoming more and more usual for PhD theses. At the same time, it makes the total time period spent on a scientific career very long, and this may conflict with family life. This is a problem particularly for recruitment of women to scientific positions in Norway today.

Another problem is that the number of medical researchers throughout the decade of rapid expansion of medical knowledge and areas of research has been constant. Should we choose broad research areas in order to cover as much as possible, or is it better to concentrate on one thing and go into depth? In practice this cannot be solved, since both needs are equally important. Limited funding, at a time when new technical equipment is appearing so rapidly on an international basis, is another limiting factor for optimal research conditions. This issue has recently been addressed by the Norwegian Government, which may result in extra support.

Traditionally, medical research has been strong in Norway, and in some respects the development is positive. At the same time some limiting forces have become more prevailing, and this is particularly evident in clinical research. The research traditions in the medical profession are therefore confronted with great challenges in the coming decade, not only connected to research itself, but also to improvement of general working conditions.

References

Amdam, R.P., and K. Sogner. *Rik på kontraster*. Oslo: ad Notam Gyldendal, 1994.

Brandtzæg, P. *Twenty-five years of research at LIIPAT 1965-90*. Oslo: Rikshospitalet, 1990.

Brunchorst, J. *Bergens Museum 1825–1900*. Bergen: Johan Griegs Forlagsekspedition, 1900.

Elster, T. *Rikets hospital*. Oslo: Aschehoug, 1990.

Evaluering av hovedinnsatsområdet helse-, miljø- og levekårsforskning (HEMIL). Oslo: NAVF, 1991.

FoU-statistikk og indikatorer. Forskning og utviklingsarbeid 1995 (R&D Statistics – Science and Technology Indicators). Oslo: Utredningsinstituttet, 1994.

Fulsås, N. *Universitetet i Tromsø 25 år*. Tromsø: Universitetet i Tromsø, 1993.

Hopstock, H. *Det anatomiske institutt, 1815–1915*. Oslo: Aschehoug Boghandel, 1915.

Kristiansen, K., and Ø. Larsen. *Ullevål sykehus i hundre år*. Oslo: Oslo kommune, Ullevål sykehus, 1987.

Larsen, I. M., *Norske universitetsforskere – kosmopolitter i forskningen? Rapport 11/92*. Oslo: NAVF utredningsinstitutt, 1992.

Larsen, Ø. *Mangfoldig medisin*. Oslo: Det medisinske fakultet, Universitetet i Oslo, 1989.

Lie, S.O. *Asbjørn Føllings sykdom*. Tidsskrift for Den norske lægeforening, 2381-5.

Madsen, S. T., and O. Sollied. *Medisinsk liv i Bergen*. Bergen: Det medisinske selskap, 1931.

Olsen, T. B., and H. Skoie (eds). *Noen forskningspolitiske spørsmål i norsk medisin. Rapport 19/91*. Oslo: NAVFs utredningsinstitutt, 1991.

Olsen, T. B., *Forskning ved norske sykehus. Rapport 5/91*. Oslo: NAVFs utredningsinstitutt, 1991.

Olsen, T. B., *Norske doktorgrader i tall – med særlig vekt på tiarsperioden 1984–93. Rapport 9/94*. Oslo: Utredningsinstituttet for forskning og høyere utdanning, 1994.

Reichborn-Kjennerud, I., F. Grøn, and I. Kobro. *Medisinens historie i Norge*. Oslo: Grøndahl & Søns forlag, 1936. Oslo: New ed Kildeforlaget, 1985.

Sivertsen, G. *Norsk forskning på den internasjonale arenaen. Rapport 1/91*. Oslo: NAVFs utredningsinstitutt, 1991.

Skodvin, O-J. *Forskerrekruttering til det medisinske fagområdet. Status og perspektiver mot år 2010. Rapport 6/91*. Oslo: NAVFs utredningsinstitutt, 1991.

Søgnen, R. *Dynamisk treghet. Endringsprosesser i NAVFs råd for medisinsk forskning (RMF) 1975-1993. Rapport 12/94*. Oslo: Utredningsinstituttet, 1994.

Ørbeck, A.L. and T. Quelprud. *Setesdalsrykkja (Chorea progressiva hereditaria)*. Oslo: J Dybwad, 1951.

CHAPTER 25

Meta-Medicine: The Rise and Fall of the Norwegian Doctor as Leader and Manager

OLE BERG

25.1. Introduction: Meta-Medicine

Physicians may, as physicians, turn their attention in three directions – toward the patient, toward society, and toward themselves and the system of which they are vital parts. When doing the first and the second, they are doctoring; they are helping individual people or groups of people (by doing something to their environment) (Freidson 1975). When doing the third, they are governing or managing those who are performing the two former functions. I shall call this function a meta-medical function.

The doctor has always been trained to perform the first two functions. The third function has generally been regarded as a continuation of the first and the second. It has been looked upon as a function that required professional insight but not much genuinely managerial training. The self-image of the doctor has thus become closely tied to the role of doctoring, and primarily in the first sense of the word: doctoring patients. This self-image is reinforced by the public image of the doctor – a person who cares for, even devotes his or her life to, the well-being of his or her individual patients.

There is little in the training of the doctor, or in his or her image, that should prompt his or her pursuing a meta-medical career. In fact, if we take a closer look at the role for which he or she is trained, we see that it is particularly anti-managerial. Personal doctoring, the mainstay of the medical role, is primarily expected to be carried out in a dyadic relationship. Each doctor has his or her own patients and is solely responsible for their treatment. The ideal-typical doctor is the solo practitioner. Few occupational roles are less likely to awaken managerial ideas in the heads of those who perform them. If anything, they are more likely to give rise to attitudes that are skeptical, even suspicious, of governance and management: Managerial functions appear to pose a threat to the most important aspect of the physician's role, that of autonomy of practice (Freidson 1970). But this is not the full picture.

Medicine has more managerial aspects and implications than those which immediately meet the eye. However, physicians have tried to define these aspects in a manner that is not inimical to the traditional role of doctor. To fathom fully the nature of medical management, it is therefore necessary to describe how this has happened.

First, personal doctoring is a partially

hierarchic activity. The doctor tries to exercise authority over patients and is conscious of it. The success of his or her practice depends on the understanding and obedience of his or her patients. The doctor is a partial manager of private lives. A sign of this is the fact that the doctor, like other managers, has a word for disobedience: non-compliance. Most doctors, though, don't give the phenomenon much systematic attention. Their socialization tells them that the managerial relation is not really a managerial one; it is a natural one. It is the relation between one who knows and one who does not know, where the knowledge of the former is used to help the latter, in the undivided interest of the latter. Thus, the managerial aspect of the relationship remains concealed from both the doctor and the patient, or should remain so. When the managerial content of the relationship is, in this way, left unrecognized, the doctor is also unlikely to use his or her clinical role to develop his or her managerial talents -at least consciously.

Second, environmental doctoring is obviously often a hierarchic activity. Whereas the personal doctor can carry out his or her treatment directly, without much assistance from the patient, the environmental doctor must work through others, often unwilling others. He or she must convince those who are responsible for a particular part the environment for example, a workplace or a leisure area that they must modify it and make it safer. He or she must also try to persuade groups of people to change their life styles and habits. It is indeed telling that environmental doctoring in the eighteenth and early nineteenth centuries was often named "medical police" (in Old German "Medicinal-Polizey"). And yet this kind of doctoring is primarily taught, and "sold" to the public, as objective, neutral, and non-managerial. "Non-compliance" is frequently met with moralizing. Much is done, though not necessarily intentionally, to conceal the managerial nature of the task.

Third, in order to achieve professional autonomy, doctors must control the conditions under which they practice. They must control the organization of the health care system of the country. And to avoid politics, doctors must control politics. Yet even this meta-medicine has been "sold" as neutral and devoid of traditional interest politics: To see what must be done organizationally to maximize medicine's ability to cure disease, alleviate pain and promote health, one must be a part of the profession Rational meta-medicine means tracing the organizational implications of professional knowledge and acumen. Only doctors are in a position to do so. The managerial role can be taken care of without loss of professional identity; the meta-doctor is primarily a doctor.

In order to understand the role of the doctor as manager over a period of time, one must realize that doctors have traditionally wanted to manage; manage patients, society and themselves, but did not see it as a management. They have wanted to see it as a continuation of the genuine physician role.

In the following I will show how the medical profession step by step succeeded in achieving acceptance for this typically medical management role. However, I shall also show how this role began to crumble after about 1970, and how the profession now struggles to find a new way of defining it.

My focus will be on pivotal events and persons and only briefly, and in broad terms, on the development. I will concentrate on three medical roles: Director General of the Public Health Services, local Medical Officer of Health ("District physician" until 1984), and Chief Physician of a hospital department ("overlege," since 1986 "avdelingsoverlege").

25.2. The Rise of Medical Management

25.2.1 The Central Medical Administration and the Role of the Director General

If medicine is to remain autonomous, it cannot be governed from without. If it is to be governed at all, it must be governed by representatives of the profession. Public medical administration must be a continuation of the clinic into the bureaucracy, rather than an extension of the bureaucracy into the clinic. Public medical authorities must be organized as a "medicracy" – a medical regime.

However, this was not how it started after the birth of a new nation in 1814. In 1815 the government, dominated by legally trained officials, abolished the professional Board of health ("Sundhedscollegium") and replaced it with an Office of Medical Affairs in the so-called Third Department. The office was headed by a pharmacist, and included no medically trained personnel. Thus, from the outset, medicine came under the direction of "laymen." The situation was all the more humiliating since the profession, as the only one of the four professions constituting the social underpinnings of the Civil Servants' state, "embedsmannsstaten," lacked a real hierarchy that could speak for it and protect its autonomy. The legal profession, by far the most powerful, had its chief justice, its prosecuters, and its police chiefs in addition to occupying most of the important administrative and political posts. The clergy had its bishops, and the army and the navy its generals and admirals. The doctors had nothing, except for three, and later four, professors. Compared to the other professions, medicine was almost acephalous. Given the selfimage of the doctor, and the dearth of medical men with real social authority, the profession was bound to have difficulties in capturing the medical part of the central administration. The profession was dependent both upon the emergence of individual doctors interested in administration and on circumstances.

The first "statesman" with a medical background was Frederik Holst (1791–1871), appointed professor of medicine in 1824. He worked indefatigably to promote his ideas about a genuinely medical administration, both through the Norwegian Medical Society (founded in 1833) and the first Norwegian medical journal (Eyr, from 1826). He found it humiliating for public doctors to have to report to authorities who did not understand the doctors' situation and way of reasoning. In 1833 the government appointed a Medical Law Commission. In 1844 the Commission, with Holst as its most influential member, proposed that a new board of health be established to administer the medical care system. Two years before, however, the first head of the medical bureau in the Ministry died and was replaced by a lawyer. Four years later Holst and his colleagues were dealt a new blow as Parliament turned down the proposal of the Minister of Internal Affairs to establish a Board of Health. This defeat revealed the double vulnerability of the medical profession. The legal establishment would always "keep tabs on" the medical profession. As the political system was democratized, the profession would also be subject to the widespread lay skepticism of medicine.

For a while the Minsitry tried to placate the doctors by appointing some of their most prominent colleagues as advisors. In 1857, however, a semi-"medicratic" solution was chosen. A medical division was established under the Minsitry of Internal Affairs, with a doctor as head. In 1875 his title was changed to Medical Director General, and in 1879 the office of the director was made into an independent state agency. A modified medicracy was about to emerge. But this emergence was more a function of general development than the result of the efforts of doctors. The modernizing society demanded a more professional and technical administration, and as a result, several specialized state agencies were organized outside the legally dominated departments (Jacobsen 1964). After the death of Frederik Holst in 1871, medicine lacked real "statesmen," and did so until the late thirties, when Karl Evang (1902–1981) entered the arena. It is no coincidence that when a public commission in 1898 proposed that a more professional board of health be established, the profession as such did not take much interest in the issue. The NMA congress in 1903 supported the proposal, leaving its organizing to the director general. However, he was not strong enough to succeed. His successors raised the issue of the organization of the central medical administration, but also they were too weak and received too little support from the rest of the profession to achieve anything.

When Karl Evang took over as Director General in 1938, the Directorate was not independent of the Department of Social Affairs. A division for medical affairs, headed by a legally trained administrator, was placed under the Department. To Evang this was unacceptable. It made him, and medicine, dependent upon men who neither could nor would understand their concerns. The medical voice, his voice, had to be presented to the Minister directly, without any kind of censorship. The medical care system had to extend into the central administration, he believed.

Evang succeeded in his efforts. His Directorate was reorganized as a combined departmental division and an independent directorate, and he himself was granted direct access to the Minister. Gradually, through the forties and into the fifties, he also succeeded in organizing the Directorate as a professional general staff. He organized the offices of the Directorate so that they, relatively directly, reflected the division of labor in the health care system. Offices were established for primary care, hospital care, dental care, psychiatric care, and so on. In this, he was assured that the ties between the clinic and the Directorate were as close as possible. He also put health experts, mostly doctors, in charge of the offices. These doctors were even given clinical, not bureaucratic, titles ("overlege"), emphasizing their affiliation to the clinic. And in order to further emphasize their clinical affiliation, doctors in the Directorate were allowed to take time off to practice medicine. (Nordby 1989.)

Locally, Evang was represented by county physicians and district physicians. He was thus able to build up the offices of these officials as local counterparts to his own central office. At the same time he was partially shielded from their immediate environments. Thus the health care system could function as a relatively independent institution. Also, Evang considered it necessary to strengthen the medical administration of the hospitals to solidify his "medicratic" edifice. Most hospital managers were too weak and needed to be replaced by managers with greater executive authority and with a combined medical and administrative training. Yet in this respect he did not achieve a great deal before he resigned from his directorship in 1972.

Like his colleagues a little less than a century earlier, Evang was helped by circumstances, even circumstances similar to theirs. The role of technical experts again became prominent.

After the Second World War, it was obvious to all that technical and professional experts were needed to reconstruct and modernize the country. Such experts were needed in industry, engineering and science, city and town planning, education, medicine and, above all, economics and economic

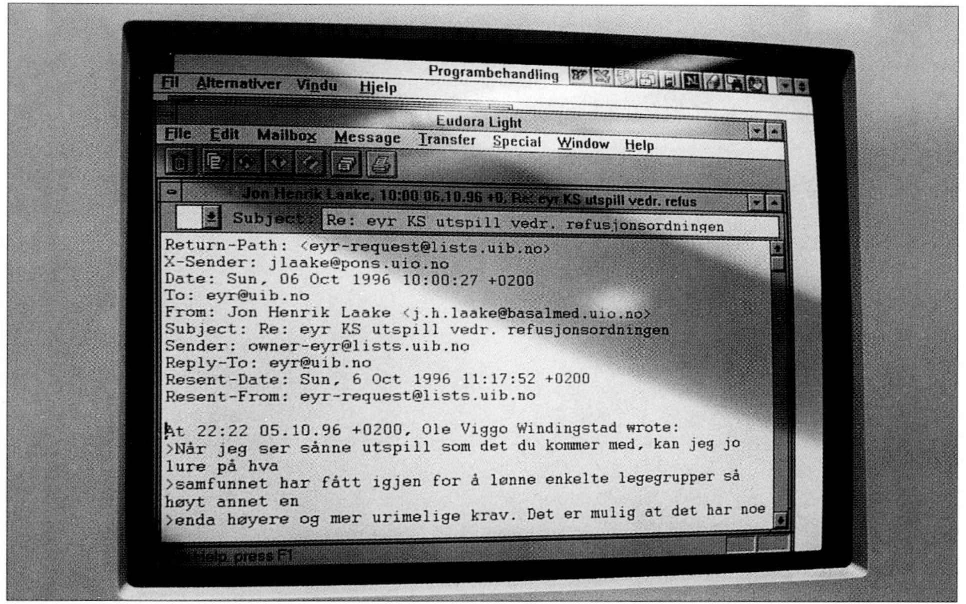

Figure 70: The first Norwegian medical journal was published 1826-1837 and named "Eyr" after the Norse goddess for healing. Editors were the professors Michael Skjelderup (1769-1852) and Frederik Holst (1791-1871); Holst as the sole editor from 1831 onward. This first arena for exchange of medical knowledge and opinion was revived in a modern form in 1996 by the Norwegian Society for Family Medicine (Norsk selskap for allmennmedisin): an e-mail list for family medicine doctors was launched and given the name «Eyr». The e-mail list has proved to be a marketplace for lively intercollegial contacts, and probably has a definite effect in strengthening professional ties. However, inherent in an e-mail information system is the lack of an editor, the most important feature that makes it different from a journal (Photo: Øivind Larsen 1996).

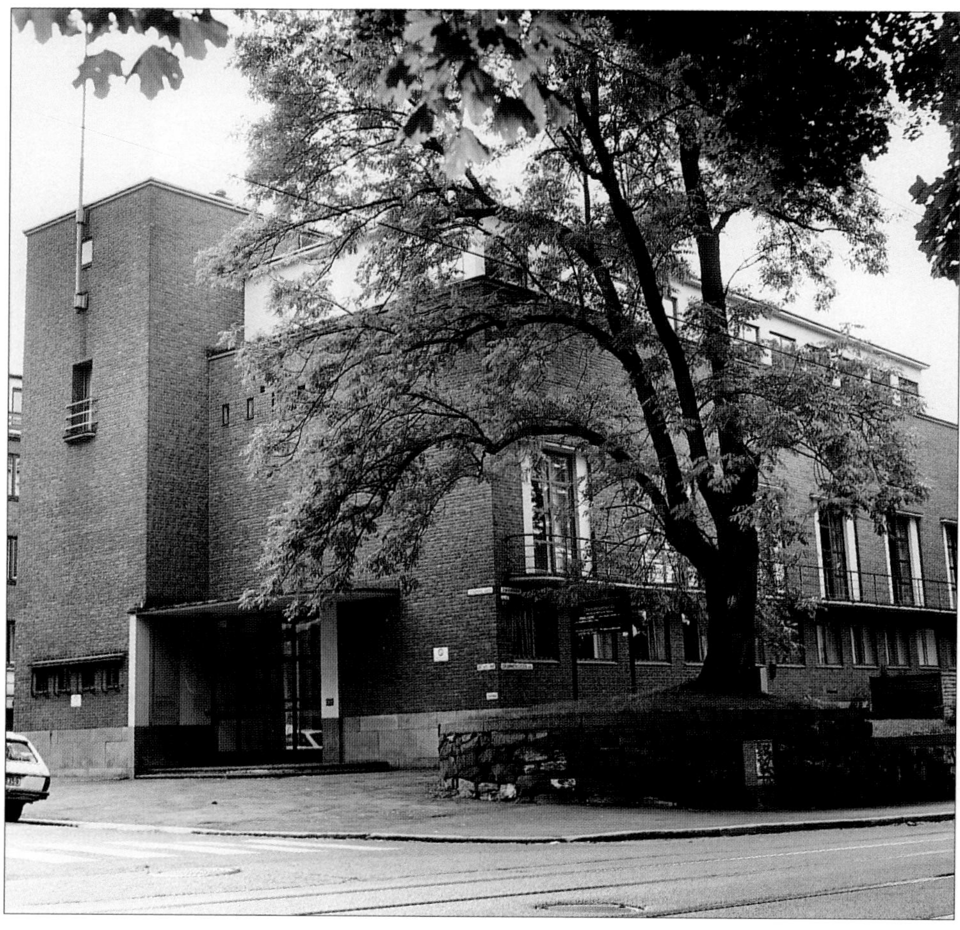

Figure 71: Medical associations and societies, but especially the Norwegian Medical Society (Det norske medicinske Selskab), founded in Christiania in 1833 after a period of more informal existence as a group of colleagues who circulated medical journals, achieved a central position in profession building and postgraduate training and updating of the profession members. By means of a bequest by the surgeon and benefactor Alexander Malthe (1845-1928), a building famous for its functionalistic architecture was erected in Oslo for the Norwegian Medical Society in 1935. Even up to 1970 the lecture hall of this building hosted the most important debates on health politics and medical matters. Later, the formalized training programs organized by the Norwegian Medical Association, its subsidiaries, and by the universities and other professional bodies reduced the need for the traditional meetings in the Society. Doctors do not attend this type of arrangements anymore to the same extent as previously. On the other hand; the responsibility for maintaining the professional norm of life-long updating has been transferred to a considerable degree from the individual doctor to his or her professional group (Photo: Øivind Larsen).

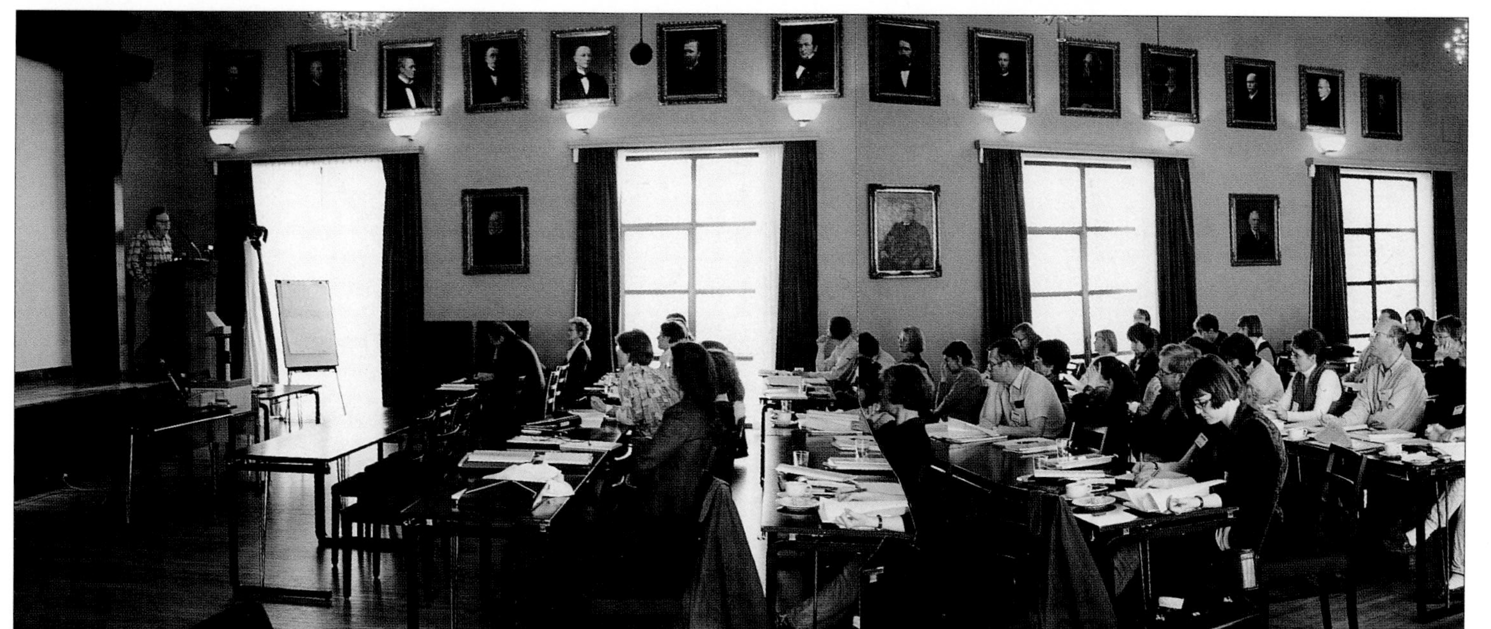

Figure 72: New tasks for the Norwegian Medical Society and similar organizations: Interdisciplinary seminars and other arrangements covering topics outside the normal training programs. The example shown here is a Nordic conference on humanistic health research, held at the premises of the Norwegian Medical Society in May 1996 (Photo: Øivind Larsen).

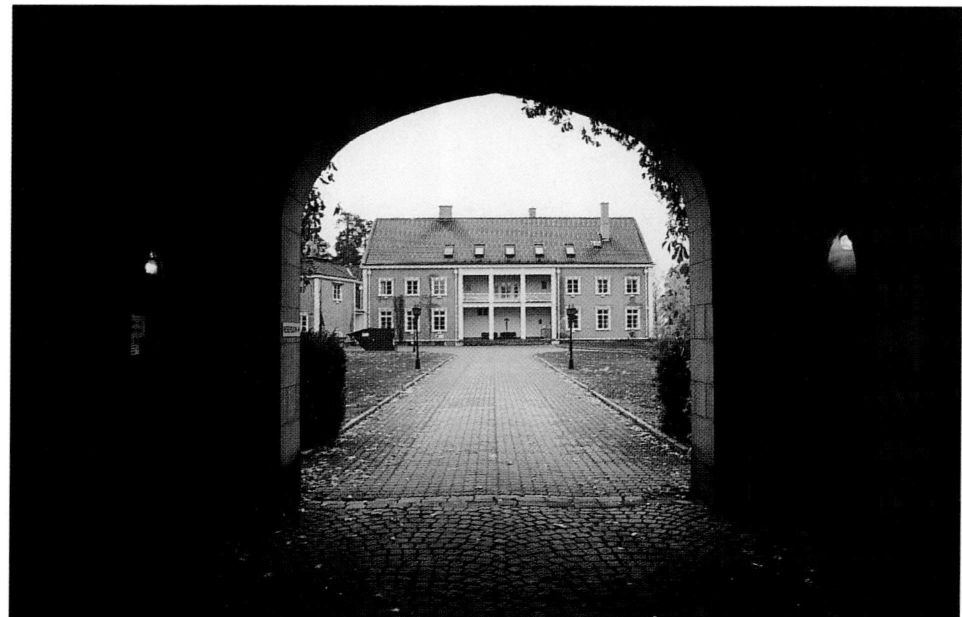

Figure 73: Since 1989 the Norwegian Medical Association has had its headquarters in the estate-like villa of a former shipowner outside Oslo. The buildings have turned out to be too cramped, and critics have also said that the architecture of these premises emitted social signals not appropriate for a professional organization (Photo: Øivind Larsen 1996).

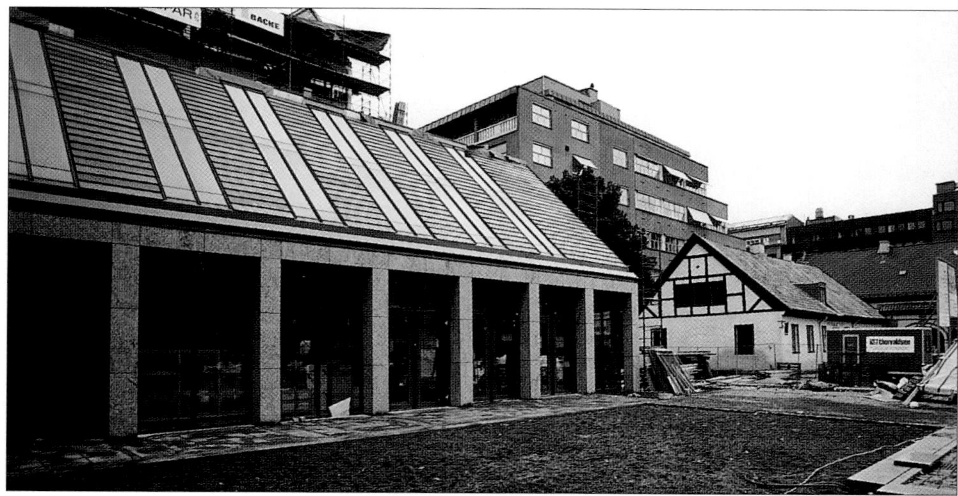

Figure 74: Still a messy construction site in October 1996, the new offices of the Norwegian Medical Association can be seen in the old marketplace of the Norwegian capital. The old building in the background, which parts of the new one are being built to match, served as an anatomical theatre in the first years of the medical faculty of the University, where teaching of medicine started in 1814 (Photo: Øivind Larsen 1996).

planning. And such experts did emerge. What is equally important, they were often entrepreneurs, pro-planning oriented, and in most cases also socially concerned. The latter is important because in this way they served the purposes of the Labor Party which reigned during almost the entire reconstruction period (1945–65). The Labor Party wanted to modernize and develop Norway and to turn her into an egalitarian welfare society (Slagstad 1995.)

Echoing his expert colleagues, Evang wrote in an article in 1952: "We live in an age of technology. In our field the expert is bound to replace the lay administrator." (Nordby 1989) However, Evang also realized that it did not follow that the expert per se would make a good administrator. He also realized that the power-wielding expert was more vulnerable to pressure from his practicing colleagues than a more distant and neutral traditional bureaucrat would be. Evang therefore emphasized the importance of educating physicians in administration. He sent his most promising people to the United States to study public health. Others were given the opportunity to attend courses at the Nordic School of Public Health (of which he was a co-founder in 1953) or to take the course in community medicine developed by the Directorate in 1948. A few words ought to be added about Evang's style of leadership.

Like most physicians, he regarded medical leadership more as a continuation of medicine than as an application of managerial principles to a medical reality. This is why he sent them abroad to give them a medical-based, not generally oriented, managerial education. Schools of public health did not emphasize modern principles of management, but took for granted rather hierarchic managerial principles. What they did emphasize was social, even radical ideas about health promotion. Thus, what public health graduates learned was to be socially radical, yet relatively authoritarian leaders. Here they deviated from their clinical colleagues in the first respect, and resembled them in the second. Evang himself was the most typical representative of this form of governance.

Evang succeeded to a great extent, but his form of governance also became the cause of his, and the profession's, demise. It did not include an understanding of the environment, and of what was to come. Its insularity became its fate.

25.2.2. The Local Medical Officer as Manager

From the very beginnings of the institution in the eighteenth century, the local medical officer had a dual role. He was both a patient doctor and an environmental doctor. In both respects he wanted to function hierarchically. He wanted to dictate, dictate to patients and to society. He wanted to do so as a medical expert. He also wanted to do so became status and hierarchy were closely related phenomena in the bureaucratic state. But he encountered problems in his managerial efforts. "Above" him the real power-wielders, the lawyers, restricted him, and "below" him the "laity" and their representatives in Parliament denied him the authority he demanded. The first general "medical police" law went into effect as late as 1860 and did not grant the district physician quite the powers he had asked for. Though he became head of the local Board of Public Health, he had to share authority with watchful laymen and (in the cities) technical experts. He never became quite the authoritarian and bureaucratic doctor he had wanted to become. He never got the uniform some doctors had demanded (Berg 1986)

The role and authority of the public health officer were vulnerable. In the 1880s agrarian parliamentarians launched a broad attack on the entire institution and proposed that it be dismantled. However, other events at that time began to the change the image of the doctor and also the public health doctor. The growth of the profession, and the increasing clinical effectiveness of emergent scientific medicine, drove a growing number of physicians into private practice. Increased market exposure gradually made the clinician change his behavior and attitudes: The authoritarian rationalist was turned into a benignly paternalistic doctor. Thus his status grew among ordinary citizens. This development also affected public health doctors. They increasingly turned their attention to their clinical tasks and away from their less typically medical responsibilities.

The introduction of public health insurance in 1911 and its gradual expansion, and the loss of status as public officials (by Royal appointment) of the public health doctors in 1912, gave more impetus to this development. The number of public doctors increased from 161 in 1900 to 400 in 1923, contributing to the same outcome: The doctor became more available.

Thus, while the public doctor earlier had relied on his formal and bureaucratic authority, that is, on borrowed authority, he now attained authority based on his own performance as a clinician and on the growing status of his profession. The authority from above that he formerly so eagerly had sought, he now loathed. It was more a burden than an asset.

Strengthened by a growing clinical authority, he could function also as an environmental doctor and as a medical manager. Now, however, he filled the other roles as extensions of his role as clinical doctor.

In a democratizing society, this change of authority was advantageous. As a manager, the role of the public health officer was not particularly hierarchic. Except in the larger cities he had few to manage. Thus he had to exercise his authority mostly in a "horizontal" way. He influenced local politicians, and indirectly local bureaucrats, through the board of public health. He influenced those who were to carry out his and the board's environmental directives. He also tried to influence his colleagues in private practice. (In addition he had the descriptive more than prespective role of monitoring the public health of his community.) Increasingly he succeeded, thanks to his professional and personal, not his bureaucratic, authority.

The public doctor's success was primarily a function of his clinical authority. For this reason he was reluctant to go very far in terms of environmental intervention. He was cautious. He did not intervene in controversial areas, or in areas where others, especially lay people, could challenge his authority. By and large he remained a hygienist. But by thus protecting himself and his authority he also protected himself from learning what he later was to need, understanding of management thinking and politics.

It was only after the Second World War that the role of public health officer was fully developed. Economic cycles influenced medicine and the status of the public health doctor. Hard-pressed politicians in the twenties and early thirties tried to balance their budgets also at the expense of the public doctor. This seldom happened after the war. Even as steady economic growth can account for this development, the growing status of the physician and the establishment of the protective medico-administrative superstructure, the Evang regime, may be an even more important source.

25.2.3. The Hospital Chief of Services as Manager

In the new hospitals, established in the wake of the scientization of medicine beginning in the last decades of the nineteenth century, doctors became very dominant. Most of these hospitals were from the outset managed by a "medical director," sometimes called only hospital physician, but relatively soon Chief Physician ("overlæge"). After the turn of the century, the undifferentiated hospitals, normally called "mixed" hospitals, began to differentiate departmental institutions (surgery, medicine, radiology). Each department in the specialized hospitals was headed by a chief of service. One of the chiefs continued as hospital director, during the interwar years often named "Medical Superintendent" ("administrerende overlæge").

Within the hospital no one could, or tried to, challenge the doctors. Socially they ranked far above all others. As an isolated and in many respects not very important social institution, people did not feel inclined to intervene in the affairs of the hospital. Thus hospitals developed, at least from the late nineteenth century, as the most medically dominated part of the health care system. Earlier in the century, however, doctors encountered some of the same bureaucratic and political skepticism as they had in the controversy over the organization of the Central Medical Administration. The National Hospital, founded in 1826, was from the outset managed by a three-member board of directors, of whom only one, the Army Surgeon General, was a doctor. But after repeated requests by the head physicians of the hospital, a medically trained doctor was appointed director of the hospital in 1874. From then and until the 1960s and 1970s Norwegian hospitals were run more or less as "medicratic" institutions.

Only a few hospitals had directors ("direktører"). They were doctors. Most hospitals were run on a part-time basis by a managing medical director, assisted by a manager ("forvalter"). As true professionals doctors could be managed only by colleagues.

Since all authority, according to the idea of professional self-governance, derives from clinical medical expertise, the specializing hospital was organized as a loosely coupled system of departments. Each department was run, in an almost autonomous way, by the clinical chief. The hospital as such existed primarily as a service institution for the departments and their chiefs (and as an external spokesperson for the institution).

To restrict outsiders' influence on their practice as much as possible, the Norwegian Medical Association decided in 1911 that doctors could not accept senior hospital positions unless the positions had been publicly advertised and the Director General of Health, i.e., a colleague, had either nominating or appointing powers. Gradually employers had to accept this. From 1936, they also accepted that the Director General in his nominating role be assisted by a specialist committee of three. Thus doctors' dependence upon colleagues was increased and their dependence on outsiders, such as employers, was further weakened.

Doctors had to accept being paid on a salary basis, but they had their working conditions defined by the profession. In 1947 the NMA adopted what was called "the normal working conditions," a set of rules defining the conditions under which doctors were willing to accept superior hospital positions. According to these rules, doctors were permitted to have out-patients in their clinics as in private practice.

This formal "medicracy" was a reflection of the status and authority physicians now enjoyed as clinicians. The existing state of affairs in hospitals was regarded as more or less natural by almost all concerned, by authorities from "above," by nurses, other subordinate personnel and patients from "below," and by the mass media and other observers from "outside."

The district physician had to face society at-large, and see patients in their own environments. The private physician had to compete with colleagues to attract and keep patients. Even if they both enjoyed high status, they had to be cautious in their approach toward others. They could not be too authoritarian. The hospital physician practiced in a secluded and protected world that he could shape as he would, a world in which others, employers, other employees, and patients, were dependent upon him. And as a specialized hospital physician, he was generally regarded as a more competent doctor than his extramural colleagues. All this made it not only possible, but also natural, to manage in an authoritarian way. If the doctor was the one who knew best, he simply had to be the primary decision-maker, and all others secondary, adaptive decision-makers.

The situation not only made it possible for the hospital chief to adopt an authoritarian style of leadership, it also rewarded him socio-culturally for doing so. He was expected to be strong, firm, decisive and unwavering – but to have those qualities in an original, personal and creative way. And he was expected to become a myth, a legend. And as an important part of his legacy, he had to leave behind a multiplicity of stories about his authoritarian and ideosyncratic ways.

25.3. The Fall of Medical Management

Up until about 1970, doctors were on the offensive, not only in society, but also as leaders and managers. They succeeded in building up the health care system based on the principle of clinical and professional autonomy and the derived principle of medical self-governance. But they succeeded also because this system did not provoke the outside society and was not too expensive.

Their success, however, also laid the foundation for their fall. Their dominance and authoritarianism made them insensitive to growing pressures from within, first from nurses and other auxiliary personnel, and later from patients. Their insularity made them insensitive to the growing, economically and legally motivated pressure from above, from politicians and bureaucrats, and from outside, from the mass media and interest organizations. This lack of sensitivity, and of willingness to learn, is all the more ironic since the forces that had mobilized the critics to a large extent were a function of the medical technology that created a great need for well-educated para-medical personnel, that is, for personnel who would recruit "rebels" from below. The same development increased the cost of medical care tremendously, also in relative terms, thus making the outside paying world increasingly suspicious of how their money was spent (a movement noted in other chapters).

25.3.1. The Central Medical Administration and the Role of the Director General

The opposition parties criticized the emergence of the bureaucratic technocracy as early at the late forties and into the fifties. They were supported by legal experts. The critics saw the development not only as a threat to the "legal state" ("Rechtsstaat"), but also as a threat to democratic governance. Labor accepted some of the criticism. In 1962 the ombudsman institution was established. In 1962 the more important Code of Administration ("forvaltningsloven") was enacted. Evang was sceptical of both reforms. They strengthened legalistic interests and weakened professional-instrumental concerns. In other words, they threatened the "medicratic" position of his directorate. Yet he was unwilling, and perhaps unable, to understand what was to come and reacted with destructive opposition.

Evang also failed to observe another important development, partly referred to above, that would seriously weaken the autonomy of the entire sector: the emerging concern over the growing costs of the welfare state. This concern would strengthen the role of the Treasury Department and become an important source of the efficiency drives that soon engulfed the health care sector. It seriously threatened the autonomy of the sector and the role of the apex of the sector, the Directorate.

The devastating attack on Evang's "medicratic" directorate was indirect, however. It started with a commission report proposing the abandonment of the local health councils and the integration of the health care into the local political and administrative system. This initiative was followed up in 1975 by a "white paper" from the government with an even more general proposal to regionalize the health care system completely (Stortingsmelding no 9 1974-75). Evang immediately sensed what was about to happen and lashed out at the proposals, particularly the ones that had the social services as their point of departure. In two articles in Oslo's major newspaper, "Aftenposten" (evening editions January 6 and 7, 1976), he rhetorically asked, "Do our authorities want a weakened health service?" He also referred to a "dangerous white paper." The Directorate and the "archbishop" of health were to be deprived of their executive arm.

The direct attack on the Directorate came later, under Evang's successor, Torbjørn Mork (1928–1992). In 1983, under the direction of the conservative State Secretary, Astrid Nøklebye Heiberg (1936–), the Directorate was moved out of the Ministry and a new division for health policy was established inside the Ministry. Mork tried to follow his predecessors "medicratic" policies. He defended the old order to the best of his abilities, only to realize that his own position and his directorate's, step by step, were becoming more and more marginal. A vying for power developed between him and the new division, a battle Mork was destined to lose. In 1991 a commission headed by the permanent secretary of the Ministry proposed that the Directorate in effect be abolished. Mork put up a valiant fight to defend his directorate and succeeded in doing so, but at a humiliating cost. The Directorate would continue as an inspectorate and an advisory body. It was placed outside the line of authority, and by now the symbolic attachments to the clinic were also gone: the clinical titles were replaced with bureaucratic ones. The old "medicratic" agency had to accept that it had become part of the general administration and was no longer the protective and authoritative apex of a medical edifice. The legal and political empire had struck back, with a vengeance (Christensen 1994.)

25.3.2.The Local Medical Officer as Manager

The old district physician had primarily been a free professional with high status and authority. He had also been hugely influential in local decision-making. With the regionalization of the health care system, the local Medical Officer of Health, as we have seen, lost this position. From 1984 on, he or she was no longer a state official and free professional but was now a municipal employee under several strata of lay administrators. Named Municipal Physician 1, Municipal Medical Director, Health Manager or the like, the former district physician very seldom had a colleague above him, such as a Director of Health and Social Affairs, for example. His or her position had in many respects become that of an ordinary bureaucratic middle-level manager.

However, some of the characteristics of the free professional continued to shape the role of the local health officer. A clause in the municipal health care act secured the doctor some independence from the local lines of authority for some time. He or she had retained a professional medical responsibility, as well as a high economic position that was inconsistent with his or her hierarchic position. The first anomaly was removed in 1995. The local health officer's authority to intervene as a professional was converted into a right to be heard as a professional (be an advisor). It remains to be seen whether the second anomaly, the economic one, will be removed too.

The role of the health officer has become more managerial and as such considerably more demanding as it has been "normalized." Schematically the health officer now has to participate in local decision-making processes above him to a much larger extent than the district physician had to. Laterally, he or she is obliged to cooperate with representatives of adjacent sectors to an extent the district physician never had to. The health officer now also has many more subordinates to relate to. In addition, many of the medical tasks now facing the local health care system have become more complex, and must be approached with more sophistication than before. Patients increasingly present problems with important psycho-social and behavioral aspects. It is also increasingly expected that preventive tasks be approached more aggressively than earlier. Therefore, the local health officer finds that he or she is forced into tackling an increasing number of challenges, managerial as well as professional, for which he or she is poorly prepared. It further weakens the doctor's ability to succeed when his or her status and authority begin to decline. Lack of success further weakens the doctor's position, and thus also his or her self-confidence. Vicious circles are often set in motion.

The organizational situation of the local medical manager has been radically altered by external conditions. Doctors have not had much influence on the shaping of their role. They have defensively, occasionally with bitter denunciations of those who are responsible for the new state of affairs, adapted to a situation they only partly understand, are poorly prepared for, and have not anticipated. This process of adaptation has in no way stopped. It still remains to be seen what kind of manager the new local health officer will become. We may also have to wait for some time, because many doctors leave this position after a short tenure. Many communities even have difficulties getting doctors to apply for bureaucratic physician positions and for other salaried, employee-type physician positions. Doctors seek "shelter" in more typically clinical positions, because they are trying to free themselves as much as possible from the local bureaucrats and politicians. They are trying to re-professionalize their roles. Paradoxically, what looks like a defensive adaptation may eventually turn out to be an expensive one. When communities, especially urban communities, respond to the situation and hire health officers under contract, they will again become more professional and independent meta-doctors.

25.3.3. The Hospital Chief of Service as Manager

Hospital development has paralleled the one we have just described for primary health care. Doctors in the managerial positions at the departmental level have step by step become middle-level managers, at the same time as doctors as a group have lost power and influence. In hospitals this development has been more gradual than in primary health care. Most public hospitals were owned and run by local (county) authorities and were thus already a part of a non-medical system. They were not so clearly a part of the Evang "medicracy" as was primary health care; but as we have already seen, in practice, hospital owners bowed to the wishes of the doctors and let them organize and run hospitals as they preferred. In the seventies this began to change. One reason was the strengthening of the county as an administrative unit. The counties had been secondary communities, politically run by an assembly of mayors, and administratively run by a County Governor ("fylkesmann"). Now (1976) counties were led by their own elected governing bodies and had their own administrations. Hospital owners were ready to begin to deal with the hospitals and their "medicrats." And so they did. They proceeded with caution, but with increasing determination.

In the county administration, a position known as County Health Care Director ("fylkeshelsesjef") was established. As a bureaucratic continuation of this position, a new and more mercantile hospital administration was established. As a bureaucratic continuation of this position, a new and mercantile hospital administration was established. The previous position of medical director was abolished and a general directorship of the hospital was established. In most cases, "lay" administrations were appointed to this position. Hospital administrators have grown more numerous gradually and have become more and more administrative in composition and in culture. The clinic has thus been brought under more stringent administration. As a result of this, doctors, including doctors in superior positions, have increasingly become ordinary employees. In 1976 the junior doctors gave up their right to treat outpatients as their private patients; their senior colleagues followed suit in 1977. Later the working conditions of hospital doctors became increasingly regulated and almost identical to employee positions. Also, senior doctors now have fixed working hours and overtime pay. They are no longer free professionals. To some extent they have developed an employee mentality and have been affected by leftist tactics at the negotiating table.

Heads of departments were previously relatively independent autocrats in almost independent departments. Now they have become, like their primary care colleagues, middle-level managers. To some extent legal provisions still secure for doctors in superior positions some independence. Increasingly, however, this independence has become restricted to the clinical performance of the doctor. Older laws provided senior doctors with managerial reponsibility for the use of auxiliary personnel, technology, and money. This is clearly stated in the Psychiatry Law of 1961. It is more obscure in the Hospital Law of 1969. In the Primary Health Care Law of 1982 there is no mention of any medical managerial responsibility. The trend now, which is most evident in employer-employee contracts, is that the organization of work in hospitals is the responsibility of the employers. In other words, as a manager the senior doctor does not have any independent authority. He or she manages solely on the basis of authority delegated from the employer. He or she has become a middle-level manager, though not yet an ordinary middle-level manager.

Other groups have begun to imitate doctors: nurses and related groups also seek recognition as professionals. To the extent that they succeed, and to some extent they do, the position of the old department chief is further weakened. He or she is no longer the department chief, but a member of a managerial team. The previously dominant medical chief of staff has become a "stunted" middle-level manager.

The role of middle-level manager is one doctors have not participated in defining. It has been imposed on them. Many department heads, like doctors in general, react with frustration, but gradually yield. The demands associated with complex legal and economic management, plus sudden political and other interventions, usurp the medical manager's time. But this is not all. Hospital departments have become independent, and department heads find that they must become coordinators and troubleshooters. They find themselves spending time as personnel managers, preparing to serve an increasingly skeptical press, tackling the problems and insecurity associated with lawsuits, and proving competence in co-operating (as the *de facto* number one) with their co-manager, the nurse. This managerial pressure devours department heads' time and attention. It turns them into administrators, or middle-level managers. Many feel they have been turned into mediocre managers who have to prove their competence on alien ground. At the same time, they are losing ground in their clinical specialties and thereby status among their medical subordinates. Mediocre managers also become mediocre clinicians. It is small wonder many become frustrated.

The head of a department at the hospital, like the municipal health officer, is still trying to define his or her new role. Some feel that they have succeeded personally, others see possibilities, and yet others just give up. The latter find, like many municipal health officers, that few are willing to succeed them. Those leaving also notice that they are not the only ones to abandon ship. As in primary health care, an increasing number of physicians refuse to be both middle-level managers and clinical functionaries. This may appear to be a continuation of a defensive adaptation. It may, however, also be an attempt to take an offensive position again.

25.4. Meta-Medicine: The Challenges

I have, in ideal-typical terms, told a story, a story about the rise and the fall of medical self-governance. The rise deals with the growing autonomy of medicine, and of medical management as an extension of the clinical role. The fall is about society's "revenge" and about the normalization of health care as service provision. The two parts are related in an interesting, but ironic, way. In its "days of glory," the medical profession insisted on defining managerial tasks as not much more than tracing the implications of clinical and environmental knowledge, making the task of learning management alien, and thus rendering the profession illprepared and unable to deal with future developments. Medicine's success became the cause of its demise.

The forceful come-back of medicine's surroundings seems destined to be more than a passing phenomenon. The health empire is growing, and will continue to grow, and thus become of increasing importance and interest to all, including the two rival regulatory systems, the state and the market. It will also become more and more complex and interdependent, demanding more determined managerial efforts. The rapid development of academic disciplines, such as economics, management theory, planning theory, logistics, operations analysis, and applied sociology, will provide outsiders, and managers in general, with the means of intervention, but also, and equally important, with the professional self-confidence they need to contend with self-confident doctors.

Will medicine continue to be politically and managerially pushed aside? Will doctors continue their retreat to the clinic, to practice an increasingly pre-programmed medicine?

If medicine is going to return to a position of influence, it must begin afresh on new premises. Clinical insight and competence alone will not suffice. Doctors must accept management as a serious professional endeavor. But they must also bring with them their medical understanding and their insight into the needs and aspirations of professional clinicians. Good management is not only a general activity, it is also a customizing activity. The effective manager must be bi-professional.

If doctors are to regain control of the clinic, they must be able to tackle the demands of bi-professionalism (and clinical multiprofessionalism). They must also be willing to accept not regaining it in full. Bi-professionalism means that there must also be room for managerial, though customizing, professionalism. The complete clinic requires that the two parties meet each other in a co-operative effort.

References

Berg, O. "Verdier og interesser – Den norske lægeforenings fremvekst og utvikling," part 3 in Larsen, Ø., O. Berg and F. Hodne: *Legene og samfunnet*. Oslo: Seksjon for medisinsk historie, Universitetet i Oslo and Den norske lægeforening, 1986.

Christensen, T. *Politisk styring og faglig uavhengighet*. Oslo: Tano, 1994.

Dingwall, R., and Lewis, P. T*he Sociology of the Professions: Lawyers, Doctors and Other*. Oxford: MacMillan Press, 1983.

Freidson, E. *Profession of Medicine*. New York: Dodd-Mead, 1970.

Freidson, E. *Doctoring Together: A Study of Professional Social Control*. New York: Elsevier, 1975.

Freidson, E. *Professional Powers: A Study of the Institutionalization of Formal Knowledge*. Chicago: University of Chicago Press, 1986.

Hafferty, F., and J. McKinlay eds., *The Changing Character of the Medical Profession: An International Perspective*. Oxford: Oxford University Press, 1993.

Jacobsen, K.D. *Teknisk hjelp og politisk struktur*. Oslo: Universitetsforlaget, 1964.

Nordby, T. *Karl Evang*. Oslo: Aschehoug, 1989.

Slagstad, R. "Den annen front – i går og i dag," *Nytt norsk tidsskrift*, 1 (1995): 12–24

Stortingsmelding no. 9, 1974-75, "Sykehusutbygging m.v. i et regionalisert helsevesen."

Strand, S. "Utenfor kirken – ingen frelse?" *Tidsskrift for Den norske lægeforening*, 115(1995): 2698-2702.

CHAPTER 26

Doctors and Migration

CHAPTER 26.1

Geographic Mobility among Early Norwegian Physicians

ANNE SOFIE FRØYSHOV LARSEN

26.1.1. Mobility with Various Backgrounds

The mobility of physicians reflects the need for medical services throughout the country, and in Norway, with its scattered population, physicians are distributed around the country as well in order to get established a reasonable coverage of medical assistance to the inhabitants. As for other professions, the mobility of physicians has varied throughout the centuries, and on the one hand reflects this need for medical services throughout the country. At least parts of Norway have always been, and still are, short of physicians, and efforts to secure health services in all parts of the country has lead to a high degree of migration. The number of relocations differ between groups of physicians, but a high mobility is often found among the physicians doing service in the periphery.

However, on the other hand, the number of relocations per physician also is dependent upon career patterns, for example, as measured by means of the number of positions held by each physician during his or her career, a number that increases with the specialization in medicine because a lot of the post-graduate medical education takes place as in-service training. In this way mobility is closely connected to career, and the mobility pattern of the individual physician is heavily dependent on which professional path the young doctor chooses to enter. And as for all other Norwegians, personal geographical preferences of course is also an important factor.

26.1.2. Biographies of Norwegian Doctors as a Source of Information

As earlier discussed in this book, the different editions of Norges Leger vary in their value as a source of information. In the three first editions (1871, 1888 and 1909, with appendix 1944), the biographies cover whole life-spans. They are therefore suited for giving us information on mobility and career patterns of Norwegian physicians in the late nineteenth and early twentieth century.

The samples selected for this study were the doctors born in the years 1810 to 1815 (n=114), in the years 1840 to 1845 (n=118), and in 1870 to 1875 (n=259). For the whole life span of these doctors, their positions and movements were encoded, using their year of graduation as the basic point. The material can thus be seen to consist of three cohorts separated by thirty years during the nineteenth century.

26.1.3. Career Patterns

Divided into groups according to their final position, the different groups of physicians followed different patterns, both in the types of positions held, the number of positions held, and in the numbers of years this process lasted. The final position can be regarded as the end of the career, when looking at the term used for it, but often the mobility continues, with the physician moving to hold the same position in another place or hospital. But this relocation may also reflect climbing further up on the professional ladder, since the same position can have different social and professional connotations in different parts of the country.

The district physician's pattern of career and mobility can be used as an example. Typically, the newly graduated physician started his career by assisting a district physician for a short period of time. Then followed two or more positions as a locum for a district physician, after which he was temporarely appointed into a position, before he finally received the title of district physician from the government. Often this appointment was followed by one or two appointments to socially and geographically better positions. Finally, the physician and his family moved on after his retirement.

The increase in numbers of positions held for all physicians is statistically significant between the last two cohorts (t-test, p=0,003) (Table 26.1). If we compare the groups of those born between 1810 and 1815, the district and city physicians held more positions than the private practitioners. Between the groups of those born 1840-45, there are no significant differences. For the last cohort the district and city physicians, the higher hospital physicians, and physicians in administrative positions held more positions than private practitioners. Also the district and city physicians and the physicians in administrative positions held more positions than the lower hospital physicians.

26.1.4. Mobility

During the nineteenth century, there were

TABLE 26.1

Average number of positions held during a career for different groups of physicians. Groups with small numbers are not included in this table. Mean values, number of physicians in brackets.

Final position (group)	Born 1810-15 n=114		Born 1840-45 n=118		Born 1870-75 n=259	
All positions	4,6	(107)	4,7	(118)	5,4	(247)
District or city physicians	5,14	(49)	4,69	(52)	6,23	(92)
Private practitioners	3	(12)	4,61	(33)	4,6	(86)
Military doctors	4,32	(22)	5,58	(12)	–	–
Lower hospital physicians	–	–	–	–	3,65	(17)
Higher hospital physicians	–	–	–	–	5,71	(17)
Administrative positions	–	–	5,88	(8)	6,73	(15)

TABLE 26.2
Median number of relocations for the physicians grouped by their final position.

	Born 1810–15	Born 1840–45	Born 1870–75
District or city physicians	4	4	5
Private practitioners	1.5	3	3
Military physicians	2	3	4
Lower hospital physicians	4	–	2
Higher hospital physicians	4	2	3
Administrative positions	4	3	5

three types of salaried posts that were most important for physicians in Norway, namely, in the armed forces, as district physicians, and in the hospitals. These three categories varyed in importance throughout the century. The military services covered all parts of Norway, as did the system of district physicians. Therefore, a lot of the salaried posts were to be found in the periphery, and many doctors in these positions were living outside the cities.

In the latter part of the nineteenth century and in the beginning of the twentieth, some of the medical institutions were located in remote places, namely the sanatoriums, which treated and isolated patients with tuberculosis; some of the asylums for psychiatric patients; and some of the spas. The towns and cities had populations large enough to feed private practitioners, and here we also found most of the hospitals, and the administration of the health care system.

The cohort born between 1870 and 1875 stayed for a shorter period of time in each place, and they relocated more often. At the same time they also settled earlier (Tables 26.2, 26.3, 26.4). This cohort differed significantly from the two earlier. Whether this reflects a trend or merely a point of change is impossible to answer from this material.

Most relocations took place in the first years following graduation. Early in the career, the physicians only stayed for a short period of time at each place, but as the physicians became more settled, both social-

TABLE 26.3
Duration of stay. Percent. Number of registered movements in brackets.

Duration	Born 1810–15 n=377		Born 1840–45 n=413		Born 1870–75 n=968	
Less than 6 months	15.1	(57)	15.7	(65)	24.7	(239)
6–12 months	15.4	(58)	15.7	(65)	19.3	(187)
1–5 years	27.3	(103)	24.7	(102)	24.4	(236)
5–10 years	18.8	(71)	13.8	(57)	10.6	(103)
More than 10 years	23.3	(88)	30.0	(124)	21.0	(203)
Mean duration of stays (months)	96.6		91.6		61.4	
Median duration of stays (months)	36		48		18	

TABLE 26.4
Number of physicians that have undertaken all their relocations within five years after their graduations.

Cohort	Number of physicians	Percent	n
Born 1810–15	40	35.1	114
Born 1840–45	48	40.7	118
Born 1870–75	119	45.9	259

ly and professionally, the frequency of relocations declined.

When we consider the relocations that take place later in the career, there can be found a tendency among the physicians to move toward the larger cities and toward the southeastern part of the country. However, the numbers of physicians in our cohorts are relatively small.

The young, newly educated physicians were responsible for the greater part of the mobility. For the three cohorts, respectively 41 (36,0 percent), 46 (39,0 percent) and 124 (47,9 percent) of the physicians relocated three times or more during the first five years after their graduation.

26.1.5. Factors Contributing to an Explanation of Physicians' Pattern of Migration

The mobility of the medical profession can be seen both as a result of the professionalization, and as a feature of the profession. Geographically, the need for medical services follows the pattern of settlement in the country. But as medicine develops, there is also a need for education and updating for the physicians, often reached by changing post or doing service at a hospital for a period of time. However, that important mobility promoting specialization was still not established as a system in the nineteenth century, and its main importance for the relocations of physicians was still to come.

Removals are influenced by a lot of push and pull factors. Physicians' relocations seem to be closely connected to a change of work that was increasingly based on professional considerations, and of course was also related to a wish for a better position than the one that was formerly held.

There were several social factors influencing physicians' mobility as well. In nineteenth-century Norway, the physicians more or less belonged to the same social category as ministers, officers, and the local law representatives (lensmenn). All three professions were more or less regarded as representatives of the authorities, somewhat above and set aside from the society in general. In addition, the physician often lived and worked in another part of the country than the one he came from, and had ties and relatives there. These and other factors also may have contributed to creating a special pattern of mobility.

CHAPTER 26.2

Doctors, Migration, and Professional Career

ØIVIND LARSEN

26.2.1. Migration: Part of Life and Part of Society

In Chapter 5 of this book, the reader will have learned how internal migration and also emigration have been a prominent trait in many periods of the history of the Norwegian population. There have been push and pull factors in abundance, and the generally increasing tendency toward relocations, based on the shift away from the traditional agrarian- to the industrial-, and lately to the post-industrial society, needs no lengthy discussion here. Education, new occupations, private and public economic growth, new personal preferences of living styles, all are among the factors which have made Norway a more unstable society than she used to be.

In the nineteenth century and well into the twentieth, hospital medicine occupied only a minor number of the physicians; in 1872 nearly nine out of ten of them worked outside hospitals and research (Table 26.5).

Formal specialization with a subsequent approval started in 1918. Specialization required the fulfillment of certain demands for practical training, which could only be obtained through service in relevant hospital departments. The major part of hospital growth in Norway is also to be found in the twentieth century.

This means that the physicians of the nineteenth century, most of them in primary

TABLE 26.5

Percentages of physicians in research, hospitals, and other types of work. (Larsen 1986, after Lindbekk 1967)

	1872	1910	1937	1953	1963
Research and university hospitals	7.6	5.8	9.0	14.3	19.2
Other hospitals	6.5	11.1	23.0	31.2	28.8
Other types of work	86.0	83.3	68.1	54.5	52.0
Total	100.1	100.2	100.1	100.0	100.0

TABLE 26.6
Removals and MD graduation. 10% sample of Norwegian physicians 1984 (Larsen 1986) (%).

Graduation year		–1949	50–64	65–74	1975+	Total
Total number of removals since	0–5	30.8	21.8	33.8	78.5	47.0
MD graduation	6+	69.2	78.2	66.2	21.5	53.0
Sum		100.0	100.0	100.0	100.0	100.0
Number		104	165	237	284	790

care, probably to a larger extent chose their place of living based on the prospects of setting up a practice, or for personal reasons, than did their successors in the following century. Not so free, of course, were those who chose a career in the public health system and applied for a position as a district physician, or those who were military physicians or had other salaried posts.

The migration waves of the demographic transition of course also affected the physicians, not least due to the fact that the mar-

TABLE 26.7
Removals and medical disciplines. 10% sample of Norwegian physicians 1984 (Larsen 1986) (%).

Discipline(s)	G	S	I	V	Total	
Total number of removal since	0–5	69.2	26.8	37.4	38.6	46.7
MD graduation	6+	30.8	73.2	62.6	61.4	53.3
Sum		100.0	100.0	100.0	100.0	100.0
Number	263	142	131	228	764	

G= General practice
S= Surgical disciplines
I= Internal medicine and related disciplines
V= Various disciplines, including psychiatry

TABLE 26.8
Birth region and region of present residence. 10% sample of Norwegian physicians 1984 (Regions, see Larsen 1986 p. 395) (%).

	Oslo	Eastern Norway	Southern Norway	Western Norway	Trøndelag	Northern Norway	Abroad	Sum (n=797)
Birth region	27.7	22.8	5.6	24.3	5.4	7.9	6.1	99.8
Region of residence	34.0	20.7	6.3	21.5	5.3	9.8	2.5	100.1

DIAGRAM 26.1
Migration in the general population 1951–1964. Net values. (Larsen and Heiberg 1983, redrawn after Bull 1979)

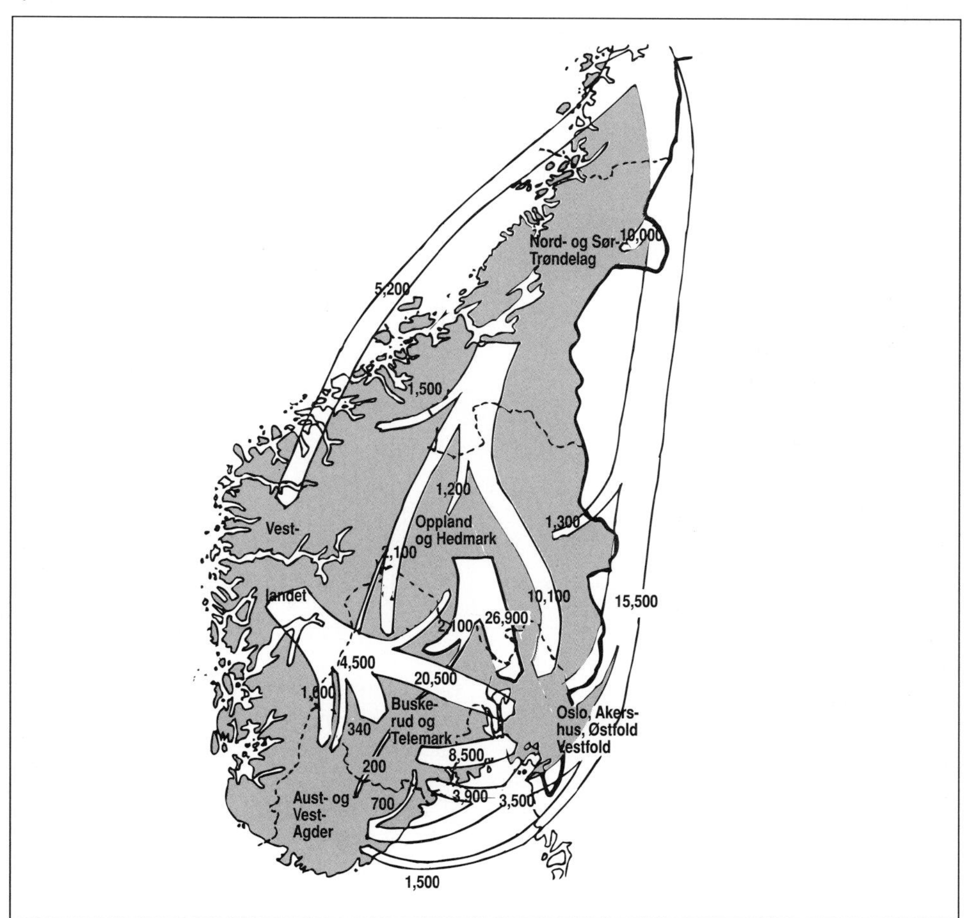

ket and the need for medical services depended on where the migrating population settled. The growth of the large cities, especially the capital Kristiania (Oslo), should be remembered in this respect.

The migration among the physicians, however, cannot be seen as an isolated phenomenon that was only connected to specialization and a greater need for hospital doctors. In later periods, a general migration also occurred, with a pattern similar to that of the demographic transition two or three generations before. Diagram 26.1. indicates some net numbers for migration in the period 1951–1964. Since moving occurred in both directions, these net values only point to a vivid demographic activity which did not calm down somewhat until 1970. In this period, as earlier, working as a physician of course included for many physicians settling down where most people lived, and many of the new hospitals of the post-Second World War period also were erected in places where there was population growth.

DIAGRAM 26.2

Number of positions. 10% sample of Norwegian physicians 1984 (Larsen 1986)

Number of removals. 10% sample of Norwegian physicians 1984 (Larsen 1986)

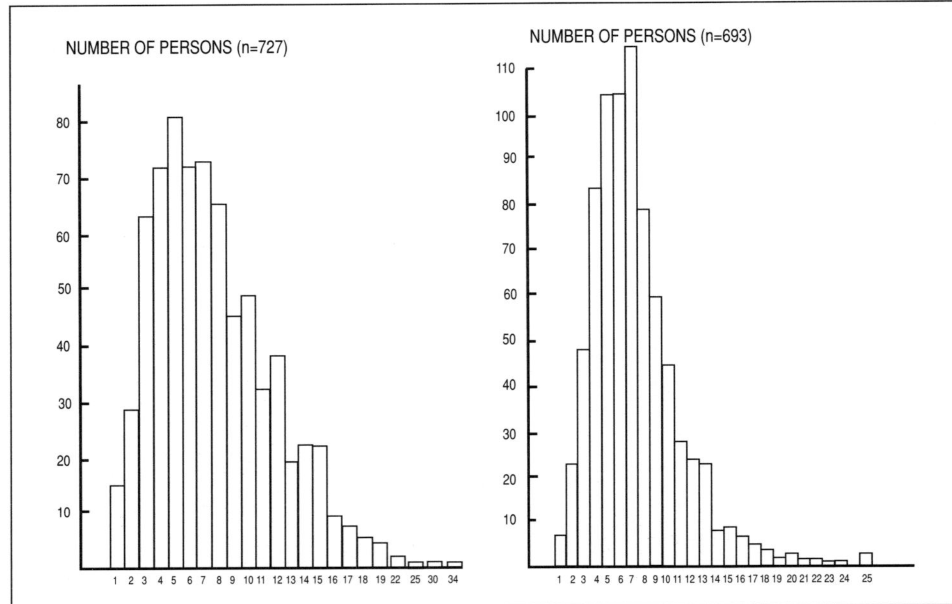

Diagram 26.2 contains two figures that were calculated from the returned questionnaires that were sent to a ten percent sample of Norwegian physicians in 1984 (Larsen 1986). In 1984, the number of physicians in Norway had steadily increased; a greater part of the corps of physicians had yet to arrive at the terminal point of their migration. In spite of this, the physicians reported having had a substantial number of jobs, and an even more impressive record of removals.

Given that the oldest group of them, those who had had their MD graduation in 1949 or before, were more likely to have finished their migration activity than their younger colleagues, Table 26.6 shows that slightly more than two-thirds of them had undertaken six or more removals. On the other hand, their colleagues who had graduated 1950–1964, and of whom probably many still were in the process of pursuing a career aiming at some desired terminal point position, the relocation activity is even greater. And the numbers for the graduation years 1965–1974 give the same indication of a high moving activity, while the numbers for the 1975 onwards group must be regarded as inconclusive in 1984.

Table 26.7 shows that the hospital physicians are the most mobile, with those belonging to the surgical disciplines at the top of the list. As a rule, the hospitals provided apartments for their physicians, often built on the hospital site and reflecting the hierarchy of the hospital, with roomy premises for the chief physicians and then progressing downward to humble lodgings for the interns. For instance, in psychiatry or tuberculosis care, this way of living could also include staying in a relatively isolated hospital community for years.

A hospital career included packing and

TABLE 26.9

Birth region and region of present residence, cross table. 10% sample of Norwegian physicians 1984 (regions, see Larsen 1986 p. 395) (%).

	Birth region, all respondents							
Region of residence, all respondents	Oslo	Eastern Norway	Southern Norway	Western Norway	Trøndelag	Northern Norway	Abroad	Sum
Oslo	57.0	29.1	27.3	20.7	34.9	23.8	18.4	34.0
Eastern Norway	17.2	43.4	11.4	9.3	11.6	9.5	28.6	20.8
Southern Norway	1.8	2.7	31.8	7.3	7.0	3.2	16.3	6.3
Western Norway	10.0	12.1	15.9	52.3	7.0	12.7	16.3	21.5
Trøndelag	4.5	2.7	0.0	4.1	30.2	4.8	6.1	5.3
Northern Norway	6.3	8.2	11.4	3.6	4.7	44.4	14.3	9.8
Abroad	3.2	1.6	2.3	2.6	4.7	1.6	0.0	2.4
Sum	100.0	99.8	100.1	99.9	100.1	100.0	100.0	100.1
Number	221	182	44	193	43	63	49	795

TABLE 26.10

Birth region and region of present residence, cross table, respondents who graduated in 1964 or earlier. 10% sample of Norwegian physicians 1984 (Larsen 1986) (%).

	Birth region							
Region of residence	Oslo	Eastern Norway	Southern Norway	Western Norway	Trøndelag	Northern Norway	Abroad	Sum
Oslo	71.2	31.9	60.0	23.0	37.5	33.3	19.8	41.7
Eastern Norway	21.9	43.5	20.0	14.8	12.5	14.3	25.0	24.7
Southern Norway	2.7	7.2	13.3	3.3	18.8	0.0	18.8	6.3
Western Norway	1.4	10.1	6.7	52.5	6.3	19.0	12.5	17.7
Trøndelag	0.0	2.9	0.0	4.9	18.8	9.5	6.3	4.1
Northern Norway	1.4	2.9	0.0	0.0	6.3	19.0	18.8	4.1
Abroad	1.4	1.4	0.0	1.6	0.0	4.8	0.0	1.5
Sum	100.0	99.9	100.0	100.1	100.2	99.9	100.2	100.1
Number	73	69	15	61	16	21	16	271

TABLE 26.11
Norwegian veterinarians 1988 (n=281, 20% sample, extracted from the biographies in Velle 1988). Birth region and region of residence 1988 (%).

	Birth region									
Region of residence	Oslo	Eastern Norway	Southern Norway	Western Norway	Trøndelag	Northern Norway	Abroad	Unknown	Sum %	n=
Oslo and Akershus	33.3	25.3	1.3	12.0	14.7	4.0	2.7	6.7	100.0	75
Eastern Norway	21.7	50.0	2.2	4.3	6.5	2.2	–	13.0	99.9	46
Southern Norway	14.3	14.3	42.9	14.3	–	–	14.3	–	100.1	7
Western Norway	6.5	14.5	1.6	54.8	6.5	1.6	4.8	9.7	100.0	62
Trøndelag	–	8.0	–	8.0	76.0	4.0	4.0	–	100.0	25
Northern Norway	–	30.4	–	13.0	4.3	30.6	–	21.7	99.8	23
Abroad	–	–	–	–	100.0	–	–	–	100.0	1
Unknown	19.0	33.3	–	21.4	7.1	11.9	2.4	4.8	99.9	42
Total %	17.1	26.7	2.1	21.4	14.9	6.4	2.8	8.5	99.9	281

unpacking, a new adjustment for the spouse, a change of school for the children, and so on. Our 1984 questionnaire inquiry, together with the additional material used (Larsen 1986), contains more comprehensive information on demographical behavior among

TABLE 26.12
Members of the Norwegian Medical Association 1996

	Physicians		Students	
	Males	Females	Males	Females
<30	307	391	1,042	1,031
30–49	5,766	2,670	135	96
50–69	3,249	619	–	1
>=70	980	156	–	–
Sum	10,302	3,836	1,177	1,128

Source: The Norwegian Medical Association

physicians, and is referred to for details. Among other topics, a recording of how this more or less forced instability was perceived by the physicians has been included. The frequent removals were ranked as a very important or important burden by approximately one-third of the respondents. But when split up into age groups, most of this resent against removals was found among the youngest doctors.

Choosing a medical discipline on the basis of a special geographical living preference, was most often reported by general practitioners, while family considerations were most frequently mentioned among the younger groups when they were selecting a career.

26.2.2. Professional Pattern and Migration

Table 26.8 indicates that approximately half of the Norwegian physicians were born in

TABELL 26.13
Members of the Norwegian Medical Association 1996. Geographical distribution.

County	Total	Working < 70 years of age		
		Sum	Males	Females
Østfold	608	545	406	139
Akershus	1,081	961	664	297
Oslo	3,371	2,957	2,032	925
Hedemark	460	404	294	110
Oppland	454	405	313	92
Buskerud	583	514	361	153
Vestfold	481	422	335	87
Telemark	447	398	302	96
Aust-Agder	258	228	179	49
Vest-Agder	434	372	291	81
Rogaland	819	760	549	211
Hordaland	1,387	1,285	938	347
Sogn og Fjordane	273	264	200	64
Møre og Romsdal	581	548	397	151
Sør-Trøndelag	820	773	550	223
Nord-Trøndelag	293	276	205	71
Nordland	566	552	383	169
Troms	642	630	420	210
Finnmark	179	179	124	55
Abroad	401	369	240	109
Sum	14,138	12,842	9,203	3,639

Source: The Norwegian Medical Association.

Oslo or Eastern Norway, and that slightly more than half of them also lived there. This fact should not be overinterpreted, as it is a part of the overall picture of the distribution of the inhabitants of Norway. However, if we go into the data presented in Table 26.9, a tendency appears indicating that the physicians either settled in the region where they were born, or they moved to Oslo. When selecting the group of physicians who graduated in 1964 or earlier (Table 26.10), and who in 1984 would presumably had had most of their mobility behind them, this tendency is even more appalling. The numbers here, however, are small, and one must be cautious in drawing conclusions.

Our project did not include the possibility of examining what this pattern looks like for other professions, but our calculations based upon a 20 percent sample of the biographies of Norwegian veterinarians (Velle 1988) indicate similar mobility tendencies as that of the physicians. Admittedly, some allowances must be made for the fact that a lot of the work of the veterinarians is carried out in rural districts. Out of a sample of 281 veterinarians, 131 reported private practice as their first job after graduation, and another 23 had had positions as veterinary assistants. When submitting their data

TABLE 26.14

Types of positions for Norwegian physicians working in 1996. (Only members of the Norwegian Medical Association.)

Divided by sex

	Sum	Males	Females	Mean age (years)
Chief Attending Physicians	3,867	3,212	655	50.0
Hospital physicians in lower positions	2,756	1,527	1,229	35.6
General Practitioners	3,331	2,389	942	42.8
Practicing Specialists	704	580	124	52.8
Occupational Health Physicians	348	232	116	45.2
Administrative positions, county and municipality	409	338	71	45.6
Administrative positions, state	63	44	19	49.6
Research and teaching	577	413	164	44.0
Other positions	526	307	219	41.1

Divided by age groups

	<30	30–39	40–49	50–59	60–66	>=67
Chief Attending Physicians	–	337	1,582	1,422	437	89
Hospital physicians in lower positions	401	1,718	557	74	4	2
General Practitioners	182	1,061	1,385	559	90	54
Practicing Specialists	–	39	234	295	80	56
Occupational Health Physicians	3	95	140	87	21	2
Administrative positions, county and municipality	4	92	192	93	26	2
Administrative positions, state	–	6	27	22	8	–
Research and teaching	23	210	171	111	48	14
Other positions	76	193	140	81	27	9

Source: The Norwegian Medical Association.

for the 1988 biography book, only 73 of the 20 percent sample were in a private practice, and none reported holding a position as a veterinary assistant. 68 held public positions such as district veterinarians and corresponding jobs, 37 were in research and teaching, 29 in food control, and 20 reported administrative positions (Table 26.11).

Another lesson learned from this superficial comparison with another profession is that the veterinarians also constitute a group in constant change: The 281 veterinarians in our sample (17,4% of them women) were born 1910–1962, and their graduated 1927–1987, but nearly six out of ten were so young that they had graduated 1970-87. Slightly less than one out of ten had completed an academic thesis.

TABLE 26.15

Types of physicians' positions 1996. (Only members of the Norwegian Medical Association.)

	Hospital physicians		Practitioners Type of practice			Administrative positions			
County	Chief Attending physicians	Lower hospital positions	General	Specialist	Occupational Health Physicians	County and municipality	State	Research and teaching	Other positions
Østfold	181	117	170	37	22	11	2	1	9
Akershus	266	218	306	82	20	21	4	9	51
Oslo	1,079	650	434	201	93	50	11	299	178
Hedemark	120	35	143	23	12	14	3	–	10
Oppland	108	91	147	14	11	20	2	–	15
Buskerud	151	107	171	35	15	14	2	–	23
Vestfold	122	86	134	48	11	10	2	1	11
Telemark	124	80	134	16	16	16	3	–	10
Aust-Agder	72	39	82	17	2	7	3	–	10
Vest-Agder	127	62	125	28	10	12	3	–	7
Rogaland	231	164	227	44	40	28	5	1	22
Hordaland	343	296	334	79	38	39	3	120	42
Sogn og Fjordane	78	66	85	5	5	19	3	–	4
Møre og Romsdal	164	124	190	11	8	31	2	–	22
Sør-Trøndelag	280	172	173	33	16	19	4	58	23
Nord-Trøndelag	85	57	89	2	7	23	2	3	12
Nordland	142	142	178	15	14	33	5	–	24
Troms	167	166	131	10	6	22	2	85	41
Finnmark	27	34	78	4	2	20	2	–	12
Sum	3,867	2,756	3,331	704	348	409	63	577	526

TABLE 26.16
Primary care physicians and specialists in this field, geographical distribution 1996. (Only members of the Norwegian Medical Association.)

County	Man-labor-years, including municipality administrative physicians and interns Data from the National Bureau of Statistics	Inhabitants per physician	Specialists in general practice	Specialists in community medicine
Østfold	167.6	1,428	89	13
Akershus	297.7	1,459	145	25
Oslo	385.1	1,255	237	33
Hedemark	152.1	1,227	82	12
Oppland	162.7	1,127	89	20
Buskerud	179.0	1,277	92	13
Vestfold	138.9	1,463	88	16
Telemark	133.9	1,218	57	8
Aust-Agder	91.6	1,088	48	11
Vest-Agder	127.1	1,176	85	13
Rogaland	239.6	1,479	146	21
Hordaland	322.9	1,309	177	24
Sogn og Fjordane	96.4	1,116	40	11
Møre og Romsdal	201.5	1,192	108	15
Sør-Trøndelag	195.3	1,312	106	20
Nord-Trøndelag	102.9	1,239	44	9
Nordland	218.6	1,104	68	13
Troms	138.1	1,091	55	12
Finnmark	90.5	847	22	8
Abroad	–	–	4	0
Unknown	–	–	–	–
Sum	3,441.5	–	1,782	297
Mean	–	1,264	–	–

Source: The Norwegian Medical Association

Also, the mobility pattern of the veterinarians seems to be steered by their personal choice of career, balanced out by society's demand for the kind of competence they have achieved in their field. This is a more or less obvious fact which, however, has to be part of the interpretation of demographic data for any profession or vocational group.

Around 95 percent of the physicians in Norway are members of The Norwegian Medical Association. On May 10, 1996, there were 14,138 members. It should be pointed out that the exact total number of physicians in the country is somewhat imperfectly documented. But for the members, the statistics are fairly accurate. As shown in Table 26.12, in 1994 25,3 percent of the doctor members and 50,9 percent of

TABLE 26.17
Specialists <70 years of age and working in hospitals, geographical distribution 1996.

	Specialists	Inhabitants per specialist	Specialists with more than one specialist approval
Østfold	236	1,010	63
Akershus	399	1,077	107
Oslo	1,580	302	438
Hedemark	144	1,301	33
Oppland	141	1,300	39
Buskerud	196	1,159	48
Vestfold	195	1,035	48
Telemark	155	1,052	39
Aust-Agder	92	1,077	26
Vest-Agder	165	900	40
Rogaland	294	1,193	78
Hordaland	557	754	157
Sogn og Fjordane	87	1,236	20
Møre og Romsdal	179	1,339	50
Sør-Trøndelag	393	650	117
Nord-Trøndelag	90	1,419	26
Nordland	168	1,433	33
Troms	236	634	67
Finnmark	34	2,249	7
Abroad	283	–	50
Unknown	121	–	8
Sum	5,745	–	1,494
Mean	–	760	–

Source: The Norwegian Medical Association

the student members were female. Tables 26.13, 26.14, 26.15, 26.16 and 26.17 show their geographical and occupational distribution.

The fact that so many physicians have educated themselves for a specialist approval, and that both specialists and hospital departments and positions required for attaining specialist approval are distributed around the country, are important elements in a migrational context. The list of specialties, presented in Tables 26.18 and 26.19, is varied and has an impressive length. Each of the specialties has an educational program of its own. All of them require service in a series of departments and institutions, and for a large part of the specialties, many of the training positions available are beyond commuting distance from each other, and therefore imply removals for the candidates.

If we examine further what we have seen in Table 26.7 as regards to specialty and migration, and compare more specifically the large specialties of general surgery, inter-

TABLE 26.18
Specialist approval, among all Norwegian physicians

Specialty	Total	< 70 years of age	Males	Females
General practice	2,142	2,087	1,704	438
Anaesthesiology	529	509	448	81
Occupational medicine	128	127	94	34
Child surgery	21	17	20	1
Child and adolescent psychiatry	117	107	53	64
Pediatrics	409	360	322	87
Haematology	41	39	36	5
Endocrinology	54	46	48	6
Gastroenterology	145	142	142	3
Rehabilitation medicine	103	89	84	19
Gynecology and obstetrics	491	446	346	145
Gastroenterological surgery	108	102	105	3
Surgery	1,025	903	987	38
Geriatrics	72	62	55	17
Cardiology	203	188	192	11
Dermatology	146	116	110	36
Immunology and transfusion medicine	56	50	45	11
Internal medicine	1,191	1,059	1,073	118
Infectious diseases	62	58	57	5
Vascular surgery	96	88	95	1
Mandicular surgery and stomatology	27	21	26	1
Clinical pharmacology	29	29	28	1
Clinical chemistry	106	87	97	9
Clinical neurophysiology	22	17	19	3
Lung diseases	184	130	165	19
Medical genetics	25	24	21	4
Medical microbiology	104	89	77	27
Neurosurgery	44	38	43	1
Neurology	219	179	180	39
Nephrology	75	73	69	6
Oncology	84	82	65	19
Orthopaedic surgery	283	260	277	6
Pathology	152	140	109	43
Cosmetic surgery	65	59	60	5
Psychiatry	872	751	628	244
Radiology	424	347	332	92
Rheumatology	126	105	102	24
Community medicine	486	455	440	46
Thorax surgery	76	66	75	1
Urology	112	102	111	1
Ear-nose-and throat diseases	277	247	263	14
Opthalmology	316	277	266	50

Source: The Norwegian Medical Association

TABLE 26.19
Approved specialists, among all Norwegian physicians, categorized by age.

Specialty	<40	40–49	50–59	60–69	Mean age Males	Mean age Females
General practice	277	1,230	474	106	47.4	45.9
Anaesthesiology	79	261	139	30	47.8	49.9
Occupational medicine	12	68	42	5	48.2	46.3
Child surgery	0	2	6	9	62.7	48.0
Child and adolescent psychiatry	6	42	35	24	52.7	54.3
Pediatrics	39	143	129	49	53.6	51.8
Haematology	1	12	18	8	53.7	48.6
Endocrinology	2	20	18	6	55.0	53.3
Gastroenterology	3	58	73	8	50.7	48.3
Rehabilitation medicine	8	34	39	8	54.9	46.9
Gynecology and obstetrics	51	179	157	59	54.1	47.5
Gastroenterological surgery	0	43	42	17	53.3	46.3
Surgery	69	349	317	168	54.3	47.1
Geriatrics	4	21	25	12	55.3	56.1
Cardiology	9	74	72	33	53.2	54.0
Dermatology	22	42	36	16	54.8	56.2
Immunology and transfusion medicine	5	19	15	11	53.8	48.0
Internal medicine	82	408	428	141	53.8	50.9
Infectious diseases	4	26	22	6	51.7	51.2
Vascular surgery	1	34	33	20	54.3	42.0
Mandicular surgery and stomatology	0	9	5	7	60.1	57.0
Clinical pharmacology	1	12	11	5	51.0	58.0
Clinical chemistry	4	24	32	27	58.8	45.8
Clinical neurophysiology	0	6	7	4	60.2	50.6
Lung diseases	6	58	55	11	59.8	55.6
Medical genetics	1	8	10	5	54.0	49.5
Medical microbiology	8	33	31	17	55.7	51.4
Neurosurgery	2	16	13	7	54.9	43.0
Neurology	21	63	63	32	56.4	49.8
Nephrology	4	25	34	10	53.1	44.8
Oncology	10	48	19	5	48.3	44.6
Orthopaedic surgery	9	110	97	44	53.1	52.6
Pathology	14	57	46	23	52.9	48.9
Cosmetic surery	2	22	23	12	54.5	50.6
Psychiatry	57	310	263	121	55.0	52.5
Radiology	48	116	138	45	56.3	49.7
Rheumatology	5	39	47	14	56.9	52.5
Community medicine	20	214	161	60	52.3	47.8
Thorax surgery	4	26	24	12	54.5	46.0
Urology	4	40	38	20	53.9	40.0
Ear-nose-and throat diseases	28	115	75	29	52.5	44.0
Ophthalmology	53	105	80	39	53.3	46.5

Source: The Norwegian Medical Association

TABLE 26.20
Removals among general practitioners, surgeons, internists, and psychiatrists. 10% sample of Norwegian physicians 1984 (Larsen 1986) (%).

		General practitioners	General surgeons	Internists	Psychiatrists	Sum
Total number of removals since	0–5	69.2	28.6	40.4	50.9	56.2
MD graduation	6+	30.8	71.4	59.6	49.1	43.8
Sum		100.0	100.0	100.0	100.0	100.0
Number		263	63	89	53	468

TABLE 26.21
Removals and gender. 10% sample of Norwegian physicians 1984 (Larsen 1986) (%).

		Males	Females	Sum
Total number of removals since	0–5	44.8	59.6	47.0
MD graduation	6+	55.2	40.4	53.0
Sum		100.0	100.0	100.0
Number		678	114	792

nal medicine, and psychiatry, the differences between the careers are even more appalling (Table 26.20). Becoming a general surgeon obviously implies a considerably larger burden in terms of migration than becoming an internist or a psychiatrist. At least in 1984, males had a larger migration activity than female physicians (Table 26.21), while, of course, the specialists ranked far above those without any specialist training (Table 26.22). However, the fact that the previously married physicians had more removals

TABLE 26.22
Removals and specialist training. 10% sample of Norwegian physicians 1984 (Larsen 1986) (%).

Specialist		No	Yes	Sum
Total number of removal since	0–5	70.7	17.5	47.1
MD graduation	6+	29.3	82.5	52.9
Sum		100.0	100.0	100.0
Number		437	348	785

DIAGRAM 26.3
Members of the Norwegian Medical Association 1920–1996

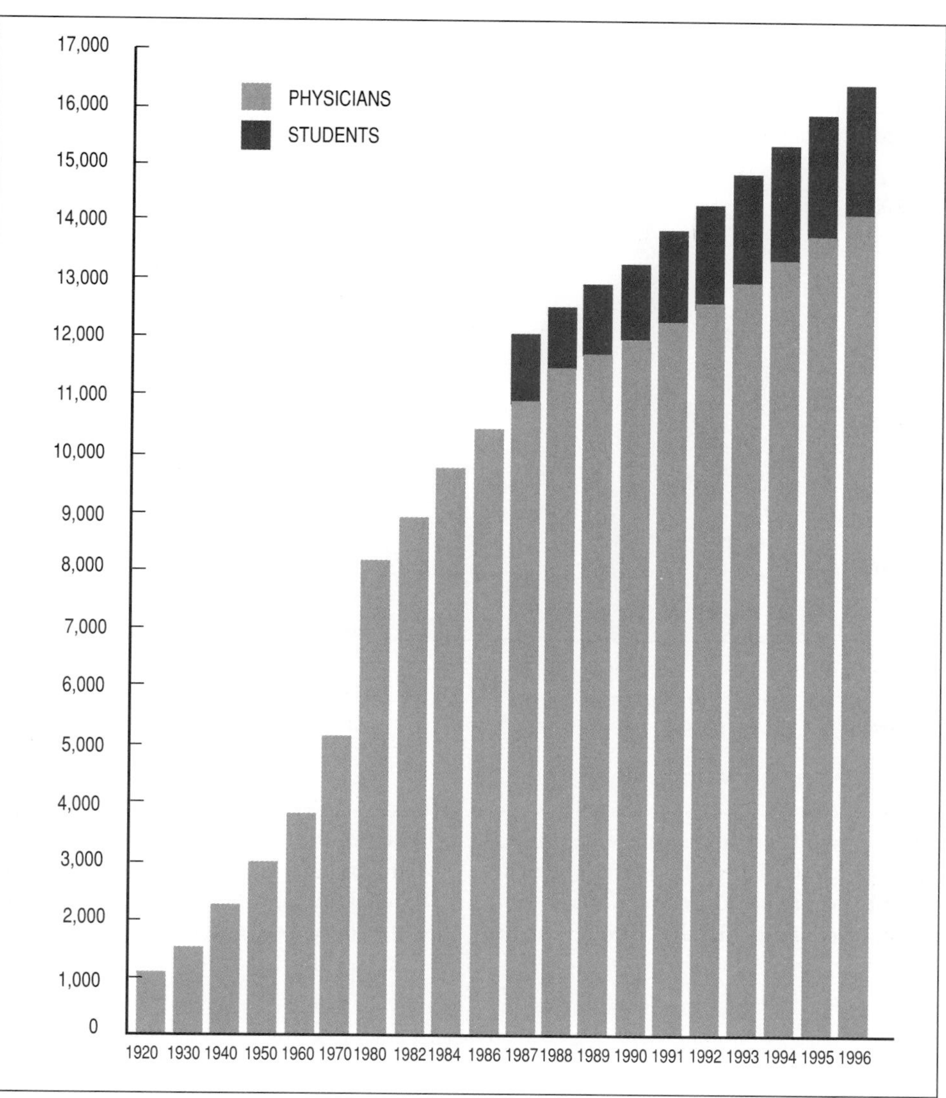

behind them than the others (Table 26.23) might be intrepreted in different directions.

26.2.3. Migratory Pattern and the Development of the Profession: Difficulties ahead?

It is intriguing to notice that most of the migration among the physicians in the last half of the twentieth century is part of an educational system and a specialization process which partially requires frequent removals. This specialization and training seems to be a necessity for maintaining and promoting the medical proficiency of the

DIAGRAM 26.4
Members of the Norwegian Medical Association 1996, divided by age and gender

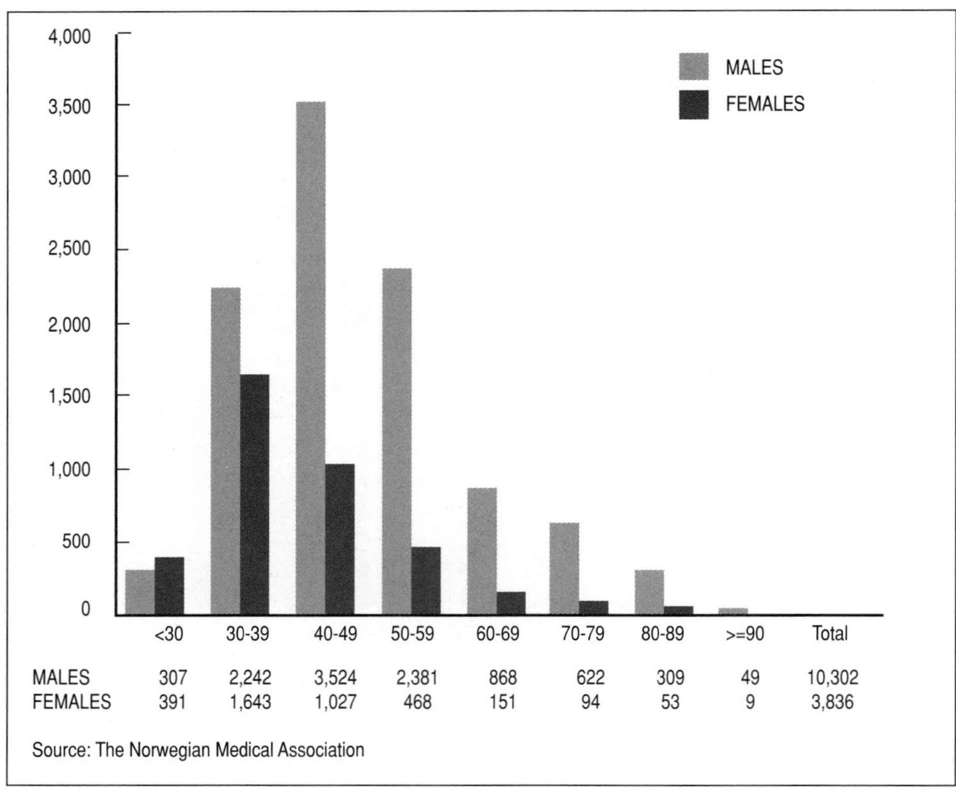

profession. This is also in general terms a more or less indispensable requirement in order to secure health services of a reasonable quality and availability throughout the country. In this respect, what we learn from Diagrams 26.3 and 26.4, and from Table 26.12, is thought-provoking: the Norwegian medical profession and the cohorts of

TABLE 26.23
Removals and marital status. 10% sample of Norwegian physicians 1984 (Larsen 1986) (%).

Previously Married		No	Yes	Sum
Total number of removals since MD graduation	0–5	47.9	33.3	46.3
	6+	52.1	66.7	53.7
Sum		100.0	100.0	100.0
Number		647	81	728

students who are recruited to it make up a young population group with increasing members. Therefore, if nothing is changed, the migration activity related to education will grow even more.

On the other hand: To rank professional and career considerations above social life seems to be increasingly less acceptable to the members of the profession.

We have no data available here to document a particular effect of this trend. An unfortunate effect on the training quality might appear when a more limited willingness to move is combined with newer working schemes in the hospitals, where for example restriction on work hours makes it difficult to gain sufficient experience in, say, complicated surgical techniques.

One would also assume that a selection effect might appear, so that specialties and positions implying social stability and few removals are favored by an increasing number of physicians, leaving behind alarming recruitment problems for important medical disciplines. The effect of the fact that modern physicians often have spouses who have their own career plans, also might exacerbate the situation.

Looking at the migration pattern of physicians, and listening to the profession members' reactions to it, might be worrying, and must be a challenge to both the health authorities and to The Norwegian Medical Association.

References

Larsen, Ø., and A. Heiberg eds., *Medisinske fag i velferds-Norge*. Oslo: Seksjon for medisinsk historie, Universitetet i Oslo, 1983.

Larsen, Ø., O. Berg, and F. Hodne. *Legene og samfunnet*. Oslo: Seksjon for medisinsk historie, Universitetet i Oslo, and Den norske lægeforening, 1986.

Velle, W. *Norges veterinærer 1988*. Bærum: Den norske veterinærforening, 1988.

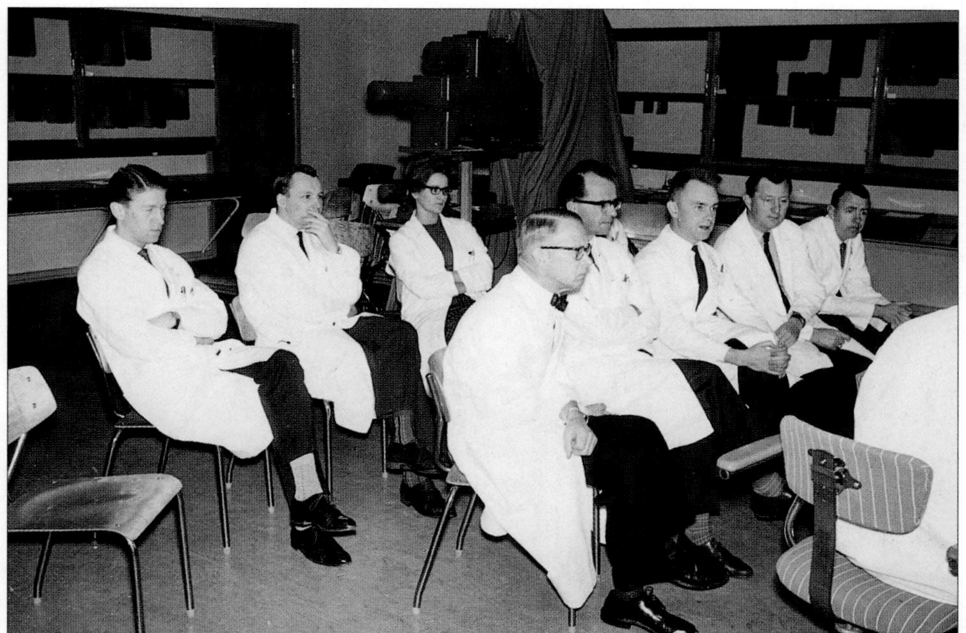

Figure 75: The history of hospital development in Norway is an important part of the history of the medical profession. The real explosion in hospital building took place in the years after World War II. The need for doctors who would work in hospitals was steadily increasing. In the course of a few decades the typical doctor became a hospital doctor. And for the doctors, work changed from relying on a single person, to becoming the work of a team. The picture shows a typical morning session in the x-ray demonstration room at the hospital in Fredrikstad in 1962. In the first row, the chief physician of the medical department Ole K. Evensen (1903-1993), Dr. Ole Rygvold (1919-), Dr. Torkjell Bru (1927-), Dr. Jens B. Andersen (1926-), and Dr. Inge Tøien (1929-). In the second row in the middle the medical student Knut Aamodt Karlsen (1939-), and at his sides two Danish students: Jens Vuust and Else Støckler (Photo: Øivind Larsen 1962).

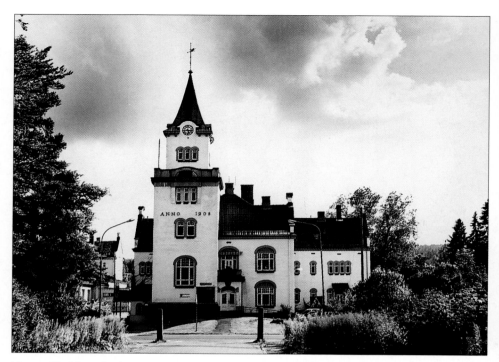

Figure 76: Often the hospitals for psychiatric diseases and the tuberculosis sanatoriums were situated in rural districts and surrounded by parks and nature. This might have been pleasant, but the disadvantage was that the hospital community became somewhat isolated, and was often separated from the rest of the local society. In addition, both patients and staff often stayed in such institutions for a long time, creating a hospital culture of its own. This is a part of medical life which nowadays by and large only belongs to history. (Dikemark psychiatric hospital outside Oslo. Photo: Øivind Larsen 1996).

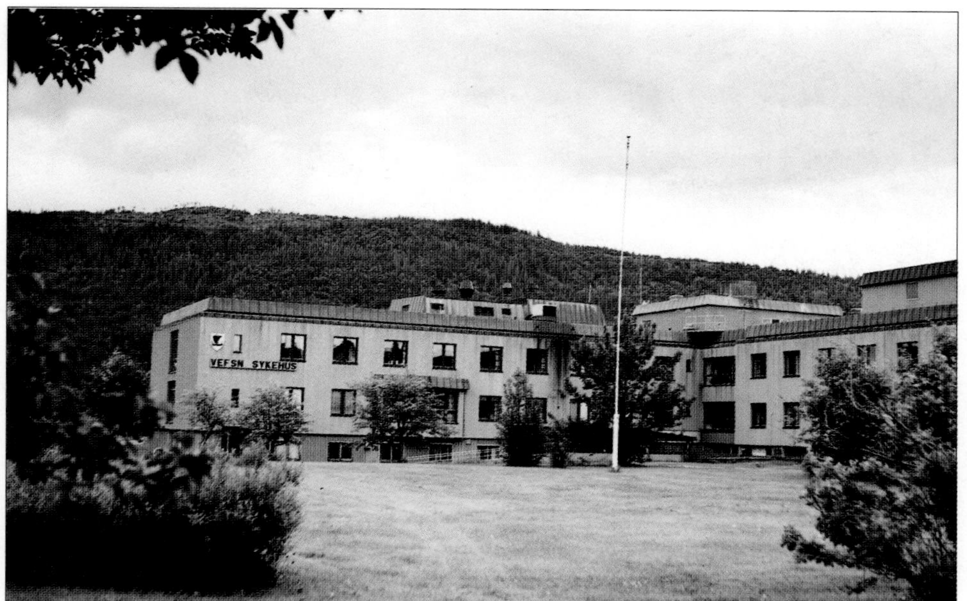

Figure 77: Local hospitals mean a lot to the local community; shown here is the hospital at Mosjøen, Northern Norway (Photo: Øivind Larsen 1996).

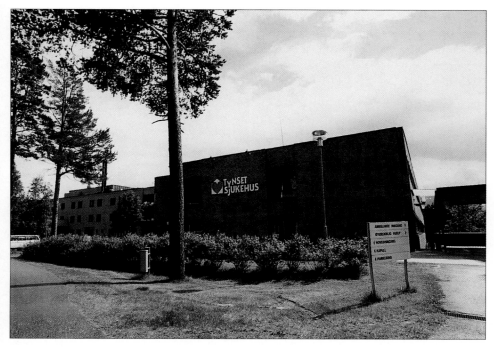

Figure 78: Tynset, a village in the Østerdalen valley, has a modern hospital (Photo: Øivind Larsen 1996).

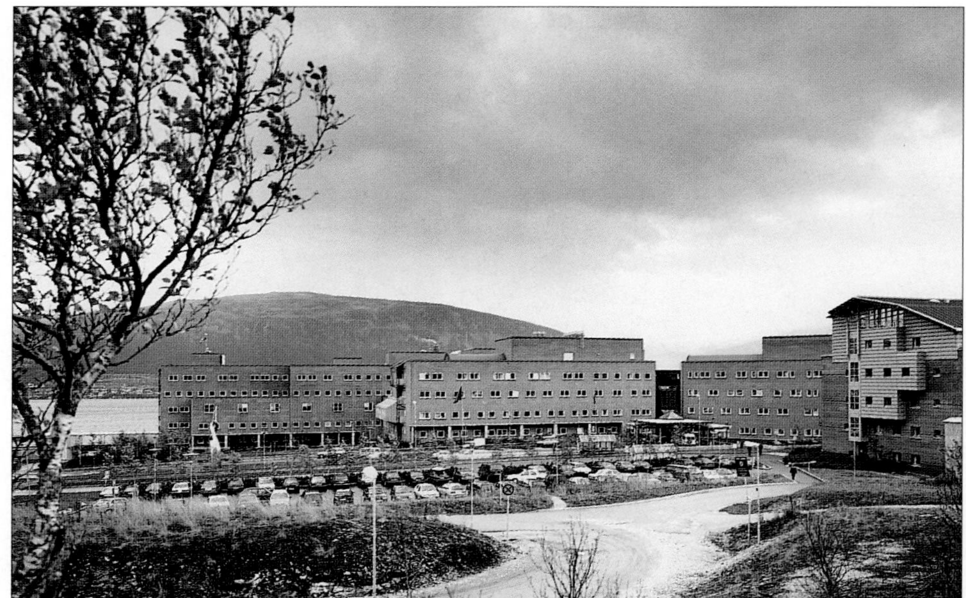

Figure 79: The Regional Hospital (University Hospital) in Tromsø in Northern Norway was inangurated in 1991. In combination with the University, an important scientific center has been created. The importance for the local society of such an investment cannot be overstated (Photo: Øivind Larsen 1996).

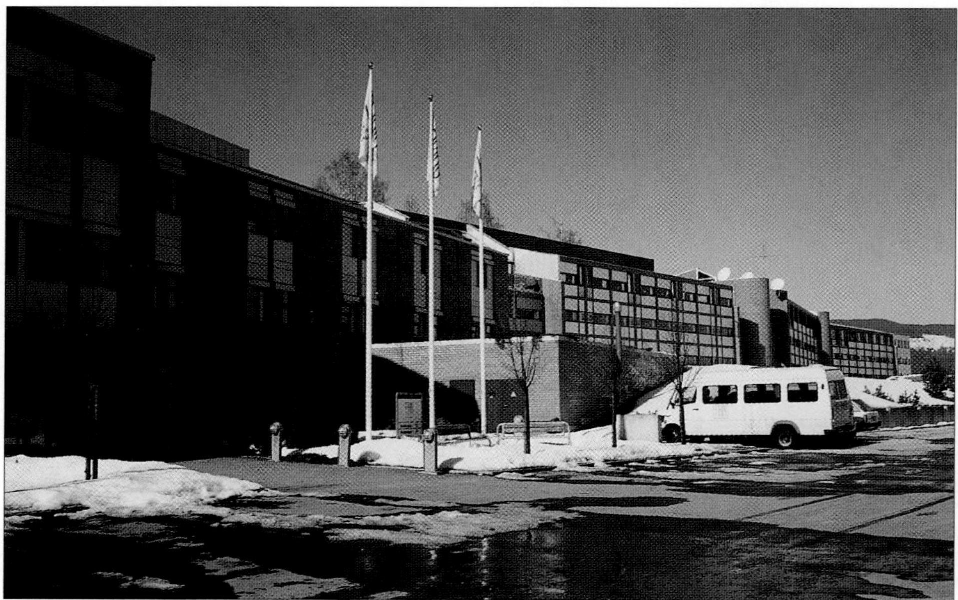

Figure 80: There are only a few private hospitals in Norway. The heart clinic at Feiring, designed to perform cardiac surgery, is one of them. It is owned by the Association for Heart and Lung Diseases and was opened in 1989 (Photo: Øivind Larsen 1996).

CHAPTER 27

Working Conditions and Standards of Life for Norwegian Physicians in the 1990s as Seen by Themselves

CHAPTER 27.1

The Norwegian Research Program on Physician Health and Welfare

OLAF GJERLØW AASLAND

The role of the modern physician has increasingly become a subject of debate. There are different approaches to this discussion. The most predominant one is based on sociological analyses of why and how the medical profession's position in society has changed over the last decades (Hafferty and McKinlay 1993), and to what extent there is a connection between the extensive change in the physician's role and status and the fact that in a number of countries the fraction of female medical students and physicians is rapidly growing (Riska and Wegar 1993).

These questions are also being investigated within the medical profession itself. There is a steadily growing body of evidence of stress and burn-out among physicians, including increased risk of clinical depression or suicide (Aasland and Falkum 1992). The medical associations in several countries have initiated various projects to assess this situation, or to offer help to individual members who experience such problems in relation to their professional activities.

Several studies of physicians' health and welfare have been made in recent years, mainly concentrating on life style and particular aspects of the work situation (Kreyberg 1954, Aarø et al 1977, Thürmer et al 1986, Aasland et al 1987, Akre et al 1992, Aarseth et al 1993, Riksaasen 1989, Buxrud 1990). A more comphrehensive study from 1986, undertaken by the Norwegian Medical Association, focused particularly on "being a doctor" (Larsen 1986). Similar limited studies have also been made in other Nordic countries (Sveriges läkarförbund 1988, Hellström 1993, Vartiovaara 1988, Kumpusalo et al 1991, Neittaanmäki et al 1993, Engsig et al 1990).

By the 1990s, however, there seemed to be a need for a comprehensive documentation of all aspects of the complicated relationship between the special work situation of the physician and the health and well-being of the profession. With this in mind, the Board of the Norwegian Medical Association decided in 1991 to initiate a large-scale research program on physician health, sickness, working conditions, and living standards.

94 percent of all practicing and retired physicians in Norway and 90 percent of all medical students are voluntary members of the Norwegian Medical Association. The total number of members in May 1995 was 15,922, of which 2,147 were medical students and 1,222 were physicians 70 years of age or older. This unique situation, with a

highly representative and at the same time not too numerous national "universe" of physicians, offered the possibility of inviting virtually all Norwegian physicians to participate in the project, in one way or another. An attempt was also made to include the physicians who were not members of the Medical Association. However, it turned out that the official register, kept by the Directorate of Health, was so incomplete that 243 of the 719 mailings were returned with "address unknown." Of the remaining 476, only 104 responded to the survey, and we do not know how many received their questionnaires.

A project director was engaged in April 1992 to plan and perform the survey, with a budget of NOK 9 mill. (USD 1.3 mill.) over a period of three years. A project organization was subsequently created, partly based on internal and partly on external research competence. A number of social scientists and physicians were invited to submit applications and study protocols, or were engaged as consultants. A statistician was engaged who also helped design the optimal survey under the given conditions.

Within one year a research program was implemented, amounting to a total of 22 man-years for the three-year program period. The program included the following areas:

1. Studies based on postal questionnaire surveys, with data comparable to both national population surveys and international studies of physicians and other relevant occupations.
2. Register-data studies (mortality and morbidity of physicians as compared to other relevant groups).
3. Studies based on qualitative data (interviews and written or audiotaped autobiographies).
4. Historical studies.
5. Prospective longitudinal studies of medical students and physicians.
6. Compilation of relevant literature.

During the planning process, it turned out that several researchers wanted to do studies based on postal questionnaire data often with similar or overlapping questions. We therefore found it convenient to combine the different protocols in one comprehensive data collection procedure. The plan was to build one central data base, and then make individual data sharing agreements between the different researchers and the owner of the data base, the Norwegian Medical Association through its project organization. An additional asset of this solution was that the individual physician would receive questionnaires from only one familiar source, namely the Norwegian Medical Association, and would probably feel more confident and willing to participate, than if different questionnaires had come from a number of different agencies.

In the spring and summer of 1993, 9,266 active physicians received four questionnaires each. After one reminder, 6,652 sets of questionnaires were returned, which amounts to a response rate of 71.8 percent.

In this process of building the extensive data base from cross-sectional survey data, an "overlapping questionnaire design" was used for collecting a large amount of data from a limited number of respondents. This technique was developed to reduce the workload for the individual physician replying to the questionnaires as well as to increase the number of estimable cross relations. Out of 16 different questionnaires, each physician received one primary questionnaire and three randomly selected secondary ones, dealing with varying topics. For a more detailed description of this method, see Aasland et al. 1995.

The two following chapters are based on data from the 1993 survey.

In 1995 the Central Board of the Norwegian Medical Association decided to channel the competence and documentation produced by the research program into a permanent research institute. During the next few years this institute will exploit the existing data from the program, follow up the longitudinal studies, and perform new studies, with special emphasis on international comparative studies and collaboration with other professional groups. It will also provide relevant background material for organizational initiatives concerning physician health and welfare.

References

Aarseth, S., S. Vatn and H.P. Aarseth. "Arbeidsmiljø og helseforhold blant sykehusleger," *Tidsskrift for Den norske lægeforening*, 113 (1993): 1864–1868.

Aarø, L.E., K. Bjartveit, O.D. Vellar, and E.L. Berglund. "Smoking Habits among Norwegian Doctors 1974," *Scandinavian Journal of Social Medicine*, 5 (1977): 127–135.

Aasland, O.G., A. Amundsen, D. Bruusgaard, J. Jervell, and J. Mørland. "Norske legers alkoholvaner," *Tidsskrift for Den norske lægeforening*, 107 (1987): 2553–2558.

Aasland, O.G., and E. Falkum. "Hvordan har vi det i dag? Om legers helse, velvære og arbeidsglede," *Tidsskrift for Den norske lægeforening*, 112 (1992): 3818–3823.

Aasland, O.G., M. Olff, E. Falkum, T. Schweder,and H. Ursin. "Health complaints and job stress in Norwegian physicians." (Submitted) 1995.

Akre, V., Å. Vikanes, and P. Hjortdahl. "Profesjonalisering uten styring? En undersøkelse om det faglige innholdet i turnustjenesten," *Tidsskrift for Den norske lægeforening*, 112 (1992): 2546–2551.

Buxrud, E.G. "Bydelshelsetjenesten – mer belastende for kvinnlige enn for mannlige leger?" *Tidsskrift for Den norske lægeforening*, 110 (1990): 3260–3264.

Engsig, A., B.Ø. Jensen, M. Johansson, K. Mogensen, M. Nordenhoft, and A. Winther. *Sosialpolitisk Arbejdsgruppe. (1990) Yngre lægers arbejds- og livsvilkår. Rapport fra Socialpolitisk arbejdsgruppe.* København: Foreningen af yngre læger, 1990.

Hafferty, F.W., and J.B. McKinlay. *The changing medical profession. An international perspective.* New York/Oxford: Oxford University Press, 1993.

Hellström, M., and G. Westlander. *Läkares arbetsvillkor inom olika specialiteter. Solna: Arbetsmiljöinstitutet, 1993.*

Kreyberg, H.J.A. *"A study of tobacco smoking in Norway," British Journal Cancer*, (1954): 8–13.

Kumpusalo, E., K. Mattila, I. Virjo, L. Neittaanmäki, V. Kataje, S. Kujala, M. Jääskeläinen, R. Luhtata, and M. Isokoski. "Medical education and the corresponding professional needs of young doctors: the Finnish Junior Physician 88 Study." *Medical Education*, 25 (1991): 71–77.

Larsen, Ø. "Å være lege," in *Legene og samfunnet*, eds Ø. Larsen, Ø. Berg, and F. Hodne. Oslo: Seksjon for medisinsk historie, Universitet i Oslo, and Den norske lægeforening, 1986.

Neittaanmäki, L., R. Luhtala, I. Virjo, E. Kumpusalo, K. Mattila, M. Jääskeläinen, S. Kujala, and M. Isokoski. "More women enter medicine: young doctors' family origin and career choice," *Medical Education*, 27(1993): 440–445.

Riksaasen, R. "Påkjenninger i legeyrket. *Tidsskrift for Den norske lægeforening*, 109(1989): 1798–1799.

Riska, E, and K. Wegar. *Gender, work and medicine.* London: SAGE Publications Ltd, 1993.

Sveriges läkarfærbund. *Läkares arbetsmiljö – en rapport från Läkarförbundets arbetsmiljögrupp.* Stockholm: Sveriges läkarfærbund, 1988.

Thürmer, H., K. Bjartveit, and A. Hauknes. "Norske legers røykevaner 1952-84," *Tidsskrift for Den norske lægeforening*, 106 (1986): 2961-2964.

Vartiovaara, I. "Stress and burnout in the medical profession. (Burnout och läkarna)," *Suomen Lääkärilehti*, 43 (1988): 1258–1259.

CHAPTER 27.2

Morbidity and Subjective Well-being

OLAF GJERLØW AASLAND

27.2.1. A Different Disease Pattern?

Doctors are known to have low rates of sick leave (British Medical Association 1993). Is this because they are more resistant to disease, or is it because they are less willing to report their illnesses, even when they would have advised their patients to do so? Not much literature exists on this topic.

As is the case with general population studies, mortality is a much more «popular» theme than morbidity, surely due to a better validity, reliability and accessibility of data. Most studies on physician mortality show that they live longer than the general population, and place themselves in the middle of social class I (Rimppelä et al. 1987, Ackermann-Liebrich et al. 1991). An important exception is death by suicide, where physicians, in a number of studies, rate higher than the general population, in comparison with other relevant groups (Ullmann et al. 1991, British Medical Association 1993).

When it comes to morbidity, the documentation is extremely scarce. A British study on morbidity among 774 consultant pathologists, 588 anatomy and pathology technicians, and 76 public mortuary technicians, with a control group of 343 police officers and coroners, found that the pathologists took significantly fewer days of sick leave than the controls, and the technicians significantly more (Hall et al. 1991). When controlling for social class, the doctors still took fewer days off. A study on certified sickness absenteeism among employees in a modern hospital in Israel found that, doctors took less sick leave than the other employees, but the duration of sickness episodes was longer, suggesting that doctors do not stay away from work for relatively minor illness, or perhaps do not certify such spells of illness (Pines et al 1985).

This tendency is paralleled in data from the National Insurance Administration in Norway (Rikstrygdeverket), which covers the whole population, including all physicians. In 1993 and 1994, 18 and 17 physicians were given disability pensions, respectively (Bjerkedal, T, personal communication). This is approximately 1.3 per 1,000 active physicians, compared to 7.0 in the general population (Rikstrygdeverket 1994).

In a Swiss study, however, 466 physicians were asked to report any diseases they might have suffered from during the last year, regardless of whether they went on sick leave or not. Almost 80 percent of the respondents reported such an incident, and the level of morbidity, evaluated by this somewhat arbitrary measure, seemed higher than in the general population (Domenighetti et al. 1984).

Morbidity studies are usually based on two different sources of data: people's own reports, often recorded in connection with general population surveys, and studies based on data from physician, hospital, or insurance records. In the first case, classification is necessarily done more on the basis of subjective experience than on actual medical diagnoses. When doctors are surveyed, however, it is possible to use a standardized system for personal reports, which, to our knowledge, has hitherto not been done.

27.2.2. The Norwegian Physician Survey

The Norwegian Physician Survey is described in the previous chapter of this book. Data on working conditions, work satisfaction, and morbidity were collected by means of a postal questionnaire survey that included 9,266 active physicians in 1993. Out of 16 different questionnaires, each physician received one primary questionnaire and three randomly selected ones, dealing with various topics.

The response rate was 71.8 percent. Female physicians had a higher response rate than males (80 and 69, respectively), and specialists in private practice, who constitute only 4 percent of the total work force, had a low response rate (50 percent). Apart from these biases, the 6,652 respondents are considered representative of active Norwegian physicians.

The primary questionnaire was returned by all 6,652 respondents. Since the Norwegian Medical Association does not have historical records of its members, the form included complete retrospective histories on cohabitational status and childbirths, places

Diagram 27.1

The Questionnaire

The following instructions were given in the questionnaire:

Enter diseases, injuries or other indispositions you have suffered from since the age of 18. List only those which led to a minimum of 14 days sick leave, but include other incidents which you feel were of conciderable significance to your well-being or job satisfaction.

Use the ICPC-classification (see p … for ICPC-codes) as far as possible, and list both description and code. Use either symptom codes or diagnostic codes. Indicate the time when the disease, injury, or indisposition started, and time recovery, if appropriate. The same incident may be listed several times.

The questionnaire layout was as follows:

Incident	ICPC-code	started when yy	started when mm	ended when yy	ended when mm
1 ______	□□□	□□	□□	□□	□□
2 ______	□□□	□□	□□	□□	□□
3 ______	□□□	□□	□□	□□	□□
.					
.					
.					
20 ______	□□□	□□	□□	□□	□□

TABLE 27.1
Prevalence and chronicity of illness leading to at least two weeks absence from work, or otherwise seriously affecting work capasity or satisfaction. ICPC-groups.

ICPC-chapter	Females		Males	
	Prevalence (per 1,000)	Chronicity (years per 100,000)	Prevalence (per 1,000)	Chronicity (years per 100,000)
A General & unspecified**	46	65	30	29
B Blood	5	17	3	6
D Digestive ***	53	79	77	124
F Eye	6	11	9	13
H Ear	6	6	3	3
K Circulatory*	13	35	22	43
L Musculoskeletal	152	336	163	305
N Neurological	29	66	24	37
P Psychological**	69	264	49	143
R Respiratory*	46	80	33	42
S Skin	10	7	11	21
T Endocrine & metabolic***	18	56	6	12
U Urology	13	32	17	22
W Pregnancy & family planning[1)]	173	378	–	–
X Female genital system	54	108	–	–
Y Male genital system	–	–	7	12
Z Social problems***	17	55	6	14
Total***	483	1,819	364	1,063
Non-gender specific	315	1,410	335	1,031

* p<05, ** p<.01, *** p<.001, chi square, gender difference of prevalence
[1)] Only pregnancies that led to sick-leave certification etc. The prevalence of having one or more children among the female physicians is 723 per 1,000.

of abode, education, jobs, and past and present illnesses of importance for work capability and work satisfaction, plus questions regarding care of minors, and pregnancies. In addition, the questionnaire included a number of health and satisfaction measures. In order to standardize the morbidity records, a short version of ICPC (International Classification for Primary Care, Lamberts et al. 1987) was printed on the back of the questionnaire. This classification system is a dual track system, mainly organized according to organ systems (blood, circulatory, digestive etc.), whereby one can choose between 16 different chapters and record either symptoms (reasons for encounter) or medical diagnoses.

The instructions given in the questionnaire are shown in Diagram 27.1.

There are several potential pitfalls with this way of collecting morbidity data. The most important is probably the fact that episodes that occurred 10 or 20 years ago may have been forgotten, or perhaps even suppressed. Also, the not-too-exact criteria (conditions which led to at least 14 days' sick leave, [or]... which you feel were of considerable significance to your well-being or job satisfaction) is clearly a major threat to the reliability of the data. We decided, however, that we had to allow these approximations, since the subjective experience of being ill is as important as the objective facts in this study.

48.3 percent of the female and 36.4 percent of the male physicians listed at least one disease incident. The numbers of incidents per person for the 16 different ICPC chapters and totally (multiplied by 1,000) are given in columns 1 and 3 (prevalence) in Table 27.1.

Since the duration of each episode is also recorded, it is possible to calculate the chronicity of the various disease groups by aggregating the durations within each group relative to the total number of exposure years (years since age 18) for each gender. This is also shown in Table 27.1. For the single chapters, only durations up to five years are included in this measure, for the summary ratios (Total and Non-gender specific), a limit of ten years is used. The few individuals who are excluded in this way have usually given only a start date of their disease, indicating a chronic state.

If we disregard chapters W and X (Pregnancy and family planning and Female genital system), chapter L (Musculo-skeletal) dominates in prevalence since the age of 18 for both females and males, with 15.2 and 16.3 percent, respectively. This disease group also dominates with respect to chronicity. The gender difference is not statistically significant. The second largest groups are chapter P (Psychological) for females, and chapter D (Digestive) for males. Both show significant gender differences.

Most dominating is chapter W (Pregnancy and family planning) with a prevalence of 17.3 percent and chronicity of 378. This means that the toll of reproductivity amounts to 15 of the approximately 3,500 man-years accounted for by female physicians in Norway every year. In addition, there are the ordinary maternity and paternity leaves, which in another study were estimated at 340 man-years in 1992 (Eskeland et al. 1995).

The Norwegian physician work force presently consists of approximately 3,500 women and 9,000 men. If we take the chronicity ratios of 1,819 and 1,063, we find that 64 female and 96 male man-years are «lost» every year to disease, which amounts to 1.8 percent and 1.1 percent of the total working time, respectively. These figures are low compared to those of the general population, where approximately 3.3 percent of all workdays are spent on sick leaves exceeding 14 days (Rikstrygdeverket 1994).

In Table 27.2., some of the major disease groups are related to gender, age, family situation, type of present job and specialty. Seven multiple logistic models are presented, where the odds ratios of having had at least one incident of the disease since the age of 18 are presented with gender and age controlled for. Only variables where at least one category is significantly or almost significantly different from the reference category are included in the table. A relationship is considered significant when the 95 percent confidence interval does not include the value 1.00.

The table shows that the significantly higher prevalence of diseases of the digestive system for males remains also when age, family and job variables are controlled for, as does the higher level of respiratory diseases and cancer among females. For psychiatric disease, however, the gender difference is no longer significant.

With respect to age, there are some interesting patterns. As expected, the age gradi-

TABLE 27.2

Prevalence and relative risk (odds ratio with 95% confidence interval) of having episodes of disease since age 18 that led to at least 14 days of absence from work, or otherwise seriously affected work capacity or work satisfaction. 6,652 *Norwegian physicians*

	Digestive system	Cardio-vascular	Musculo-skeletal	Psychiatric	Respiratory	Cancer	All diseases
Prevalence (%)	7.5	1.9	16.2	5.5	3.6	2.0	42.7
Gender							
female	1.0	1.0	1.0	1.0	1.0	1.0	1.0
male	1.28 (1.00-1.65)	0.96 (0.60-1.54)	0.86 (0.73-1.01)	0.82 (0.64-1.04)	0.62 (0.46-0.84)	0.54 (0.36-0.80)	0.45 (0.40-0.51)
Age							
<31	1.0	1.0	1.0	1.0	1.0	1.0	1.0
31-40	1.88 (1.07-3.30)	2.12 (0.48-9.47)	1.24 (0.90-1.71)	1.16 (0.75-1.78)	2.07 (1.08-3.99)	2.43 (0.72-8.18)	1.40 (1.31-1.73)
41–50	2.55 (1.40-4.63)	2.93 (0.63-13.8)	1.86 (1.31-2.64)	1.75 (1.08-2.84)	2.09 (1.01-4.30)	3.06 (0.86-10.9)	1.90 (1.49-2.42)
51–60	3.58 (1.93-6.66)	8.33 (1.76-39.4)	2.22 (1.53-3.23)	1.23 (0.70-2.15)	3.20 (1.50-6.82)	4.48 (1.21-16.5)	2.33 (1.79-3.04)
61+	4.88 (2.49-9.57)	32.1 (6.73-1.53)	2.19 (1.41-3.40)	1.07 (0.49-2.32)	5.12 (2.25-11.7)	9.40 (2.47-35.8)	3.85 (2.76-5.36)
Family							
alone				1.0	1.0	1.0	
cohab				0.72 (0.46-1.13)	1.75 (0.88-3.50)	0.74 (0.27-2.02)	
married				0.46 (0.33-0.66)	1.38 (0.77-2.49)	0.88 (0.43-1.80)	
separated				0.97 (0.25-2.09)	3.17 (1.26-7.98)	3.55 (1.26-9.96)	
divorced				1.38 (0.80-2.41)	1.46 (0.58-3.68)	1.27 (0.45-3.56)	
widowed				2.47 (0.90-6.77)	3.45 (0.89-13.5)	1.02 (0.12-8.71)	
Job							
hospital	1.0		1.0				1.0
PHC	0.87 (0.61-1.24)		0.87 (0.69-1.10)				1.06 (0.90-1.26)
OHS	1.94 (1.18-3.19)		0.77 (0.50-1.19)				1.22 (0.89-1.26)
private	1.01 (0.74-1.38)		1.04 (0.84-1.29)				0.96 (0.82-1.13)
other	1.36 (0.93-1.98)		1.31 (1.00-1.70)				1.28 (1.03-1.59)
inactive	1.32 (0.39-4.47)		0.84 (0.32-2.19)				1.52 (0.78-2.95)

(Table 27.2 continued)

	Digestive system	Cardio-vascular	Musculo-skeletal	Psychiatric	Respiratory	Cancer	All diseases
Specialty							
nospec		1.0	1.0	1.0			1.0
GP		2.22 (1.10-4.46)	1.44 (1.13-1.84)	1.35 (0.95-1.92)			1.55 (1.29-1.86)
laboratory		1.03 (0.39–2.75)	0.99 (0.69-1.42)	0.66 (0.34-1.27)			0.98 (0.75-1.29)
medicine		1.40 (0.69-2.84)	1.37 (1.07-1.75)	0.67 (0.43-1.03)			1.27 (1.05-1.53)
surgery		1.28 (0.61-2.69)	1.30 (1.01-1.75)	0.59 (0.37-0.95)			1.18 (0.98-1.44)
psychiatry		1.81 (0.81-4.06)	1.54 (1.14-2.08)	1.67 (1.08-2.58)			1.74 (1.36-2.21)
publ.health		2.53 (1.02-6.26)	1.98 (1.39-2.83)	1.07 (0.61-1.89)			1.64 (1.22-2.19)
Hosmer-Lemeshow chi square (8 df)	5.87 (p=0.682)	7.021 (p=0.534)	7.522 (p=0.482)	5.740 (p=0.676)	6.736 (p=0.565)	14.052 (p=0.80)	14.59 (p=0.068)

ent is strong for cardiovascular disease and cancer, whereas psychiatric illness peaks in the age group 41–50, which is the only group significantly different from the reference group (30 and younger). For musculoskeletal conditions, there is also a tendency for the oldest physicians to have a lower prevalence than the middle-aged ones.

Family situation affects diseases, respiratory diseases and cancer, in different ways. Being married clearly decreases the probability of psychiatric disorders, as compared to living alone, and being separated increases the risk of respiratory diseases as well as cancer. This may partly be explained by the (not significantly) higher prevalence of daily smokers among the separated physicians, which is 25 percent, as compared to 12 percent in the total sample (data not shown).

The present job situation is not a very good predictor of disease after the age of 18, in this sample. There is a tendency for occupational health service physicians to suffer more from digestive problems than hospital employed physicians, and the heterogeneous group «other»- which consists mainly of physicians who, for a period, have taken positions as project leaders etc., or who are working as full-time researchers – has an increased risk of having had musculoskeletal problems. Maybe this is a reason why they decided to «step out of the line» in the first place? The column at the right shows that this group also has an increased risk of having had any disease.

With regard to specialty, general practitioners and public health specialists have increased risks of cardiovascular and musculoskeletal diseases when compared to nonspecialists. Specialists in internal medicine, surgery, and psychiatry also have a moderately elevated risk of musculoskeletal diseases, compared with the non-specialists, while psychiatrists in addition have a higher risk for psychiatric disorders. Interestingly, all specialty groups, except laboratory

DIAGRAM 27.2A

Total duration of disease episodes relative to the number of years passed since the age of 18 (means and 95% confidence intervals, logarithmically transformed) by gender and age among Norwegian physicians. Only physicians who have at least one disease incident are included.

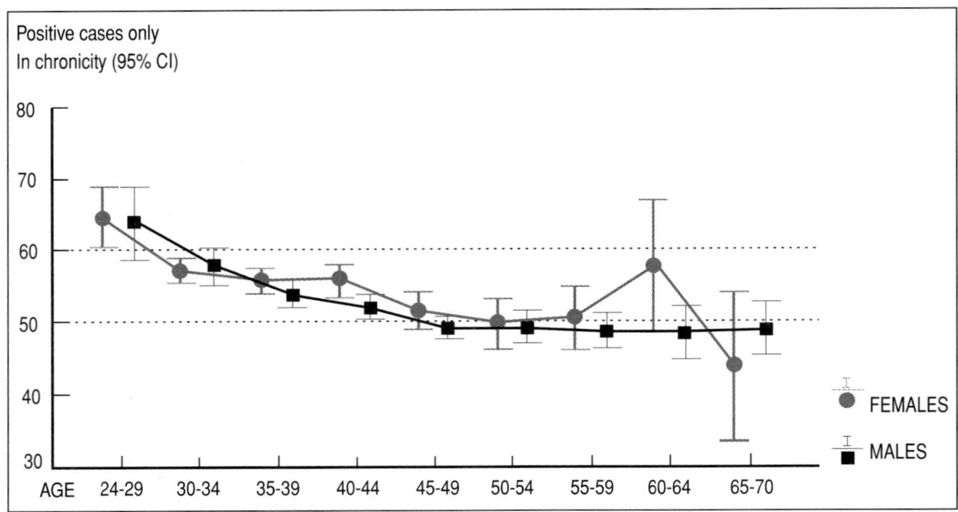

DIAGRAM 27.2B

Total duration of disease episodes relative to the number of years passed since the age of 18 (means and 95% confidence intervals, logarithmically transformed) by gender and age among Norwegian physicians. All physicians, including those who did not report any disease episodes.

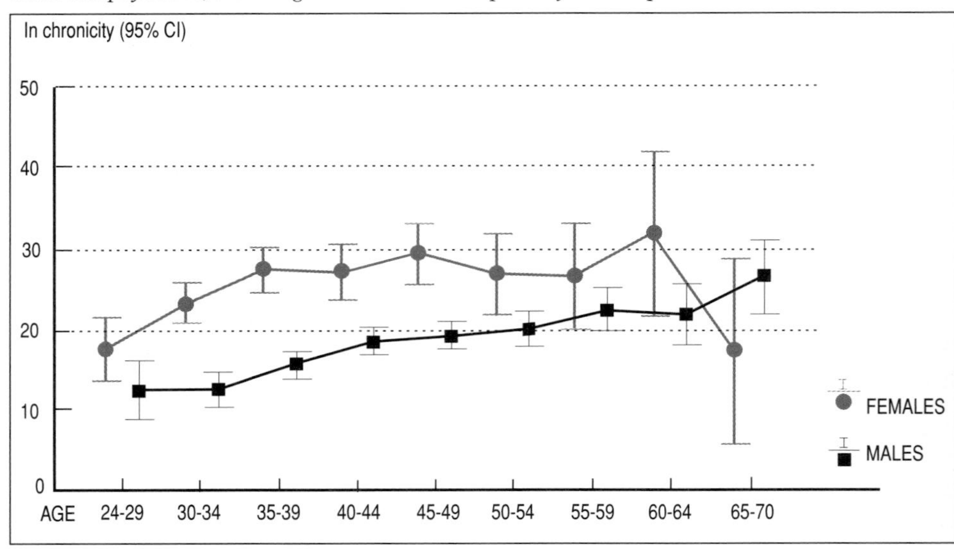

physicians, have a higher probability of having had a disease, compared to the non-specialists, although surgeons do not quite reach significance level.

Are young physicians today privileged with the same low morbidity as their older colleagues? This question is relevant with respect to medical student recruitment, and is often brought forward in discussions about whether young doctors today have a harder time than their seniors, when they were fresh from medical school. There is anecdotal evidence that today's internship candidates (interns) experience a more strenuous and less supportive work atmosphere, which could easily lead to a higher morbidity, reflected in, for instance, more sick days per year.

Diagrams 27.2a. and 27.2b. show the relationship between age, gender and morbidity, as measured by a chronicity ratio (total sickness divided by number of years since the age of 18 for each respondent). Since this ratio is very skewed, with the majority having zero or low values, a logarithmic transformation was performed before doing a simple comparison of means across five year age groups, for females and males separately. Diagram 27.2a. shows the results when only the positive cases are included, that is, those who reported at least one disease incident. This can be interpreted as an indication of the seriousness of disease incidents, as measured by the individual cumulative duration. There is no gender difference, but a significantly higher score among the youngest physicians.

In Diagram 27.2b. the mean chronicity ratios are calculated for the whole group. This measure can be interpreted as the relative contribution of a particular gender and age group to the total amount of sickness incidents among the physicians. Females are significantly higher than males from age 30 to age 50, and there is a moderate increase with age for both genders, with the possible exception of the oldest females.

The conclusion must be that the young doctors' sickness periods last longer than those of their older colleagues, but there is no indication that the total morbidity (the risk of having to take sick leave) is higher among younger physicians today than it used to be when their older colleagues were young.

27.2.3. Subjective Well-being

In addition to the attempt at measuring objective morbidity described above, the Norwegian Physician Survey included a large number of subjective measures of health and well-being. One of the questions on subjective well-being was: «When you think about your life today, would you say that you are, by and large, satisfied with life, or are you mostly dissatisfied?»

Besides being included in the Norwegian Physician Survey (Aasland and Falkum 1994), this question has been used in a number of general population surveys (Hol-

TABLE 27.3

Response to the question: "When you think about your life today, would you say that you are by and large satisfied with life, or are you mostly dissatisfied?" Original response scale 1 to 7. Percent

Response alternative	Physicians n=6,580	Population n=62,475
Very satisfied (response 1)	11	14
Satisfied (response 2 to 4)	76	83
Dissatisfied (response 5 to 7)	13	3

TABLE 27.4
Probability of being extremely satisfied among 6,305 active Norwegian physicians, expressed as odds ratio (OR) with 95% confidence interval (CI)

variable	OR (95% CI)
Gender	
female	1.0
male	0.66 (0.55-0.79)
Age	
24-30	1.0
31-35	0.99 (0.68-1.42)
36-40	0.77 (0.52-1.12)
41-45	0.82 (0.55-1.21)
46-50	1.08 (0.74-1.60)
51-55	1.13 (0.74-1.74)
56-60	1.32 (0.84-2.06)
61-65	1.73 (1.05-2.87)
66-70	3.90 (2.29-6.64)
Job	
hospital	1.0
community health	0.93 (0.72-1.20)
occupational health	1.44 (0.95-2.19)
private practice	1.62 (1.31-1.99)
other	2.27 (1.73-2.99)
Number of children	
0	1.0
1	1.58 (1.10-2.27)
2	1.87 (1.36-2.56)
3	1.71 (1.23-2.39)
4	1.95 (1.33-2.86)
5 or more	2.89 (1.83-4.58)

men et al. 1990) as well as in assessments of quality of life, in various groups of patients (Moum et al. 1992).

The possible scores, with the distribution of the 6,580 respondents in percent, compared with a population sample of 62,475 inhabitants from the Norwegian county of Nord-Trøndelag, were:

	Physicians	Population
1 Extremely satisfied	11	14
2 Very satisfied	40	35
3 Fairly satisfied	24	33
4 Yes and no	12	17
5 Fairly dissatisfied	8	1
6 Very dissatisfied	4	0
7 Extremely dissatisfied	1	1

There is a significant difference between physicians and the general population, and we see that three percent fewer physicians are extremely satisfied, and 11 percent more physicians are dissatisfied (options 5.6 and 7 taken together). A closer analysis (data not shown) reveals that it is particularly the youngest physicians who are dissatisfied.

We have taken a look at the 11 percent of the physicians who expressed their extreme satisfaction with life, to see to what extent they could be identified by way of gender, age, family situation, number of children, specialty, and type of work. Excluding a small group who were presently not active, we entered the variables into a logistic model with being extremely satisfied or not as the dependent variable. Specialty and family situation did not have any significant effect, and were not included in the final model, presented in Tables 27.3 and 27.4.

Somewhat unexpectedly, we see that female physicians are much more likely to be in the extremely satisfied group than male physicians. With regard to age, only the two oldest categories are significantly more likely to be extremely satisfied than the reference group, the youngest physicians. The pattern is interesting, however, with the 36 to 40 year olds being least likely to be extremely satisfied. The reference category for job situation is the hospital physicians. Two groups with a significantly higher probability are private practioners and the group «other.» As mentioned above, this is a heterogeneous group comprised of physicians who are doing unusual physician's work, such as being project organizers or full time researchers.

References

Aasland, O.G., and E. Falkum. «Legekårsundersøkelsen. Reponsen på spørreskjemaundersøkelsen», *Tidsskrift for Den norske lægeforening*, 114 (1994): 3052–3058.

Ackermann-Liebrich, U., and S. M. Wick. «Survival of female doctors in Switzerland,» *British Journal of Medicine*, 302 (1991):959.

Balarajan, R. «Inequalities in health within the health sector,» *British Journal of Medicine*, 299 (1989): 822–825.

British Medical Association. *The morbidity and mortality of the medical profession.* London: British Medical Association, 1993.

Domenighetti, G., and S. Berthoud. «Les medicins sont-ils aussi malades?» *Schweizerische Medizinische Wochenschrift*, 114 (1984): 858–873.

Engsig, A., B.Ø. Jensen, M. Johansson, K. Mogensen, M. Nordentoft, and A. Winther. *Yngre lægers arbejds- og livsvilkår. Rapport fra Socialpolitisk arbeidsgruppe.* København: Foreningen af yngre læger, 1990.

Eskeland, M., S. Fønnebø Knutsen and A. Forsdahl. «Legekårsundersøkelsen 1993: Legemangel – svangerskaps- og omsorgspermisjoner,» submitted 1995

Hall, A., T.C. Aw, and J.M. Harrington. «Morbidity survey of post mortem room staff.» *Journal of Clinical Pathology*, 44 (1991): 433–435.

Hellström, M., and G. Westlander. *Läkares arbetsvillkor inom olika specialiteter*. Solna: Arbetsmiljöinstitutet, 1993.

Holmen, J., K. Midthjell, K. Bjartveit, P.F. Hjort, P.G. Lund-Larsen, T. Moum, S. Næss, and H.T. Waaler. *The Nord-Trøndelag Health Survey 1984–86*. Verdal: Folkehelsa (SIFF), 1990.

Kumpusalo, E., K. Mattila, I. Virjo, L. Neittaanmäki, S. Kujala, M. Jääskeläinen, R. Luhtata, and M. Isokoski. «Medical education and the corresponding professional needs of young doctors: the Finnish Junior Physician 88 Study.» *Medical Education*, 25 (1991): 71–77.

Lamberts, H., and M. Wood, eds. *ICPC – International classification of primary care.* Oxford: Oxford University Press, 1987.

Moum, T., T. Sørensen, S. Næss, and J. Holmen. «Gir diagnosen høyt blodtrykk endret livskvalitet? Resultater fra en medisinsk masseundersøkelse i Nord-Trøndelag», *Tidsskrift for Den norske lægeforening*, 112(1992): 18-23.

Neittaanmäki, L., R. Luhtala, I. Virjo, E. Kumpusalo, K. Mattila, M. Jääskeläinen, S. Kujala, and M. Isokoski. «More women enter medicine: young doctors' family origin and career choice,» *Medical Education*, 27(1993): 440–445.

Pines, A., K. Skulkeo, E. Pollak, E. Peritz, and J. Steif. «Rates of sickness absenteeism among employees of a modern hospital: the role of demographic and occupational factors,» *British Journal of Industrial Medicine*, 42(1985): 326–335.

Rikstrygdeverket. *Trygdestatistisk årbok 1994. Rikstrygdeverket.* Oslo: Utredningsavd. Rikstrygdeverket, 1994.

Rimpelä, A.H., N.M. Nurminen, P.O. Pulkkinen, M.K. Rimpelä, and T. Valkonen. «Mortality of doctors: do doctors benefit from their medical knowledge?» *Lancet*, 1(1987): 84–86.

Sveriges läkarförbund. *Läkares arbetsmiljö – en rapport från Läkarförbundets arbetsmiljögrupp*. Stockholm: Sveriges läkarförbund, 1988.

Ullmann, D., R.L. Phillips, L. Beeson, H.G. Dewey, B.N. Brin, J.W. Kuzma, C.P. Mathews, and A.E. Hirst. «Cause-specific mortality among physicians with differing life-style,» *The Journal of the American Medical Association*, 265(1991): 2352–2359.

Vartiovaara, I. «Stress and burnout in the medical profession (Burnout och läkarna),» *Suomen Lääkärilehti*, 43(1988): 1258–1259.

Vikanes, Å., V. Akre, and P. Hjortdahl. «Medisinsk utdanning i utakt. Grunnutdanninga slik turnuskandidaten opplever ho. (Norwegian basic medical education from the intern's point of view.),» *Tidsskrift for Den norske lægeforening*, 112 (1992): 2541–2545

CHAPTER 27.3

Psychosocial Work-Environment and Job Satisfaction

ERIK FALKUM

27.3.1. Stress and Overload – an Important Problem

An increasing amount of literature on physician stress and job satisfaction has demonstrated that work overload is a prevalent problem among physicians. The internationally most commonly reported frustration is lack of time to do a proper job, and at the same time to lead a normal family life (Cartwright et al. 1981a, Cartwright et al. 1981b). The main focus of a considerable part of these workload studies is on the supposed relation between workload and quality of care (Groenewegen et al. 1991).

As early as 1968, Mechanic stated that the average doctor responded to the increasing demands on his time by practicing at the pace and style of the assembly line (Mechanic 1968). The time pressure supposedly shortens consultations and reduces the quality of communication between patient and physician, thereby increasing the risk that important patient problems are left unaddressed. The overall result is a lower quality of care (Melville 1980). If these conclusions are correct, work stress and job satisfaction among physicians are important issues, not only to the physicians themselves, but also to health administrators and planners, and to the total population of present and future patients.

Based on data from the Norwegian Physician Survey, which has been described in detail in the preceding chapters, this chapter presents some of the results of the research into the interrelations between job satisfaction, perceived stress and autonomy among Norwegian doctors.

27.3.2. Job Stress

Workload can be measured in "objective" and "subjective" ways. Various studies in this field have used number and length of consultations, total work hours, frequency of overtime, and so on, as measures of workload (Groenwegen et al. 1991). However, there is evidence that even though such "objective" measures are correlated positively with job strain and negatively with work satisfaction, the associations tend to be relatively weak (Payne & Firth-Cozens 1987, Lazarus & Folkman 1984). This does not preclude that very long work hours add to the physician's strain, but it means that measures of perceived workload or stress tend to be stronger predictors of both satisfaction and the various strain variables, probably because they are more direct indicators, that is, their effects are not diluted by the fact that some people thrive on a brisk pace and long hours, while others are strained by them.

The measures of perceived workload range from direct single questions as to whether physicians feel overworked (Wilkin et al. 1986, Statistisk sentralbyrå 1985), to rather comprehensive measures of job stress (Makin et al 1988). Our survey posed four questions about how often the physicians felt that their work situation was too fast-paced, the pressure unacceptable, and the number of tasks and disturbances prevented them from working effectively.

The internal consistency of the questions proved to be quite good (Cronbach's alpha=0.83), and they were combined to a sum score ranging from four to nineteen (mean=11.67, st.dev.=3.31), as shown in Diagram 27.3.

Subjects who consequently chose response categories indicating high levels of perceived job stress scored 15 or more. 21.4 percent of the total sample belongs to this group.

Table 27.5 displays the prevalence of high job stress in three demographical subgroups of physicians. High job stress is more common in men than in women, while the distribution according to age seems to be curvilinear, with the highest prevalence among doctors between forty and fifty. Interestingly, the highest percentage of subjects feeling stressed is found among the chief physicians, while only a few of the respondents working as researchers score above the high stress threshold. The correlation between this perceived stress measure and the respondent's total work hours (the sum of the scheduled work hours and overtime) was not higher than 0.1, a result in line with the above reasoning on this relationship.

27.3.3. Job Control

The pioneers of stress research studied the demand dimension in isolation. This proved problematic, because on the one hand, demands (be they long work hours, number of patients, patients' expectations, length of consultations, interruptions, administrative tasks, or technically complex procedures), challenge and mental arousal are necessary conditions for effective learning, development and coping, but on the other hand, they can induce the experience of strain. The relation between psychological demands and stress seems to be illustrated by a U-shaped curve, indicating the existence of a demand

DIAGRAM 27.3

Perceived stress among Norwegian physicians. (n=2,600)

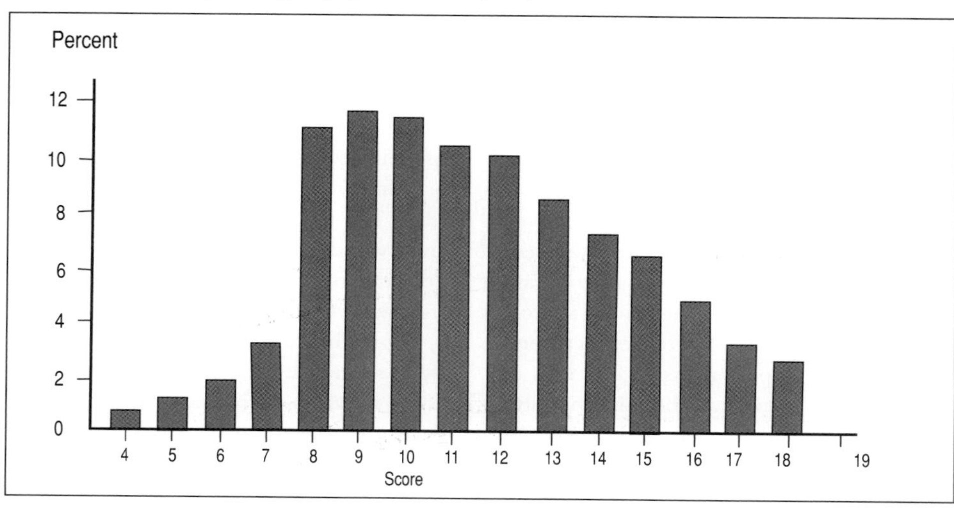

TABLE 27.5
Norwegian physicians with high perceived job stress according to sex, age, and position. Percent. (n= 2,600)

Sex	Men	Women					
	23.0	17.5	p=.002				
Age	25-30	31-40	41-50	51-60	61-69		
	17.4	20.2	24.5	23.2	11.8	p=.004	
Position	Outside hospital work	Chief physician	Consultant	Resident	Intern	Researcher	
	20.4	29.2	25.2	18.0	22.4	6.5	p=.000

optimum, around which stress will increase on both sides (Selye 1976). A growing body of evidence now indicates that the so-called decision latitude dimension acts as a moderator, strongly influencing the extent to which the demands produce learning and coping or strain (Karasek 1979, Karasek & Theorell 1990).

The decision latitude or control concept has two highly correlated dimensions: autonomy and task variety. The learning of new skills over time is a central condition for the increase of autonomy, that is, the surgeon or the experienced family physician tend to experience a broader decision latitude than the intern or the resident.

We measured perceived autonomy among the doctors by six questions on whether they themselves could decide about work speed and order of tasks, discuss the organization of their own work, influence decisions on planning, and postpone scheduled tasks if

TABLE 27.6
Norwegian physicians with low perceived autonomy according to sex, age, and position. Percent. (n= 2,309)

Sex	Men	Women					
	14.4	23.9	p=.000				
Age	25-30	31-40	41-50	51-60	61-69		
	32.2	21.2	13.5	8.4	6.3	p=.000	
Position	Outside hospital work	Chief physician	Consultant	Resident	Intern	Researcher	p=.000
	11.5	5.5	16.4	33.6	53.2	1.3	

DIAGRAM 27.4
Perceived autonomy among Norwegian physicians. (n=2,309)

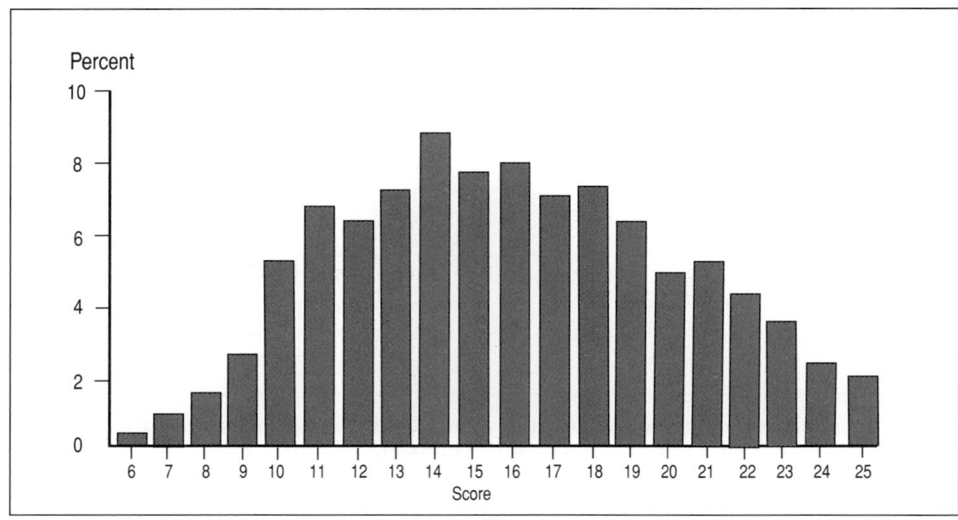

required or desirable. The internal consistency among these questions also proved to be satisfactory (Cronbach's alpha=0.83), and their sum score was used as an overall measure of perceived autonomy, ranging from six to twenty-five (mean=16.05, st.dev.=

TABLE 27.7
Predictors of low perceived autonomy among Norwegian physicians. Logistic regression. (n=2,295)

Variable	Category	Odds ratio	Wald	p
Sex	women	1.49	10.18	.001
	men	1.00		
Age	25-30	3.28	6.25	.01
	31-40	2.61	4.68	.03
	41-50	2.08	2.78	ns
	51-60	1.29	0.29	ns
	61-69	1.00		
Position	outside hospital work	1.00		
	chief physician	0.66	1.43	ns
	consultant	1.84	14.43	.0001
	resident	3.22	60.44	.0000
	intern	6.00	34.44	.0000
	researcher	0.09	5.97	.02

4.34). The distribution of perceived autonomy scores in the total sample is shown in Diagram 27.4.

Doctors who consequently chose response categories indicating low perceived autonomy scored less than twelve. 17.2 percent of the respondents belonged to the low autonomy group.

Table 27.6 shows that there are relatively more women than men in this subsample. There is also a clear age gradient, with larger shares of low autonomy among younger physicians than among older. Most of the young physicians were residents or interns and, as expected, the prevalence of low perceived autonomy is clearly higher among them than among more experienced physicians. Almost none of the respondents working as researchers belong to this low autonomy group. In order to evaluate the relative predictive importance of sex, age, and position, we included these variables in a logistic regression analysis with autonomy (low=1, medium or high=0) as the dependent measure. The results are displayed in Table 27.7.

One could hypothesize that the sex and age ingredients would disappear when position was controlled for, because residents and interns are young and because the number of female doctors has increased rapidly over the last two decades. However, both sex and age remain significant predictors of low perceived autonomy: the chance that female respondents belong to the low autonomy group is about one and a half times that of males, and the risk also clearly increases with decreasing age. The chance that interns belong to the low autonomy group is six times that of doctors working outside the hospital.

TABLE 27.8

Predictors of high perceived stress among Norwegian physicians. Logistic regression. (n=2,292)

Variable	Category	Odds ratio	Wald	p
Sex	women	0.61	14.96	.0001
	men	1.00		
Age	25-30	1.26	0.35	ns
	31-40	1.87	3.44	ns
	41-50	2.31	6.59	.01
	51-60	2.34	6.20	.01
	61-69	1.00		
Position	outside hospital work	1.00		
	chief physician	1.69	6.68	.01
	consultant	0.90	0.63	ns
	resident	0.53	15.38	.0001
	intern	0.69	1.13	ns
	researcher	0.59	1.41	ns
Autonomy	low	8.0	160.45	.0000
	medium	2.97	47.40	.0000
	high	1.00		

The correlation (Pearson) between perceived stress and autonomy was -0.43 (p=0.000), that is, stress increases with decreasing autonomy scores. Table 27.8 displays the results of a logistic regression analysis in which high perceived stress (high perceived stress=1, medium/low perceived stress=0) was predicted by sex, age, position, and autonomy. The latter variable was included as a trichotomy with approximately equal subject numbers in each category (low, medium, high).

The chance that the respondents belong to the high stress group was about eight times higher among subjects with low than among subjects with high perceived autonomy. Furthermore, all the three demographical variables maintained their significant predictive values when autonomy was controlled for. The chance that female doctors belong to the high stress group is clearly smaller than that of males, the risk of high stress remains highest among physicians between forty and sixty, and only the chief physicians feel more stressed than doctors working outside the hospital. The chance that residents belong to the high stress group is particularly small, only about half that of the subjects in the reference category.

27.3.4. Job Satisfaction

Various empirical findings support the demand/decision latitude model: exhaustion, depression, pill consumption, and job dissatisfaction increase with increasing demands and decrease with increasing control in American, Swedish, German, and Finnish studies (Kasl 1989, Ganster 1989, Kauppinen-Toropainen et al. 1983, Braun & Hollander 1988, Karasek 1979), and the associations do not seem to be substantially reduced when demographic variables such as sex and age are controlled for. In a study of English general practitioners, Makin and colleagues (Makin et al. 1988) applied a 32-item scale developed from interviews with general practitioners. Factor analysis produced four job stress dimensions: interruptions, emotional involvement, administrative involvement and the home/work interface, and routine medical work. The first three of them were significant predictors of job satisfaction. Cooper a.o. (Cooper et al. 1989) and Sutherland and Cooper (Sutherland and Cooper 1992) reproduced most of these results in large general practioner samples, and also demonstrated that female general practitioners had higher job satisfaction than their male counterparts. Branthwaite

TABLE 27.9
Mean scores (in order of importance) for ten job satisfaction indicators among Norwegian physicians. (n=2,295)

Variable	Mean	St.dev.
Overall job satisfaction	5.37	1.26
Amount of variety	5.36	1.29
Fellow workers	5.35	1.23
Opportunity to use ability	5.34	1.38
Freedom to choose method of working	5.26	1.40
Physical working conditions	5.12	1.46
Amount of responsibility	4.95	1.42
Recognition for good work	4.82	1.52
Rate of pay	4.49	1.75
Hours of work	4.25	1.73

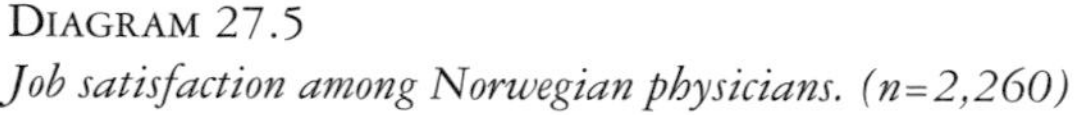

DIAGRAM 27.5
Job satisfaction among Norwegian physicians. (n=2,260)

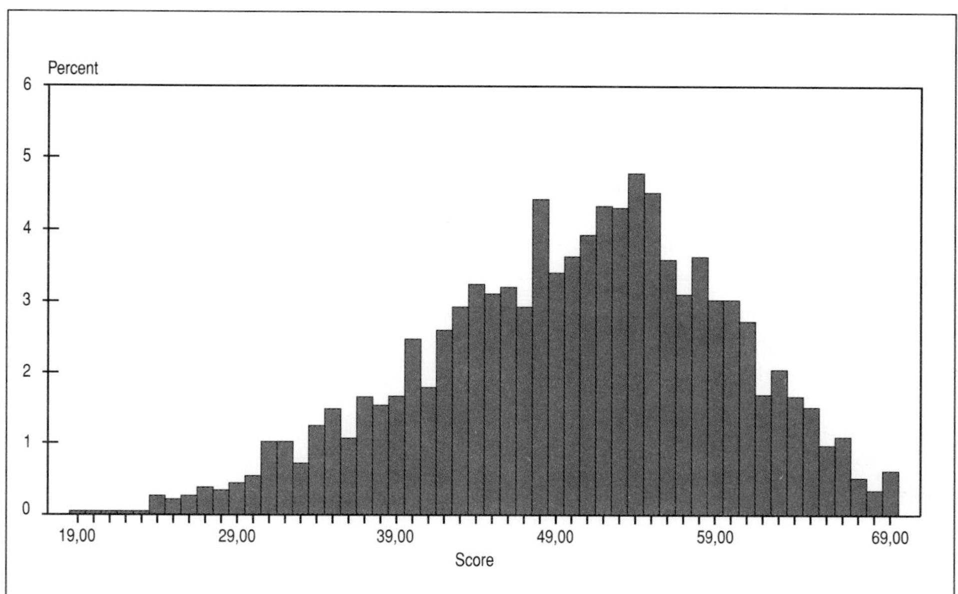

and Ross (Branthwaite et al. 1988) focused on uncertainty and insecurity as sources of pressure among general practitioners. The latter finding favors the hypothesis that job satisfaction among physicians increases with age, since professional insecurity is probably more common in inexperienced doctors. However, previous studies are not conclusive on this point (Wilkin et al. 1986).

In line with earlier findings, we hypothesized that male doctors are more often dissatisfied than female ones, that younger, inexperienced doctors are more often dissatisfied than older ones, and that the risk of being dissatisfied increases with increasing stress and decreasing autonomy. During the last decade, extensive retrenchments have increased the time pressure and bureaucratic control in Norwegian hospitals, and the complaints among hospital physicians are many. Even though the demand-resource imbalance in hospitals tends to spread to practitioners outside, because patients often are discharged before treatment has been completed, we hypothesized that job dissatisfaction is more common among hospital doctors than among those working in outpatient clinics. We also looked for gradients according to position in the hospital hierarchy.

Our primary questionnaire included a ten-item job satisfaction instrument developed by Warr and colleagues (Warr et al. 1979). Satisfaction was assessed for nine different job dimensions: freedom to choose working methods, amount of responsibility, amount of variety, physical working conditions, fellow workers, opportunity to use ability, rate of pay, recognition for good work, and hours of work. The inventory also included a question about overall job satisfaction. Each item was scored on a seven point Likert scale.

Table 27.9 displays the sample means for each item. The lowest scores were obtained for the question about satisfaction with work hours and wages, while the highest item

TABLE 27.10
Norwegian physicians with low job satisfaction according to sex, age, position, stress, and autonomy. Percent. (n= 2,552)

Sex	Men	Women					
	15.6	11.5	p=.005				
Age	25-30	31-40	41-50	51-60	61-69		
	26.0	15.0	11.0	6.3	3.3	p=.0000	
Position	Outside hospital work	Chief physician	Consultant	Resident	Intern	Researcher	
	11.0	8.7	11.9	18.2	38.8	9.2	p=.0000
Stress	Low	Medium	High				
	4.5	10.0	24.5	p=.0000			
Autonomy	Low	Medium	High				
	29.8	9.3	2.2	p=.0000			

mean concerns general job satisfaction. Differences along the demographic categories exist for some of the items. For instance, doctors working outside hospitals (mostly general practitioners) are clearly more satisfied with their rate of pay than are consultants, residents, interns, and researchers in hospitals. Contrary to the situation in many other Western countries, pay rates have long been higher among general practitioners (especially among those in private practice) than among hospital doctors. The reliability of the instrument proved to be good (Cronbach's alpha=0.86), and an unweighted sum score of all items, theoretically ranging from ten (extremely dissatisfied) to seventy (extremely satisfied), was computed. Diagram 27.5 shows the distribution of overall job satisfaction scores among Norwegian doctors.

The mean value for the whole sample was 50.98 (st.dev.=9.54, range=11–70), meaning that most physicians are quite satisfied with their work. On the seven point Likert scale, four may be considered the "neutral" item score, and subjects with a sum score below 40 may be classified as "dissatisfied." 13 percent of the sample scored less than 40.

Table 27.10 displays the prevalence of job dissatisfaction in the various demographical subgroups. Female physicians are somewhat less often dissatisfied than male ones, and older physicians are clearly less often dissatisfied than younger ones, while interns and residents display the highest figures among the position categories. There are also substantial gradients according to perceived stress and autonomy in the hypothesized directions.

TABLE 27.11
Predictors of job dissatisfaction among Norwegian physicians. Logistic regression. (n=2,251)

Variable	Category	Odds ratio	Wald	p
Sex	women	1.08	0.29	ns
	men	1.00		
Age	25-30	5.08	6.22	.01
	31-40	3.03	3.14	ns
	41-50	2.68	2.54	ns
	51-60	1.86	0.93	ns
	61-69	1.00		
Position	outside hospital work	1.00		
	chief physician	0.90	0.11	ns
	consultant	0.94	0.10	ns
	resident	0.94	0.15	ns
	intern	1.23	0.36	ns
	researcher	2.58	4.54	.03
Stress	low	1.00		
	medium	1.57	3.92	.05
	high	3.92	36.60	.0000
Autonomy	low	12.40	71.35	.0000
	medium	3.58	18.10	.0000
	high	1.00		

Table 27.11 shows the results of the multivariate analysis of job dissatisfaction. Autonomy is clearly the strongest predictor: the chance that a subject with low perceived autonomy belongs to the group of dissatisfied doctors is more than twelve times that among respondents with high perceived autonomy. Correspondingly, the risk that a physician with high perceived stress is dissatisfied with his job is nearly four times that among doctors with low perceived stress. The youngest doctors (25–30 years old) belong to the dissatisfied group five times more often than do their oldest colleagues (61–69 years old). Only the group of physicians doing research has a significantly higher risk of being dissatisfied with their jobs than doctors working outside the hospital, a finding which is probably based on their low salaries, the often intense competition for attractive academic positions, and the fact that many physicians in this group are working in relative isolation. Thus, most of the differences according to sex, age, and position seem to be based on gradients along the stress and autonomy dimensions.

Naturally, several other variables should be considered in order to produce a more complete picture of the factors predicting job satisfaction among doctors. However, the above analysis indicates that health administrators, planners, and the various professional organizations should seriously consider the impacts of psychological demands and work autonomy on the physician's satisfaction, coping and development, and consequently on the quality of his or her medical work.

References

Brainthwaite, A., and A. Ross. "Satisfaction and Job Stress in General Practice," *Family Practice*, 5(1988): 83–93.

Braun, S., and R.B. Hollander. "Work and depression among women in the Federal Republic of Germany," *Women and Health*, 14(1988): 5–24.

Cartwright, A., and R. Anderson. *Changes in the frequency and nature of doctor-patient contacts.* In *General Practice Revisited.* London: Tavistick Publications, 1981. (a)

Cartwright, A., and R. Anderson. *General Practice Revisited. A second study of patients and their doctors.* London: Tavistock Publications, 1981. (b)

Cooper, C. L., U. Rout, and B. Faragher. "Mental health, job satisfaction, and job stress among general practitioners," *British Journal of Medicine* 298(1989): 366–370.

Ganster, D. "A review of research in the workplace," in *Job control and worker health*, eds. S.L. Sauter, J.J. Hurrell, and C.C, Cooper (New York: Wiley, 1989), pp 3–23.

Groenewegen, P.P., and J.B.F. Hutten. "Workload and job satisfaction among general practitioners: A review of the literature," *Social Science and Medicine* 32(1991): 1111–1119.

Karasek, R. A. "Job demands, job decision latitude, and mental strain: Implications for job redesign," *Administrative Science Quarterly* 24 (1979): 285–308.

Karasek, R., and T. Theorell. *Healthy work. Stress, productivity, and the reconstruction of working life*. Basic Books/Harper Collins Publ, 1990.

Kasl, S.V. "An epidemiological perspective on the role of control in health." In S.L. Sauter, J.J.Hurrell, and C.C.Cooper (eds.), *Job control and worker health*, (pp.161-189), 1989.

Kauppinen-Toropainen, K., I. Kandolin, and P. Mutanen. "Job dissatisfaction and work-related exhaustion in male and female work," *Journal of Occupational Behaviour*, 4(1983): 193–207.

Lazarus, R.S., and S. Folkman. *Stress, appraisal, and coping*. New York: Springer Publishing Company, 1984.

Makin, P.J., U. Rout, and C.L. Cooper. "Job satisfaction and occupational stress among general practitioners – a pilot study," *Journal of the Royal College of General Practitioners*, 38(1988): 303–306.

Mechanic, D. "General medical practice in England and Wales; its organization and future," *New England Journal of Medicine* 279(1968): 680–689.

Melville, A. "Job satisfaction in general practice: Implications for prescribing," *Socal Science and Medicine*, 14A(1980): 495–499.

Payne, R., and J. Firth-Cozens. *Stress in health professionals*, New York: John Wiley & Son, 1987.

Selye, H. *The stress of life.* New York: McGraw-Hill, 1976.

Statistisk sentralbyrå. *Helseundersøkelse 1985*. Oslo: Statistisk sentralbyrå, 1985.

Sutherland, V.J., and C.L. Cooper. «Job stress, satisfaction, and mental health among general practitioners before and after introduction of new contract,» *British Journal of Medicine*, 304(1992): 1545–48.

Warr, P., J. Cook, and T. Wall. «Scales for the measurements of some work attitudes and aspects of psychological well-being,» *Journal of Occupational Psychology*, 52(1979): 129–148.

Wilkin, D., P. Hodgkin, and D. Metcalfe. «Factors affecting workload: Is received wisdom true? In P. Gray (ed.), *The medical annual, 1986, The yearbook of general practice (pp.185–196).* Bristol: Wright, 1986.

CHAPTER 28

Reluctant to Be Perceived as Ill – The Case of the Physician

VIGDIS MOE CHRISTIE AND BENEDICTE INGSTAD

28.1 Introduction

We know little about how physicians experienced the fact of getting ill in the old days. But as shown in Chapter 10, at least more than half of the physicians' illnesses at the end of the last century were caused by their work. Today, a hundred years later, the picture of illness has changed drastically; the awareness of "self-inflicted" illnesses is growing, creating in the patient more self-reproach and feelings of guilt than might have been the case in the earlier days. Maybe the physicians were then looked upon more as "heroes," getting ill as they attempted to help others?

This chapter will be concentrated on these four statements:

1. The physician who gets ill has difficulties in admitting his illness.
2. The physician who is ill experiences a role conflict or dilemma – that is, to what extent the physician or the patient role is to be played, in contact with a physician/colleague.
3. The physician/colleague, on his side, experiences a conflict between playing the role of the physician and playing the role of a colleague.
4. These dilemmas illustrate the important aspects involved in this encounter. They can tell us something of general interest about the role of the patient, the role of the physician, as well as the patient/physician relationship in general, in our society.

28.2. The Project, Material, and Methods

The Norwegian Medical Association has approximately 15,000 members. Ninety-five percent of all physicians are members. Of these members, a random sample of 1,200 physicians were asked to participate in this project. However, as we were interested only in those between the ages of 30 and 60 who were, or had been seriously ill during the last five years, we do not know how many of the 1,200 fullfilled these criteria.

The material for this chapter was gathered in the period from autumn 1993 until summer 1994.

In brief: this is a qualitative research project, based on 88 case stories. Thirty-nine physicians who live in the Oslo region have been interviewed face to face. Forty-nine other physicians who are practicing in different parts of Norway have themselves written or taped their case stories, five of them more briefly.

The 39 interviews lasted from 1 1/2 to 4 1/2 hours. They were open interviews, during which we tried to get the physicians to tell about their illnesses without interruption. A theme-guide was used at the end of the interviews to cover the topics they had not mentioned during their story.

The 49 physicians who sent in their written or taped case stories also received this theme-guide. Nearly all of the stories are told in a very conscientious manner. One of them consists of 37 pages, but mostly they are four to ten pages long. Five of these physicians have answered by filling in the theme-guide only. If we include them in our material, we have a total of 88 cases of illness.

Sixty-seven percent of the physicians are men and thirty-three percent are women. Considering their age and workplace, this is about the same proportion as for the members of the medical association.

The physicians report a wide range of illnesses, from serious depression, "burn out," cancer, ischia, to different sorts of heart troubles and so on.

To be concise, we have only provided one example for each point.

28.3. Statement 1: The Physician Who Becomes Ill has Difficulties in Admitting His Illness

28.3.1. Physicians Themselves are not supposed to Become Ill

In several instances the literature mentions that physicians often wait for a long time before seeking help when they are ill (Murray 1978, Scheiber and Doyle 1983, Langsley 1983, Marzuk 1987, Wise 1991), something that our material confirms. After all, a physician isn't supposed to be ill himself.

It is a well-known fact that medical students often believe that they suffer from the diseases they read and learn about. As one of the informants said: "In the beginning of our medical education we thought something was wrong as soon as we had a vague presentiment. We did a biopsy to make sure."

After a while, physicians almost have to force themselves into thinking that they do not have this or that particular illness. Something like that could not possibly happen to them. The result, however, might easily be that they start believing that they cannot become ill at all, that they are invulnerable.

Physicians are also often exposed to the danger of attracting infections, but should they constantly be in fear of this, it could affect their work negatively.

In addition, physicians are naturally confronted with so much illness, suffering, and death that deep inside they are afraid of getting ill. Maybe this is the reason why they try to minimize their own illnesses. They so desperately hope that the discovered symptoms are not signs of serious illness that they, in the end, decide that it is nothing to worry about. Many patients also think in this way, although some physicians may not believe it.

We must remember that during their education, physicians are taught to take care of other people. During the six years of medical training in Norway, the fact that they also should remember to take care of themselves, is hardly mentioned.

In addition, some physicians see getting ill as a defeat, since they know, better than most, that many illnesses could have been avoided (Stevensen 1952).

Considering all of these factors, it is perhaps only natural that they seem astonished when forced to acknowledge their own illnesses: "Becoming ill suprised me, since I was not used to it. I have always been the healthy one in the family, and I honestly did not believe that I could get ill." Another physician expressed it in this manner: "My belief – that illness and death would not touch me – was crushed."

This phenomenon is well known, in scientific literature as well as in fiction (AMA Council of Mental Health 1973, Marzuk 1987, Richards 1989, Wise 1991, Fyrand 1992, among others). Peter M. Marzuk writes: "Many physicians are masters at denying their own illnesses, and they often ignore the warnings they give to patients about signs and symptoms. As a result, they seek treatment much later in the course of a disease than other patients do" (p. 409).

28.3.2. A Physician should be Strong and Tough, not Feeble or Squeamish.

One of the physicians we interviewed said: "I am not working in a squeamish environment. We have to be tough and keep our noses to the grindstone. The one among us with the lowest fever must take the watch. Beyond this, there is a contempt for weakness. Maybe this could be the result of the fact that we are so used to playing the role of the giving physician, that when we suddenly become the one lying on our back, we feel weak.... I do not know."

"We are reluctant to show weakness," said several of the questioned physicians. One of them put it like this: "One has to be tough and clever, and one has to try hard the whole time."

Sargent et al. 1977, Scheiber and Doyle 1983, Rutle et al. 1988, Fugelli and Malterud 1989 wrote about this phenomenon. Douglas A. Sargent et al. reported: "Physicians tend to regard personal illness as weakness, a narcissistic injury which triggers defensive psychic regression and impairs reality-appreciation, allowing the physician to deny a suicidal danger that would be quickly detected in the patient. This denial is often supported by the physician's fantasy that he or she is a miraculous healer, immune to diseases" (p.144).

28.3.3. Minimizing or Belittling, Playing Down

One of the reasons why many physicians wait so long before seeking help is the fear that they are overdramatizing the situation, and that medical help really is not necessary. In general, physicians often make fun of patients who run to see a physician for the meerest problems, and have no wish to resemble these people. A physician, who turned out to have cancer, said: "I put the thought out of my mind, although it was painful when I ran in the corridors at the hospital. I had felt this way for several weeks, but the thought that it could be cancer never occurred to me. I thought that it would heal by itself." Another physician said: "I have learnt a lot about the dangers of ignoring one's own body, playing it down, denying one's own illness, and setting one's own needs aside.

I think it was in the autumn of 1988 that I first noticed a small sore on my throat. I cleaned it regularly – but time passed – and it would not heal. For almost two years I had this sore that grew, stung, and would not heal, without doing anything about it or seeking medical help. The last six months, I began suspecting that it might be cancer, and I thought of going to the policlinic to do a biopsy.

However, I did not get the time to think of my own needs until the summer of 1990, when I went to see a physician. He immediately made the diagnosis – cancer – and sent me to a surgeon.

The surgeon was angry and disgusted that I, a physician, had not come to see him before. I felt ashamed.

Afterwards I was shocked by the fact that I had ignored myself and my own health. I realized that I took my own health as a matter of course, and was primarily focused on work, duties and responsibility."

28.3.4. Afraid that Someone might Learn about it

We will briefly mention another finding, which is that physicians are often afraid that someone will learn about their illness. This also strengthens the statement that physicians are reluctant to be perceived as ill. It might be the family that they are trying to hide their illness from, their neighbors, their patients, or their colleagues. For instance, in the case of this physician: "I did not want my colleagues to know that I had heart problems. I was afraid that they then would no longer consider me as a worthy colleague."

One of the physicians wrote to us that he was totally "burned out" at the time he became ill, and he continued: "I was very annoyed at the fact that I was becoming severely ill. I did not mention it to anybody. I lost weight at a rapid speed. When people asked me if I was seriously ill, I answered: 'Oh no, I've just been exercising to get fit.' In the end I went to see a colleague who found a duodenal ulcer. Tests were taken from the wound. I guess it was then that I decided that it was time to let my wife and children know about the problem. My office was only told that I had a gastric ulcer."

Some of the physicians in our material were especially afraid that their patients would find out about their illnesses. This can be due to several factors. One of the most important is perhaps the fear that, in learning of a physician's illness, patients might be skeptical of the physician's ability to cure others.

A psychiatrist, who was troubled by an obsessive neurosis, said: "I have been so afraid that people would find out about it. But mainly, I would definitely not want my patients to know. I want them to relate to me as a therapist."

Many of our subjects told us that they had felt very alone when it came to their illness. They had had few, if any, friends or relatives to share their secret with; and they were grateful for the possibility this project gave them to share it with another person. The fact that we ourselves are not physicians may have made it easier for them to overcome their fear of talking about their disease.

28.4. Statement 2: The Ill Physician Experiences a Conflict in Entering Into the Treatment of Another Physician/Colleague, Namely, What Part He Should Play – The Role of the Competent Physician, or That of the Patient

28.4.1. Change of Roles – a Dilemma

As shown earlier, it is difficult for physicians to admit to themselves that they are ill. When they finally seek help, or are hospitalized, it is difficult for most of them to switch roles from that of the physician to that of the patient. It is not easy to accept this deprivation of status. The fact that they are familiar with the difficulties concerned when a practicing physician receives a colleague as a patient contributes to making the experience still more difficult.

28.4.2. Some Physicians Continue Treating Themselves, Even After They Have Been Hospitalized.

"I was in the intensive care ward for three days," one of the physicians told us. Serious complications had arisen after childbirth, and she was operated on three times: "I was listless, could hardly lift a finger, and much less hold the baby when he was placed beside me. My blood count was 50, but all the time I felt that I had to check up on the people looking after me. I had to make sure that the nurses did what they were supposed to do. I was really afraid. I paid attention to their every move. 'What sort of medicine are you giving me?' I asked. They would not tell me, and just shot the medicine into my arm without telling me what it was. I thought that was very bad."

A surgeon was operated on for a polyp. He writes that he was not allowed to leave the hospital two hours after the operation, as is customary for the patients he himself operated on: "I was alert after the operation, and I was thinking of myself as I usually think about any of my patients. When my wife came and was very upset, I tried to comfort her as I usually comfort my patients' family members. . .

None of the staff would let me go home, in spite of the fact that I was the only specialist in this field in the hospital.

In the end I pulled off all the tubes, put my clothes on, and went to the ward's office and told them that I was going home."

Osmond and Siegler (1977) write about this very incident by quoting the old saying: "The one who treats himself has a fool for a patient and an even greater fool for a physician."

28.4.3. Not being Believed Despite the Fact that you are a Physician.

"I started getting frustrated when the assistant physician, who admitted me at the hospital, did not believe my indications about the mobility of my hands and feet. I had to tell him that I knew whether or not my left hand was functioning normally. He thought it was, but I knew that it used to be much stronger. I ended up tiptoeing into the ward's office the next day, and correcting my case record with a blue pen, on all the points I thought were wrong! The staff did not comment."

Another physician we interviewed said: "Sometimes I wondered whether I had to drive off the road or slash my wrist, or something like that, to make people believe that my illness was serious. I also felt that there were very few colleagues I could turn to."

This story resembles stories told by patients with fibromyalgia (Lilleaas 1991).

28.4.4. Not being Allowed to be a Patient

"Subsequently, it has occurred to me that, as a physician, I'm not allowed to be a patient. Even when you are in such a life-threatening situation, you still don't stop being attentive to what is happening around you. On the other hand, you also wish to be a little more passive than you are allowed to be, when it comes to treatment. To me that was a strange experience.

However, the nurses in the intensive care ward put their foot down and actually threw my colleagues out of my room, and told them to discuss the case outside."

Several authors have written about this problem. Alex Cohen (1984) writes that a physician treating another physician tends to perceive his patient as still occupying the physician's role.

28.4.5. Not being Allowed to Participate

A few of the physicians we questioned complained that they were completely ignored and left out of the discussion concerning their treatment, as if they themselves had no medical education whatsoever. Some perceived this as very difficult.

"The discussions went on behind my back. I was not allowed to participate in the discussion about my own condition at all. That was indeed difficult. At that time, I was working at the hospital, in the same department and in the very same ward, where I had now become a patient."

28.4.6. Psychiatric Symptoms or Diagnosis are the Worst of All

As a physician, becoming a patient due to some form of physical illness is bad enough. Receiving a psychiatric diagnosis, however, is undoubtably experienced as a much greater threat to the physicians we interviewed. They were afraid they would be stigmatized: "No, I have not tried to hide this from anybody. After all this was a clear somatic illness."

Another one said: "It is not difficult to talk about one's own somatic illness, but it is, however, in my experience, much more difficult talking about a mental illness. A physical illness does not stigmatize one in the same way, so there was no reason to keep it secret."

Another physician expressed it in this way: "I am very concerned about the fact that they did not offer any psychiatric treatment. I have clear changes on the electrocardiogram (ECG) so there was no suspicion of a mental illness. However, I read in my own case record that: 'She works rather hard because she often becomes depressed when she has nothing to do.'

I had a daughter who died some years ago, and my work has been a good medication. However, when I saw that my case record said that I was depressed, I thought: 'Aha, they might think that I am depressive.'

When I was alone with my case record, I therefore added: 'In connection with her daughter's death' to it. This was so they would not dare to classify me as a psychiatric patient. For such is the way of the world, you see."

In international literature, it is a well-known fact that physicians are especially afraid of receiving a psychiatric diagnosis. Thomas N. Wise (1991) writes: "Physicians fear being labelled with a psychiatric diagnosis. The fear of the reactions from colleagues, as well as a sense of personal failure, can hinder the physician from seeking psychiatric care. Physicians who have a need to be in control of their environment may rationalize their depression as their own fault, and therefore avoid proper treatment. The fear of stigmatization being cited as one reason why family practitioners do not refer their patients to psychiatrists, it is not suprising that they are reluctant in seeking treatment for their own problems" (p. 458).

A few of the physicians in our material, however, relaxed completely in the role of the patient: "I thought it was a relief to be taken care of, to receive thoughtful consideration, get the right medicine, go on sick-leave, and just be able to lie in bed. It really was a relief."

28.4.7. Convalescence

We shall now briefly consider the matter of convalescence. "After I was discharged from the hospital, I became my own physician. This was for the best considering the sickness I had, at least as far as the treatment of it was concerned. Only the patient himself can say: 'I can take so much, but no more.' No one has a better knowledge of how much a patient can endure than the patient himself."

Others were disappointed with the lack of help they received after the diagnosis was given: "It was a drawback being a physician, since you are expected to actively take part in the treatment of yourself. I not only had to estimate my need for blood tests myself, I also had to requisition them, as well as analyze them. I did not receive appointments for check-ups, and had to ask for a five minute consultation in the corridor, between the X-rays and the morning meeting. I myself had to remember the time and place of the examination etc. The estimation of the effects my medicine was having on me, was also assigned to me.

Had I been an ordinary patient, I would have been hospitalized. Since I was a physician, that was obviously not considered necessary."

28.4.8. There are no Discussions about the Illnesses of Fellow Physicians.

Some of the physicians I interviewed also mentioned the fact that, when they finally went back to work after being away on sick-leave, neither their illness nor their absence was even mentioned: "I experienced the strangest thing when I came back to work after six weeks of sick-leave due to depression. Judging from my colleagues' reaction, my illness did not even exist. It was completely ignored. I do not know whether this was for my sake, or for theirs.

Family and friends handled it better, by showing interest and concern. They were easy to talk to.

I think that maybe physicians are so afraid of becoming ill themselves that they refuse to see a physician in such circumstances."

Another one says: "When I went back to work after my daughter's death, only one physician commiserated with me, a woman of course, who patted me on the shoulder. Apart from that not a word was said about it. There was no offering of condolences or anything.

Seeing how helpless physicians are in such a situation, it makes me wonder how they, of all people, can help the world around them at all?"

Robert Hahn (1995) gives several examples of this phenomenon. He has read books physicians have written about their own experiences with illness. He writes: "Several of these physicians are troubled and surprised by the reactions they get from both friends and strangers among their colleagues. When they are severely afflicted, many of their colleagues turn away. The afflicted physicians sometimes refer to this phenomenon as 'shunning.' They also discover that their colleagues often are not nearly as helpful as they might have been. They offer several explanations for the range of the collegial responses they have experienced, as well as descriptions of some quite striking exceptions" (p.244).

28.5. Statement 3: The Physician/Colleague Experiences a Conflict Between Playing the Part of the Physician and Playing the Part of the Colleague

Of course, it is not only the physician/patient who experiences a conflict in the role he should play. This is also true for the physician's physician. We have shown a variety of problems concerning the physician/patients in their relationship with their physician/colleagues. It is, however, just as difficult for the physician's physician to decide to what extent he should play the part of the physician, and to what extent he should remain the colleague.

His point of view may vary, depending on the seriousness of the disease, the physician/patient's specialty, and so on, and even if both parties are sure about the role they wish to take in this cooperation, it is not sure that their views are concurrent. In some cases, it may develop into what we can call a real conflict. At least that is how it may seem to the patient who may be touchy, as is often the case when one is ill. He can feel underestimated and powerless. This is a common feeling for ordinary patients as well (Christie 1991).

It is repeatedly being stated that openness between the physician and the patient is important and that the solutions required will vary for each particular case.

Sometimes the meeting between the two physicians can, happily enough, be completely successful and harmonious: "I want to praise the physician who treated me. He made it clear to me, maybe even more explicitly than the psychiatrist did, that 'when you are ill, you are my patient, it is I who make the decisions about the therapy, and there is not going to be any discussion about that.'

Later he even told me that the biggest

mistake physicians make is to put themselves on the same footing as their patient/colleague and start discussing. My physician took the lead."

28.6. Statement 4: These Dilemmas Can Tell Us Something of General Interest About the Role of the Patient, the Role of the Physician, as well as the Patient/Physician Relationship in General, in Our Society

The authority the physician had in the old days was based mostly on the big difference there was in the amount of knowledge physicians had compared with people in general. The growing medical specialization, not least in the field of high technology, has, to a certain extent, contributed toward maintaining this authority. At the same time, the higher educational level, health information in general, and not least the data revolution have brought some changes.

Many patients today, more often than before, are in the same situation as the physician/patients. They read about their illness in medical journals and periodicals, and find out which medicines or treatment are appropriate. It is also more common to be able to use databases for information. There are patient organizations as well, where the patients can obtain information.

The informed patients will, in the same way as many physician/patients, want to discuss the different treatment alternatives with their physician. They will feel the need for a dialogue with the physician where their knowledge and experience of their illness can be considered and where they are treated as a partner in a process in which important decisions for the patients' future are being made. (Christie 1991).

Many practicing physicians think they do not have the time to engage in this kind of dialogue, or find it an unnecessary interference. They may also feel that it indicates a lack of confidence in their competence.

As an example of how physician/patients, as well as other patients, search the available literature for information on their illnesses, we can quote one of our interviewees who had been operated for cancer: "They told me at the hospital: 'You have been lucky, you have a form of cancer where the chances of survival are very good'. . . One has something of a scientific attitude and likes to see for oneself. It is an advantage to be able to look into the literature. I went to the United States, afterwards, and I remember spending a lot of time in the library there, looking up literature for a better picture of what I in fact had been through, what sort of possibilities I had."

28.7. Conclusion

Even though physicians, when they become ill, may have easier access to health services through their knowledge and networks, they are at the same time in a more difficult position than people in general. They know more about the weaknesses of the health system and the insecurities of medicine and find it difficult to relax in the ordinary patient role. As patients, they feel a loss of status and are reluctant to admit to themselves and the people around them that they are ill.

They experience a difficult role conflict with regard to how they should use their medical knowledge in relation to their physician/colleagues. In extreme cases, this may lead to their getting no help at all and ending up being their own physician.

Neither does the physician/colleague have an easy job. He is in a position which puts his empathy and flexibility to an unusual test. We have seen that this is a problem that is present in many more situations than the one in which the patient is a physician.

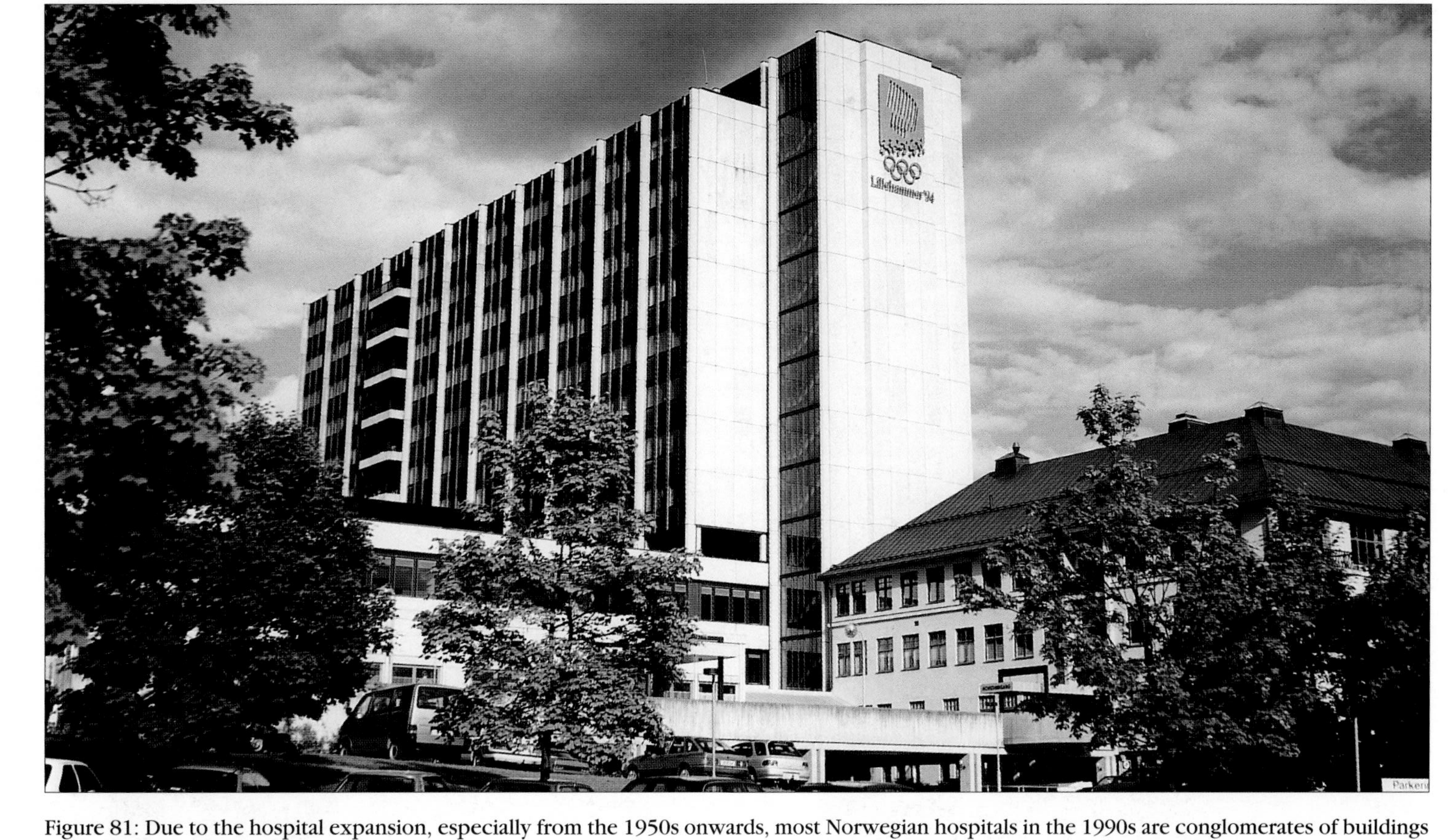

Figure 81: Due to the hospital expansion, especially from the 1950s onwards, most Norwegian hospitals in the 1990s are conglomerates of buildings from different periods. This example is from Lillehammer. The hospitals as a rule offered apartments for the staff, often situated on the hospital site. This, combined with the frequent relocations and change of workplace during a hospital career, made the hospital even more a closed and separated community for many physicians (Photo: Øivind Larsen 1996).

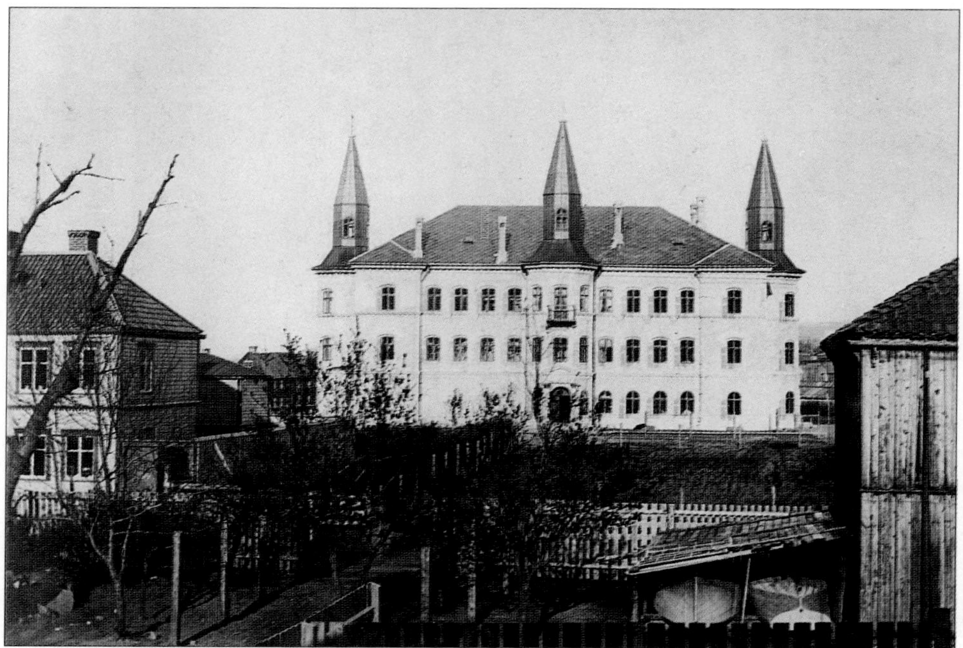

Figure 82: St. Elisabeth Hospital, Trondheim in the 1870s (Photo: P.O.Næss. Courtesy University Library, Trondheim).

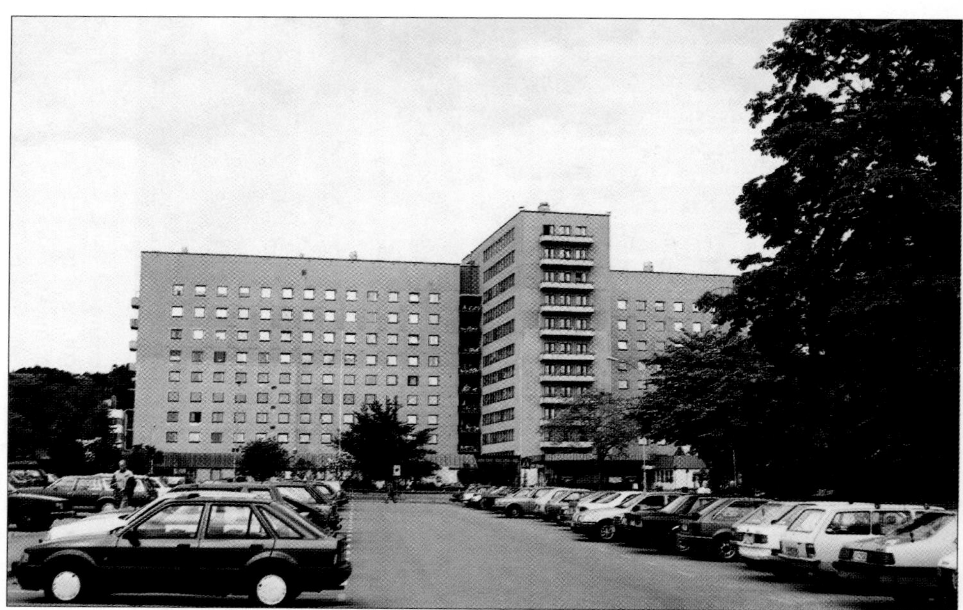

Figure 83: The Regional Hospital in Trondheim is also the University Hospital of the city (Photo: Øivind Larsen 1996).

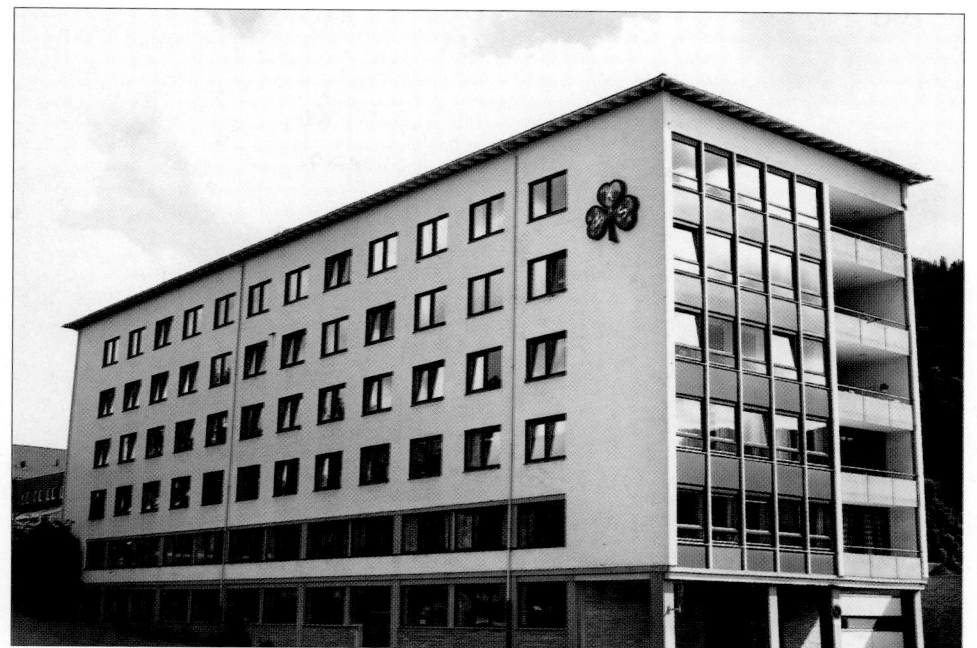

Figure 84: The hospital at Orkdal southwest of Trondheim (Photo: Øivind Larsen 1996).

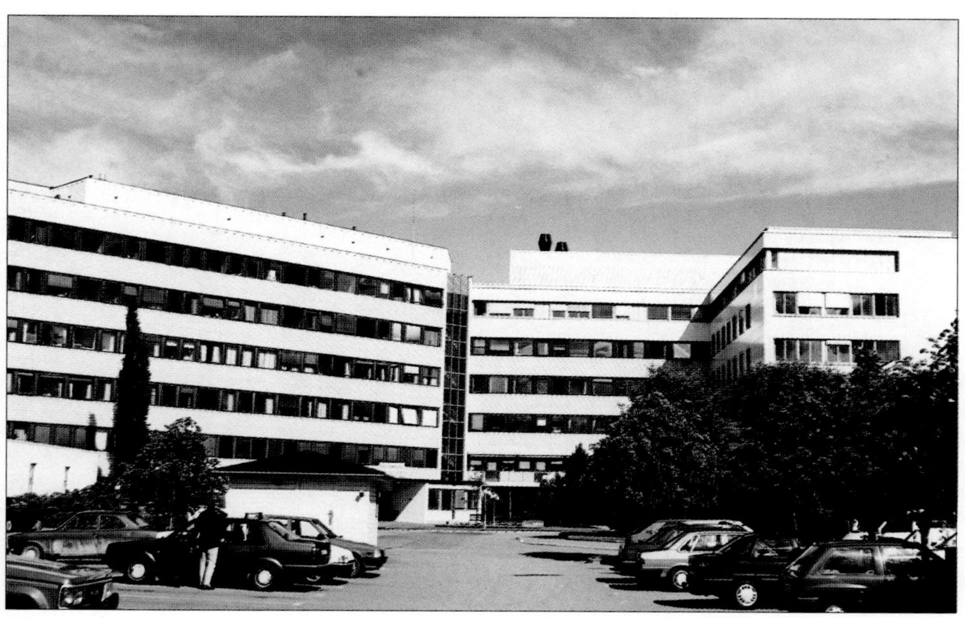

Figure 85: A modern hospital in the city of Levanger, north of Trondheim (Photo: Øivind Larsen 1996).

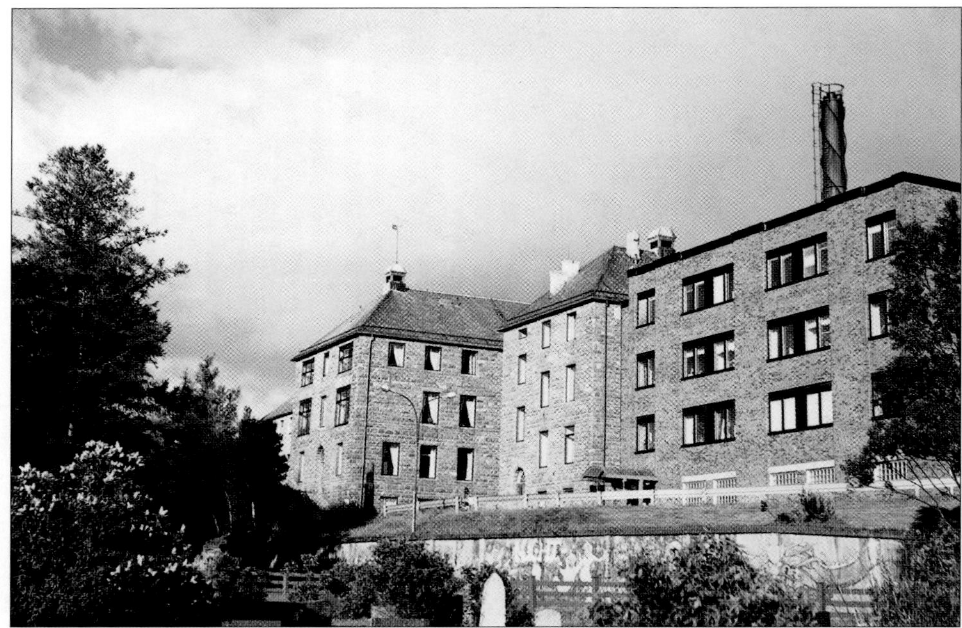

Figure 86: The hospital in Sandnessjøen, Northern Norway: various part of the building are from different periods (Photo: Øivind Larsen 1996).

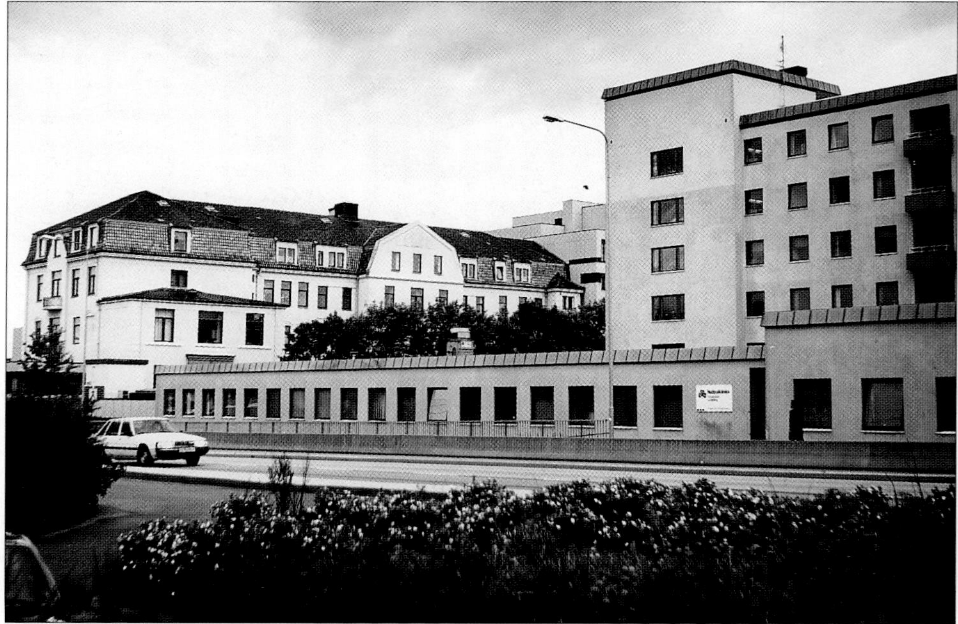

Figure 87: The hospital complex in Haugesund, Western Norway, reflects building activity that has occurred through the decades (Photo: Øivind Larsen 1996).

The old manuscript for the role of the patient as well as the role of the physician will, perhaps, have to be rewritten?

References

AMA Council of Mental Health. "The ill physician. Impairment by psychiatric disorders, including alcoholism and drug dependence." *JAMA* 223, 6(1973): 684–687.

Christie, V. M. *Den andre medisinen.* (The other medicine) Oslo: The University press, 1991.

Christie, V.M. "Hesitant about being seen as ill – The case of the doctor," lecture given at the British Sociological Association's medical sociology group conference at York University, September 1995.

Cohen, A. "Care of the care-givers". *Medical Journal of Australia*, 1(1984): 520–523.

Fugelli, P., and K. Malterud. *Den utbrente legen. Medicinsk Årbog.* (The burned-out physician) København: Munksgaard, 1989.

Fyrand, O. *Legen – i teknikkens eller menneskets tjeneste?* (The physician – in the duty of the technic or the humanity?) Oslo: Gyldendal, 1992.

Hahn, R.A. *Sickness and healing. An anthropological Perspective.* Chapter 9. "Between two worlds: Physicians as Patient." London: Yale University Press, 1995.

Jerome, J.K. *Three men in a boat.* New York: Viking Penguin, 1978.

Langsley, D. *Foreword. In The impaired physician.* eds. Scheiber and Doyle. New York and London: Plenum Medical Book Comp., 1983.

Lilleaas, U.-B. *Før var jeg et arbeidsjern. Kvinner med muskelsmerter i et kjønnsrolleperspektiv.* (I used to be a workaholic. Women with muscularpains in a gender perspective) Oslo: Institute for Preventive Medicine, University of Oslo, 1991.

Marzuk, P.M. "Sounding board. When the patient is a physician." *The New England Journal of Medicine*, 317, 22(1987): 1409–1411.

Murray, R.M. "The health of doctors. A review." *Journal of the Royal College of Physicians*, 12,5(1978): 403–415.

Osmond, H., and M. Siegler. "Doctors as patients." *The Practitioner*, 218(June 1977): 834–839.

Richards, C. "The health of doctors. King Edvard's Hospital Fund for London." *KF project paper nr.* 78, 31(October 1989).

Rutle, O., et al. "Den oppbrukte legen." (The warnout physician) *Tidsskrift for Den norske lægeforening*, 108, 23 (1988): 1819–1824.

Sargent, D.A., et al. "Preventing physician suicide. The role of family, colleagues, and organized medicine." *JAMA*, 237, 2(1977): 143–145.

Scheiber, S.C., and B.B. Doyle. "Conclusions and Recommendations," in *The impaired physician*, eds. Scheiber and Doyle (New York and London: Plenum Medical Book Comp., 1983), pp. 169–172.

Stevensen, J. "Observations on illness from the inside," in *When doctors are patients*, eds. M. Pinner and B.F. Miller, New York: Norton and Comp., 1952, pp. 223–235.

Wise, T.N. "Depression and fatigue in the primary care physician." *Primary Care*, 18, 2(1991): 451–464.

CHAPTER 29

Modern Doctors and Modern Technology

FRODE LÆRUM

29.1. General Problems and Attitudes

Society's most modern and prestigious technology of the past was often associated with religion, as expressed in advanced church architecture, or in military arms and weapons. During the twentieth century, health has gradually found such a central place in society that medical technology now may be said to have acquired a similar standing and prestige, perhaps replacing the previous standing of the Church. The jogging craze of the 1980s, the flourishing of new health-food shops and health studios, the doctors' columns in the popular press and the focusing on health and the environment in daily newspapers can be interpreted as a steadily increasing fixation on the body and health which has occurred during the second half of the twentieth century. Medicine and health-related studies have become the most popular among young people applying for further education.

Medical equipment and health technology have also acquired a similar interest and prestige. Medical equipment has been characterized by high price and steadily more complicated technology. For example, the price of diagnostic ultra-sound equipment has tripled over the last ten to fifteen years, even though data technology has become cheaper in relation to performance. Such machines have increased in complexity, and the number of control buttons or menu options on the control panel have increased. Equipment of this type has reflected high professional competence among health personnel and has satisfied the need of patients to feel that they are subject to examinations that are performed by the most advanced methods.

The interest and prestige of doctors and industry have often coincided, since equipment has often been both highly advanced and very expensive, but this has sometimes been at the cost of distribution and availability. Up until the last decade, there were few objections that advances in health technology were justified, if they could in any way be shown to have any effect. There was what might be called an autonomy of medical machinery (Berg 1987). This attitude has now changed to a more critical view, one that is more steered by economic arguments, is changed due to shifts in decision-making within the medical services, and to changes in socio-political attitudes.

Machines are tools that make diagnosis

and treatment of patients by health personnel more effective and systematic. However, patients also need attention from doctors, and they need to feel that there is interaction and trust at the human level. The greatest danger lies within the technological disciplines. Patients can feel as though the health professional hides behind the machines, that they are deserted in magnetic or computer tomography, with neither enough information about the method, nor about the results. In the doctors surgery, it can often seem as though the PC wins the battle for the attention of the health professional. Many patients feel that the dialogue between the doctor and the machine or the screen is given precedence, while they and their health problems play second fiddle. Such alienation is probably often the result of the health professionals' uncertainty and lack of routines in relation to the new tools. But registering data, choosing options and searching for data take up much of the operator's time, and as a rule the amount of time allocated to each consultation is very limited. As health services become more and more characterized by machines and technology, we must be more conscious of the ethical issue that people must take precedence over machines.

However, medical technology is not synonymous with machines, but also includes techniques and procedures based on basic biological and medical knowledge. In Norway, a committee was set up in 1986 under the auspices of the Norwegian Research Council for Science on the development and consequences of medical research and technology. In their report (Norges almenvitenskapelige forskningsråd 1986), they give definitions of low, medium, and high technology, which are more comprehensive than the definitions which we normally associate with these concepts.

Low technology is primarily based on provision of nursing care, often in connection with diseases for which there is no really effective intervention. The level of medium technology is where we find most medical treatment. Diseases which are included at this level are characterized by limited insight into the cause of the disease, and thus limited possibilities for direct curative treatment or real prevention. Examples of medium technology in this context are cardiac surgery, haemodialysis, and advanced treatment of rheumatic conditions. Endoscopic surgery and intervention, radiological treatment, surgery with catheters guided by X-rays and similar procedures are also included in this group. These are procedures with high cost and high tech, advanced machines which demand a high level of knowledge of the procedure, and which are often associated in layman's language with high-tech treatment (Lærum and Stordahl 1991). However, high technology also is characterized by thorough knowledge of the basic causes of the disease, and therefore may give special possibilities for prophylactic or curative measures. Vaccination programs and specific antibiotic treatment are examples of such treatment. Requiring minimum resources to implement them, such medical measures either make the patient healthy or maintain the patient in a healthy state (Norges almenvitenskapelige forskningsråd 1986).

According to the definitions, the greatest medical resources are used in the middle technology group, and it is in this group that controversial procedures and priorities lie. For a long time, it was generally believed that the Norwegian health services were among the best in the world. However, despite a long period of growth in the health services, from the 1970s on there was increasing dissatisfaction over lack of resources, long hospital waiting lists, and a general feeling that people did not get the service which they believed they were entitled to. The reason for this was probably that a smaller proportion of gross national product was used on health services in Norway than in other comparable countries. In addition, changes in policy on health and safety at work, such as shorter working hours and a reduced number of maximum permissible shifts, probably have led to poorer continuity and availability of doctors for individual patient treatment, at least in relation to many patients expectations.

Investment in equipment led to frustration, particularly among health personnel. New and advanced medical technology was often purchased only a few years after it had been developed. But renewal of old, worn-out equipment was continually neglected. As a result of budgeting and investment policy, without provision for depreciation, resources were not continually allocated to updating and renewing technical equipment. When a piece of machinery finally fell apart, it had to be renewed on an ad hoc basis. Long-term planning and resource allocation for renewal of technical equipment still seems not to be generally accepted by hospitals, in contrast to the usual procedure in other high-technology industries in society. Many worn-out machines which are twenty to thirty years old, and which are essential for central hospital services, are still to be found in hospitals, even in radiography departments and other departments which are characterized by high-technological development. Automobiles of a similar age have a vintage status in Norway.

New and particularly advanced equipment has often been acquired through the efforts of enthusiasts, sometimes coming in from an unexpected direction. The first magnetic resonance imaging machine in Norway was installed in the Central Hospital in the county of Rogaland in 1986, as the result of an initiative from the director of a hotel and a subsequent fund-raising campaign and co-operation with the oil industry. Use of this technology in Norway began three to five years later than in many other countries, and came in a period of accumulated interest within the health services. In the course of a short time, many magnetic resonance imaging machines were acquired in Norway, until Norway had a top position internationally, in terms of the number of such machines related to the population. A research center of international proportions was established in Trondheim. This high level of investment in a national professional environment which had not yet been built up led to strong negative reactions from other sectors of the health service. In 1987, the governmental committee for priorities within the health service used magnetic resonance imaging as an example of high-technology medicine which had no priority and no documented beneficial effect. Expansion of this technology in Norway was therefore immediately stopped, despite a rapidly increasing scientific documentation of the method from centers in other countries. It took five years before Norway came into line again with the other countries, in terms of the development and spread of technology in this field (Lærum 1993). A roller-coaster trip within the spread of technology on a national basis had finally become stabilized.

The national system functioned better in other ways. The first extra-corporeal kidney stone crusher was installed as early as 1985, under the initiative of professor Sten Sander. This machine was installed at Ullevål Hospital, and made it possible to treat many kidney stone patients without surgery. The method proved to be very useful, both clinically and practically, and the different health regions in Norway generally seem to have managed to co-operate well in order to utilize and expand the capacity of this patient-friendly method, with a perspective of national economy.

Sometimes Norway has chosen to be on the outside. Positron emission tomography is an expensive advanced technology for studying metabolic processes in the body. It was developed at the beginning of the 1970s by, among others, pioneers in medical centers in Sweden. Now, at the beginning of the 1990s, there are eight such machines in Scandinavia, but none in Norway. However, this technology seems to have limited clinical application, but has great research interest (Innstilling om PET 1994). Still, the conditions for international co-operation should be present, so that Norwegian researchers should also be able to participate.

29.2. Norwegian Achievements before World War II

At the end of the nineteenth century, Norwegian doctors had close contact with leading medical centers, primarily in Germany and Austria. Radiographic investigations were introduced as early as 1897, just shortly after the discovery of X-rays. The first scientific reports in this field were by Severin A. Heyerdahl (1870–1940) in 1899. Heyerdahl founded the radiography department of the National Hospital, and was one of the people involved in fund-raising and the erection of the Norwegian Radium Hospital in 1932. This hospital became an important center for the treatment of cancer and cancer research, and Heyerdahl was the hospital's first director (Larsen 1989).

Lister's antiseptic principles were introduced in the National Hospital in Oslo in 1870, three years after Joseph Lister's publication of his method. Surgical treatment of gallstones was introduced in the 1880s by Hagbart Strøm (1854–1912). His presentation of the method in 1895 led to heated discussions with the doctors of internal medicine, who believed that this condition "belonged" to their area. "Battles" of this kind have taken place in Norway, just as in other countries. Thoracic surgery was limited to incisions and empyemic drainage until Edvard Bull (1845–1925), a doctor of internal medicine, carried out the first operations for lung abscess about 1880. Certain medical instruments have been known by their Norwegian name in the medical world. The eye specialist Professor Hjalmar August Schiøtz (1850–1927), together with Doctor Javal of the University of the Sorbonne in Paris, developed an ophthalmometer for measuring distortion of the cornea, which was in use for a long time. In 1905, Schiøtz demonstrated his ingeniously simple tonometer for measuring intra-ocular pressure in glaucoma.

The obstetrician Jørgen Løvset (1896–1981) constructed a new birth forceps, which was widely used in Europe. Arne Thorkildsen (1899–1968) achieved international attention by introducing ventriculcisternostomy for stenosis of the aqueduct of Sylvius in the 1940s (Thorkildsen's shunt).

29.3. Achievements and Trends after 1945

The greatest developments in Norwegian medicine have taken place since 1945 (Kristiansen and Larsen 1991). There are many factors which have contributed to this. Antibiotics and immuno-suppressants have been introduced. A greater understanding has been obtained of local and general reactions to trauma and medical intervention. Great steps forward in anaesthesia and intensive care have led to improved patient survival. Better medication and a range of new diagnostic and therapeutic tools became available. Some examples which can be mentioned are digital subtraction angiography, computer tomography, magnetic tomography, various ultrasound techniques, and flexible and rigid endoscopes with video techniques. New materials for implantation, laser techniques and other technical developments have led to an explosion in knowledge, which can be mastered only through continuously increasing specialization and interdisciplinary communication and co-operation.

As an illustration of how Norwegian doctors adopted new techniques, we can mention heart surgery, an area of high prestige which is given much public attention. Suturing of the heart following a knife wound was attempted in 1896 and 1900, but both patients died. In the 1940s, surgical ligature of patent ductus Botalli was introduced, and in the 1950s, transatrial closed commisurotomy for mitral stenosis was carried out. Leif Efskind (1904–1987) performed the first open-heart surgery to close an atrial septal defect in 1957. Extracorporeal circulation became possible from 1959 on, and in 1969 Karl-Victor Hall (1917–) carried out the first coronary bypass operation. Hall, together with the American R. Kaster (1928–) and the physicist Arne Wøien (1931–) also developed the "Hall-Kaster" heart valve, which was widely used over large parts of the world.

Transplantation surgery has held a high position in Norway. The first kidney transplant was carried out by Leif Efskind in 1956, and the graft functioned for 4 weeks. In 1963, the first kidney transplant from a living relative was carried out at Ullevål Hospital. In the wake of introduction of Cyclosporin A in 1983, during the recent years, there have been 45 transplants per million inhabitants in Norway. The one-year survival rate for transplants has been 90 percent with kidneys from living donors, and 80 percent with kidneys from cadavers. An important factor in Norway's early progress in this area, in relation to other Scandinavian countries, was probably the foresighted Act on Transplantation of 1973, which regulated the criteria for donors and organ availability, with complete cerebral infarction as the criterion for death.

Liver transplantation has been a well-established procedure since 1984, after two unsuccessful attempts on children with atresia of the gall duct in the beginning of the 1970s. Transplantations of lung, heart, and pancreas have been carried out to a varying extent from the middle of the 1980s. The National Hospital in Oslo is Norway's transplantation hospital. At this hospital, there is a prominent immunology environment at the hospital's tissue typing laboratory, headed by Erik Thorsby (1938–).

The first heart transplantation in Scandinavia was carried out at the National Hospital in 1983, by a team led by Tor Frøysaker (1929–1994). An important condition for open heart surgery was haemodilution, which was developed by the anaesthetist Per Lilleåsen (1933–). He published a paper on this in 1979.

The physicist Odd Dahl (born 1889), developed and built the first high-voltage unit for treatment of cancer at Haukeland Hospital in Bergen in the 1950s. The unit was early for units of its kind, both nationally and internationally.

Norway has also made an impact in the field of apparatus development in cardiac diagnostic ultrasound and Doppler technique, led by the technological group in Trondheim, with the company Vingmed as an industrial partner. Norway also gained a leading position in this area of ultrasound development in the 1980s. A liquid current cytometer was invented at the beginning of the 1970s. This apparatus, developed with the company Kontron, could determine the number and size of particles (cells and bacteria) in suspension, and it became widely used. In this way, Norwegian researchers attained a high international position within analytic cytology during the first half of the 1970s.

Aasmund Lærdal was running a toy factory in Stavanger. In the 1960s he began to produce life-size dolls, which could be used for practicing life-saving mouth to mouth resuscitation, and he produced teaching equipment with advanced electronic technology. This product was also a success as an export article.

Fredrik Kiil (1921–) developed an artificial kidney and led a very active research group at Ullevål Hospital in Oslo from the 1960s on. Professor Paul A. Owren (1905–1990) at the National Hospital was leader of an active haematology research group, and he invented the widely-used coagulation tests "normotest" and "trombotest." Lorentz Eldjarn (1920–) developed a range of sera for use in clinical biochemistry.

In 1978, the radiologists Professor Ivar Enge (1922–) and Staal Hatlinghus (1945–) were the first in Scandinavia to carry out balloon dilatation of arteries, at Aker Hospital in Oslo. In 1994,Staal Hatlinghus (1945–) and Hans Olav Myhre (1939–) introduced the first percutaneous stent graft in Norway for treatment of abdominal aortic aneurism.

29.4. Present State and Future Out-look

In the 1990s there is an increasing interest in so-called minimal invasive treatment methods as alternatives to open surgery. An interdisciplinary organized interventional center has been established at the National Hospital, where advanced, open magnetic tomography is concentrated on, in addition to state-of-the-art radiography and endoscopy.

Certain particularly important specific niches of medical/technological research and development have become prominent in Norway during recent years. Norwegian deep-sea diving is one of these areas, supported by extensive activities in the Norwegian oil industry in the North Sea.

Extensive medical/technological research and development take place in the technical university environment in Trondheim and Oslo. Norwegian pharmaceutical technology holds a strong position, with the intravascular contrast medium of Nycomed Imagings, which at the moment dominates much of the world market in its field. Monodispersion particles (Ugelstad spheres, named after John Ugelstad, born 1921) are gaining an increasing area of application, particularly within treatment of cancer. The particles are covered by a Norwegian patent, and the researchers at the Norwegian Radium Hospital in Oslo have a central position in the clinical development of the method.

Norway, with just over four million inhabitants, might be said to have had an international position within technology, which reflects the size of the country and the resources which have been utilized for medical research.

References

Berg, O. *Medisinens logikk: studier i medisinens sosiologi og politikk*. Oslo: Universitetsforlaget, 1987.

Innstilling om PET. Oslo: Rikshospitalet, 1994.

Kristiansen, K., and Ø. Larsen. "Surgical science, general surgery and superspecialization. The development of surgery in Norway in the 20th century," *Acta Chirurgia. European Journal of Surgery* Suppl 565 (1991).

Larsen, Ø. *Mangfoldig medisin*. Oslo: Det medisinske fakultet, Universitetet i Oslo, 1989.

Lærum, F., and A. Stordahl. *Intervensjonsklinikk*. Oslo, Aker sykehus, 1991.

Lærum, F. Magnetic resonance imaging in Norway. Government policies. *Invest Radiol* 28(1993) Suppl 3, 46–47.

Norges almenvitenskapelige forskningsråd. *Medisinens forskning og teknologi. Utvikling og konsekvenser (Del 1)*. Rådet for medisinsk forskning. Oslo: 1986.

C H A P T E R 3 0

The Tradition of the Physician's Professional Ethics – from Hippocrates to the Ethical Rules for Physicians of the Norwegian Medical Association

NAIDI ENGELSKJØN

30.1. The Long Traditions of Physicians' Professional Ethics

Physicians have a tradition of professional ethics which is more than 2,000 years old, a period by far exceeding the history of the Norwegian medical profession. The shaping of a modern profession of physicians in Norway also includes an adoption of the prevailing ethics. The local adoption and interpretation of the traditional code are of interest in order to understand the history of the profession.

The first ethical rules for physicians that we know of in the Western world are expressed in the Hippocratic Oath, a part of the Hippocratic Corpus. It is generally assumed that these writings were authored by several different persons, probably members of a group of physicians living on the island of Kos 500–400 BC. This historical basis of physicians' ethics is remarkable, but it is even more surprising to see that its contents have changed so little throughout history. The Norwegian Medical Association's Ethical Rules for Physicians of 1989 (ER–89) express ideas virtually identical with those expressed in the Hippocratic Oath. However, in 1994 Ethical Rules for Physicians were revised (ER–94) in an attempt to incorporate completely new principles with the old ones.

It was necessary to revise the rules, but the new principles are in many ways in conflict with the traditional Hippocratic ones. The following is an attempt to show that the new rules only with great difficulty will be able to serve as guidelines for practical actions.

Professional ethics directs the members of the profession and should help them to realize the objectives of the medical vocation. Ethics is supposed to promote good practice and protect against the bad one. Of course, professional ethics also has other functions, which probably are less pronounced: it gives the members of the profession a common frame of reference, and may contribute to a strengthening of solidarity and identity within the group. Some people will say that the most important task of ethics is to express ideal objectives. People outside the profession (and a few rebels within) often claim that its most important function is to secure the profession's privileges, and to impress – at worst, to oppress – those who are not members of the profession. All aspects mentioned above are central, but professional ethics that cannot work as a guideline for actions will soon perish.

30.2. Medical Ethics, Physician's Ethics, and Medical Practice

In everyday speech, including conversations between physicians, the terms "medical ethics" and "physician's ethics" are used interchangeably. There is nothing strange about this. Through much of history they have meant the same thing, but that is no longer the case.

"Medical ethics" could be seen as the application of general ethics to ethical questions in the medical sphere. The phrase "general ethics" could be understood as any kind of set of values or system of norms.

"Physician's ethics" is a more specific matter, and pertains to the norms and rules concerning the physician's acts *as physician*, in other words, standards which are specific to that role. The part of the physician is acted out in a certain context, viz. the medical practice. Aristotle pointed out that the traits and norms which are the basis for right actions must be decided on in accordance with the practice they are to be applied to. A good soldier has qualities different from those of a good philosopher. What then characterizes the medical practice, the stage upon which the physician's part is enacted?

Medical practice has health as one of its objectives. However, to understand the concept of "health" without a context is impossible. The meaning of the concept will to a great extent be determined by society, time, and place. The context will shape the criteria concerning what is to be considered healthy. Medical science will then be able to ascertain absence or presence of these criteria.

Nevertheless, despite the relativity of the concept of health per se, the view that medicine's central task is to move a person from sickness to health, from deviation to normality, seems to be a constant element in the self-understanding of medicine, no matter how "sickness" and "health" are defined.

Hence medical practice is normative on several levels. First, the maintenance or the restoration of health, seen as the "normal" state, demands that the standards of normality be determined. Second, medical practice is characterized by explicit and implicit directives concerning what is the correct action, what could be called a professional ethics. Third, people both outside and inside the medical profession will have opinions about medicine based on more general norms, what has here been called "medical ethics" in a wide sense.

As a result of the emergence of social sciences and social medicine in the nineteenth century, the normative aspects of the concepts of health and sickness have been systematically problematized. Academic philosophical reasoning concerning medical ethics came into vogue in the 1950s. Some people, somewhat irreverently, claim that at that point moral philosophers had become redundant, and that the ethical questions raised by new medical science and technology literally saved the life of ethics as a philosophical discipline (Toulmin 1973).

On the other hand, the earliest known ethical rules for physicians were codified more than 2,000 years ago, and these have been the origin of a tradition which has stayed virtually unchanged up to the present. What then are the characteristics of this tradition?

30.3. The Hippocratic Tradition

As mentioned at the beginning, the Hippocratic tradition's origin is the Hippocratic Oath, which probably was written down in the fifth century BC. The oath reads as follows:

> I swear by Apollo Physician and Asclepius and Hygieia and Panaceia and all the Gods and Godesses, making them my witnesses, that I will fulfil according to my ability and judgement this oath and this covenant:
>
> To hold him that has taught me this art equal to my parents and to live my life in

> partnership with him, and if he is in need of money to give him a share of mine, and to regard his offspring as equal to my brothers in male lineage and to teach them this art – if they desire to learn it – without fee and covenant; to give a share of precepts and oral instructions and all the other learning to my son and to the sons of him who has instructed me and to pupils who have signed the covenant and have taken an oath according to the medical law, but to no one else.
>
> I will apply dietetic measures for the benefit of the sick according to my ability and judgement; I will keep them from harm and injustice.
>
> I will neither give a deadly drug to anybody if asked for it, nor will I make a suggestion to this effect. Similarly I will not give to a woman an abortive remedy. In purity and holiness I will guard my life and art.
>
> I will not use the knife, not even on sufferers from stone, but will withdraw in favor of such men as are engaged in this work.
>
> Whatever houses I may visit, I will come for the benefit of the sick, remaining free of all intentional injustice, of all mischief and in particular of sexual relations with both female and male persons, be they free or slave.
>
> What I may see or hear in the course of this treatment or even outside of the treatment to the life of men, which on no account one must spread abroad, I will keep to myself holding such things shameful to be talking about.
>
> If I fulfil this oath and do not violate it, may it be granted to me to enjoy life and art, and being honored with fame among all men for all the time to come; if I transgress it and swear falsely, may the opposite of all this be my lot (Translation in Beauchamp and Childress 1983).

The Hippocratic Corpus was known in ancient Rome; perhaps the Oath's compatibility with Christianity secured its survival as Christianity's power and influence grew in the Middle Ages. A Christian version of the Oath dates back to the 12th or 13th century AD. The Hippocratic Corpus was taught in the first universities. Several translations of parts of the Corpus were made in the 1500s and 1600s.

The interest which the Oath raised in the Renaissance probably had more to do with the general interest in the writings of Antiquity than with a practical need for rules for a physicians' ethics. However, this changed at the end of the eighteenth century: one of the first known attempts at drawing up a modern version of the Oath was a result of professional dissension in a small hospital in Manchester in 1789. A serious epidemic caused a conflict between surgeons, physicians, and apothecaries concerning the distribution of responsibility and duties, and the respected physician Thomas Percival was given the task of formulating an ethical code which could contribute to solving the conflict. The resultant set of rules showed a strong Hippocratic influence. Percival's code in its turn became a source of inspiration to several of the sets of rules that were drawn up at the foundation of medical associations throughout the nineteenth century.

There may be a point in emphasizing the profession shaping and the protective aspects of the professional ethics. At any rate, there is little doubt that these considerations were present when the first modern codifications of physicians' ethics were formulated; the Hippocratic demand of profession loyalty was more important than the relationship with the patient.

The disclosure of the horrid part played by the Nazi doctors in the Second World War necessitated a confirmation of the part of the Hippocratic Oath which ensures that the physician always acts in the best interest of the patient. This is exemplified in international codes like the Geneva Declaration of 1948, and in national codes like the Norwegian Ethical Rules for Physicians.

30.4. The Hippocratic Oath and Ethical Rules for Physicians of 1989

The Hippocratic Oath opens with regulating the relationship between physicians, and then puts forward norms which define the physician's tasks and his relationship with the sick.

Ethical Rules for Physicians (the 1989 edition is from Yearbook of the Norwegian Medical Association 1990-91; the 1994 edition is from the Yearbook of 1995) consist of five parts. The first two show similarities to the Oath. Part I, "General Regulations," treats the physician's tasks and his relationship with his patients. Part II carries the title "Rules for the Relationship between the Physician and his Colleagues and Co-Workers." Parts III, IV, and V deal with advertisements for and information about medical services, rules for issuing certificates and statements, and observance of the ethical rules. These latter three parts will not be discussed here.

What values should characterize the relationship between physicians? In the Hippocratic Oath the physicians swore the following:

> To hold him that has taught me this art equal to my parents and to live my life in partnership with him ... to give a share of precepts and oral instruction and all the other learning to my son and to the sons of him who has instructed me and to pupils who... have taken an oath according to the medical law, but to no one else.

As has been mentioned earlier, the physicians of ancient Greece were members of a religious cult just as much as they were physicians. The oath meant a declaration of absolute loyalty, secrecy, and respect, and special concern for other members of the cult. What has all this got to do with Norwegian physicians of today? According to ER-89 obviously a lot:

> A physician must not voice degrading or criticizing remarks about a colleague's activities to patients, their relations or other members of the laity. Criticism of co-workers and subordinates must not be made in such a way that it will break down respect for the person concerned. It must not take place in the presence of patients and their relatives. Disagreement between physicians ... must be kept at a factual level and not be brought to the public in such a way that it is liable to damage the prestige and the interests of the medical profession. Fees should not be demanded from physicians, their spouses, or those of their children who live at home. (ER-89, part II, clauses 1, 2, 3, and 8)

Except for the vows to Apollo and the other gods, all the central elements of the Hippocratic Oath are retained. The demand of keeping conflicts hidden from the public, unconditional loyalty within the profession, and special concern for colleagues and their families are in 1989 still seen as a central part of the physician's ethics.

A similar correspondence is found in the norms defining the physician's duties and relationship with his patient. According to the Oath, the physician swears:

> I will apply dietetic measures for the benefit of the sick according to my ability and judgement: I will keep them from harm and injustice ... Whatever houses I may visit, I will come for the benefit of the sick.

ER-89 states that:

> The duty of a physician is to secure man's health. He is to practice his work painstakingly and conscientiously, help the sick to regain his health and the healthy to keep it. A physician must not use methods that unnecessarily expose the sick to harm... the well-being of the sick should always be his aim. (Ibid. part I, clauses 1 and 6)

30.5. The Ethical Basis of the Tradition

The basis of the professional ethics expressed above may be formulated in two fundamental ethical principles: the principle of not harming (non-maleficence), and the principle of doing good (beneficence). These two principles form the core of the Hippocratic tradition. They are both based on a consequential ethics. Consequential theories claim that the choice of and the assessment of actions should be made on the basis of an evaluation of the probability and the value pertaining to possible consequences.

The relativity of the concept of health makes it difficult to define the notion of good and bad in the Hippocratic tradition. The fixed and constant part of the tradition is the idea that deeds are done and evaluated according to how well they realize the motion away from sickness, defined within a certain context, towards what is in this context considered to be normal.

Consequential ethical theories are often contrasted to deontological theories. The latter holds that an act is right if it satisfies some principle of obligation or fulfills a duty. Moral standards exist independently of good and bad consequences. These standards can be expressed in norms of obligations and norms of rights. Deontological ethics will maintain that under certain circumstances obligations and duties must have priority over the considerations of consequences, that is, they must be followed no matter how bad their consequences are. Adherents of consequential theories may also accept obligations and rights as essential parts of morality, but their validity depends on the positive consequences in the long run, not on inherent value.

ER-89 deals with the physician's duties and obligation, but these are supposed to make him able to do good and ease pain, and thus have a basis in consequential ethics. With one exception, there is no reference to the patient's rights; they are not even implied, which produces a clear asymmetry. One person's duties usually correspond to another person's rights. It is perhaps too much to ask that the patient's rights should be mentioned explicitly in a physician's code of ethics, but they ought to be implicit. The one exception in ER-89 is clause 13 of part I, where the physician is recommended to give the patient information about his health condition. This right to information naturally follows the patient's right to autonomy.

"Autonomy" is often seen as equal to the patient's right to self-determination; that is, the patient can make decisions about himself, and his wishes concerning treatment, information, and so on, must be respected. The patient's right to autonomy presupposes that he, in both a legal and a real sense, is capable of making a choice, that the choice is made on the basis of correct information, that the patient's choice is thought through and not the result of a sudden impulse, and that he is not exposed to external pressure (Førde 1995).

In ER-89 the patient's autonomy must give way to the physician's right to withhold information he believes will harm the sick. As long as the autonomy is for the patient's benefit or, at least, does not hurt him, he may have information. If the information is harmful, this right can be disregarded – and the physician is the person who decides whether the information is harmful or not. The physician's right to make this decision is based on what may be called the "paternalism" of the Hippocratic tradition.

The term "paternalism" describes an asymmetric relationship between people, where one person has the authority to make decisions for another person. This presupposes that the exercise of authority is done with care and consideration, in the best interest of the person in question, analogous with the authority a father exercises over his child. How may this paternalism be justified in the physician-patient relationship?

If it is agreed upon that the physicians have a duty to act in the best interest of the patient (the premise of consequential ethics), and if it is presupposed that the physician knows what is best for the patient (the paternalistic premise), then it necessarily follows that the physician's decision is the best one, regardless of what the patient may wish. But is it correct to assume that the physician is the one who knows what is best for each individual patient?

It may be the case that the physician, as a result of his medical competence, is able to predict consequences directly related to the disease. He will know about the possibility of survival, subsequent medical conditions, and so on. But he has no special competence that makes him able to decide what *value* these possible consequences have for the patient in question. Robert Veatch writes:

> If total benefits are the relevant consideration, then physicians seem to be in no position to assess them, since they have no particular expertise in economic, spiritual, intellectual or other non-medical dimensions of benefit to the patient. Alternatively, if health benefits are the relevant concern, it is hard to see why decisions should be made on that basis alone, excluding all other dimensions of benefit and harm. (Veatch 1981)

The assumption that the physician always knows what is best for the patient is the aspect of the Hippocratic tradition that has been the most criticized. On a purely factual level, it is not reasonable to assume that the physician is the person who is best suited to decide what is good and valuable for the individual patient.

It is perhaps not surprising that the person who has traditionally been seen as guardian of the medical practice has obtained such an elevated position. As has been shown, medical practice is normative on several levels, but this normativity has not always been acknowledged. The physician has been seen as a practitioner of a neutral technology based on scientific "truths." Because he possesses scientifically based knowledge, it has been assumed that he should make the decisions. This assumption seems unreasonable today, among other things because of the recent focus on the medical practice's complexity. The Norwegian Medical Association has seen this as well. The following is a presentation of the changes of the 1994 revision of Ethical Rules for Physician.

30.6. The Revision of Part II – The Relationship Between Colleagues and Co-workers

Part II of ER-94 opens with the request that physicians are to show colleagues and co-workers respect, help, advise, and guide them (ER-94, Part II, clause 2). Further, a physician is to be careful with criticism of colleagues and co-workers addressed to patients and their relations, but must nevertheless always act in the best interest of the patient (Ibid. Part II, clause 4).

The new edition emphasizes that showing each other respect is something with inherent value. The old rules, on the other hand, continually stress the medical profession's outward prestige: one is not to criticize while members of the laity are present, or in such a way that respect is diminished with patients present. The tendency of ER-89 is that respect for the physician as a physician should be protected, to prevent the detriment of the respect for the profession. The tendency of ER-94 is that colleagues should be shown respect because they are human beings, and thus are entitled to respect. And despite the fact that one is to be cautious when criticizing colleagues, one is always to look after the patient's interests.

This consideration is not mentioned at all in ER-89.

The revision of Part II is a turning away from the physician's position as a member of a cult-like society whose purpose is to keep the "laity" in ignorance of conflicts; it represents a formulation of standards for co-operation built on mutual respect, which can be seen in relation to the patient's interests. This step was necessary, and probably occurred in due time after 2,000 years. However, the revision of Part I, General Regulations, is not equally unproblematic.

30.7. The Revision of Part I – The Physician's Duties and his Relationship with the Patient

Clause 1 of both editions states that the physician's duty is to look after man's health, help the sick to regain it, and the healthy to keep it. The revised edition in addition requests that the physician should "heal, soothe, and comfort," and that "the physician should base his actions on respect for basic human rights, and on truth and justice in his dealings with man and society." The references to human rights, truth, and justice are completely new. Moreover, the commitments to society are emphasized far more than in the old edition.

The new edition also contains important additions in the clauses regulating the physician's relationship with his patient (Ibid. Part I, clause 2). The patient is to be treated with compassion, consideration, and respect. The collaboration is to be based on mutual trust and, if possible, informed consent. In ER-89 reciprocality and consent are not mentioned at all (ER-89, Part I, clause 11).

According to ER-89, physicians should as a rule inform the patient about his health condition, but the physician was given the right, following a scrupulous assessment, to keep back facts which could harm the sick (Ibid. Part II, clause 13). ER-94 emphasizes that the patient should be given information if he so desires, and provides no rights to withhold particularly charged information; on the other hand, it is stressed that this should be conveyed with prudence (ER-94, Part I, clause 3).

30.8. The Ethical Foundation of the Revision

The criticism of the Hippocratic tradition which has been voiced the last twenty to thirty years has mainly claimed that there must be greater emphasis on the patient's rights and on his autonomy. At the same time, there has been a wish to keep the focus on the principles which constitute the core of the Hippocratic tradition, that is, the request to do good and to ease pain.

This has led to a tendency in modern medical ethics that claims that medical ethical evaluations in general, and evaluations concerning physician's ethics in particular, are to be based on central principles drawn from *different* ethical traditions and theories. The rationale seems to be that all the different systems can contribute something valuable. It is neither possible nor necessary to choose between them. The approach has been called "Principlism" (Clouser and Gert 1990), and means that in moral reasoning emphasis is put on "principles." "Principles" can be seen as intermediaries of abstract moral theory and concrete rules of action (Beauchamp and Childress 1983).

This is quite different from the kind of principles that summarize an ethical theory. Examples of such summarizing principles are the principle of utility, which holds that one always should seek the greatest happiness of the greatest number, or Rawls's principle of justice, which claims that in a just society social and economic differences must be arranged so that they benefit the least advantaged. Principles like these are "short versions" of uniform and systematic theories. If you commit yourself to act according to one of them, you commit yourself to reject something else at the same time. If you follow utilitarianism, you must reject Kant's absolute prohibition against treating individuals as a means. If you are a Rawlsian, you must reject complete economic liberalism.

The principles of "principlism," on the other hand, are inclusive, and do not depend on a specific moral foundation. In one situation one principle must be applied, in another situation another one; and sometimes one principle must be weighed against another in one and the same situation.

In one of the most influental works on modern medical ethics, Principles of Biomedical Ethics (Beauchamps and Childress 1983), the following central principles are emphasized:

- The principle of autonomy
- The principle of non-maleficence
- The principle of beneficence
- The principle of justice

During recent years, a great deal of the literature on medical ethics has discussed these four principles. And "principlism" has perhaps acquired an even greater impact outside academic circles. Most reports from public boards and committees, lower level textbooks, seminar reports, and so on, follow the same pattern: there is a general introduction on ethics in which a couple of different competing theories, usually consequential and deontological, are presented. Then there follows an expression of the importance of stressing principles from both. Eventually, recommendations and evaluations are given. These are presented as if they follow from the introductory reflections on ethics.

The popularity of "principlism" can best be seen against the background of the ethical pluralism of our times. It seems like an excellent tool by which to reach agreement within groups consisting of people of different religious, political, and ethnic backgrounds.

ER-94 is a typical example of "principlism" in practice:

The principle of beneficence is expressed in the request that the physician is to promote health and remove disease, to heal, alleviate, and comfort (I.1), and to show compassion and care (I.2).

The principle of justice is expressed in the request that the physician is to base his actions on truth and justice in his dealings with his patient and with society (I.1), and to properly take the economy of society into consideration (I.12).

The principle of autonomy is expressed in the request that the physician is to respect basic human rights (I.1), and to look after the patient's interests and integrity. The treatment is to be based on mutual trust and informed consent (I.2), the patient has a right to receive information (I.3), and the patient's right to self-determination at the end of his life is to be respected (I.5).

The principle of non-maleficence is implied in the prohibition against applying untried methods which may put the patient in unnecessary danger (I.9).

Accordingly, all the central principles of "principlism" are incorporated, sometimes even into the same clause. Most people agree that the values which are expressed are good and important. The good thing about "principlism" is that everyone can agree. But does this necessarily make a good physician's ethics?

30.9. Criticism of "Principlism"

"Principlism" has been criticized not only for its lack of philosophical consistency and its low level of abstraction, but also because it ignores the long empirical tradition in physicians' ethics, a tradition which stresses the importance of individual practical judgement. It is consequently attacked by two different schools of moral philosophy, the rationalistic one (Clouser and Gert 1990), and the empiristic one (Toulmin 1981).

The main objection of the rationalist school is that "principlism" lacks a theoretical foundation. The problem is not that the principles are drawn from different traditions, but that they are not organized in a systematic and coherent way. If individual principles are disconnected from their theoretical basis, a new foundation and a new connection has to be constructed if the principles are to be valid. This has not been done in the case of "principlism." Principles which originally belonged to different theories are put together, and since the composition is not systematized, conflicts will unvariably arise between them. No help is offered to decide how to act, because there are no rules for setting priorities and choosing between the principles.

The question arises: Are these rationalistic demands reasonable? Does any ethical system offer clear, concise, complete, and specific rules for action? Is this the task of a physicians' ethics?

The introductory remarks stated that a professional ethics should express the duties specific to the physician's role. It is supposed to define the physician's tasks in relation to the medical practice as a whole. It should regulate the relationship with the patients and protect against bad practice. It should draw lines and give direction for actions. But it will hardly ever be able to command individuals to act in specific ways in concrete practical situations. This is not a defect or a flaw in the ethical rules, but a consequence of the necessary universality of rules in general. Rules are supposed to give a general framework and foundation for individual decisions, but the application of general rules to individual actions can never be done automatically. The application demands not only insight into all relevant aspects of the concrete situation, both factual and moral, but also a power of practical judgement, experience, and prudence. The demand for reasonable use of prudence applies to all ethical considerations, not only to those concerning physicians' ethics.

And this is the basis of another kind of criticism of "principlism." Rather than being attacked because it is not based on theory, it is attacked because it is not adequately connected to tradition and the individual's practical power of discernment. Stephen Toulmin writes:

> Moral wisdom is exercised by ... those who understand that in the long run no principle – however absolute – can avoid running up against another equally absolute principle: and by those who have the experience and discrimination needed to balance conflicting considerations in the most humane way. (Toulmin 1981)

Medicine is an example of a type of profession where the members like to consider themselves as individuals with experience, overview, and practical judgement. Individuals who, after a scrupulous assessment, make their decisions based on a long tradition, namely the Hippocratic one. The geneticist Kåre Berg writes on clinical ethics :

> ... an analytical consideration of what treatment will result in the greatest good or the least evil for the patient is a central point in the use of clinical ethics. To take into consideration the individual situation and to prioritize on the basis of this gain central importance ... the consideration of an existing emergency situation must have higher priority than the consideration of ideal demands and stipulated rules. (Berg 1979)

It may be that the principles formulated in the Hippocratic Oath are more like the kind of principles which have here been called "short versions" of a unified moral platform than the principles of "principlism." An acceptance of the Hippocratic principles means a rejection of other principles. They are excluding, not including; and they commit you to a rather specific basis. However, this basis is not formulated in a systematic theory; very little is made explicit. It has rather been handed down and internalized for thousands of years, by socialization, model-learning, and experience, more than by textbooks and lectures. Perhaps this implies that the revised edition of Ethical Rules for Physicians contains two different types of principles, and therefore is not arranged in such an unsystematic way after all. The old Hippocratic principles, the duty to do good and to ease pain, seem to be rooted in quite another manner than the modernist principles of rights and autonomy. The following is an attempt at illustrating this.

30.10. Autonomy or…

In 1995, legal charges against a physician were considered because he had respected his patient's wish not to have a blood transfusion during an operation. The patient, an elderly woman, was a Jehovah's Witness. She satisfied all the requirements which are usually demanded of an autonomous person. She had been informed of all possible consequences of refusing treatment. Her decision was an integrated part of her system of values, not a sudden impulse. This was not an emergency situation, but an elective operation. Consequently, the patient's autonomy had to be respected. An agreement had been reached between physician and patient.

By respecting his patient's wish, the physician maintained her integrity, and what she herself defined as being in her own interest. The requirement for informed consent and mutual trust had been fulfilled. All this is completely in line with clause 2 of ER-94.

This was not good enough for the Department of Justice and the National Medical Board. They stressed clause 6 of ER-94, the duty to give immediate help. This is not only an ethical duty but also a legal one, founded on clause 7 of the medical code, and on clause 387 of the penal code.

The head of the Norwegian Medical Association announced his support of the physician. Under the title "The Patient's Right to Co-Determination" (Eldjarn 1995), he defends the patient's right to refuse treatment. He first states that this right rests on the competence of the patient. If the physician is sure of the patient's competence, then the right to refuse treatment must be respected. He then refers to the fact that giving treatment without regard for the situation is incompatible with "the humanistic tradition of medicine." He sees the present case as analogous to far more common cases, where old and chronically sick patients refuse treatment for acute complications and die as a consequence. The head of the Medical Association believes the physician should not intervene where: "… life-saving treatment is in principle possible, but does not give the patient a life he finds worth living."

The reasoning here takes a turn which this author finds surprising. The age and the current health condition of the patient are of course included in the assessment of whether or not treatment is to be carried out. This is because age and health condition influence the assessments of risks and possibility of complications. In other words, factors like these concern the assessments of consequences probability, not of their value for the patient. Are age and health conditions relevant in this situation? Would the situation have been different if the patient in question had been a formerly healthy thirty-year-old?

It cannot be stated with certainty, but based on the comparison made by the head of the Medical Association, it seems that age and health condition form a morally relevant difference. And the physician in question stated during a TV debate that he himself would not have been able to reach such an agreement with a young and healthy patient.

The question then arises whether the patient's autonomy is really respected at all. Neither an eighty-year-old nor a thirty-year-old Jehova's Witness want to live with another person's blood in their veins. This is because of their religious conviction, which to some of us may seem absurd. We nevertheless respect the wish of the eighty-year-old woman. But is this a result of our respect for her autonomy, which includes her right to make seemingly absurd decisions? Or do we respect her because, in her case, treatment could lead to a painful end of life, while refusal of treatment avoids this, and thus can be accepted from a consequential moral basis? Is it because of this circumstance that we accept her wish, while if she had been thirty years old, we would have trouble accepting it?

It is difficult to decide what would be right or wrong here. The point is that assessments are seemingly based on one principle, while they are in reality based on another one. We may think there is a principle called "patient's autonomy," firmly established and justified. We may think that it guides our actions, but then it is revealed that our decisions are based on principles of good deeds after all.

30.11. Norms without Norms?

The problems relating to blood transfusions make ethical questions come sharply into focus. But a practicing physician will meet similar problems every day, naturally on a smaller scale, with less serious consequences. Ethical considerations are not supposed to be easy. But ethical guidelines ought to offer some help when one tries to make a difficult choice. It is doubtful whether the revised ethical rules for physicians meet this demand.

This chapter has emphasized that a professional ethics should draw boundaries and give guidelines for actions. As was mentioned in the opening remarks, it has many other important functions as well, functions which may have been overlooked here. Perhaps the revised rules for physicians are meant to be ideal requirements, which should always be aspired to, but can never be reached – The Sermon on the Mountain does not become morally irrelevant even though no person here on earth has ever been able to live up to its commands. If this is the intention, it is a beautiful thought, but the person searching for perfection will probably benefit more from reading Plato or the Bible than from reading ER-94. If there is to be a point in formulating ethical rules for physicians, it is that they ought to carry a certain relevance to the physician's everyday work.

Actually, the rules do not appear to be meant to be unreachable aims. For example, in the current debate on euthanasia, the clause that prohibits active euthanasia is presented as an absolute and concrete duty, not as an aim to reach for.

The problem is whether the attempted synthesis between Hippocratic principles and principles with a totally different basis can give a set of good and applicable ethical rules for physicians, or if the attempted synthesis just covers up underlying conflicts. The latter is most likely the case. This author finds that the 1994 edition of ethical rules for physicians is a mixture of norms with variable status: some are founded in the Hippocratic tradition, some are drawn from the modern rights school; some have the character of absolute duties, while others seems more like ideal aims. The relations between the different principles are not problematized. The lack of philosophical consistency may be a problem only to philosophers, but the potential for a conflict between the rules when put to practical use is a problem for practicing physicians.

What has been exemplified here is one type of conflict, that is, between the physician's duty to do what in his opinion is good, and the duty to respect the patient's autonomy; but numerous other conflicts spring to mind: conflicts between justice and mercy; conflicts between concern for the patient and concern for society; conflicts between compassion and the duty to save lives.

No rules for physicians can eliminate these types of conflicts. But they ought to offer some help to solve them. As long as this help is not offered, physicians will most likely always return to Hippocrates whenever they think the patient does not take his best interests into account.

And normally this will work out well. Hippocrates is important to keep in mind. Nevertheless, the strong criticism of the tradition launched during the last decades is not completely baseless. The medical profession has to take the demand for an incorporation of other types of principles seriously. Physicians' professional ethics needs a revision. But if the medical profession is to meet the challenges of a changing society and a changing medical practice, it has to understand that a moral principle is not something you can tear from its theoretical basis and just decide to use as a supplement to an already existing traditional code, just because it sounds nice and politically correct. In that case principles will never be anything but empty ideas.

References

Beauchamp, T.L., and J.F. Childress. *Principles of Biomedical Ethics*. Oxford: University Press, 1983.

Berg, K. "Prenatal diagnostikk: Praktiske og etiske aspekter," *Kirke og Kultur*, 8(1979): 476–478.

Clouser, K.D., and G. Bernard. "A Critique of Principlism," *The Journal of Medicine and Philosophy*, 2(1990): 219–236.

Eldjarn, K. "Pasienters rett til medbestemmelse," *Tidsskrift for Den norske lægeforening*, 29(1995): 3663.

Førde, R. "Pasientautonomi," *Tidsskrift for Den norske lægeforening*, 20(1995): 2568–2570.

The Norwegian Medical Association, *Yearbook 1990-91*.

The Norwegian Medical Association, *Yearbook 1995*.

Toulmin, S. "The Tyranny of Principles," *Hastings Center Report* (December 1981): 31–39.

Toulmin, S. "How Medicine Saved the Life of Ethics," *Perspectives in Biology and Medicine*, 25(1973): 735–750.

Veatch, R. *A Theory of Medical Ethics*. Basic Books Inc. Publishers, 1981.

CHAPTER 31

Modern Times – The Socio-cultural Shaping of Doctors and Patients

PER FUGELLI

31.1 Of Children

Last Saturday afternoon, I stood, as on all Saturday afternoons, and combined two pleasures: I ironed the next week's white shirts and listened to children's hour on the radio. A woman reporter interviewed four-, five- and six- year-olds about being frightened, about scary things. One boy had been terrified for a month now. Each evening, when he lay under the duvet and his mother had said goodnight, a monster which had hidden under the bed crawled out, and the boy said: "And then the monster gobbled me up (a short, dramatic pause); without chewing!"

This little boy had obviously been well brought up, indoctrinated every day: You must chew your food. It was bad enough being gobbled up by a monster, but worst of all, judging by the intensity of his voice, was to be eaten by a monster who did not chew his food.

31.2 Declaration of Intent

What can medical society learn from children's hour? That diseases do not exist, only the experience of disease. That health and disease consist of amino acids and self-image, cell membranes and human ideals, body and politics. That health and disease spring up on earth, grow by means of politics, social climate and culture.

Medicine is inclined to believe that it is alone in the world. The medical profession is inclined to believe that it has created itself. We are inclined to forget that traditions, political forces, and the flow of culture influence patients' health behavior and experience of disease, as well as the role of physicians and the way they practice. In the west, including Norway, it is the custom to have an absolute and biomedically determined concept of health and disease (Helman 1991, Lock and Gordon 1988, Malterud 1990, Meland and Fugelli 1991). But health, disease, and patient-physician relationship are relative phenomena, which take form from the social climate and color of health culture – from the medically valid thoughts, feelings, values, and manners which prevail at the time (Kleinmann 1980, Helman 1990, Patcher 1994).

Elements of contemporary health and challenges for physicians are culturally determined, in Norway as elsewhere (Fugelli 1994, Evang 1991, Guldvog 1993).

In this chapter I will:

- present ten case stories in order to arouse curiosity about the connection between modernity and medicine
- identify ten characteristics of modernity which mold physicians and patients in Norway today
- outline the values which can be conveyed to public health and the medical profession through improved medico-cultural competence.

31.3 Case Stories

Case 1

Two weeks ago, I was at the health center in Uranienborg (a district of Oslo). On the bulletin board in the waiting room was a notice inviting pregnant women, actually the little person-to-be in the womb, to attend Foetus School, arranged in association with the Norwegian Association for Upbringing before Birth. At Foetus School, according to psychological-educational models developed in Japan and in the United States, systematic stimulation of the senses and the brain of the foetus in the womb is undertaken, so that the new-born baby shall have a head start as soon as he or she is pressed out into competitive society.

Case 2

During the fishing season in Lofoten in 1995, I was at Røst, and was walking along the road to the cottage hospital, when a voice from behind me said:

"Tell me now, is that you, Fugelli, I see before my eyes?"

Along came Arne Røstgård, 77 years old, cycling against the wind on his way home to Laurine and dinner, after a tough day on the sea.

"I wish I was as fit as you!" I said, and triggered off this story: Two weeks ago, he came home from the sea, sat at the kitchen table and browsed through the local newspaper, while Laurine finished making dinner. Suddenly, the newspaper fell on the floor, his head hit the table and Laurine shouted:

"Oh no, Arne! Have you been drinking?"

Arne answered: "Don't fuss, woman, I have been on the sea you know."

Laurine: "You are lop-sided, we must ring for the doctor."

Arne: "Don't fuss, woman. We will eat dinner now, then I will lay down and have a little rest. If I am still lop-sided afterwards, then you can ring for the doctor."

He then ate, climbed up and fell down the attic stairs three times, slept for three hours – and was just as lop-sided as before. The physician came, Arne was examined in hospital and was told about hardening of the arteries and aspirin. Now he was back on the sea, with just one difference. He had installed a safety line, because if he should have another stroke out on the sea, then not only an empty fishingboat would be washed up on land. Laurine should have a body to bury.

Arne has never been off sick because God, his parents and local culture have given him good health, good nerves, good ability and good working morale. He belongs to the generation of fishermen who say that: "During the fishing season in Lofoten, you are either out in the fishing grounds or in the coffin, but never sick in bed."

Case 3

At a conference in the United States last year, I met Professor Limestone, Chief Director of Climate Medicine Programme Inc. Professor Limestone and his team are building a medical industrial imperium based on the King of Risk Factors: that is to say, THE WEATHER. The weather has everything a mega risk factor ought to have: it threatens everyone on earth, all the time. Professor Limestone has developed sophisticated climatic-epidemiological models, which show risk scores for people who are fat and thin, old and young, people with heart disease, lung disease, allergy, and so on, for different meteorological compositions. And while we cavemen in Norway are looking at the thermometer outside the window to see whether we should wear long underpants or not, more and more wealthy Americans now buy Professor Limestone's health-weather planner for $4,800. The health-weather planner consists of an exterior component which contains assorted high-technology sensors which are mounted on the wall of the house to register temperature, humidity, wind, UV rays, pollen, air-pollution, and so forth. This information is fed into a computer which is programmed with your personal health data. Every morning you can print out your health-weather plan, which tells you whether you can allow the sun to shine on your skull or whether you should wear a hat today, whether it is safe to play tennis this afternoon or not, and other similar information.

Case 4

A while ago, I was contacted by an old friend who is the director of an insurance company. He had pains in his chest. There was nothing to indicate that he had heart disease, but he was frightened, so I referred him to a cardiologist. He came back to me, disappointed and just as frightened, because all the heart specialist had done was to take a working ECG, and he and all the other leaders in the firm took that test routinely, twice a year, as part of the health package which they bought from Medical Personal Investment Company. He had expected a thorough examination.

Case 5

Dear Per Fugelli,

My mother is 72 years old and is a widow. She lives in a block of flats which has been modernized, and the rent suddenly went up by NOK 1,700 per month. My mother cannot manage this expense on her pension. Much against her will, she went to the social security office, but she did not get any help there, because she told them that she had NOK 23,000 in the bank. Mother explained that this is money which she has saved for 10 years, and is not to be touched, because she will pay for her own funeral. The social security office will not budge. No social security benefits as long as you have money in the bank. Mother is now threatened with eviction. She who used to be so happy and proud now feels crushed.

With compliments, the daughter.

Case 6

In one of the states of America, two children died in 1991 by falling from a chair onto the floor. The two children, eight and ten months old, were placed in highchairs to eat dinner with their mother and father. Suddenly the telephone rang or something boiled over on the stove, the child was alone, climbed out of the chair, fell, hit his head on the floor and died. The events were blown up in the newspapers, radio and television. Panic was sown. Demands for safety measures came from all quarters. The health authorities, the Association of Pediatricians, industry and the media joined forces in a huge campaign. Now, in 1995, all parents who want to be good parents put a helmet on their baby when he or she eats at the table with mother and father.

Case 7

In Stavanger, about a month ago, a young father telephoned the health visitor to ask whether it was alright if he and his wife took a 2-weeks holiday on the Island of Reunion in the Indian Ocean. They wanted to celebrate the birth of their first son, who was now six weeks old and could stay with his grandmother. When the health visitor could not answer one hundred percent yes or no, the young father became angry, accused her of incompetence and said that she was typical of the public health service.

Case 8
On my way home from the National Hospital, I pass the newly opened Skin Care Academy in Rosenkrantz gate. There are queues of young, well-off men who have recently read the distinguished report in Aftenposten (a newspaper) about Norway's first skin therapy/beauty center for men. In the report, Adrienne Holmes recommends two visits per week at NOK 175 for the following reason: "That men should take proper care of themselves is absolutely natural, most men are actually more in need of skin care than women. Daily shaving puts a great strain on the skin – in addition, men are more often in close contact with wind and rain."

Case 9
In Boston one afternoon, I suddenly saw a shiny, gleaming bus, right in the middle of a slum district, with crumbling buildings, stinking rubbish and people living under poor social conditions. "Free Medical Van and Screening for Cholesterol and Blood Pressure" was written on the outside. Inside were physicians and technicians in smart uniforms and electronics that could have belonged to a medium-sized space-ship terminal. Prostitutes and schizophrenics staggered in, drug addicts and homeless people tottered out.

Case 10
In Røst, last summer, a 65-year-old fisherman came to the health center with a painful back and a more and more pressing request to be examined with computer tomography at Nordland Central Hospital. I said no, and explained the medical inappropriateness of such an examination. Then the fisherman put forward his ultimate argument: "Yes, but Fugelli, I've never been in CT."

Now we must either call the overdose team, or else move further on from anecdotal raw material to an attempt at analysis. Hopefully, these examples give food for thought. They are in line with the title of a book by Heinrich Böll: *Something Has Happened.* But what? In order to understand more, we shall search for special features in the development of society which can mold the concept of health, the experience of disease, and therefore the work of physicians.

31.4 Modern Trends

The iron cage of rationality

Rationality and secularization characterize modern society. Leading philosphers highlight purposive-rational action (Zweck Rationalität) as the steering principle, both in capitalist economy and in the modern state (Weber 1971, von Wright 1986, Habermas 1987). Intellectualization and rationalization characterize politics, bureaucracy, production, and the professions. We cultivate science, and reckon that it is always possible to attain goals through internally-controlled and quality-assured professional input. Illich believes that the picture of man at the transition from the twentieth to the twenty-first century is reduced to "homo economicus." (Illich 1995) He polemicizes against the spirit of time which "reduced persons born for suffering and delight to provisionally self-sustaining information loops."

The growth of science can induce megalomanic expectations in people. Advances in science and technology give people the illusion of mastering the universe: life can be calculated, society can be designed, danger can be overcome. Since science is all-powerful, why accept disease, suffering, risk, injury? Science is God's terminator, which brings us to the next symptom of modernity: the fall of religion.

Religion probably promoted health by:

– giving basic security
– giving order and meaning to life

- giving hope in the face of disease and suffering
- providing rituals for life's entrance and exit
- providing moral norms, which act to promote health.

Religion brought peace to a threatened humanity by fostering the concept of destiny. Belief in destiny made disease and accidents tolerable. Doris Day extracted an effective tranquillizer from all the religions of the world when she sang: "Whatever will be, will be." Predetermined, religiously-defined opinions and patterns brought a certain humility into humanity's struggle towards the good life. God and destiny have, to a large extent, withdrawn from modernity. It is possible that this motivates a search for security surrogates, in the form of medical science and technology on the one hand, and new-age resembling sub-cultures, that which Illich calls neo-witchcraft (Illich 1995) , on the other.

Modern medicine can do a lot, but it cannot resusciate God. We should learn from Machiavelli, who writes in The Prince:

Many have held, and still hold the opinion that the things of this world are, in a manner, controlled by fortuna and by God, that men in their wisdom cannot control them, and, on the contrary, that men can have no remedy whatsoever for them; and for this reason they might judge that they need not sweat much over such matters but let them be governed by fate ... I judge it to be true that fortuna is the arbiter of one half of our actions, but that she still leaves the control of the other half, or almost that, to us ..."

Machiavelli understood that the rational human being is science fiction belonging to the year 2000. We will never be successful with medicine as long as we image that the unit we work with is a rational being. Human beings are not robots, whose behavior can be programmed. We often flirt with danger; we throw caution to the wind; we rebel against the healthy life and sing along with Leonard Cohen: "They sentenced me to twenty years of boredom." We are warm-blooded, passionate, bizarre, unpredictable hominids, closer to animals than to health visitors, steered more by basic instincts than by the Board of Health. A wise health service must accept and respect that which Americans call "the counterfactual irrationality of man."

The growth of science and the fall of religion can have an adverse influence on health culture, but can also have positive potential. A population steered by rationality can possibly take more responsibility for its own health and adopt more rational patient roles. Myths, prejudice, fright and other metaphorical elements of disease can perhaps be weakened.

31.5 Colonization of the Life-world (Lebenswelt) by Expert Systems

Habermas points out another trend which is relevant to health: the colonization of the life-world (Lebenswelt) by professional systems (Habermas 1987). Bureaucratic, technological and professional systems become more and more dominating, while at the same time they distance themselves more and more from their original justification, that is to say, people's everyday life.

Medicine is one of modernity's most potent expert systems. Medicine influences people's health culture in a way which is full of contradictions: expansive medicine can remove people's ability to master situations, and lead them into a fixation with being a client. Medicine can induce helplessness in people, by converting more and more biological variation, natural stress and life's own trouble into diagnoses, with demands for specialized investigation and therapy. Earlier, Carling (1975) warned against a development where responsibility is replaced by causality, and where problems are transferred from people to professions. Fløgstad (1991) has given an eloquent description of the expansion of expert systems:

> Behind every child, a commissioner for children. Behind every refugee, an immigration expert. Behind every bus, a bus of crisis psychiatrists. Behind every elderly person, a support service. Behind every boat, a boat of bananas.

Another consequence of highly specialized expertise is reduced capacity to have a comprehensive view. Medical experts have a tradition of uncritically promoting their own risk factor, their own disease, their own technology, their own medication. Altogether, the impression that medicine is omnipotent can be created. Disease simply means that insufficient medical-technical resources have been invested in your cure.

By believing in a limitless concept of health, medicine becomes susceptible to a concept of disease that lacks content. By accepting the World Health Organization's definition of health, that health is not just the absence of disease, but a state of complete physical, mental and social well-being, medicine creates an enormous need for itself. Medicine cultivates a worry culture, where smaller and smaller trivialities and more and more distant dangers trigger off the need for clarification and prevention (Fugelli 1994). Medical self-support and social mutual support seem to disappear. Tolerance of bodily variation, subjective inconvenience, and threats to functioning probably becomes less. Fear of disease and desire for tests and guarantees probably becomes greater.

On the other hand, what modern medicine can offer is to make people understand that diseases which one previously just had to accept can now be prevented, and that suffering which one previously just had to tolerate can now be alleviated. Medicine which is too invasive can damage health culture, by making people obsessed with health, frightened of disease, and dependent on experts. Medicine which is too defensive can end up by leaving too much to "natural spheres," and can be responsible for unnecessary illness and suffering.

Medicine can also influence peoples' health culture through the way in which it manages the metaphor of health. Through its reductionist science and biomedical practice, medicine can distort the relationships between politics and disease, economy and disease, culture and disease, the environment and disease. Modern medicine makes people experience disease as a kind of "alien phenomenon," as a rocket from outer space which only medical super-men in a medical "Star Wars" program can fight against.

Medical measures can turn out to have a moral, economic or political motivation or effect. Turner (1984) and Bull (1990) point out that moral control over individuals and groups of people is gradually being transferred from religion to medicine. Rules for living and forms of co-existence are now justified according to health. Conduct which is conducive to health is seen as a duty, both to oneself, to one's employer, and to society: "medicine has replaced religion as the dominant moral ideology of advanced capitalist society" (Bull 1990).

Conscious or unconscious misuse of medicine for moral or political purposes will also mold people's perception of health, their experience of disease, and their trust in and use of health services.

The trend for medicine to be dominated by experts and characterized by social engineering is now being counteracted by clear opposition. The growth of alternative medicine can, to some degree, be seen as a protest by the people against medicine which is authoritarian and orientated towards medication and technology. But also, within classical medicine, there is a trend towards critical self-investigation. Within family medicine, new models of communication are being worked with, both scientifically and practically, with the aim of transferring power, language, and reality from the physician to the patient (McWhinney 1989, Malterud 1990). Within public health, new methods of health promotion are being tested, with the emphasis on the local population itself directing and participating in the process (Hancock 1993, Fugelli 1995).

31.6 Bureaucracy

The health/social/national insurance sectors have greatly expanded during the last few decades. This growth has been accompanied by a logical increase in medical bureaucracy. Bureaucratization can influence health culture through several mechanisms.

The health sector is Norway's largest work-place, with more than 200,000 employees. It is also the country's "most expensive" area of public production, with over NOK 50 billion allocated to it from the national budget in 1995. Concepts and methods from the manufacturing sector are being used to an ever-increasing extent, in order to measure effectiveness, quality, and cost/benefit in the health sector. An editorial in the British Medical Journal (Morrison and Smith 1994) highlights "the power of big, ugly buyers," whether they are public health authorities or private insurance companies, as one of the most important elements of change for medical practice in the twenty-first Century. Patients are redefined as units of production. Diagnoses and treatment are given a price. The interest of investing in treatment procedures is calculated in quality-adjusted life years. The economic/administrative process of making patients into things can lead to a weakening of the humanistic tradition in the health sector, in favor of purposive-rational action (Zweck rationalität).

The possibility of earning a living from one's own work varies according to health, education, place of residence, and what is offered and demanded by the manufacturing sector. Only rarely is one of these factors the deciding factor. However, health is selected as the criterion for allocating social security benefits. There seems to be increasing demand for the credibility and dignity which a medical diagnosis gives. When disease is made into the formally valid and psychologically worthy entrance ticket to attractive social security benefits, even the concept of disease can be changed. Consciously or unconsciously, patients and well-meaning helpers can translate adverse life situations, psycho-social problems, difficulties associated with work and economy to diagnoses of disease. This can be unfortunate in two ways:- by camouflaging problems, conflicts and oppression, which should be combatted on the political, social or familial arena; – by obscuring the demarcation between the troubles of life and disease, and thus the demarcation between the need for self-help and the need for medical help.

Legal values and methods are gaining more and more entry into the health sector. The number of complaints and cases of compensation have greatly increased. The health services ombudsman system is to be expanded. A separate act on patient rights is imminent. It is difficult to predict whether further formalization of patient rights can come to have an influence on health culture. However, the increase in numbers of matters regarding compensation can lead to a situation where diagnosis and treatment become orientated towards legal safeguards and away from clinical evaluation. An over-cautious attitude can lead to a formal clinical practice with overuse of laboratory tests, special medical examinations, pharmacotherapy, and control consultations – just in case. Such a medico-legal perfectionism can, in turn, influence patients' expectations and demands for that which they experience as a reassuring examination and treatment arrangement.

31.7 Democratization

People are becoming better and better educated. With increased knowledge follows greater ability and willingness to have insight and to participate in decision-making. This also applies to the health field. Modern man is not willing to be treated as a passive object, but will be a well-informed, responsible, and co-operating subject. The population meets the health care sector with greater independence, demands for respect, and ability to judge than before (Morrison and Smith 1994). Both within preventive health work and in clinical practice, medicine must re-orientate itself from an authoritarian to a democratic model of communication (McWhinney 1989, Hancock 1993).

Pluralism, open markets, and freedom of choice characterize the development of society. The right of consumers to choose from a variety of goods and services is highly valued. The editorial in the British Medical Journal, mentioned previously (Morrison and Smith 1994), predicts "the rise of sophisticated consumers" as a driving force behind the development of health services in the years to come. The patients of the future will not tolerate rationing and regulation of such an essential good as medical services. Those who have knowledge, drive, and purchasing power will assert their consumer freedom in the medical field, as elsewhere.

31.8 Free Market Economy

Liberalization of economic policy probably influences health culture. The signs can be seen most clearly internationally (Leufkens 1994, Smith et al. 1990, Davey Smith and Blande 1990), but can also be detected in Norway (Fugelli 1994).

Advertising probably creates an unnatural ideal of body image. Deviation from this can be experienced as disease with the need for correction. Advertising probably also creates unrealistic expectations of what constitutes a normal human condition. The result can be feelings of being different and the search for conditions which are within normal biological, psychological, or social variation

The economic system can lower the threshold for illness by demanding maximum functioning from people. The more performance-orientated industry becomes, the less tolerant it becomes of reduction in ability to perform, even before this becomes stigmatizing or else regarded as illness.

Finally, economic forces can alter health culture by transforming health and safety into "goods." Commercialization of health can particularly be seen in two areas:

– In "the comfort zone," where an attempt is made to redefine lack of well-being and deviation from idealized beauty to disease. The health food branch, health studios, training institutes, solarium studios, the cosmetics industry, and part of the fields of plastic surgery and orthodontics are participants in this market.

– In "the fear zone," where natural risks, variety in life, and healthy dangers become medicalized. Examples are sophisticated medical checks at short intervals, private mammography screening clinics, costly preventive technology and pharmacotherapy, and promotion of do-it-yourself diagnostic tests. The concept of risk is fashionable at the moment, as indicated by the title of a recent article in Social Science and Medicine: The risk epidemic in medical journals (Skolbekken 1995). Focusing on risks is not only commercially-determined. It also has its roots in socio-psychological trends and technological innovations (Hayes 1992, Beck 1992).

We are now seeing a new social gradient:

the medical well-being and security industry directs what it has to offer at the well-to-do, comfort, and security-seeking majority. In the free market, there are few who ask the question: How safe is safe enough? On the contrary, we detect a development where part of the medical/industrial complex develops more and more costly solutions for subtle health needs, which have been created by itself (Nichter 1994). Leufkens and his co-workers (Leufkens et al. 1994) assert that when commercialization becomes extreme enough, then this will trigger off a "red/green" countermovement characterized by social and ecological values.

31.9 Deviation from Solidarity

Policy can also alter health culture, reversing social equality. Galbraith (1992) has introduced the concept of the three-quarter society, where the Content Majority, those who are well-educated, have a good income, good health, and low risk, become increasingly perfectionistic in their search for greater well-being, comfort, security, and health. On the other side live the losers in this "winners' society": the unemployed, the poor, the disabled, ethnic minorities, often in inner-city ghettoes with an accumulation of violence, injury, and disease. The moral philosopher Harald Ofstad says in his book "Our contempt for weakness" (Ofstad 1991): "It is more important to reduce suffering than to increase happiness." One can imagine an opportunistic health and social policy which gives priority to needs of the Content Majority, and neglects the risks and suffering of those who are weak in terms of health, money, and political appeal. Such a policy can give us a health culture divided in two and the pathology of a divided society (Fugelli 1994, Leufkens 1994, Smith et al. 1990, Davey Smith and Egger 1993).

One suspects the growth of a refined health culture among the Content Majority who are willing to invest huge resources in health checks, early diagnosis, preventive medication, beauty medication, and anti-ageing medication. One suspects the growth of a nihilistic health culture among the minority group of losers, who are characterized by laissez-faire attitudes and self-destructive life-styles.

Policy has an influence on health culture not only by influencing the distribution of living conditions, but also by creating a social climate: a winner culture or solidarity, the value of production or the value of human beings, comfort in the present or responsibility for the future. The experience of disease is not only biologically determined, but also determined according to how sick people are accepted by healthy people and how sick people view themselves. A social climate characterized by acceptance, respect, and caring makes it easier to be sick. On the contrary, a social climate characterized by a competitive mentality and individualism makes it harder to be sick. A social morality which places the individual in focus, with personal responsibility for individual life-style, individual success or misery, in the field of health, can add to the burden of patients and groups at risk. A "blaming the victim" tendency, which does not distinguish between responsibility and blame, can worsen the experience of illness and stigmatization.

Policy can also influence health culture through the availability of social services. Some people maintain that the Scandinavian welfare model promotes a regressive health culture, which weakens people's own medical and social strength, and makes them dependent on and demanding of public care.

31.10 The End of Nature

The anthropologist McKibben (1990) argues that the occupation of nature by modernity is so radical that we can now refer to "the end of nature."

Along with the eradication of "the wild," it may be that we will experience that people's ability to meet and to master danger gradually diminishes. Technology and culture work together in the health field, as in other fields. The impressive advances in medical technology may contribute to the expectation that medicine is omnipotent: the risk of disease can be replaced. The expansion and perfection of modern technology can create a collective conception that we have the right to a diagnosis and the right to treatment, in order to free us from danger and suffering. More and more people seem to demand this divine service from medicine. Violation of this right can lead to frustration and aggression directed towards the physician.

New creations within medical technology can also lead to changes in people's perception of what constitutes a natural or an artificial body (Haraway 1991). Experiences of life and of our body can be transferred from the natural sphere, which is characterized by risk, uncertainty, and variation, into the technical sphere, which is characterized by gene technology, predictive tests, lifestyle designing, health check programming, replacement of old or diseased organs, and use of more and more sophisticated technological aids (data-programmed robots, etc). More and more people will consist of both natural and artificial chemicals, natural and artificial skills, natural and artificial expectations of life and the health sector.

31.11 The Rapidity of Change

Freud urged us never to forget that: "Das Mensch ist ein Tier." Man is an animal, an animal of habit. To feel secure, man needs predictable structures. Modernity is characterized by a rapid momentum of change (Giddens 1992, Douglas 1992). Modern times suck us out of our local habitats and expose us to a mobile world system with new challenges, strange threats, and fresh stress every day (Douglas 1992). Rapidity of change outstrips our capacity to adapt and to cope. It makes lessons of yesterday invalid tomorrow. The devaluation of experience creates profound insecurity, and may contribute to the collective demand of an all-mighty medicine.

31.12 The Media

The media have probably had a favorable effect on that part of people's health culture which involves their relationship to the professional medical apparatus. Medicine represents a relatively authoritarian tradition and an autonomous structure. The media have played a part in laying medicine open to scrutiny from society, and to criticism from consumers. The media have probably contributed to reducing inferiority and increasing independence in the way in which people relate to health services.

But the media also have unfavorable effects on health culture:

- the media build up unrealistic expectations, by making medical supermen into heroes and by heralding the approach of new miracle cures.
- the media create medically terrified people, by producing shock reports of the type: "meat-eating bacteria" and "carcinogenic data screens."

The last modern megatrend which eats gigabytes of people's health is:

31.13 The Environment

Global environmental developments contribute to collective anxiety. The ecological risks which have serious consequences are (Giddens 1992, McMichael 1994):

- a global increase in temperature
- thining of the ozone layer

- air, water and soil pollution
- the danger of radiation from 110,000 tonnes of highly radioactive atomic waste
- the division of the world into a more and more impoverished, desperate southern hemisphere, and a more and more protectionistic, over-consuming northern hemisphere.

These risks paint an ongoing, threatening picture for every person, everywhere on earth, every day, without the protection of land, money, knowledge, skills, or power. The media industry world-wide now exposes modern man, particularly through pictures, to a continuous bombardment of terror and catastrophe. It is no longer possible to hide oneself away in a cosy place, blissfully ignorant of all the horror. Living in such a pre-apocalyptical scenario can lead people into a state of chronic existential anxiety.

The influence on health culture can follow two paths, possibly both at the same time:

- the threat to the environment can trigger off "environmental hypochondria," where fear for the environment is transformed into medical forms of expression, with associated demands for medical solutions (Shrader-Frechette 1995).
- the threats to the environment can trigger off clearer consciousness of and greater responsibility for the environment, and thus for the health of the individual.

31.14 The Usefulness of Increasing the Level of Health Culture Competence within Medicine

I have tried to demonstrate how certain trends in socio-cultural development at large seem to be manifested in medicine.

Experiences from trend-setting countries, particularly the United States, indicate that macro-cultural, commercial, and technological forces can distort the development of health culture in the near future. It hardly helps to meet these threats with defensive prohibitions and by extinguishing the flames only in emergency situations. There is probably only one reasonable solution in the long run: to build up the power of patients and physicians to judge medico-cultural issues. In order to promote such a development, a broader cultural perspective must be taken in medical research and in the post- graduate training of physicians.

We must improve our understanding and interpretation of Norwegian health and illness culture. Medical anthropology has traditionally focused on exotic cultures. We have limited scientifically documented knowledge about health and illness culture in our own country. In 1995, the Institute of General Practice and Community Medicine at the University of Oslo proposed to the Norwegian Research Council that a Reseach Program on Norwegian Health and Illness Culture should be established (Fugelli 1995). Better knowledge about Norwegian health and illness culture can be useful, both in clinical practice and in public health.

31.15 Clinical Work

The importance of cultural competence becomes particularly obvious when we encounter patients from foreign cultures (Austveg 1994, Hylland Eriksen and Sørheim Arntsen 1994, Mull 1993, Krau 1990). But Norwegian health culture also has clinical relevance. Hafting (1995) has recently shown that local culture in a rural district in Hardanger influences self-help and seeking the physician. In diagnostic practice, it is important to be familiar with the mechanisms which lie behind the cultural construction of disease (Fabrega 1979, Angel and Thoits 1987). Chronic fatigue syndrome (Abbey and Garfinkel 1991) and hypoglycaemia (Hunt and Browner 1990) are examples of conditions which can partly be understood from a cultural background. Whiplash, fibromyalgia, candida syndrome, amalgam syndrome, and the "allergy epidemic," are examples of health problems in Norway, that can have a cultural element.

In medical anthropology, the concepts of illness and disease are central (Kleinman 1980, Eisenberg 1977). Illness means the subjective experience of disease, including the patient's personal interpretation of causes, fear of consequences, and expectations of treatment, and so on. Disease stands for the medical/scientific concept of the same condition, influenced by the physician's professional knowledge and conception. There is increased awareness that the concept of disease is inadequate. The physician must also integrate illness, the patient's own experience of disease, into examination and treatment. This double approach, most clearly formulated by McWhinney and his co-workers (McWhinney 1989), is called the patient-centered method.

Secure and effective communication is crucial if clinical work is to be of high quality. There are several promising examples of how anthropological approaches and interpretations can enrich clinical communication (Wood 1991, Borkan 1992, Cole-Kelly 1992). Malterud (1990) has shown that good communication must be built on insight into and respect for the patient's socio-cultural premises.

Familiarity with and consideration of the patient's health culture are also important when providing treatment. A relationship between the patient's expectations and myths about the disease, and follow-up of the treatment regime, has been shown, for example, for hypertension, diabetes, and after organ transplantation (Heurtin and Resin 1992, Hawthorne et al. 1993, Washington 1993).

31.16 Health Education

Increased insight into Norwegian health culture can be of benefit to health education in two ways:

- Increased knowledge about people's attitudes, feelings and expectations with regard to injuries, diseases, choice of lifestyle, and so on raises the possibilities for effective health education (Cella et al. 1992, Wang 1992, Lee et al. 1993).
- Greater focus on health and illness culture can contribute to re-orientating health education away from technical information and in the direction of having a more fundamental influence on concepts, attitudes, expectations, and relationships of responsibility and power.

We should go in for health education which provides cultural norms concerned with:

- generous limits to normality
- tolerance of biological and social variation
- respect for nature's command over human life
- motivating people to make a contribution to promoting health and caring for the sick themseles, outside the domain of medical experts
- curing people from having unrealistic expectations
- pointing out the limits of medication.

31.17 Public Health Work

Internationally, a new concept is being launched: the New Public Health (Fugelli 1995). The characteristics of this concept are:

- emphasis on knowledge from anthropology and ecology, not just epidemiology
- emphasis on dissemination of knowledge and responsibility for health and the environment to other sectors: agriculture, traffic, schools, and town planning
- emphasis on mobilizing people themselves to be engaged in health and the environment, both in their workplace and

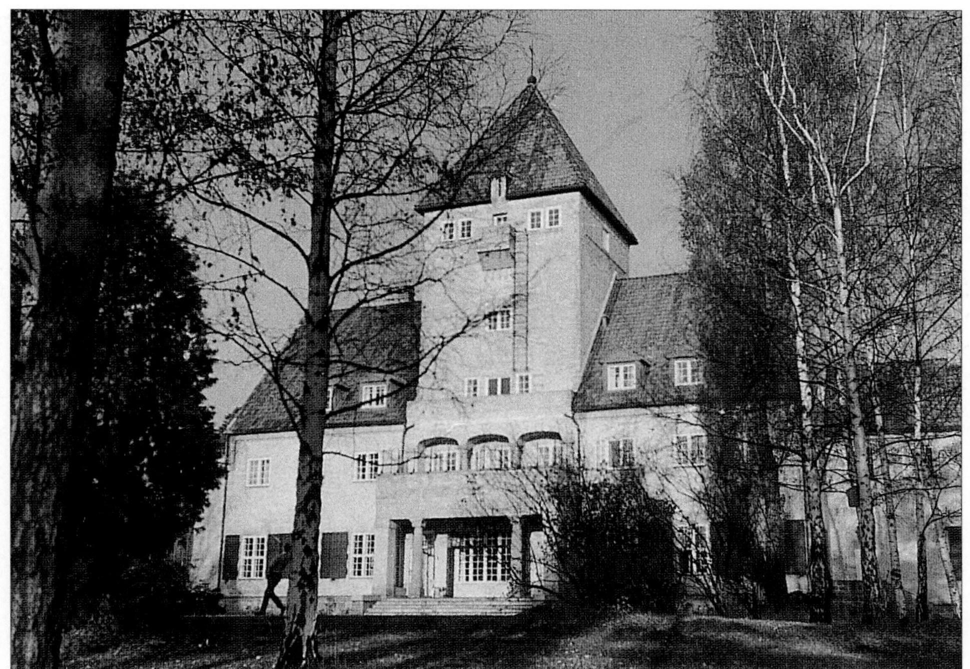

Figure 88: The idea the integrating of education of health personnel, an important issue in a profession history perspective, is not new in Norway. After World War II, a center for training different kinds of health personnel was established in the villa on the peninsula of Bygdøy outside Oslo, where the wartime Nazi "ministerpresident" Vidkun Quisling (1887-1945) had had his residence. The courses for district physicians were given here for many years (Photo: Øivind Larsen 1964).

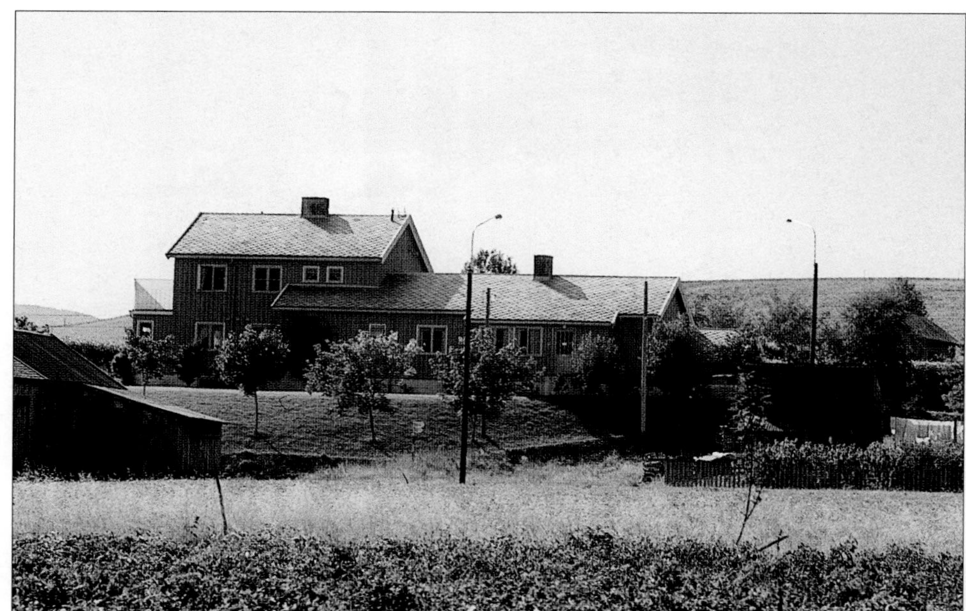

Figure 89: This house contained a district physician's home and offices in the 1960's. To the left, facing the garden, was the roomy two-story apartment for the district physician and his family. The right wing contained a waiting-room for patients, a reception room, and offices for the physician and his assistant, the intern (turnuskandidat). In the middle was a humble and diminutive one-room abode for the intern (Kyrksæterøra, Sør Trøndelag. Photo: Øivind Larsen 1963).

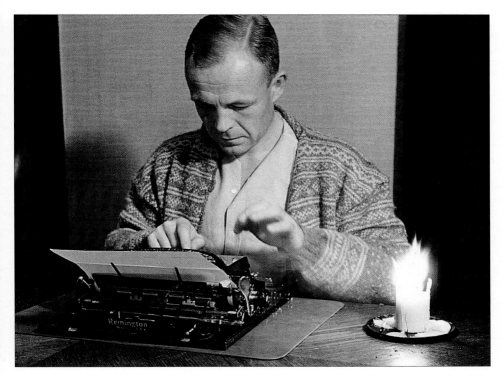

Figure 90: For the busy district physician it has always been a problem that much of the paperwork has to be postponed to the late evenings (Self-portrait, Dr. Knut A. Schrøder [1905-1988], 1930s. Courtesy Aina Schiøtz).

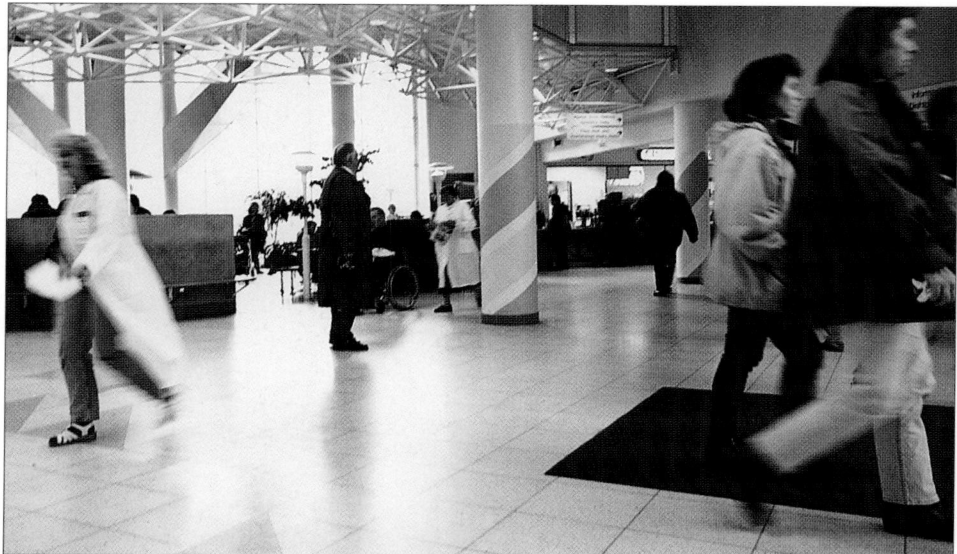

Figure 91: The medicalization of the society has given medicine, physicians, health services, and health institutions new roles: Among these, the hospital lobby often has taken over the part of the church or the marketplace as the site where people meet. And the hospital with its staff is the institution that you trust when you are sick, and criticize when you are healthy again. In Norway is there also a certain chance that the hospital or the health services is your employer. (Entrance area, Regional Hospital, Tromsø, Northern Norway. Photo: Øivind Larsen 1996).

in the area in which they live
- emphasis on pointing out and doing something about damage to health which can be attributed to political and economic power structures.

Acquiring more knowledge about how the socio-cultural environment influences patients and physicians can strengthen the New Public Health into two ways.
- by showing how health and culture, to a large extent, are formed by forces outside medicine. In this way, motivation can be increased, for transferring responsibility for health and transferring health work to people themselves, to local communities, to work places, to voluntary organizations, to other public bodies, political levels and political parties.
- by creating a new body of knowledge which can provide a firmer foundation for a knowledge-based public health practice.

31.18 Giving Nuances to the Biomedical Model

Medical science and practice are strongly characterized by the scientific way of thinking, by biological ways of explaining things, and by chemical/technical ways of finding solutions. By focusing more on the cultural shaping of patients and physicians, a humanistic stimulus can be provided to the monotonous biomedical culture.

Physicians, as a part of their professional task, should take a look at the socio-cultural framework surrounding the picture of illness which patients present. Physicians can mold health culture by omission: by giving political, commercial, and technological forces a free hand. Or else they can play an offensive role, and actively contribute to molding people's health and illness culture, and thus the content of their own profession, according to norms of medical quality.

References

Abbey, S.E., and P.E. Garfinkel. "Neurasthenia and chronic fatigue syndrome: the role of culture in the making of a diagnosis," *American Journal of Psychiatry*, 148(1991): 1638–46.

Angel, R., and P. Thoits. "The impact of culture on the cognitive structure of illness," *Culture, Medicine and Psychiatry*, 11(1987): 465–94.

Austveg, B. *Helsearbeid og innvandrere. Mangfold, sunnhet og sykdom.* Oslo: TANO, 1994.

Beck, U. *Risk society. Towards a new modernity.* London: Sage Publications, 1992.

Borkan, J.M., W.L. Miller, and S. Reis. "Medicine as storytelling," *Family Practice*, 9(1992): 127-9.

Bull, M. "Secularization and medicalization," *British Journal of Sociology*, 41(1990): 245–61.

Carling, F. *Skapt i vårt bilde.* Oslo: Gyldendal Norsk forlag, 1975.

Cella. D.F., D.S. Tulsky, B. Sarafian, C.R. Thomas Jr, and C.R. Thomas Sr. "Culturally relevant smoking prevention for minority youth," *Journal of School Health*, 62(1992): 377–80.

Cole-Kelly, K. "Illness and patient care in the family practice setting," *Family Medicine*, 24(1992): 45–8.

Douglas, M. *Risk and blame.* London: Routledge, 1992.

Eisenberg, L. "Disease and illness: distinction between professional and popular ideas of sickness," *Culture, Medicine and Psychiatry*, 1(1977): 9–23.

Evang, A. *Verdier som kompass. Om personlighet, samfunn og fremtid.* Oslo: J.W. Cappelen forlag, 1991.

Fabrega, H. "The ethnography of illness," *Social Science and Medicine*, 13A(1979), 565–76.

Fløgstad, K. *Kniven på strupen.* Oslo: Gyldendal Norsk Forlag, 1991.

Fugelli, P. "Med Rudolf Ludwig Karl Virchow som veiviser inn i den nye samfunnsmedisinen," *Tidsskrift for Den norske lægeforening*, 115(1995): 1091–4.

Fugelli, P., B. Ingstad, and Ø. Larsen. *Den norske helse- og sykdomskulturen. Argumenter for og skisse til et forskningsprogram.* Oslo: Instituttgruppe for samfunnsmedisinske fag, Universitetet i Oslo, 1995.

Fugelli, P. *Pasienten Norge*. Oslo: J.W. Cappelen forlag, 1994.

Galbraith, J.K. *Den tilfredse majoritet*. Oslo: Gyldendal Norsk forlag, 1992.

Giddens, A. *The consequences of modernity*. Cambridge: Polity Press, 1992.

Guldvog, B. "Bunner helsetjenestens krise i ressurs- eller teorimangel?" *Tidsskrift for Den norske lægeforening*, 113 (1993): 624–9.

Habermas, J. *The philosophical discourse of modernity*. Cambridge: Polity Press, 1987.

Hafting, M. *Et eple om dagen – eldre småforbrukere av helsetjenester*. Oslo: TANO, 1995.

Hannock, T. "Healthy development and the community ecosystem: three ecological models," *Health Promotion International*, 8(1993): 41–6.

Haraway, D.J. *Simians, cyborgs, and women. The reinvention of nature*. London: Free Association Books, 1991: 149-81.

Hawthorne, K., M. Mello, and S. Tomlinson. "Cultural and religious influences in diabetes care in Great Britain," *Diabetic Medicine*, 10(1993): 8–12.

Hayes, M.V. "On the epistemology of risk: language, logic and social science," *Social Science and Medicine*, 35(1992): 401–7.

Helman, C.G. "Limits of biomedical explanation," *Lancet* 337(1991): 1080–3.

Helman, C.G. *Culture, health and illness*. London: Wright, 1990.

Heurtin-Roberts, S., and E. Reisin. "The relation of culturally influenced lay models of hypertension to compliance with treatment," *American Journal of Hypertension*, 5(1992): 787–92.

Hunt, L.M., and C.H. Browner. "Hypoglycemia: Portrait of an illness construct in everyday use," *Medical Anthropology Quarterly*, 4(1990): 191–210.

Hylland Eriksen, T., and T. Sørheim Arntsen. *Kulturforskjeller i praksis. Perspektiver på det flerkulturelle Norge*. Oslo: Ad Notam Gyldendal, 1994.

Illich, I. "Pathogenesis, immunity and the quality of public health," *Qual Health Res* 5(1995): 7–14.

Kleinman, A. *Patients and healers in the context of culture*. Berkeley: University of California Press, 1980.

Krau, A.M. "Healers and strangers. Immigrant attitudes towards the physician in America – A relationship in historical perspective," *JAMA*, 263(1990): 1807–11.

Lee, K.L., E. Schwarz, and K.Y.K. Mak. "Improving oral health through understanding the meaning of health and disease in a Chinese culture," *Int Dent Journ*, 43(1993): 2–8.

Leufkens, H., F. Haaijer-Ruskamp, A. Bakker, and G. Dukes. "Scenario analysis of the future of medicine," *British Medical Journal*, 309(1994): 1137–40.

Lock, M., and D. Gordon, eds. *Biomedicine examined*. Dordrecht: Kluwer, 1988.

Malterud, K. "Medisinens hjelpeløshet I. Allmektige ambisjoner," *Nordisk Medicin*, 105(1990): 27–9.

Malterud, K. *Allmennpraktikerens møte med kvinnelige pasienter*. Oslo: TANO, 1990.

McKibben, B. *The end of nature*. London: Viking, 1990.

McMichael, A.J. *Planetary overload. Global environmental change and the health of the human species*. Cambridge: Cambridge University Press, 1994.

McWhinney, I.R. *A textbook of family medicine*. Oxford: Oxford University Press, 1989.

Meland, E., and P. Fugelli. "Perestrojka – i medisinen også," *Tidsskrift for Den norske lægeforening*, 11(1991): 354–6.

Morrison, I., and R. Smith. "The future of medicine," *British Medical Journal*, 309(1994): 1099–100.

Mull, D.J. "Cross-cultural communication in the physician's office," *West Journal of Medicine*, 159(1993): 609–13.

Nichter, M., and N. Vukovic. "Agenda for an anthropology of pharmaceutical practice," *Social Science and Medicine*, 39(1994): 1509–25.

Ofstad, H. *Vår forakt for svakhet*. Oslo: Pax Forlag, 1991.

Pachter, L.M. "Culture and clinical care. Folk illness beliefs and behaviors and their implications for health care delivery," *JAMA* 271(1994): 690–4.

Schrader-Frechette, K.S. "Comparative risk assessment and the naturalistic fallacy," *Tree*, 10(1995): 50.

Skolbekken, J.A. "The risk epidemic in medical journals," *Social Science and Medicine*, 40(1995): 291–305.

Smith, G.D., M. Bartley, and D. Blande. "The Black report on socioeconomical inequalities in health 10 years on," *British Medical Journal*, 301(1990): 373–3.

Smith, G.D., and M. Egger. "Socioeconomic differentials in wealth and health," *British Medical Journal*, 307(1993): 1085–6.

Turner, B.S. *The body and society*. Oxford: Basil Blackwell, 1984.

Wang, C. "Culture, meaning and disability: injury prevention campaigns and the production of stigma," *Social Science and Medicine*, 35(1992): 1093–1102.

Washington, A.W. "Moving toward cultural competence in the transplant milieu," *Transplantation Proceedings*, 25(1993): 2499–501.

Weber, M. *Makt og byråkrati*. Oslo: Gyldendal Norsk Forlag, 1971.

Wood, M.L. "Naming the illness: the power of words," *Family Medicine*, 23(1991): 534–8.

Wright, G.H. von. *Vetenskapen och förnuftet*. Stockholm: Bonnier, 1986.

CHAPTER 32

The Dynamics of a Profession: Some Concluding Comments on Being a Norwegian Physician

ØIVIND LARSEN

32.1. An Issue for Discussion

To try to pull the lines together, and to see if contours of some general conclusions come into view from the many historical and present-day details which have been covered in the preceding chapters, seems to be such an ambitious task that it probably would be better to abstain from it. Moreover, it is recognized that the reader's interpretation will always be a personal one. However, the dynamics inherent in the development and life of a profession are an issue that arouses interest. If more ideas for personal consideration are required, especially pertaining to Norwegian conditions, newer literature which could be recommended is at hand (Torgersen 1994, Kringlen 1996).

32.2. The Medical Profession – Some Markers

We have been discussing the profession of the physicians, mainly looking at what has happened during the last two hundred years, and we have taken into account some of the theories which have been launched about the phenomenon of professional development; these, however, were hampered by having a substantial part of their base in just the same history as we have been describing and want to discuss.

And we have undertaken some comparisons to vocational groups with similar professional traits: dentists, theologians, law candidates, and veterinarians. But what about the apothecaries? Medical history and the history of pharmacy are traditionally close to one another (Sverre 1982). The pharmacists constitute a professional, health-related group with a long history in Norway. The first royal privilege to run a pharmacy was issued to the Bergen merchant Nicolaus de Freundt on December 13, 1595. The year of 1595 is thus regarded as the birth year for apothecaries in Norway (Johannessen and Skeie 1995). However, for reasons based in profession theory, it might be argued that this part of the history of Norwegian professional groups is not quite comparable. To be a pharmacist, running a dispensary, seems to have more to do with business than with medicine. In the other professions mentioned, the weight of some overruling commitment seems more important and justifies their being grouped together.

A greater share of the public image of profession members, and the public expectations of them, relates to such overruling abstract elements: for the doctors and dentists such matters as health and well-being; for the clergy, belief and morality; for the lawyers, the notion of justice; for the veterinarians, animal welfare and public hygiene. A commitment of this type is a general professional marker which admittedly has a varying visibility, but which ties some of the vocational groups together and gives medicine, dentistry, theology, law, and veterinary medicine a special character. It is possible that the perception by the public of this sort of higher-ranking values has a provoking effect. It may add to that criticism of the health services, and of the physicians as part of them, which almost daily appears in Norwegian media in the 1990s, and which in most cases is experienced as unjust by the professionals concerned.

However, there is another marker too. If you look at the contents of the physician's work, the skills she or he has been trained to use, and the role the physician has been socialized into, there is an important element of making swift decisions, often of substantial importance for the other parties involved, normally the patients. Such decisions often have to be made when the basis for them and the information available are preliminary and incomplete, but when the situation requires immediate action. Decisions cannot wait, and sometimes even a suboptimal decision is better than none. This is part of daily life for many physicians. The first position as a licensed physician, especially in a local hospital, or in a rural general practice can be frightening. The physician has to cope with such things as car accident victims, acute and instable heart attack patients, violent psychotic individuals, and threatening epidemics. During the years in medical school, by means of practical in-service training, and in spare-time jobs as a student, the new candidate has been trained to handle such situations. The setup of the health care system provides a professional backing for most young physicians when they are working as an intern in a hospital or in the practice of a district physician for example, but the burden of personal responsibility is heavy anyhow. And even if work takes place as part of a team, most medical decisions are laid on the physician. If the young medic was not a grown-up person before, she or he definitely will be after having endured the stress and passed through the first year as a licensed physician.

However, this gradually developing decision-prone attitude perhaps does something to the personality. The problem-oriented attitude, and the internalized way of thinking about a diagnosis before embarking on a treatment plan are parts of medical working methods. The capacity to sort the important from the less important, to look through exaggerations, to find out what the realities are in confusing and messy situations, is gradually trained and becomes a personal trait of the doctor. And this trait is a definite professional marker.

When some physicians are accused of being arrogant, and experience resentment because of this, of course it simply might be true to them, because they really do display arrogant and disgusting behavior, as measured by any standard. In such cases, most people will say that they deserve the resentment, and feel that their behavior does not call for any theoretical interest. But what is more important is that professional decisiveness in medical matters may be misinterpreted and experienced as arrogance.

There obviously is a historical aspect here, which also touches on the term "paternalism". When you are sick or in distress, you often need, and accept as well, someone who will take over responsibility and act as a father toward you, someone who will express a paternalistic attitude toward you. The same applies to a society with public health problems: threatening or ravaging epidemics are suitable examples. From the early years of a modern, national medicine in Norway in the nineteenth century and onwards, paternalism seems to have been an important tool for the medical profession, both in its work with patients and in public health matters.

But nineteenth-century Norway was accustomed to paternalism. And in addition: Although the medical knowledge and skills held by the members of the medical profession were less than in later periods, the knowledge gap between the physicians and the public was so marked that paternalistic decisions were accepted, even when the scientific base for them was more than questionable.

The general attitudes towards paternalistic behavior have changed. But still people fall sick, are in dispair and distress, and have a psychological need for a fatherly doctor. On the other hand, many not so serious conditions are presented to the doctor of the 1990s. And the gradual extension of the range of what is considered to be medical problems leads to the fact that it is not necessarily the fatherly decision by a physician which is the appropriate way to a solution. Paternalism as a tool for the physician probably is still important in the 1990s, but for the physician it is crucial to reserve it for the right situations, and to use the paternalistic approach only then, to avoid understandable adverse reactions from the surroundings.

A marker which is rather strong for Norwegian physicians, and which probably shows some difference from the conditions in other comparable countries, is the social consciousness which is expected of the physician. In a way, the expectations of a good physician have a close resemblance to the ideology of what may be called the Scandinavian brand of social democracy. But even if this social conciousness is part of the accepted ethical codes, it is not necessarily accepted by the general population in the same way, at least not when it comes to priorities, for example in the case of expensive, non-documented medical treatment.

And to fulfill an expectation to be the advocate and the solicitor on behalf of a patient, for example versus the national health insurance system or versus the authorities, is not necessarily in compliance with the prevailing ethical standards, even if just that is what the patients want from their doctor. An attorney in court may elaborate his evidence to the extreme, to the benefit of his client and to achieve a successful solution of the case. It is a different matter for physicians. In the eyes of the medical profession as such, it is not a morally clear asset for a Norwegian doctor if he has argued in such a way that his patient, say, gets financial support from the national health insurance system on dubious premises. Responsibility to the society is a strong professional requirement which may be difficult to maintain.

Another marker, typical for the Norwegian medical profession, seems to have been the ethical norm of universality: When a new procedure based on advances in medicine, and with a sufficiently documented effect, is to be implemented in practical medicine, it should be possible to offer it to everyone. In the 1990s, there obviously is a general agreement within the profession that this norm should be upheld, although difficult cases appear in the media at regular intervals and attract considerable public interest.

But there have also been more general problems that have occurred when pursuing this principle: The establishment of the occupational health services and the introduction of health screening programs for selected groups of the population have become main issues in the professional and public debate, because such arrangements may imply that a medical service is offered only to a part of the population, at least for an introductory period, and not to every Norwegian citizen. Needless to say, such discussions may both take off from the ground and become endless and unproductive.

32.3 The Medical Profession – an Entity?

As we have seen in Chapter 26, around 95 percent of all Norwegian physicians of the 1990s are members of the Norwegian Medical Association, and in recent years the greater part of the medical students, too. No wonder that in the eyes of the rest of the population, the corps of physicians might give the impression that it is a closed community, a movement, a brotherhood, or a league.

The development of the strong and unifying position of the Norwegian Medical Association over a period of more than one hundred years was discussed in depth in connection with the one hundredth anniversary of the Association in 1986 (Larsen, Berg, Hodne 1986).

This unity, however, probably must not exclusively be regarded as the result of a proficient policy on the part of the leaders of the Association: The Norwegian physicians in the nineteenth and twentieth century have very much in common, because they have been through a very homogenous process of socialization in the medical schools. The tight curriculums often give a strong class feeling, when the groups of students are stable through many years. Even from the very outset, from the time of admittance to a medical school, the medical profession has a distinct flare of exclusiveness, which is a marker. And this marker may spark adverse feelings.

The accompanying strong forces of inclusiveness inherent in the corps of physicians may also be a psychologically understandable provoking trait, and a certain later resentment on the part of the many applicants who were not admitted to the medical schools may be a factor of some importance.

But the structure of medical knowledge may also add to the unifying forces. The theoretical background which has been taught in basic medical sciences has always been heavy, even in the years before more or less internationally accepted standards for the contents and scope of medical education were established at the beginning of the twentieth century. The vivid Norwegian discussions over the years about the objectives of the medical curriculum: should it primarily be aimed at practical work, or should the science be emphasized, and where the University for a long time played the conservative part and saw to it that basic sciences were defended, can be interpreted in a professional context: The weight on science both unified the students and made their professional profile distinctively different from that of other vocational groups in the health services.

Alternatively the ever ongoing process in favor of practical skills and patient orientation may also constitute a threat to the profession of physicians, and to the use of the practical tool which their professionalism can be. Practical medical procedures may be performed by people who are not physicians, and who do not have the basis in medical science acquired by the medical students. But, to act like a good physician in an encounter with a patient, is not the same as being a good physician. What separates the physicians from other groups of health personnel is their theoretical knowledge. Even if specialized knowledge outside what is taught in the medical curriculum is held by other actors on the health care stage, the physicians as a rule have the most comprehensive background. Anything that weakens this upper hand in general medical knowledge will also weaken the power of professionalism.

Reviewing the history of the Norwegian

medical profession gives a definite impression that the unifying forces have been strong, and that they have only to a very limited degree been challenged from the inside of the profession, and they have withstood attacks from the outside.

32.4. *Professionalization within the Profession*

The tables presented in Chapter 26 on the distribution of the Norwegian physicians in the different specialty groups show that there is a substantial diversity within the profession. And all the specialties have their own long-lasting training programs which socialize the physicians into subgroups, into what might be called sub-professions. It seems, however, that by and large it has been a successful policy on the part of the Norwegian Medical Association to harmonize the varying interests of the different groups without violating the strong cohesive entity.

One of the most important sub-professionalizations is that of the general practitioners. In the 1960s, when this process gained in force, experiences with the professional development of the physicians as a total group were at hand; and the first influential scientific works on professions had already appeared or were in preparation (Palmstrøm 1935, Lindbekk 1967, Torgersen 1972).

The upgrading of family medicine and general practitioners seems to have implemented the knowledge of the time that had been systematized by the professional sociologists. For example, there emerged a quest for their own knowledge production and for their own research as a strong objective, together with the other elements of professionalization which had been identified and discussed. The general practitioners used professionalism as a way of lifting themselves, and obviously with success, albeit with some periods of setback as well.

Another group has some theoretical interest in this respect, although it is by far a smaller group: the industrial medical officers. The historian Hilde Ibsen (Ibsen 1996) has studied the industrial health services in three large industrial companies in Norway. Among her conclusions on why workplace-based welfare systems, including health services, never gained real strength in Norway are that conflicting interests opposed the policy of the dominating Labour party, and that there was a reluctance to implement workplace welfare because it could tie the employees too closely to the employers and hamper the development of workplace democracy. However, from 1977 on, a new professionalization process started for the industrial physicians, and this process showed similarities to, but also important differences from, that of the general practitioners (Larsen 1990).

The industrial medical services with preventive objectives covered a larger part of Norwegian workplaces in 1977, when a new worker's protection act was put into force. Industrial physicians would now be part of a more comprehensive system for surveying and controlling working conditions.

Till then, a typical model for industrial medicine had been the local doctor, the district physician, or a local practitioner, who, with some additional training and based on his insights into the prevailing conditions in the community, had a part-time job in a factory or in other private or public workplaces. Of course, large companies for a long time had employed full-time doctors, but this would from now on be the rule, even when geography and industrial structure were unfit for such a reform and called for special arrangements: ambulatory offices, separate industrial health centers, and so forth. New industrial physicians would replace the physicians of the old system. This expelling process met with heavy resistance in many local communities, where faith in the local doctor was well established. The introduction of the new system was launched by the Factory Inspectorate (Arbeidstilsynet), and caused many a conflict, which probably has been unfortunate for both occupational medicine and to the medical profession as such, before the situation calmed down somewhat after some years had passed.

The important issue here, from the viewpoint of professionalization, was that the formation of a new sub-profession among the colleagues included the replacement of other colleagues, and this could hardly be carried through without an argument that the work hitherto performed was of an unacceptably low quality, an impression which was not generally shared, either by the physicians or by the public. This situation, as seen from a professional perspective, is a striking contrast to family medicine, where the upgrading of the general practitioners did not require that others be pushed out.

Another point must also be mentioned: The upgraded general practitioner fitted very well into the general image of a doctor. The new industrial medical officer did not. A so-called basic course in occupational medicine had as one of its main objectives to socialize the new industrial physicians into a new professional role, in which the single patient was not the focus anymore, and in which the working conditions were supposed to be the prime objective. The industrial physician was to be a member of a team which studied working conditions in cooperation with personnel with other vocational backgrounds. This demand for a shift of the role triggered much resistance on the part of the physicians, which may be interpreted as the reaction to a threat to their professionalism. Likewise, a postgraduate, high-level course in occupational health, based on the same principles, and launched at the University of Oslo in 1989, encountered substantial difficulties, partly as the result of the mixup of professional roles. It was forced to close down temporarily in 1993 in order to be reorganized. As a contrast, a new institute for occupational medicine at the University of Bergen, inaugurated in 1990, seemingly became a success because it concentrated on research and the conveying of knowledge to the existing vocational groups of the industrial medical system.

The quest for deprofessionalization of the traditional doctor's autonomy, the establishing of a new role, a physician's role in an advisory position, and in a system which in many places needed legal enforcement to be adopted and maintained by the workplaces, is of core interest when looking at professional development in general. It demonstrates the forces which normally are concealed, but which may be released when the image and the role of the physician in the eyes of the profession and the public is challenged. In the case of occupational medicine: In a way, the authority and the prestige of the physicians were taken hostage when the new system for industrial medicine in Norway was introduced.

A similar development may be seen in, say, modern hospital organizations, where the status of the physicians has been and still is attacked from many sides. The professional role is gradually altered when the responsibility is narrowed and the management to a larger extent is transferred to other personnel groups.

It seems as if the core point in professional status and prestige, and in fact for professionalism as a tool in the practical work, is a close connection between high-level knowledge and skills, responsibility, and authorization to take action, independently, and based on the same knowledge, skills, and responsibility. When these connections are broken or weakened, the profession is at stake. This is an obvious challenge.

32.5. Images and Objectives

In the introductory chapter of this book, some hypotheses were launched, and a framework for discussion of them was suggested.

It seems to be well documented through our historical and present-day survey that the importance of the three roles of the physician: the life saver, the caring supporter, and the gate-keeper, undergo historical variations.

Changes, both in morbidity and in the organization of the health services, probably have weakened the general notion of the physician as the strong and fatherly life saver who enters the stage at the critical moment. Most clinical situations of the 1990s do not imply life saving. When they think of emergencies, what comes to peoples' minds usually are pictures of helicopters, ambulances, and proficient paramedics in orange suits, and not a physician.

However, the caring medical tasks have increased in importance. Good health seems to a considerable degree to be looked upon as a human right. To take over a mother's supporting role in what might be perceived as an uphill fight against biology and death, against the inevitable end-point of a human life, is complicated. It may be especially exhausting when the tool of paternalism and authority has been weakened.

It is a fact, here documented by figures in Chapter 26, that more and more of the physicians are women. Perhaps it should be considered whether there is a risk ahead that the female doctors, as a result of still prevailing opinions and traditions in the population, to an even larger extent than their male colleagues will be confronted with unfulfillable demands for mothering?

The gate-keeper role of the doctor has increased throughout history, as economy has become more important and visible in health matters. Paperwork related to health insurance, social security, and so forth has increased in amount and complexity. On the other hand, it has become clear that the word of the doctor in many cases is regarded as only a recommendation: the real gatekeepers sit on an higher level, and are not necessarily doctors at all.

Through the texts, tables, diagrams, and pictures of this book, sufficient clues should have been presented to support the hypothesis that the expectations of the physician, and of hers or his different roles, have been, and still are, of paramount importance to the attitudes towards the medical profession. Further it seems, for the individual physician, that hers or his willingness, skills, or also the real, perhaps even dubious, chances to meet such expectations, are crucial for the relationship to patients and society.

Our introductory chapter has already touched on the variations in the objectives in the practical work of a doctor. Why choose to become a doctor? And after one has become a doctor, what are the most important elements of the profession to emphasize?

The "serve the sick" objective is an ethical obligation for all physicians, and is also strongly tied to the notion of social responsibility, but with slight, but important differences in the practical consequences.

As a prime objective, however, the strength of the "serve the sick" objective may be questioned when the sick whom the doctor has an obligation to are not always that sick anymore; many of them may present to their general practitioner rather diminutive problems. After a consultation, instead of being filled with satisfaction that yet another human being could be helped, the physician may instead feel tired of wasting time and efforts on just another luxury problem.

To distinguish between what is important and what is not becomes a prime issue in first line medicine, and it will be a new challenge to the physician to handle and to feel comfortable even with the less important problems.

The problem of the not-so-sick of course also looks different from the viewpoint of, say, a physician on a fixed salary in a hospital policlinic, a private practitioner, or an industrial medical service doctor who is working in one of those private occupational health services which sell medical services to companies for their employees, and who are to a large extent dependent on living up to the expectations of the customer company.

The second objective discussed in our introduction was the "serve the society" attitude, the strong norm of social responsibility hailed by many of the old district physicians. Although preventive medicine and a community medicine approach is still put forward as important by the population, the politicians, and the medical profession itself, an active commitment within this field in many ways was easier in a climate where the general authority of the doctor had more weight. But the legislation of the past was of paramount importance. Difficult medical problems such as leprosy, insanity, tuberculosis, and epidemic diseases were covered by legislation regulating the efforts against them, and the physicians had a special role (Boye and Angell 1927).

The health care system of the Evang period was also a system heavily based on medical competence, not on political decisions: medicine was a medical matter. In light of the historical development of the potentials for the individual doctor to pursue goals and objectives of social responsibility on the local level, the legislation introduced in 1984, when the state-commissioned district physician was converted into a municipality employee, can be regarded as a setback.

The "serve the science" objective, the internalized norm to participate in the buildup of the medical base of knowledge, has experienced varying circumstances. When more and more of the doctors are on fixed salaries, and the size of these salaries becomes increasingly important, delicate negotiation skills will be required from the medical side if time and resources for scientific work are not to be completely lost.

In The Norwegian Medical Association, the maintenance of this requirement probably should be discussed and it should be agreed upon that the pursuit of scientific work in principle is a requirement which should be insisted on beyond negotiation. When looking at history, there are reasons to say that the key to keeping the upper hand in the medical services has been, and still is, the superiority in medical knowledge. Time and money for updating and further education is a frequently mentioned requirement by many vocational groups, and is based on the same reasoning. But to nurture also the norm of participation in the development of the base of knowledge keeps the profession of physicians a step ahead.

The objective of serving oneself, to work as a doctor with the prime objective to make a living, preferably a good living, of course may be defended without criticism. When considering Norwegian medical history, however, it seems that many physicians for a long time have evaluated the other objectives mentioned to be more worthwhile. Clues for such a conclusion are found in the migration patterns for example, where a vivid moving activity seems to be a consequence of a desired career pattern. Especially the investigations referred to in our Chapters 26 and 27 explore these problems.

However, in our 1986 study (Larsen 1986), both questionnaire replies and key in-depth interviews indicated that there was a time gradient: personal objectives became more important for the younger generation than they had been before. This is a finding with bearings for the future.

Potentials for conflicts obviously are at hand: To keep up with the professional standards requires frequent changes of workplaces, while altered family patterns and new sets of basic demands make this requirement ever more uncomfortable.

Even if privatized medicine has flourished for periods in Norway, it mostly has been, and still is, only a supplement to the publicly run and publicly financed health services. One of the reasons for this is that generations of Norwegians have been accustomed to a public system, in which the costs more or less invisibly have been folded into the taxation system, and the amounts paid for medical services have been low. A private service calculated on real cost therefore competes with the lower-cost, public system.

For most modern Norwegian doctors, their career will imply holding positions or arrangements with the public health services, with the economic terms offered there. But still, to leave the medical profession, to quit medical work, is very rare, even if conditions could be better elsewhere. When looking through the biographies of Norwegian physicians, it of course is difficult to assess what the working day of the biographee is really like, and the establishment of reliable statistics as to this point was not included in our project. But titles indicating jobs outside the range of the health services are rare. A lawyer may go into a wide variety of positions without offending his professional image and loyalty; a theologist seeking work outside the clergy probably is somewhat more unusual; and a doctor leaving his profession even more so. Again a marker of a profession appears!

Perhaps this special trait of the medical profession also should be regarded as a sort of indicator: When unrest develops, and colleagues start thinking of fleeing the career pattern they seemingly have chosen, warning signals should flash in the professional organizations. Stability and loyalty to the profession seem to be so strong a marker, and so specific for physicians, that any deviation should cause concern. Then something is probably wrong with the working conditions. And this of course not only relates to the profession of physicians as such, but as much, and perhaps even more so, to the sub-professions within the ranks of Norwegian doctors.

In the introductory chapter, the reader was recommended to consider the development of the medical profession in light of the images and the objectives of the doctor. Recalling and interpreting what has happened in the years that lie behind us might be a useful tool for the task which lies ahead: The active discussion and interpretation of the experiences related to the ever ongoing *Shaping of a Profession.*

References

Boye, T., and T. Angell. *Norsk medicinallovgivning*. Oslo: Aschehoug, 1927.

Ibsen, H. *Mellom profitt og moral*. Oslo: Tano Aschehoug, 1996.

Johannessen, F.E., and J. Skeie. *Bitre piller og sterke dråper. Norske apotek gjennom 400 år 1595–1995*, Oslo: Norsk farmasihistorisk museum, 1995.

Kringlen, E. *Medisin og samfunn*, Oslo: Universitetsforlaget, 1996.

Larsen, Ø., O. Berg, and F. Hodne. *Legene og samfunnet*, Oslo: Seksjon for medisinsk historie, Universitetet i Oslo and Den norske lægeforening, 1986.

Larsen, Ø. "Arbeidsmedisinens utvikling i Norge." *Norsk bedriftshelsetjeneste* 1990; 11:140–52.

Lindbekk, T. *Mobilitets- og stillingsstruktur innenfor tre akademiske profesjoner 1910–1963*, Oslo: 1967.

Palmstrøm, H. "Om en befolkningsgruppes utvikling gjennom de siste 100 år," *Statøkonomisk tidsskrift*, 49(1935):161–370.

Sverre, N.A. *Et studium av farmasiens historie, 2. ed.* Oslo: Norges Apotekerforening, 1982.

Torgersen, U. *Profesjonssosiologi*. Oslo: Universitetsforlaget, 1972.

Torgersen, U. *Profesjoner og offentlig sektor*. Oslo: Tano, 1994.

CHAPTER 33

Bibliography

References and Suggestions for Further Reading

Aall, H. C. "Kvaksalver-annonser og lægers avertisementer i dagsaviserne," *Tidsskrift for Den norske lægeforening*, (1903):631–632.

Aamodt, A. "Medorg – et Oslo fenomen," *Æsculap*, 2(1980):13–14.

Aarflot, V., B. Dybdahl, M. Falke, T. H. Michelet, E. C. Egebakken, T. Kumar, H. Haukeland, and E. Lærum. "Vet legen om pasienten er tilfreds?" *Tidsskrift for Den norske lægeforening*, 114(1994):3579–3582.

Aarseth, S., S. Vatn, and H. P. Aarseth. "Arbeidsmiljø og helseforhold blant sykehusleger," *Tidsskrift for Den norske lægeforening*, 113(1993):1864–1868.

Aarø, L. E., K. Bjartveit, O. D. Vellar, and E. L. Berglund. "Smoking Habits among Norwegian Doctors 1974," *Scandinavian Journal of Social Medicine*, 5(1977):127–135.

Aasland, O.G. and E. Falkum. "Legekårsundersøkelsen. Responsen på spørreskjemaundersøkelsen." *Tidsskrift for Den norske lægeforening*, 114(1994):3052–3058.

Aasland, O.G. "Helter og skurker – og faren ved å være lege." *Tidsskrift for Den norske lægeforening*, 113(1993):1837–1838.

Aasland, O. G. and E. Falkum. "Hvordan har vi det i dag? Om legers helse, velvære og arbeidsglede," *Tidsskrift for Den norske lægeforening*, 112(1992):3818-3823.

Aasland, O. G., M. Olff, E. Falkum, T. Schweder, and H. Ursin. "Health complaints and job stress in Norwegian physicians," *(Submitted to Social Science and Medicine* 1996).

Aasland, O. G., A. Amundsen, D. Bruusgaard, J. Jervell, and J. Mørland. "Norske legers alkoholvaner," *Tidsskrift for Den norske lægeforening*, 107(1987):2553–2448.

Abbey, S. E. and P. E. Garfinkel. "Neurasthenia and chronic fatigue syndrome: the role of culture in the making of a diagnosis," *American Journal of Psychiatry*, 148(1991):1638–1646.

Abbott, A. "The Order of Professionalization: An Empirical Analysis," *Work and Occupations*, 18(1991):355–384.

Abbott, A. "The Future of Professions: Occupation and Expertice in the Age of Organization," *Research in the Sociology of Organizations*, 8(1991):17–42.

Abbott, A. "Professional Ethics," *American Journal of Sociology*, 88(1983):855–885.

Abbott, A. "The new Occupational Structure: What Are the Questions?" *Work and Occupations*, 16(1989):273–291.

Abbott, A. "Status and Status Strain in the

Professions," *American Journal of Sociology*, 86(1981):819–835.

Abbott, A. "The Sociology of Work and Occupations," *Annual Review of Sociology*, 19(1993):187–209.

Acker, J. "The problem with patriarchy," *Sociology*, 23(1989):235–240.

Ackerknecht, E. H. *A Short History of Medicine*. Baltimore: Johns Hopkins University Press, 1968.

Ackerman-Liebrich, U. and S. Wick, M. "Survival of female doctors in Switzerland." *British Journal of Medicine*, 302 (1991):959.

Adams, S. "Origins of American Occupational Elites," *American Journal of Sociology*, 70(1957):360–368.

Adams, J.W. "Patient discrimination against women physicians." *Journal of the American Medical Womens Association*, 32 (1977): 255–261.

Adams, O. "Canada's doctors who they are and what they do: lessons from the CMA's 1986 manpower survey. " *Canadian Medical Association Journal*, 140 (1989):212–221.

Adams, P. G. *Travellers and Travel Liars 1660-1800*. Berkeley and Los Angeles: University of California Press, 1962.

Adcock, C. J. and L. B. Brown. "Social class and the ranking of occupations," *The British Journal of Sociology*, 8(1957): 26–32.

Adorno, T. "Sociology and Psychology," *New Left Review*, 46(1967):67–80.

Adorno, T. "Sociology and Psychology – II," *New Left Review*, 47(1968):79–97.

Akre, V. and Å. Vikanes. *Turnuskandidaten, menneskets beste venn? En kartlegging av turnustjenesten*. Lagåsen: Den norske lægeforening, 1991.

Akre, V., E.Falkum, B. O. Hoftvedt, et al. "The communication atmosphere among physicians-colleagues: competitive perfectionism or supportive dialogue? A Norwegian Study." *Social Science and Medicine* (1996) In press.

Akre, V., Å. Vikanes, and P. Hjortdahl. "Profesjonalisering uten styring? En undersøkelse om det faglige innholdet i turnustjenesten," *Tidsskrift for Den norske lægeforening*, 112(1992):2546–2551.

Album, D. and G. Midre. "Mellom idealer og realiteter. Studier i medisinsk sosiologi." Oslo: ad Notam, 1991.

Album, D. "Sykdommers og medisinske spesialiteters prestisje," *Tidsskrift for Den norske lægeforening*, 111(1991):2127–33.

Album, D. "Sykdommers og medisinske spesialiteters prestisje," *Nordisk Medicin*, 106(1991):232–236.

Alfsen, G.C. and C. Haug. "På kvinners premisser" *Tidsskrift for Den norske lægeforening*, 114(1994):3050–3051.

Allen, I. *Doctors and their careers: a new generation*. London: Policy Studies Institute, 1994.

Allen G. Freeman, *Railways. Past, Present & Future*, London: Orbis Publishing, 1982.

Alsvik, O. *"Friskere, sterkere, større, renere". Om Carl Schiøtz og helsearbeidet for norske skolebarn*. Hovedoppgave i historie. Oslo: Universitet i Oslo, 1991.

Alvarez-Dardet, C. and M.T. Ruiz. "Thomas McKeown and Archibald Cochrane: a journey through the diffusion of their ideas." *British Journal of Medicine*, 306(1993):1252–1254.

Alvestad, M. "Problembasert læring i Trondheim," *Tidsskrift for Den norske lægeforening*, 115(1995):2131.

AMA Council of Mental Health. "The sick physician. Impairment by psychiatric disorders, including alcoholism and drug dependence," *Journal of the American Medical Association*, 223(1973):684–687.

Amdam, R. P. and K. Sogner. *Rik på kontraster*. Oslo: ad Notam Gyldendal, 1994.

Andersen, E. "Innlegg i diskussionen om det offentlige civile lægevæsen," *Tidsskrift for Den norske lægeforening*, (1935): 365–371.

Andersen, E. "Udtalelse om revision av det civile lægevæsen," *Tidsskrift for Den norske lægeforening*, (1927):366-377,633–636, 876–877, 980–981.

Andresen, R. *Fra norsk sanitets historie.* Oslo: NKS forlaget, 1986.

Angel, R. and P. Thoits. "The impact of culture on the cognitive structure of illness," *Culture, Medicine and Psychiatry*, 11(1987): 465–494.

Anstensen, T. "Til diskussion om taushetspligten," *Medicinsk Revue*, (1916):108–110.

APLF 1938–1988. *Tidsskrift for Den norske lægeforening,* 108(1988)(29b).

APLF OLL. *Tanker om morgendagens primærlegetjeneste,* Oslo: Den norske lægeforening, 1977.

Armstrong, D. "Medicine as a profession: times of change," *British Medical Journal*, 301(1990):691–693.

Armstrong, D. "The Patient's View," *Social Science and Medicine*, 18(1984):737–744.

Arnesen, H. "Sindsykelægernes kaar og utdannelse," *Tidsskrift for Den norske lægeforening*, (1912):308–312.

Arndt, K. A. "Information excess in Medicine", *Alch Delmatol,* 128(1922):1249–56.

Arnetz, B. White collar stress: What studies of physicians can teach us." *Psychoterapy and psychosomatics*, 55(1991):197–200.

Arnetz, B. "Klart høg självmordsrisk bland kvinnliga läkare. Svensk rapport visar overrisk också hos män." *Läkartidningen* 83(1996):2022–2023.

Atkinson, P. "The Reproduction of the Professional Community," in *The Sociology of the Professions: Lawyers, Doctors and Others*, eds. Dingwall, R. and P. Lewis. London: Macmillan, (1983):224–241.

Atkinson, P. "Training for certainty," *Social Science and Medicine*, 19(1984):949–956.

Atkinson, P., M. Reid, and P. Sheldrake. "Medical Mystique," *Sociology of Work and Occupations*, 4(1977):243–280.

Aubert, A. "Lægeforeningens rolle i utviklingen av helsevesenet." *Tidsskrift for Den norske lægeforening* 106(1986): 1209–1219.

Aubert, V., U. Torgersen, K. Tangen, T. Lindbekk, and S. Pollan. "Akademikere i Norsk samfunnsstruktur 1850–1950", *Tidsskrift for samfunnsforskning*, 1 4 (1960):185–248.

Austveg, B. *Helsearbeid og innvandrere. Mangfold, sunnhet og sykdom.* Oslo: TANO, 1994.

Azzarto, J. "Medicalization of problems of the elderly," *Health Soc Work*, 11 (1986): 189–195.

Bach, S. "Managing a pluralist health system: The case of health care reform in France." *International Journal of Health Services*, 24(1994):593–606.

Backer, J. E. *Dødeligheten og dens årsaker i Norge 1856–1955.* Oslo: Statistisk Sentralbyrå, Samfunnsøkonomiske studier nr. 10, 1961.

Backett, K. and C. Davison. "Lifecourse and lifestyle: The social and cultural location of health behaviours," *Social Science and Medicine*, 40(1995):629–638.

Bain, M. H. *"I hine haarde dage". Legeberetninger fra Lurøy legedistrikt.* Lurøy: 1979.

Balarajan, R. "Inequalities in health within the health sector," *British Journal of Medicine,*229(1989):822–825.

Bankowski, Z. "Etics and Health." *World Health Forum*, 16(1995):115–125.

Banwell, S.S and J.M. Paxman. "Health law and ethics. The search for meaning: RU 486 and the law of abortion." *American Journal of Public Health*, 82(1992):1399–1406.

Barber, B. "Some problems in the sociology of professions," *Dædalus*, (1963):669–688.

Barr, D.A. "The professional structure of Soviet medical care: the relationship between personal characteristics, medical education, and occupational setting for Estonian physicans." *Am J Public Health*, 85(1995):373–378.

Bartholin, Thomas. *On the Burning Of His Library*, Copenhagen: Petrus Haubold, 1670 and *On medical Travel,* Copenhagen: Daniel Paulli, 1674. *On The Burning of His Library and On Medical Travel*, translated by Charles D O'Malley, Lawrence: The University of Kansas Libraries, 1961.

Bartrip, P. W. J. *Mirror of medicine*. Oxford: Claredon, 1990.

Barzun, J. "The professions under siege: Private practice versus public need," *Journal of the American Dental Association*, 98 (1979):672–677.

Barzun, J. *Clio and the Doctors. Psycho-History, Quanto-History & History*. Chicago: 1974.

Baszanger, I. "Professional socialization and social control: From medical students to general practitioners," *Social Science and Medicine*, 20(1985):133–143.

Bauman, Z. "The scandal of death," *New Statesman & Society*, 6(1993):20–21.

Beatty, W. K. "Medical care for Norwegian immigrants in the Chicago area," *Proc Inst Med Chgo*, 36(1983):147–150.

Beauchamp, T.L. and J.F. Childress. *Principles of Biomedical Ethics.* Oxford; University Press, 1983.

Beck, U. *Risk society. Towards a new modernity*. London: Sage Publications, 1992.

Beck, U. "From Industrial Society to the Risk Society: Questions of Survival, Social Structure and Ecological Enlightenment," *Theory, Culture & Society*, 9 (1992):97–123.

Becker, H. S. and J. W. Carper. "The development of identification with an occupation," *The American Journal of Sociology*, 61(1956):289–298.

Becker, H. S. and J. Carper. "The elements of identification with an occupation," *American Sociological Review*, 21(1956): 341–348.

Becker, H., B. Geer, E. Hughes, and A. Strauss. *Boys in White. Student Culture in medical School*. Chicago: University of Chicago Press, 1961.

Becker, H. S. "The Nature of a Profession," in *Sociological Work*, Chicago: Aldine, 1970.

Becker, M. "The tyranny of health promotion," *Public Health Revue*, 14(1986):15–25.

Begun, J. W. "Economic and Sociological Approaches to Professionalism," *Work and Occupations*, 13(1986):113–129.

Beitrusten, G. *Husmannsvesenet under avvikling. Hovedoppgave i historie*. Oslo: Universitet i Oslo, 1976.

Bell, S. E. "Changing ideas: the medicalization of menopause," *Social Science and Medicine*, 24(1990):535–542.

Ben-David, J. "Professions in the class system of present-day societies," *Current Sociology*, 12(1964):247–330.

Ben-David, J. *The Scientist's Role in Society*. New Jersey: Prentice-Hall, Inc. 1971.

Ben-David, J. "Scientific growth: A sociological view," *Minerva*, 2(1963):455–476.

Ben-David, J. and A. Zloczower. "Universities and Academic Systems in Modern Societies," *Archives Europeénnes de Sociologie*, 3(1962):45–84.

Ben-David, J. "The Profession of Science and its Powers," *Minerva*, 10(1972):362–383.

Ben-David, J. *Centers of Learning: Britain, France and the United States*. New York: 1977.

Ben-David, J. "Scientific productivity and academic organization in nineteenth century medicine," *American Sociological Review*, 25(1960):828–843.

Benjamin, W. "Paris – Capital of the Nineteenth Century," *New Left Review*, 48 (1968):77–88.

Benneche, O. "Det civile lægevesens omordning," *Tidsskrift for Den norske lægeforening*, (1909)

Bennett, D. "Explanation in Medical Geography: Evidence and Epistemology," *Social Science and Medicine*, 33(1991):339–346.

Bensing, J. "Doctor-patient communication and the quality of care." *Social Science and Medicine*, 32(1991):1301–1310.

Benson, K. R. "Science and the Single author: Historical reflections on the problem of authorship." *Cancer Bull,* 43 (1991):324–331.

Bentsen, B. G. ICPC–ICHPPC–Defined—IC–Process–PC. *Klassifikasjoner og definisjoner for primærhelsetjenesten. WONCAs internasjonale klassifikasjoner og definisjoner tilrettelagt for Norge.* Oslo: TANO, 1991.

Bentsen, B. G. *Illness and general practice.* Oslo, Bergen and Tromsø : Universitetsforlaget, 1970.

Bentsen, N. "Prioritering i sundhedsvæsenet." *Ugeskrift for læger*, 155(1993): 4113–4116.

Bentzen, F. "De kollegiale bestemmelser og kringkastningen," *Tidsskrift for Den norske lægeforening*, (1936):684–685.

Benum, E. *Statsadministrasjonens historie.* Oslo: Universitetsforlaget, 1979.

Beretning om Rigets økonomiske Tilstand 1861–65. Christiania: Departement for det Indre, 1867–68.

Berg, O. "Verdier og interesser – Den norske lægeforenings fremvekst og utvikling," in *Legene og samfunnet*, eds. Larsen, Ø. O. Berg, and F. Hodne. Oslo: Seksjon for medisinsk historie, Universitetet i Oslo og Den norske lægeforening, 1986.

Berg, O. *Medisinens logikk. Studier i medisinens sosiologi og politikk.* Oslo: Universitetsforlaget, 1987.

Berg, O. "Medikrati, hierarki og marked. Noen historiske betraktninger om regulering av medisinsk yrkesutøvelse." *Mellom idealer og realiteter. Studier i en medisinsk sosiologi.* Eds. Album, D. and G. Midre. Oslo: ad Notam, 1991. PP. 147–175.

Berg, K. "Prenatal diagnostikk: Praktiske og etiske aspekter," *Kirke og Kultur,* 8 (1979):476–478.

Berg, O. and P. Hjortdahl. *Medisinen som pedagogikk. En studie av pasienters erfaringer med leger.* Oslo: Universitetsforlaget, 1994.

Berglund, J. *In interview with Bertelsen, T.* 23. october 1995.

Bergsjø, P. "Acta seventy years ago," *Acta Obstet Gynecol Scand*, 70(1991):5–7.

Bergsjø, P. "Tidsskrift for Den norske lægeforening – status presens og veien videre," in *Kunnskap er makt – og bør deles med andre*, eds. Fugelli, P. and M. Nylenna. Oslo: Universitetsforlaget, 1987.

Berkner, L. K. "The Use and Misuse of Cencus Data for the Historical Analysis of Family Structure," *Journal of Interdisciplinary History*, 5(1975):721–738.

Berlant, J. *Profession and Monopoly: a study of medicine in the United States and Great Britain.* Berkeley: University of California Press, 1975.

Berner, J. H. ed. *Den norske lægeforening 1886–1936.* Oslo: Centraltrykkeriet, 1936.

Bertelsen, I. *Kampen for et medisinsk fakultet i Tromsø.* Bergen: 1991.

Birenbaum, A. "Reprofessionalization in pharmacy," *Social Science and Medicine*, 16(1982):871–878.

Biørn-Hansen, E. "Lægernes skysshold, utgifterne dertil ved offentlige og private reiser," *Tidsskrift for Den norske lægeforening*, (1922):528–530.

Bjercke, O. "Lægeforeningens sekretariat gjennom 75 år," *Tidsskrift for Den norske lægeforening*, 81(1961):646–658.

Bjørnsson, B. "Legesituasjonen i Norge," *Sosialt Arbeid*, 39(1965):34–44.

Bjøro, K., B. Berg, K. Kjærheim, B. Hem, and T. Negaard. *Jordmorutdanning gjennom 175 år.* Oslo: Jordmorhøgskolen, 1993.

Bjøro, K., and P. E. Børdahl. *Fødselshjelp gjennom 175 år.* Oslo: Kvinneklinikken Rikshospitalet, 1993.

Blackburn, R.T. and T.G. Fox. "Physicians' values and their career stage." *Journal of Vocational Behavior*, 22(1983):159–173.

Blackwell, E. and R. Blackwell. "Medicine as a Profession for Women," *English Women's Journal*, 5(1860):145–156.

Blaikie, P., T. Cannon, I. Davis, and B. Wisner. *At Risk: Natural hazards, people's vul-*

nerability, and disasters. London and New York: Routledge, 1994.

Blegen, T. C. *Norwegian migration to America 1825–1860*. Northfield, Minn. The Norwegian-American Historical Association, 1931.

Blegen, T. C. *Norwegian migration to America. The American transition*. Northfield, Minn. The Norwegian–American Historical Association, 1940.

Blegen, T. C. ed. *Land of their choice. The immigrants write home*. St. Paul, Minn. The University of Minnesota Press, 1955.

Blindheim, S. *Nordmenn under Hitlers fane.* Oslo: Noregs boklag, 1977.

Blom, I. "Sykehusfødsler i Norge på 1800-tallet," *Historisk Tidsskrift*, 3(1987):324–344.

Blomberg, W. "Vannkurer og medisinsk entreprenører i galebransjen," *Sosial Trygd*, 79(1991):15–20.

Bloom, S. "The Process of Becoming a Physician," *The Annals of The American Academy of Political and Social Science: Medicine and Society*, 346(1963):77–87.

Bloor, M., M. Samphier, and L. Prior. "Artefact explanations of inequalities in health: an assessement of the evidence," *Sociology of Health & Illness*, 9(1987):231–264.

Bluestone, N.R. "The future impact of women physicians on American medicine." *American Journal of Public Health*, 68(1978):760–763.

Bonner, T. N. *To the Ends of the Earth: Womens Search for Education in Medicine*. Cambridge and London: Harvard University Press, 1992.

Bonnevie, P. and H. Theorell. "Nordisk Medicin – historia och nutid," *Nordisk Medicin*, 87(1972):1.

Bonnevie, P. "Nordisk Medicin 50 år. En epoke er endt, men den videnskablige kontinuitet sikret," *Nordisk Medicin*, 95(1980):26–28.

Bonsdorf, B. v. *The History of Medicine in Finland*. Helsinki: 1975.

Boorstin, D.J. *The Exploring Spirit*, New York: Random House, 1975.

Booth, C. C. "Medical communication: the old and the new," *British Medical Journal*, 285(1982):105–108.

Booth, C. "Is British medicine European?" *Transactions of the Medical Society of London*, 108(1992):79–91.

Borchrevink, O. J. "Ansettelsesvikår for sykehuslægen," *Tidsskrift for Den norske lægeforening*, (1919):250–254.

Borkan, J. M., W. L. Miller, and S. Reis. "Medicine as storytelling," *Family Practice*, 9(1992):127–129.

Bourdieu, P. "The specificity of the scientific field and the social conditions of the progress of reason," *Social Science Information*, 14(1975):19–47.

Bourdieu, P. "The social space and the genesis of groups," *Theory and Society*, 14(1985): 723–744.

Bourdieu, P. "The Peculiar History of Scientific Reason," *Sociological Forum*, 6(1991): 3–26.

Boye, T. and A. Angell. *Norsk medicinallovgivning.* Oslo: Aschehoug, 1927.

Bradburn, N. M., L. J. Rips, and S. K. Shevell. "Answering Autobiographical Questions: The Impact of Memory and Inference on Surveys," *Science*, (1987): 157–161.

Bradford Hill, A. "The reasons for writing," *British Medical Journal,* 2(1965):870–2.

Brainthwaite, A. and A. Ross. "Satisfaction and Job Stress in General Practice," *Family Practice*, 5(1988):83–93.

Bramness, J. G., T. C. Fixdal and P. Vaglum. "Effect of medical school stress on the mental health of medical students in early and late clinical curriculum," *Acta Psyciatrica Scandinavia*, 84(1991):340–345.

Bramness, J.G., T.C. Fixdal, and P. Vaglum. "Sosialisering til legerollen i studiets kliniske del. Del I: Studentens vurdering av egne ferdigheter," *Tidsskrift for Den norske lægeforening*, 112(1992): 2207–2210.

Bramness, J. G., T.C. Fixdal and P. Vaglum. "Sosialisering til legerollen i studiets kliniske del. Del II: Studentenes identifisering med legerollen," *Tidsskrift for Den norske lægeforening*, 112(1992):2211–2213.

Brandtzæg, P. *Twenty-five years of research at LIIPAT 1965–1990*. Oslo: Rikshospitalet, 1990.

Brante, T. "Sociologiska föreställningar om professioner," in *Den sociologiska fantasin – teorier om samhället*, ed. Bergryd, U. Rabön & Sjögren, 1987.

Brante, T. "Sociological Approaches to the Professions," *Acta Sociologica*, 31(1988): 119–142.

Brante, T. "Professioners identitet och samhälleliga villkor," in *Kampen om yrkesutövning, status och kunskap*, ed. Selander, S. Lund: Studentlitteratur, 1989.

Brante, T. "Teori och typologi: Om forhålandet mellan makrosociologi, institutionella sfärer och social handling," *Sociologisk Forskning*, 31(1994):3–25.

Brantenberg, G. *Sangen om St. Croix*. Oslo: Aschehoug, 1979.

Branthwaite, A. and A. Ross. "Satisfaction and Jobb Stress in General Practice," *Family Practice*, 5(1988):83–93.

Bratt, J. F. "Beretning om Nationalforeningens diagnosestasjons virksomhet under Lofots- og Finnmarksfisket," *Medd f D n nationf*, (1932).

Braun, S. and R. B. Hollander. "Work and depression among women in the Federal Republic of Germany," *Women and Health*, 14(1988):5–24.

Brazier, M., J. Lovecy, M. Moran, and M. Potton. "Falling from a Tightrope: Doctors and Lawyers between the Market and the State," *Political Studies*, XLI(1993): 197–213.

Brekke, D., O. Iversen, and O. Ødegaard. Helsetjenester i Møre og Romsdal gjennom hundre år. Tingvoll: Bettens Trykkeri, 1986.

Bretteville-Jensen, P. "Realartium for læger," *Tidsskrift for Den norske lægeforening*, (1940):672–674.

Brieger, G. H. "The History of Medicine and the History of Science," *Isis*, 72(1981):537–540.

Brint, S. "Eliot Freidson's Contribution to the Sociology of Professions," *Work and Occupations*, 20(1993):259–278.

Britannica Book of the Year 1996. Chicago: Encyclopœia Britannica Inc., 1996.

British Medical Association. *The morbidity and mortality of the medical profession*. London: British Medical Association, 1993.

Broch, B. E. "Aarsakerne til lægernes ufri økonomiske stilling og forslag til veier til at avhjælpe denne," *Norsk Magazin for Lægevidenskaben*, (1912): 60–67, 154–167.

Broch, B. E. "Lægenes livsbetingelser og arbeidsvilkår," *Norsk Magazin for Lægevidenskaben*, (1912): 571–575, 617–624, 870–875, 972–973, 1014–1020

Broch, O. J. *Le Royaume de Norvége et le peuple Norvegien*. Christiania: Steen, 1878.

Brochmann, S. W. "Lægenøden i Nord-Norge og dens avhjælp ," *Norsk Magazin for Lægevidenskaben*, (1920): 174–175, 806–808, 839.

Brock, H. H. "Lægernes stilling ligeoverfor sundhedskommissionerne," *Ugeskrift for læger*, (1892):306–309.

Brockliss, L. W. B. "The development of the spa in seventeenth-century France," *Medical History*, (1990):23–47.

Brodal, P. "Er kvalitetssikring integrert i grunnutdanningen av leger?" *Tidsskrift for Den norske lægeforening,* 112(1992): 3592–3593.

Brodman, E. *The development of medical bibliography*. Baltimore: 1954.

Brown, E. R. "He Who Pays the Piper: Foundations, the Medical Profession, and Medical Education," in *Health Care in America. Essays in Social History*, eds. Reverby, S. and D. Rosner. Philadelphia: Temple University Press, 1979.

Brown, M.C. "Do physicians locate as spatial competition models predict? Evidence from Alberta." *Canadian Medical Association Journal*, 148(1993): 1301–1307.

Brunchorst, J. *Bergens Museum 1825–1900*. Bergen: Johan Griegs Forlagsekspedition, 1900.

Bruusgaard, D. and T. Gjestland. *Medisinske kandidater fra norske og utenlandske universiteter 1959–1966*. Oslo: Universitetet i Oslo, Institutt for allmennmedisin og Sekretariatet for utenlandsmedisinere, 1976.

Bruusgaard, D., A. Hatland, and A. Syse. *Et nødvendig gode. Folketrygdens plass i Velferds-Norge.* Oslo: ad Notam Gyldendal, 1994.

Bucher, R. and J. Stelling. "Characteristics of Professional Organisations," *Journal of Health and Social Behavior*, 10(1969):3–15.

Bucher, R. and A. Strauss. "Professions in process," *The American Journal of Sociology*, 66(1961):325–334.

Bucy, P. C. ed. *Modern Neurosurgical Giants*. New York: 1986.

Budde, C. "Beretning om en med Stipendium foretagen videnskabelig Reise," *Norsk Magazin for Lægevidenskaben*, (1859):889–914.

Bugge, J. *På tokt med korvetten Nordstjernen 1869/70*, Oslo: J Johan Grundt Tanum, 1943.

Bull, E. *Nordmenn før oss.* Oslo: Tanum Norli, 1976.

Bull, E. *Klassekamp og felleskap 1920–1945*. Norges historie, bd 13. Oslo: Cappelens forlag, 1979.

Bull, M. "Secularization and medicalization," *British Journal of Sociology*, 41 (1990): 245–261.

Bunker, J.P. "Can professionalism survive in the marketplace? Government and management need to recognise doctors as equal partners in health care." *British Journal of Medicine* 08 (1994): 1179–1180.

Bunton, R., S. Nettleton, and R. Burrows. "The sociology of health promotion. Critical analyses of consumption, lifestyle and risk." London: Rouledge, 1995.

Burger, W. E. "The Decline of Professionalism," *Proceedings of the American Philosophical Society*, 137(1993):481–487.

Börkle de la Camp, H. *Chirurgenverzeichnis*. Berlin: 1969.

Burman, K. D. ""Hanging from the masthead": Reflections on autorship," *Ann Intern Med*, 97(1982):602

Burnham, J. C. "Will Medical History Join the American Mainstream," *Reviews in American History*, 6(1978):43–49.

Burnham, J. C. "The Reception of Psychoanalysis in Western Cultures: An Afterword on Its Comparative History," *Comparative Studies in Society and History*, 24(1982):603–610.

Burnham, J. C. "American Medicine's Golden Age: What Happened to It?" *Science*, 215(1982):1474–1479.

Burnham, J. C. "The evolution of editorial peer review," *JAMA*, 263(1990):1323–9.

Burnham, J. C. "The Past of the Future of Medicine," *Bulletin of the History of Medicine*, 67(1993):1–27.

Burnham, J. C. "How the Concept of Profession Evolved in the Work of Historians of Medicine," *Bulletin of the History of Medicine*, 70(1996):1–24.

Burrage, M. and R. Torstendahl. eds. *Professions in Theory and History. Rethinking the Study of Professions*. London: SAGE, 1990.

Bury, M. R. "Social constructionism and the development of medical sociology," *Sociology of Health & Illness*, 8(1986): 137–169.

Buxrud, E. G. "Er helsetjenesten en god arbeidsplass for kvinner?" *Tidsskrift for Den norske lægeforening*, 133(1993):1869–1872.

Buxrud, E. G. "Bydelhelsetjenesten – mer belastende for kvinnelige enn for mannlige leger?" *Tidsskrift for Den norske lægeforening*, 110(1990):3260–3264.

Bynum, W. F. "Health, disease and medical care," in *The ferment of knowledge. Studies in the Historiography of Eighteenth-Century Science*, eds. Rousseau, G. S. and R. Porter. Cambridge: Cambridge University Press, 1980.

Bynum, W. F. and R. Porter. eds. *Medicine and the five senses*. Cambridge: Cambridge University Press, 1993.

Bynum, W. and R. Porter. eds. *Companion encyclopedia of the history of medicine*. London: Routledge, 1993.

Bærheim, A., *Lower urinary tract infections in women. Aspects of pathogenesis and diagnosis. Thesis.* Bergen: Division for General Practice, Department of Public Health and Primary Health Care, University of Bergen, 1994.

Bø, O. *Folkemedisin og lærd medisin: nordisk medisinsk kvardag på 1800-tallet*. Oslo: Samlaget, 1972.

Bø, O. "Folkemedisinen – signekjerringer og bygdedoktorer," in *Norsk Kulturhistorie, Vol 5.*, Oslo: Aschehoug, 1980.

Calhoun, D. H. *Professional Lives in America: Structure and Aspiration, 1750-1850*. Cambridge, Mass. Harvard University Press, 1965.

Calman, K. "The profession of medicine." *British Journal of Medcine*, 309(1994): 1140–1143.

Calnan, M. "Images Of General Practice: The Perceptions of the Doctor." *Social Science and Medicine*, 27(1988):579–586.

Cantor, D. "The contradictions of specialization: Rheumatism and the decline of the spa in inter-war Britain," *Medical History*, (1990):127–144.

Carling, F. *Skapt i vårt bilde*. Oslo: Gyldendal Norsk Forlag, 1975.

Carlsen, S. "Kvaksalveri og arkana-uvæsen." *Tidsskrift for Den norske lægeforening*, (1909):605–609.

Carpenter, E.S. "Women in male-dominated health professions." *International Journal of Health Services*, 7(1977):191–207.

Carr-Saunders, A. M. and P. A. Wilson. *The professions*. Oxford: Clarendon Press, 1933.

Cartwright, A. and R. Anderson. "Changes in the frequency and nature of doctor-patient contacts," in *General Practice Revisited. A second study of patients and their doctors*, eds. Cartwright, A. and R. Anderson. London: Tavistock Publications, 1981.

Carøe, K. ed., *Den danske Lægestand. 1786–1838.* København og Kristiania: Gyldendalske Boghandel og Nordisk Forlag, 1905.

Carøe, K. red. *Den danske Lægestand. Kirurger eksaminerede ved Theatrum anatomico – chirurgicum 1738–1785.* København og Kristiania: Gyldendalske Boghandel og Nordisk Forlag, 1906.

Carøe, K. ed. *Den danske Lægestand. Doktorer og Licentiater 1479–1788.* København og Kristiania: Gyldendalske Boghandel og Nordisk Forlag, 1909.

Carøe, K. *Studier til dansk medicinalhistorie. Dansk-norsk-svenske læger og kirurger.* København og Kristiania: Gyldendalske Boghandel og Nordisk Forlag, 1912.

Carøe, K. "Kirurger i Norges købsteder 1720". *Tidsskrift for Den norske lægeforening,* (1917):486–493.

Carøe, K. "Norges kirurger 1776". *Tidsskrift for Den norske lægeforening,* (1918):1–13.

Casey, E. S. "The Place of Space in The Birth of the Clinic," *The Journal of Medicine and Philosophy*, 12(1987):351–356.

Castberg, F. *Minner om politikk og vitenskap fra årene 1900–1970.* Oslo: Universitetsforlaget, 1971.

Castiglioni, A. *A History of Medicine.* Translated and edited by E. B. Krumbhaar. New York: Alfred A. Knopf, 1941.

Cella, D. F., D. S. Tulsky, B. Sarafin, C. R. Thomas Jr, and C. R. Thomas Sr. "Culturally relevant smoking prevention for minority youth," *Journal of School Health*, 62(1992):377–380.

Chadwick, E. *Report of an Inquiry into the Sanitary Conditions of the Labouring Population of Great Britain.* Edinburgh 1842. Quoted in Rethinking Community Medicine, London: Department of Community Medicine, Guy's Hospital Medical School, 1979.

Chapman, C. B. "The Flexner Report by Abraham Flexner," *Dædalus*, 103(1974): 105–117.

Cherniss, C. *Professional burnout in the human service organizations.* New York: Praeger, 1980.

Cherniss, C. *Staff burnout: Job stress in the human services.* Beverly Hills: Sage, 1980.

Chernomas, R. "An Economic Basis for the Proletarianization of Physicians," *International Journal of Health Services*, 16(1986): 669–674.

Cherry, S. "The Hospitals and Population Growth: The Vouluntary General Hospitals, Mortality and Local Populations in the English Provinces in the Eighteenth and Nineteenth Centuries, Part 1" *Population Studies*, 34(1980):59–75.

Cherry, S. "The Hospitals and Population Growth: The Vouluntary General Hospitals, Mortality and Local Populations in the English Provinces in the Eighteenth and Nineteenth Centuries, Part 2," *Population Studies*, 34(1980):251–265.

Cherubini, A. *Medici Scrittori d'Europa e d'America*. Roma: 1990.

Child, J. and J. Falk. "Maintenance of Occupational Control: The Case of Professions," *Work and Occupations*, 9(1982):155–192.

Chitnis, A. C. "Medical education in Edinburgh, 1790–1826, and some Victorian social consequences," *Medical History*, 17(1973):173–185.

Christensen, T. *Politisk styring og faglig uavhengighet*. Oslo: TANO, 1994.

Christie, V.M. *Hesitant about being seen as ill – The case of the doctor*, lecture given at the British Sociological Association's Medical sociology group conference at York University September, 1995.

Christie, V. M. *Den andre medisinen*. Oslo: Universitetsforlaget, 1991.

Christoffersen, N. "Distriktslægerne, særlig nordpaa." *Tidsskrift for Den norske lægeforening*, (1918):414–416.

Christoffersen, N. "Distriktslægers bopæl i eller utenfor by," *Tidsskrift for Den norske lægeforening*, (1920):188–190.

Christoffersen, N. "En fylkeslæges gjøremål," *Tidsskrift for Den norske lægeforening*, (1938):1031–1033.

Christophersen, H.O. *Eilert Sundt, en dikter i kjensgjerninger.* Oslo: Gyldendal Norsk forlag, 1962.

Clarke, E. ed. *Modern Methods in the History of Medicine*. London: Athlone Press, 1971.

Clemente, F. "The measurement problem in the analysis of an ecological concept: the division of labor," *Pacific Sociological Review*, 15(1972):30–40.

Clendering, L. *Source Book of Medical History*. New York: 1942.

Clouser, K.D. and G. Bernard. "A Critique of Principlism," *The Journal of Medicine and Philosophy*, 2(1990):219–236.

Coburn, D. "State authority, medical dominance and trends in the regulation of the health professions: the Ontario case." *Social Science and Medicine*, 37 (1993): 841–850.

Cochrane, A. *Effectiveness and Efficiency: Random Reflections on Health Services*. London: Nuffield Provincial Hospitals Trust, 1972.

Cogan, M. L. "Toward a Definition of Profession," *Harvard Educational Review*, 23 (1953):35–50.

Cohen, A. "Care of the care-givers," *Medical Journal of Australia*, 1(1984):520–523.

Coker, R. E., J. Kosa, B. G. Greenberg, K. W. Back, T. G. Donnelly, N. Miller, and F. S. McConnell. "Medical Careers in Public Health," *Milbank Memorial Fund Quarterly: Health and Society*, 44(1966): 143–258.

Cole-Kelly, K. "Illness and patient care in

the family practice setting," *Family Medicine*, 24(1992):45–48.

Collins, R. "Functional and conflict theories of educational stratification," *American Sociological Review*, 36(1971):1002–1019.

Collins, R. *The credential society*. New York: Academic Press, 1979.

Condrau, F. "Lungenheilstätten im internationalen Vergleich. Zur Sozialgeschichte der Tuberkulose im 19. und fröhen 20. Jahrhundert," *Historia Hospitalium*,19 (1996):221–235.

Conk, M. A. "Occupational Classification in the United States Census: 1870–1940," *The Journal of Interdisciplinary History*, 9(1978):111–130.

Conrad, P. "Types of medical social control," *Sociology of Health & Illness*, 1(1979): 1–11.

Conrad, P. "Medicalization and social control," *Annual Review of Sociology*, 18 (1992):209–232.

Conrad, P. and R. Kern. ed. *The Sociology of Health and Illness*. New York: St. Martin's Press, 1986.

Conrad, P. and J. Schneider. "Looking at levels of medicalization: a comment of Strong's critique of the thesis of medical imperialism," *Social Science and Medicine*, 14A(1980):75–79.

Conrad, P. and J. Schneider. *Deviance and Medicalization: From Badness to Sickness*. St. Louis: Mosby, 1980.

Conrad, P. and D. C. Walsh. "The new corporate health ethic: lifestyle and the social control of work," *International Journal of Health Services*, 22(1992):89–111.

Conradi, A. C. "Cholera i Christiania og Omegn 1853," *Norsk Magazin for Lægevidenskaben*, (1854):433–460.

Conradi, A. C. "Om Sykelighetsforholdene og Sygdomsconstitutionerne i Christiania". *Norsk Magazin for Lægevidenskaben*, (1860).

Conrads, N. "Politische und staatsrechtlichte Probleme der Kavalierstour," in *Reiseberichte als Quellen europäischer Kulturgeschichte. Aufgaben und Möglichkeiten der historischen Reiseforschung*, eds. Maczak, A. and H. J. Teuteberg. Herzog August Bibliothek Wolfenbüttel, 1982.

Cooper, C. L., U. Rout, and B. Faragher. "Mental health, job satisfaction, and job stress among general practitioners," *British Journal of Medicine*, 298(1989): 366–370.

Corfield, P. "Georgian Bath: The Magical Meeting Place," *History Today*, 40(1990): 26–33.

Couburn, D. "Freidson Then and Now: An "Internalist" Critique of Freidson's Past and Present Views of the Medical Profession," *International Journal of Health Services*, 22(1992):497–512.

Cousins, N. ed. *The Physician in Medicine*. Philadelphia: Saunders, 1982.

Crawford, R. "Individual Responsibility and Health Politics in the 1970s," in *Health Care in America. Essays in Social History*, eds. Reverby, S. and D. Rosner. Philadelphia: Temple University Press, 1979.

Crawford, R. "Healthism and the medicalization of everyday life," *International Journal of Health Services*, 10(1980): 365–388.

Crow, G. "The Use of the Concept of "Strategy" in Recent Sociological Literature," *Sociology*, 23(1989):1–24.

Curtoni, S. *European investigation on the number of medical doctors and of students admitted in the faculties of medicine,* AMSE Newsletter, April: 1994.

Dahl, H.F. *Vidkun Quisling – En fører for fall. Vol II.* Oslo: Aschehoug, 1992.

Dahle, R. "Inntrengere eller nyskapere. Flere kvinnelige leger?" *Tidsskrift for Den norske lægeforening*,113(1993):2597–2600.

Dahle, T. "Om utdannelse og lønsforhold for amtsykehusenes pleiepersonale," *Medicinsk Revue*, (1913):586–591.

Dahle, R. Arbeidsdeling – makt – identitet. Trondheim: Institutt for sosialt arbeid, Universitetet i Trondheim, 1990.

Danchertsen, J. C. "Febris recurrens i Vadsø Lægedistrikt i 1858–1861," *Norsk Magazin for Lægevidenskaben*, (1865): 746–751.

Dannevig, L. H. "Det militærmedisinske selskap i Oslo 1923–1932," *Norsk Tidsskrift for Militærmedisin*, (1930):45–53.

Davey Smith, G. and M. Egger. "Socioeconomic differentials in wealth and health," *British Medical Journal*, 307 (1993):1085–1086.

Davies, C. "Professionals in Bureaucracies: the Conflict Thesis Revisited," in *The Sociology of the Professions: Lawyers, Doctors and Others*, eds. Dingwall, R. and P. Lewis. London: Macmillan, 1983.

Davison, C., S. Frankel, and G. D. Smith. "The limits of lifestyle: Re-assessing "fatalism" in the popular culture of illness prevention," *Social Science and Medicine*, 34(1992):675–685.

Dawe, A. "The two sociologies," *The British Journal of Sociology*, 21(1970):207–218.

De Beer, E. S. "The Development of the Guide-Book until the Early Nineteenth Century," *Journal of the British Archaelogical Society*, 15(1952):35–46.

Dedichen, H. A. T. "Lægen før og nu," *Tidsskrift for Den norske lægeforening*, (1932):720–725.

Dedichen, H. G. "Norsk helsetjeneste i Storbritannia under krigen 1940–45", *Nordisk medicinhistorisk årsbok* (København 1945):189–198.

Degré, M. et al. (eds). *Medisinsk mikrobiologi.* Oslo: Universitetsforlaget, 1994.

Delamothe, T. "Social inequalities in health." *British Medical Journal* 303 (1991): 1046–1050.

Den norske Patologforening. *Årsrapport for 1994.* International Academy of Pathology, Norwegian Division.

Dent, K. S. "Travel as Education: the English Landed Classes in the Eighteenth Century," *Educational Studies*, 1(1975): 171–180.

Denzin, N. K. and C. J. Mettlin. "Incomplete professionalization: the case of pharmacy," *Social Forces*, 46(1968):375–381.

Derber, C. "The proletarianization of the professional: A review essay," in *Professionals as workers: Mental labor in advanced capitalism*, ed. Derber, C. Boston: G. K. Hall, 1982.

Derber, C. "Sponsorship and the control of physicians," *Theory and Society*, 12(1983): 561–601.

Derber, C., W. A. Schwartz, and Y. Magrass. *Power in the Highest Degree: Professionals and the Rise of a New Mandarin Order.* New York: Oxford University Press, 1990.

de Solla Price, D. J. "The development and structure of the biomedical literature," In: Warren K. S., ed. *Coping with the biomedical literature.* New York: Praeger, 1981:3–16.

de Solla Price, D. J. *Science since Babylon.* New Haven, Connecticut: Yale University Press, 1961.

Det medisinske fakultet, Universitetet i Oslo. *Orientering vedrørende spørsmål om medisinsk studium i utlandet med henblikk på å oppnå tillatelse til å utøve legevirksomhet i Norge,* 1. October 1954.

Det medisinske fakultet, Universitetet i Tromsø, "Opptaksstatistikker 1976–96."

Deutche Akademi der naturforscher Leopolding zu Halle (Saale). Gegn 1652 in Schweinfurt. Struktur und mitgliederbestand vom 1. Januar 1987. Mit einem alphabetichen Mitgleiderverzeichis 1652–1986. 1987.

Dibble, V. K. "Occupations and Ideologies," *The American Journal of Sociology*, 68(1962):229–241.

Digby, A. *Making a medical living.* Cambridge: Cambridge University Press, 1994.

Digby, A. "Quantitative and Qualitative Perspectives on the Asylum," in *Problems and Methods in the History of Medicine*, eds. Porter, R. and A. Wear. Beckenham: Croom Helm Ltd, 1987.

Dingwall, R. "Introduction," in *The Sociology of the Professions: Lawyers, Doctors and*

Others, eds. Dingwall, R. and P. Lewis. London: Macmillan, 1983.

Dingwall, R. "Accomplishing profession," *Sociological Review*, 24(1976):331–349.

Dingwall, R. ed. *Health Care and Health Knowledge*. London: Croom Helm, 1977.

Dingwall, R. "'In the Beginning Was the Work...' Reflections on the Genesis of Occupations," *Sociological Review*, 31 (1983):605–624.

Dingwall, R. and P. Fenn. ""A respectable profession"? Sociological and economic perspectives on the regulation of professional services," *International Review of Law and Economics*, 7(1987):51–64.

Dingwall, R. "Atrocity Stories" and Professional Relationships," *Sociology of Work and Occupations*, 4(1977):371–396.

Dodd, P. "The Views of Travellers: Travel Writing in the 1930s," in *The Art of Travel. Essays on Travel Writing*, ed. Dodd, P. London: Frank Cass & Co. Ltd, 1982.

Dolby, R. G. A. "The transmission of science," *History of Science*, 15(1977):1–43.

Domenighetti, G. and S. Berthoud. "Les medicins sont-ils aussi malades?" *Schweizerische Medizinische Wochenschrift*, 114(1984):858–873.

Donnison, J. *Midwives and Medical Men. A History of Inter-Professional Rivalries and Women's Rights*. London: 1977.

Douglas, M. *Risk and blame*. London: Routledge, 1992.

Dowe, A. "The two sociologists," *British Journal of Sociology*, 21(1970)

Drachman, V.G. "The limits of progress. The professional lives of women doctors 1881–1926." *Bulletin of the History of Medicine* 60 (1986): 58–72.

Draper, P. and T. Smart. "Social science and health policy in the United Kingdom: some contributions of the social sciences to the bureaucratization of the National Health Service," *International Journal of Health Services*, 4(1974)

Drejer, P.M. "Om dødelighet på barselseng i Norge", *Norsk Magazin for Lægevidenskaben*, (1907):600–627.

Drobniewski, F. "Why did Nazi doctors break their "hippocratic" oaths?" *Journal of the Royal Society of Medicine*, 86 (1993): 541–543.

Dublin, L. I. and M. Spiegelman. "The Longevity and Mortality of American Physicans, 1938–1942: A Preliminary Report." *The Journal of the American Medical Association*, 134(1947):1211–1215.

Duman, D. "The creation and diffusion of a professional ideology in nineteenth century England," *Sociological Review*, 27(1979):113–138.

Dumesil, R. and H. Schadewaldt. *Die Berühmten Ärzte*. Köln: 1989.

Dupree, M. W. and A. M. Crowther. "A profile of the medical profession in Scotland in the early twentieth century: The Medical Directory as a historical source," *Bulletin of the History of Medicine*, 65 (1991):209–233.

Eade, J. "Pilgrimage and tourism at Lourdes, France," *Annals of Tourism Research*, 19(1992):18–32.

Ebbesen. "Om en Hösten 1855 foretagen videnskabelig Reise til en Deel af Tysklands Bade samt en Sammenstilling mellem disse og Sandefjords Bad," *Norsk Magazin for Lægevidenskaben* (1856):217–249.

Eckhoff, T. "Vitenskap, profesjoner og klienter," in *Nordisk Forum 1967*, Roskilde: Roskilde Universitetsforlag, 1967.

Edvardsen, P. *Ortopediens historie i Norge*. Helsingfors: Nordisk Ortopedisk Förening 1919–1979, ky Printaes Kb, 1978.

Edwards, G. M. Encyclopaedia Britannica. *Britannica Book of the Year*. Chicago, Auckland, London, Madrid, Manila, Paris, Roma, Seoul, Sydney, Tokyo and Toronto, 1996.

Egeland, M. *Med kunnskap skal landet bygges. Universitetsforlaget 1950–1990*. Oslo: Universitetsforlaget, 1996.

Ehrenrich, B. and D. English. *Witches, mid-*

wives & nurses. London: Writers and Readers Publishing Coopertive, 1976.

Einbu, S. and O. Skotte. *Lesja. Litt frå den kommunale soga 1838–1938.* Lesja: Lesja kommune, 1949.

Eisenberg, L. "Disease and illness: distinction between professional and popular ideas of sickness," *Culture, Medicine, and Psychiatry*, 1(1977):9–23.

Ekman, S. and Grimnes, O. K. *Broderfolk i ufredstid.* Oslo: Universitetsforlaget, 1991.

Eknes, K. G. and I.S. Kristiansen. "Tilgang på leger i Norge. Bør vi øke utdanningen av medisinere?" *Tidsskrift for Den norske lægeforening*, 111(1991):723–726.

Eldjarn, K. "Pasienters rett til medbestemmelse," *Tidsskrift for Den norske lægeforening*, 29(1995):3663.

Elling, R.H. "Theory and Method for the cross-national study of health systems." *International Journal of Health Services* 24 (1994): 285–309.

Elliot, P. *The sociology of professions.* London: Macmillan, 1972.

Elliot, P. "Professional ideology and social situation," *Sociological Review*, 21(1973): 211–228.

Elstad, J. I. "Legene og samfunnet," *Tidsskrift for Samfunnsforskning*, (1987):290–302.

Elstad, J. I. "Health Services and Desentralized Government: The Case of Primary Health Services in Norway," *International Journal of Health Services*, 20(1990):545–559.

Elstad, J. I. "Tre konstruksjonistiske teser i helse- og sykdomssosiologien," *Sosiologisk tidsskrift*, 1(1993):69–76.

Elster, T. *Rikets hospital.* Oslo: Aschehoug, 1990.

Elston, M. A. "Women doctors in a changing profession: the case of Britain," in *Gender, Work and Medicine: Women and the Medical Division of Labour*, eds. Riska, E. and K. Wegar. London: SAGE, 1993.

Emblem, T., T. Syvertsen and Ø. Stenersen. *Cappelens historieverk.* Oslo: Cappelens Forlag, 1983.

Engelhardt, H. J. "The disease of masturbation: values and the concept of disease," *Bulletin of the History of Medicine*, 48 (1974)

Engelsen, R. "Mortalitetsdebatten og sosiale skilnader i mortalitet," *Historisk Tidsskrift*, (1987):161–202.

Engelstad, F. "Arbeidet," in *Det norske samfunn*, eds. Alldön, L., N. Rogoff Ramsøy and M. Vaa. Oslo: Gyldendal Norske Forlag, 1986.

Engle, R. L. and B. J. Davis. "Medical Diagnosis, Present, Past and Future," *Archives of Internal Medicine*, 102(1963):512–519.

Engsig, A., B. Ø. Jensen, M. Johansson, K. Mogensen, M. Nordentoft and A. Winther. *Yngre lægers arbejds- og livsvilkår.* Rapport fra Socialpolitisk arbeidsgruppe. København: Foreningen af yngre læger, 1990.

Erichsen, S. Morgenbladet, 12. april 1934.

Erichsen, V. "State traditions and medical professionalization in Scandinavia," in *Health professions and the state in Europe*, eds. Johnson, T. G. Larkin, and M. Saks. London: Routledge, 1995.

Ericsson, K. *Den tvetydige omsorgen. Sinnsykevesenets utvikling – et sosialpolitisk eksempel.* Oslo: Universitetsforlaget, 1974.

Eriksen, L. *Oslo Sanitetsforenings Revmatismesykehus 1938–1988.* Oslo: NKS, 1988.

Eriksen, T.B. "Hippokrates i dag?" *Samtiden* 5 (1991): 2–14.

Eriksen, T. B. "Helse i hver dråpe. Innspill om Etikk, kunnskap og omsorg." Oslo: Universitetsforlaget, 1995,

Ertesvaag, E. *Bergen bys historie, bind 3.* Bergen: Universitetsforlaget, 1982.

Eskeland, M., S. Fønnebø Knutsen and A. Forsdahl. "Legekårsundersøkelsen 1993: Legemangel – svangerskaps- og omsorgspermisjoner," submitted 1995.

Eskerud, J. R. *Studies on fever: Clinical aspects in general practice, perception, self-care, and information. Thesis.* Oslo: Department of

General Practice, and Department of Pharmacotherapeutics, University of Oslo, 1995.

Esmarch, L., and J. Utheim. *Oversigt over Det norske civile Lægevesens historiske utvikling og nuværende ordning.* Supplements to Odelstingsprop. 39, 1911. Ministry of Justice 1911.

Eulner, H.H. *Die Entwicklung der medizinischen Spezialfächer an den Universitäten des deutschen Sprachgebietes.* Stuttgart: Enke, 1970.

Evaluering av hovedinnsatsområdet helse-, miljø- og levekårsforskning (HEMIL). Oslo: NAVF, 1991

Evang, A. *Verdier som kompass. Om personlighet, samfunn og fremtid.* Oslo: J.W.Cappelen forlag, 1991.

Evang, K. "Noen aktuelle oppgaver ved gjenreisningen av den norske folkehelsen og det norske helsevesen," *Tidsskrift for Den norske lægeforening*, 8(1945).

Evang, K. "Public Health" – sosial og administrativ medisin," *Tidsskrift for Den norske lægeforening*, 20(1953).

Evang, K. "Helsestellets utvikling i Norge i 75 år," *Tidsskrift for Den norske lægeforening*, 2(1955).

Evang, K. *Health Service, Society, and Medicine.* London: Oxford University Press, 1960.

Evang, K. "Den spesialsakkyndiges plass i helseadministrasjonen," *Läkartidningen*, 36(1965).

Evang, K. *Helse og samfunn.* Oslo: Gyldendal, 1974.

Evang, K. "Følger medisinutdannelsen med i samfunnsutviklingen?" *Nordisk Medicin*, 91(1976):137–139.

Evang, K. *Health Services in Norway.* Oslo: Universitetsforlaget, 1976.

Fabrega, H. "The ethnography of illness," *Social Science and Medicine*, 13A(1979): 565–576.

Fabritius, H. F. "Sanitetsarbeidet i Sverige under krigen", *Nordisk Medicin,* 37 (1948):545.

Falkenberg, J. E. "Lægevesenets eventuelle omordning," *Tidsskrift for Den norske lægeforening*, (1901):1368–1372.

Falkenberg, J. E. "Omordningen av det civile lægevesen," *Tidsskrift for Den norske lægeforening*, (1903):571–581.

Falkenberg, J. E. "I diskussionen om "Lægevesenets omordning"," *Tidsskrift for Den norske lægeforening*, (1904):185–186.

Falkum, E. *Sykdomsoppfatning, helseomsorg og samfunn.* Oslo: Universitetsforlaget, 1978.

Falkum, E. "Helsebegrepet i spenningsfeltet mellom deskripsjon og vurdering." *Tidsskrift for Den norske lægeforening*, 113(1993): 3470–3474.

Falkum, E. and Ø. Larsen. *Helseomsorgens vilkår. Linjer i medisinsk sosialhistorie.* Oslo: Universitetsforlaget, 1981.

Farnes, O. *Lege på mange fronter.* Oslo: Dreyer, 1982.

Farr, R. M. "Heider, Harré and Herzlich on health and illness: Some observations on the structure of 'représentations collectives'," *European Journal of Social Psychology*, 7(1977):491–504.

Fauske, H. "Profesjonene – Bremsekloss eller syndebukk," *FAFO*, 118(1991).

Faye, F.C. "Om Forholdene ved flere af Udlandets Hospitals-Indretninger, hovedsagelige dem for Qvinder og Börn." *Norsk Magazin for Lægevidenskaben*, 4 (1850)1–43 and 65–112.

Faye, F.C. "Om de hygieniske Forholde vedkommende Fødsel og Barselseng med særligt Hensyn Resultaterne i flere af Udlandets Fødselsstiftelser". *Norsk Magazin for Lægevidenskaben,* 22 (1868) 193–227 and 265–312.

Faye, F.C. "Nogle Bemærkninger i Anledning af et i Magazinets Novemberhefte f. A. optaget Brev fra Udlandet vedkommende Læren om Fødsel og Födselshjelp," *Norsk Magazin for Lægevidenskaben*, (1869):109–124.

Fee, E. and D. Porter. "Public health, preventive medicine and professionalization:

England and America in the nineteenth century," in *Medicine in society. Historical essays*, ed. Wear, A. Cambridge: Cambridge University Press, 1992.

Fichtner, G. and H. Siefert. *Medizinhistoriche Reisen. 2: Padua*. Stuttgart: 1978.

Fiorentine, R. and S. Cole. "Why Fewer Women Become Physicians: Explaining the Premed Persistence Gap," *Sociological Forum*, 7(1992):469–496.

Fischer, A. *Grundriss des sozialen Hygiene. Zweite Auflage.* Karlsruhe: C.F. Möller, 1925.

Fischer, A. *Geschichte des deutschen Gesundheitswesens I–II.* Berlin: Urban & Schwarzenberg, 1933, new edition: Hildesheim: Olms, 1965.

Fischer-Homberger, E. "Hypochondriasis of the eighteenth century – neurosis of the present century," *Bulletin of the History of Medicine*, 46(1972):391–401.

Fletcner, A. *Medical Education in the United States and Canada.* New York: Carnegie Foundation, 1910. (Bulletin No. 4)

Flexner, A. *Medical Education in Europe.* New York: Carnegie Foundation, 1912. (Bulletin no. 6).

Flexner, A. *Medical Education: A Comparative Study*. New York: The Macmillan Company, 1925.

Flexner, A. *Universities: American, English, German*. New York: Oxford University Press, 1930.

Flood. A.B. and M-L- Fennell. "Through the lenses of organizational sociology: The role of organizational theory and research in conceptualizing and examining our health care system." *Journal of Health and Social Behavior*, (1995):154–169.

Florelius, S. "Sanitetsoppsetningene ved de norske polititroppenes' feltavdelinger i Sverige", *Sanitetsnytt,* 11(1965).

Florelius, S., and J. H. Berner. *Norsk Militærmedisinsk Forening, Festskrift – 100 års jubileum 1882–1982.* Oslo:1982.

Flottorp, S. "Kvinnelige leger – Valg av spesialitet og karriere," *Tidsskrift for Den norske lægeforening*, 113 17(1993):2111–2116.

Fløgstad, K. *Kniven på strupen*. Oslo: Gyldendal Norsk Forlag, 1991.

Folkow, B. "History of physiology in Scandinavia," *Acta Physiol Scand,* 138(1990): 5–12.

Foreningen av yngre lægers socialpolitiske arbeidsgruppe. "Danske underordnede lægers arbejds- og livsvilkår," *Nordisk Medicin*, 106(1991):279–280.

Forhandlinger i Odelstinget, (1959–60):331–332.

Forsdahl, A. *Sunnhetstilstanden, hygieniske og sosiale forhold i Sør-Varanger 1869–1975 belyst ved medisinalberetningene. ISM skriftserie nr. 2.* Tromsø: Universitetet i Tromsø, Institutt for samfunnsmedisin, 1977.

Forsdahl, A. *Utdrag av medisinalberetninger fra Finnmark 1863–1929*. Fylkeslegen i Finnmark, 1991.

Forsdahl, A., "Utdrag av medicinalberetninger fra Sulitjelma 1891–1990". *ISM Skriftserie nr. 27,* University of Tromsø, Institute for Social Medicine, Tromsø, 1993.

Forster, M. M. "Mineral springs and miracles," *Canadian Family Physician*, 40 (1994):729–737.

FoU-statistikk og indikatorer. Forskning og utviklingsarbeid 1995 (R&D Statistics – Science and Technology Indicators). Oslo: Utredningsinstituttet, 1994.

Foucault, M. *Power/Knowledge: Selected Interviews and Other Writings*. New York: 1972.

Foucault, M. *The Birth of the Clinic*. London: Tavistock, 1973. Fox, D. M. "The Decline of Historicism: The Case of Compulsory Health Insurance in the United States," *Bulletin of the History of Medicine*, 57(1983):596–610.

Fox, J. and C. Suschnigg. "A note on gender and the prestige of occupations," *Canadian Journal of Sociology*, 14(1989):353–

360.

Fox, R. C. "Training for uncertainty. The Student-Physician," in *Introductory studies in the Sociology of Medical Education*, eds. Merton, Reader, and Kendall. Harvard: Harvard University Press, 1957.

Fox, R. C., E.E.W. Goss, M.J. Huntington, et al. "The Student-Physician. Introductory studies in the socilogy of medical education." Cambridge: Harvard University Press, 1957. 1–360.

Fox, R. C. "The medicalization and de-medicalization of American society," *Dædalus*, 106(1977):9–22.

Fox, R. C. *Essays in Medical Sociology: Journeys Into the Field*. New York: John Wiley & Sons, 1979.

Fox, R. C. "The Evolution of Medical Uncertainty," *Milbank Memorial Fund Quarterly: Health and Society*, 58(1980):1–49.

Fox, R. C. "The sociology of medicine: A participant observer's view." Prentice – Hall, Inc. 1989.

Fra *Norsk Etnografisk Samlings* spørreskjemaer: "Folkemedisin" (emnenr. 80, 1960) Questionnaires.

Frank, J.P. "Biography," in *History of Medicine*, ed. Rosen, 3(1948):11–46 and 279–314.

Frank, J.P. *System einer vollständigen medisinischen Polizey.* I: Mannheim: Schwan, 1779. II: Mannheim: Schwan, 1780. III: Mannheim: Schwan, 1783. IV: Mannheim: Schwan, 1788. V: Töbingen: Cotta, 1813. VI: Wien: Schaumburg, 1817.

Frankenau, R. *Det offentlige Sundhedspolitie under en oplyst Regiering*. Kiøbenhavn: S. Poulsen, 1801.

Freddi, G. and J. W. Björkman. eds. *Controlling Medical Professionals: The Comparative Politics of health Governance*. Newbury Park CA: Sage, 1989.

Freedman, M. *Labor markets: Segments and shelters*. Montclair, NJ: Allanheld, Osmun, 1976.

Freidson, E. ed. *The Professions and Their Prospects*. Beverly Hills, CA: Sage, 1973.

Freidson, E. *Professional Dominance: The Social Structure of Medical Care*. New York: Atherton Press, 1970.

Freidson, E. "Professionals and amateurs in the welfare state," in *Applied Research and Structural Change in Modern Society*, ed. Kjølsrød, L. Oslo: Institute of Applied Research, 1987.

Freidson, E. "Knowledge and the Practice of Sociology," *Sociological Forum*, 1(1986): 684–700.

Freidson, E. *Professional Powers: A Study of the Institutionalization of Formal Knowledge*. Chicago: University of Chicago Press, 1986.

Freidson, E. *Profession of Medicine: A Study in the Sociology of Applied Knowledge*. Chicago: University of Chicago Press, 1970.

Freidson, E. *Profession of Medicine.* New York: Dodd-Mead, 1970.

Freidson, E. *Doctoring Together: A Study of Professional Social Control*. New York: Elsevier, 1975.

Freidson, E. "The Theory of Professions: State of the Art," in *The Sociology of the Professions: Lawyers, Doctors and Others*, eds. Dingwall, R. and P. Lewis. London: Macmillan, 1983.

Freidson, E. "Viewpoint: Sociology and Medicine: A Polemic," *Sociology of Health & Illness*, 5(1983):208–219.

Freidson, E. "The changing nature of professional control," *Annual Review of Sociology*, 10(1984):1–20.

Freidson, E. *Professionalism Reborn. Theory, Prophecy and Policy.* UK: Polity Press, 1994.

Freidson, E. "Are professions necessary?" in *The authority of experts: Studies in history and theory*, ed. Haskell, T. L. Bloomington, IN: University of Indiana Press, 1984.

Freidson, E. "Occupational autonomy and labor market shelters," in *Varieties of work*, eds. Stewart, P. and M. Cantor. Beverly Hills, CA: Sage, 1982.

Freidson, E. "The division of labour as social interaction," *Social Problems*, 23(1976): 304–313.

Freidson, E. "The deprofessionalization of everyone?" *Sociological Focus*, 3(1975): 197–213.

Freidson, E. "Professionalization and the organization of middle-class labor in post-industrial society," *Sociological Review Monograph*, 20(1973):47–59.

Freidson, E. "The Reorganization of the Professions by Regulation," *Law and Human Behavior*, 7(1983):279–290.

Freidson, E. "The Reorganization of the Medical Profession," *Medical Care Review*, 442(1985):11–35.

Frich, O. "Fra et studieopphold i Kønigsberg in/Pr," *Norsk Magazin for Lægevidenskaben*, (1900):1273–1283.

Fruton, J. S. *A Bio-bibliography. For the History of the Biochemical Sciences Since 1800*. Philadelphia: American Philosophical Society, 1982.

Frølich, A. *Norges første kvinnelige leger 1893–1920*. Bergen: Universitetet i Bergen, 1984

Fugelli, P. *Pasienten Norge*. Oslo: J.W. Cappelen forlag, 1994.

Fugelli, P. "Med Rudolf Ludwig Karl Virchow som veiviser inn i den nye samfunnsmedisinen," *Tidsskrift for Den norske lægeforening*, 115(1995):1091–1094.

Fugelli, P., B. Ingstad, and Ø. Larsen. *Den norske helse- og sykdomskulturen. Argumenter for og skisse til et forskningsprogram*. Oslo: Instituttgruppe for samfunnsmedisinske fag, 1995.

Fugelli, P. and K. Johansen. eds. *Langsomt blir faget vårt eget*. Oslo: Universitetsforlaget, 1984.

Fugelli, P. and K. Malterud. "Den utbrente legen," in *Medicinsk årbog*, København: Munksgaard, 1989.

Fugelli, P. and M. Nylenna. eds. *Kunnskap er makt – og bør deles med andre*. Oslo: Universitetsforlaget, 1987.

Fulsås, N. *Universitetet i Tromsø 25 år*. Tromsø: Universitetet i Tromsø, 1993.

Furre, B. *Norsk historie 1905–1940*. Oslo: Det Norske Samlaget, 1972.

Furre, B. *Soga om Lars Oftedal*. Oslo: Det Norske Samlaget, 1990.

Fye, W. B. "Medical authorship: Traditions, trends, and tribulations," *Ann Intern Med*, 113(1990):317–325.

Fye, W. B. "The History of Medicine: An Annotated List of Key Reference Works," *Annals of Internal Medicine*, 118 (1993):59–62.

Fyrand, O. *Legen – i teknikkens eller menneskets tjeneste*. Oslo: Gyldendal, 1992.

Førde, R. "Pasientautonomi", *Tidsskrift for Den norske lægeforening*, 20(1995):2568–2570.

Førde, R. "Har Illich fått rett? Skaper risikofokuseringen i medisinen uhelse?" *Norsk Medicin*, 111(1996):113–115.

Gabe, J., M. Calnan, and M. Bury. eds. *The Sociology of the Health Service*. London: Routledge, 1991.

Galbraith, J. K. *Den tilfredse majoritet*. Oslo: Gyldendal Norsk Forlag, 1992.

Galdstone, I. "Diagnosis in historical perspective," *Bulletin of the History of Medicine*, 9(1941):367–384.

Galdstone, I. *Social Medicine – Its Derivations and Objectives*. New York: The Commonwealth Fund, 1949.

Gallagher, E. B. and B. Ferrante. "Medicalization and social justice," *Social Justice Research*, 1(1987):377–392.

Ganster, D. "A review of research in the workplace," in *Job control and worker health*, eds. Sauter, S. L. J. J. Hurrell, and C. C. Cooper. New York: Wiley, 1989.

Garrison, F. H. *An Introduction to the History of Medicine*. 4th ed. Philadelphia and London: W.B. Saunders, 1960.

Gaustad, I. *Arbeiderklassen på Hedemarken 1850–1900*. Hovedfagsoppgave i historie. Oslo: Universitetet i Oslo, 1935.

Gay, R. "A Spa in Germany: Tepida, Tenuissima, Simplicissima," *American Scholar*, 56(1987):549–556.

Gedde-Dahl, T. M. "På helsa løs. En leges opplevelser i det tyvende århundre." Manuskript owned by the family, Oslo 1991.

Geirsvold, M. "Europeiske kvarantæneanstalter," *Norsk Magazin for Lægevidenskaben*, (1900):1248–1272.

Geirsvold, M. "Bergens sundhetsvæsen," in *Bergen 1814–1914*, eds. Geelmuyden, C. and H. Shetelig. Bergen: John Griegs Forlag, 1914.

Geison, G. L. ed. *Professions and the French State, 1700–1900*. Philadelphia: University of Pennsylvania Press, 1984.

Gelfand, T. "Medical Professionals and Charlatans," *Histoire sociale*, 11(1978): 62–97.

Gelfand, T. "The Annales and Medical Historiography: Bilan et Perspectives," in *Problems and Methods in the History of Medicine*, eds. Porter, R. and A. Wear. Beckenham: Croom Helm Ltd, 1987.

Gelfand, T. "The history of the medical profession," in *Companion encyclopædia of the history of medicine*, eds. Bynum, W. F. and R. Porter. London: Routledge, 1993.

Gerhardt, U. "The Parsonian paradigm and the identity of medical sociology," *Sociological Review, 27(1979):229–251.*

Gerhardt, U. "Toward a critical analysis of role," *Social Problems*, 27(1980):556–569.

Gerhardt, U. *Ideas about Illness. An Intellectual and Political History of Medical Sociology.* New York: New York University Press, 1989.

Gerhardt, U. "Models of illness and the theory of society: Parsons' contribution to the early history of medical sociology," *International Sociology*, 5(1990):337–355.

Gerhardt, U. "Women's Role and Role Theory: A View from the Federal Republic of Germany," *Research in the Sociology of Health Care*, 9(1991):249–277.

Gerson, E. "The Social Character of Illness," *Social Science and Medicine*, 10(1976):219–224.

Gesler, W. M. "Therapeutic Landscapes: Medical Issues in light of the New Cultural Geography," *Social Science and Medicine*, 34(1992):735–746.

Getz, B. ed. *Norges Læger 1947–1951.* Oslo: H. Aschehoug & Co. (W. Nygaard), 1956.

Getz, B. ed. *Norges leger 1967.* Oslo: Den norske lægeforening, 1968.

Geyer-Kordesch, J. "Cultural habits of illness: The Enlightened and the Pious in eighteenth century Germany," in *Patients and practitioners. Lay perceptions of medicine in pre-industrial society*, ed. Porter, R. Cambridge: Cambridge University Press, 1985.

Geyer-Kordesch, J. "Georg Ernst Stahl's radical Pietist medicine and its influence on the German Enlightenment," in *The medical enlightenment of the eighteenth century*, eds. Cunningham, A. and R. French. Cambridge: Cambridge University Press, 1990.

Geyer-Kordesch, J. "Geschlecht und Gesellschaft: Die erste Ärztinnen und sozialpolitische Vorurteile," *Berichte zur Wissenschaftsgeschichte*, 10(1987):195–205.

Geyer-Kordesch, J. "Court physicians an State Regulation in Eighteenth-century Prussia: The emergence of medical science and the demystification of the body," in *Medicine at the Courts of Europe, 1500–1837*, ed. Nutton, V. London: Routledge, 1990.

Giddens, A. *The consequences of modernity*. Cambridge: Polity Press, 1992.

Gilb, C. L. *Hidden Hierarchies: The Professions and the Government*. New York: Harper & Row, 1966.

Gilje, N. and H. Grimen. *Samfunnsvitenskapenes forutsetninger. Innføring i samfunnsvitenskapenes vitenskapsfilosofi.* Oslo: Universitetsforlaget, 1993.

Gillon, R. "Medical ethics: four principles plus attention to scope." *British Medical Journal*, 309(1994):184–188.

Gjerset, K. and L. Hektoen. "Health conditions and the practice of medicine among the early Norwegian settlers, 1825–1865," *The Norwegian-American Historical Association: Studies and records*, I(1926): 1–59.

Gjersøe, N. W. "Skyds og diæt," *Tidsskrift for Den norske lægeforening*, (1895): 180–185, 275–278.

Gjersøe, N. W. "Om distriktlægers forhold til fattigpraksis etc." *Tidsskrift for Den norske lægeforening*, (1899):697–701.

Gjestland, H. "Voss pleiehjem for tuberkuløse," *Tidsskrift for Den norske lægeforening*, (1904):70–71.

Gjestland, H. "Om skyds og diæt," *Tidsskrift for Den norske lægeforening*, (1895): 413–414.

Gjør, H. "Beretning om en med Stipendium foretagen videnskabelig Reise," *Norsk Magazin for Lægevidenskaben*, (1859):857–889.

Gogstad, A. C. *Helse og hakekors*. Bergen: Alma Mater, 1991.

Gogstad, A. C. *Slange og Sverd*. Bergen: Alma Mater forlag, 1995.

Goldfinger, S. E. "A Matter of Influence," *New England Journal of Medicine*, 316(1987):1408–1409.

Goldner, F. H. and R. R. Ritti. "Professionalization as Career Immobility," *American Journal of Sociology*, 72(1967):489–502.

Goode, W. J., Jr. "Encroachment, charlatanism, and the emerging profession: psychology, medicine and sociology," *American Sociological Review*, 25(1960):902–914.

Goode, W. J. "Community within a community: The Professions," *American Sociological Review*, 22(1957):194–200.

Goodwin, C. "Professional Vision," *American Anthropologist*, 96(1994):606–633.

Göransson, S. *De svenska studieresorna och de religiösa kontrollen: Från reformationstiden till frihetstiden.* Uppsala: Appelbergs Boktryckeriaktiebolag, 1951.

Gotfredsen, E. *Medicinens Historie*. København: Nyt Nordisk Forlag Arnold Busck, 1973.

Gottstein, A. *Geschichte der Hygiene.* Berlin: F. Schneider & Co, 1901.

Goubert, J.-P. "Twenty Years On: Problems of Historical Methodology in the History of Health," in *Problems and Methods in the History of Medicine*, eds. Porter, R. and A. Wear. Beckenham: Croom Helm, 1987.

Gran, J. *Skizzer af Bergenske Forholde fra ældre og yngre Tid*. Bergen: 1873.

Granovetter, M. "Economic Action and Social Structure: The Problem of Embeddedness," *American Journal of Sociology*, 91(1985):481–510.

Granshaw, L. "The Hospital," in *Companion Encyclopœdia of the History of Medicine, Vol 2.*, eds. Bynum, W. F. and R. Porter. London: Routledge, 1993.

Granshaw, L. and R. Porter. eds. *The Hospital in History*. London and New York: Routledge, 1989.

Granshaw, L. "The rise of the modern hospital in Britain," in *Medicine in society. Historical essays*, ed. Wear, A. Cambridge: Cambridge University Press, 1992.

Gray, P. eds. *The medical annual, 1986. The yearbook of general practice*. Bristol: Wright, 1986.

Greenwood, E. "Attributes of a Profession," *Social Work*, 2(1957):45–55.

Grimnes, O. K. *Et flyktningesamfunn vokser frem*. Oslo: Aschehoug, 1969.

Grimnes, O. K. *Hjemmefrontens ledelse*. Oslo: Universitetsforlaget, 1977.

Groenewegen, P. P. and J. B. F. Hutten. "Workload and job satisfaction among general practitioners: A review of the literature," *Social Science and Medicine*, 32(1991):1111–1119.

Grotjahn, A. *Soziale Pathologie. Versuch einer Lehre von den sozialen Beziehungen der menschlichen Krankheiten als Grundlage der sozialen Medizin und der sozialen Hygiene.*

Berlin: August Hirschwald, 1912.

Grundt, E. "Hospiterende læger," *Tidsskrift for Den norske lægeforening*, (1913):76–78.

Grundt, E. "Hospiterende læger ved sykehus," *Tidsskrift for Den norske lægeforening*, (1912):924

Grøn, A.F. "Indberetning til Collegium academicum om en med Stipendium foretagen Reise til Paris og Wien i Aarene 1849 og 1850". *Norsk Magazin for Lægevidenskaben,* 4 (1852) 65–84.

Grøn, F. *Det Norske Medicinske Selskab 1833–1933. Festskrift til selskapets 100-års jubileum.* Oslo: 1933.

Grøn, F. "Konjunkturskatten og lægerne," *Tidsskrift for Den norske lægeforening*, (1920):122–123.

Grøn, F. *Det norske medicinske Selskab 1833–1933*. Oslo: Steenske boktrykkeri Johannes Bjørnstad a/s, 1933.

Grøn, F. "Den norske lægestand og utstillingen i 1914," *Tidsskrift for Den norske lægeforening*, (1912):835–836.

Guldvog, B. "Bunner helsetjenestens krise i ressurs- eller teorimangel?" T*idsskrift for Den norske lægeforening,* 113(1993):624–629.

Gundersen, G. "Influence of Norwegian Medicine in the United States during the past seventy-five years," *Tidsskrift for Den norske lægeforening*, Jubileumsnummer (1955):113–115.

Gussow, Z. *Leprosy, Racism, and Public Health. Social Policy in Chronic Disease Control.* Boulder, San Francisco, and London: Westview Press, 1989.

Gustin, B. H. "Charisma, Recognition, and the Motivation of Scientists," *American Journal of Sociology*, 5 78(1973):1119–1134.

Haas, J. and W. Shaffir. *Becoming Doctors: The Adoption of a Cloack of Competence*. Greenwich, Connecticut: Department of Sociology, McMaster University, 1987.

Habenstein, R. W. "Critique of "Profession" as a Sociological Category," *Sociological Quarterly*, 4(1963):291–300.

Habermas, J. *The philosophical discourse of modernity*. Cambridge: Polity Press, 1987.

Hafferty, F. W. "Theories at the Crossroads: A Discussion of Evolving Views on Medicine as a Profession," *Milbank Quarterly*, 66(1988):202–225.

Hafferty, F. W. and F. D. Wolinsky. "Conflicting characterizations of professional dominance," *Current Research on Occupations and Professions*, 6(1991):225–249.

Hafferty, F.W. and J.B. McKinlay. *The changing medical profession. An international perspective.* New York/Oxord: Oxford Univercity Press, 1993.

Hafferty, F. W. and J. B. McKinlay. *The changing character of the medical profession: An international perspective.* New York and Oxford: Oxford University Press, 1993.

Hafferty, F.W. and D.W. Light. "Professional dynamics and changing nature of medical work." *Journal of Health and Social Behavior* (1995): 132–153.

Hafstad, C. "Advarsel mot det medicinske studium," *Tidsskrift for Den norske lægeforening*, (1923):137–138.

Hafting, M. *Et eple om dagen – eldre småforbrukere av helsetjenester*. Oslo: TANO, 1995.

Hägerstrand, T. *Innovation diffusion as a spatial process*. Chicago: The University of Chicago Press, 1967.

Hahn, R. A. and D. G. Atwood. eds. *Physicians of Western Medicine: Anthropological Approaches to Theory and Practice*. Dordrecht: D. Reidel, 1985.

Hahn, R. A. *Sickness and healing. An anthropological Perspective*. London: Yale University Press, 1995.

Hall, O. "The stages of a medical career," *American Journal of Sociology*, 53(1948): 327–336.

Hall, O. "Types of medical careers," *American Journal of Sociology*, 55(1949):243–253.

Hall, A., T.C. Aw and J.M. Harrington. "Morbidity survey of post mortem room staff." *Journal of Clinical Pathology*, 44(1991):433–435.

Hall, R. H. "Professionalization and bureaucratization," *American Sociological Review*, 33(1968):97

Halpern, S. A. "Medicalization as a Professional Process: Postwar Trends in Pediatrics," *Journal of Health and Social Behavior*, 31(1990):28–42.

Halpern, S. A. and R. R. Anspach. "The Study of Medical Institutions: Eliot Freidson's Legacy," *Work and Occupations*, 20(1993):279–295.

Halvorsen, S. *På ungenes parti*. Oslo: Nikolai Olsens Trykkeri a.s., 1994.

Hamilton, B. "The medical professions in the Eighteenth century," *The Economic History Review*, 4(1951):141–169.

Hamlin, C. "Chemistry, medicine, and the legitimization of english spas, 1740–1840," *Medical History*, Supplement No.10(1990):67–81.

Hancock, T. "Healthy development and the community ecosystem: three ecological models," *Health Promotion International*, 8(1993):41–46.

Hansen, F. H. "Helsesektoren i velferdsstaten: kjempevekst og fordelingskrise," *Tidsskrift for Samfunnsforskning*, 20(1979).

Hansen, K. *Om Levemaaden under Lofotfisket*. Beretning om Sundhedstilstanden m.m. i Norge, 1864.

Hansen, K. *Bemærkninger i Anledning af Storsildfisket i Nordlands Amt og de hygiæniske Forholde derunder.* Beretning om Sundhedstilstanden m.m. i Norge, 1886.

Hansen, K. ed. *Lesebuch für Ärzte*. Berlin: 1950.

Hansen, L.I. K. *Koleraen i Christiania i 1853.* Oslo: 1986. Thesis.

Hansen, L. K. "Helsetidsskrifter," *Historisk Tidsskrift*, 3(1987):391–399.

Hanson, J. *Bidrag til Oplysning om Byen Christiansands medicinske Topographi og Historie.* Beretning om Sundhedstilstanden m.m. i Norge, 1858.

Hansson, R. S. "Den norske lægestand og Norges lægevæsen i hundredaaret 1814–1914," *Tidsskrift for Den norske lægeforening*, (1914):1137–1164.

Haraway, D. J. *Simians, cyborgs, and women. The reinvention of nature.* London: Free Association Books, 1991.

Harbsmeier, M. "Reisebeschreibungen als mentalitätsgeschichtliche Quellen: Überlegungen zu einer historisch-antropologischen Untersuchung frühneuzeitlicher deutscher Reisebeschreibungen," in *Reiseberichte als Quellen europäischer Kulturgeschichte. Aufgaben und Möglichkeiten der historischen Reiseforschung*, eds. Maczak, A. and H. J. Teuteberg. Herzog August Bibliothek Wolfenbüttel, 1982.

Harlem, O. K. "Tidsskriftet. En målsettingskavalkade," 106(1986):1269–1271.

Harley, D. "A sword in a madman's hand: Professional opposition to popular consumption in the waters literature of Southern England and the Midlands, 1570–1870," *Medical History*, Supplement No.10(1990):48–55.

Harré, R. "Knowledge," in *The ferment of knowledge. Studies in the Historiography of Eighteenth-Century Science*, eds. Rousseau, G. S. and R. Porter. Cambridge: Cambridge University Press, 1980.

Hart, N. "Inequalities in Health: The Individual versus the Environment," *Journal for the Royal Statistical Society*, 149(1986): 228–246.

Hauan, T. (MD. born 1909, cand.med. 1936) in interviews with Aina Schiøtz 27.06., 14.09., 03.12.94 and 03.08.95.

Haug, C. "Myter og forventninger. Konsekvenser av økt kvinneandel i legeyrket." *Tidsskrift for Den norske lægeforening*, 113 (1993):3225–3226.

Haug, K. "Distriktlægeembedernes lønningsforhold," *Tidsskrift for Den norske lægeforening*, (1911):458–459.

Haug, M. R. "Deprofessionalization: An alternative hypothesis for the future,"

Sociological Review Monograph, 20(1973): 195–211.

Haug, M. R. "The Deprofessionalization of Everyone?" *Sociological Focus*, 8(1975): 197–213.

Haug, M. R. "A Re-examination of the Hypothesis of Physician Deprofessionalization," *Milbank Quarterly*, 66(1988): 48–56.

Haug, M. R. "The Erosion of Professional Authority: A Cross-cultural Inquiry in the Case of the Physician," *Milbank Quarterly/Health and Society*, 54 (1976): 83–106.

Haug, M. R. and B. Lavin. "Practitioner or Patient: Who's in Charge?" *Journal of Health and Social Behavior*, 22(1981): 212–229.

Haug, M. R. and B. Lavin. *Consumerism in Medicine: Challenging Physician Authority*. Beverly Hills: Sage, 1983.

Haugholt, K. "Mor Sæther," *St Hallvard*, (1958):270–287.

Haugseth, K. "Avancementsforholdene for vore sykehuslæger," *Tidsskrift for Den norske lægeforening*, (1925):884–885.

Haukeland, J. V. *Internasjonal turisme. Historiske tilbakeblikk på – og noen drøftinger av – turismens utviklingstrekk*. Molde: Møre og Romsdal distriktshøgskole, 1986.

Haukeland, J. V. "Non-Travelers: The Flip Side of Motivation," *Annals of Tourism Research*, 17(1990):172–184.

Hawthorne, K., M. Mello, and S. Tomlinson. "Cultural and religious influences in diabetes care in Great Britain," *Diabetic Medicine*, 10(1993):8–12.

Hayes, M. V. "The Risk Approach: Unassailable Logic?" *Social Science and Medicine*, 33(1991):55–61.

Hayes, M. V. "On the Epistemology of Risk: Language, Logic and Social Science," *Social Science and Medicine*, 35(1992): 401–407.

Hearn, J. "Notes on patriarchy, professionalization and the semi-professions," *Sociology*, 16(1982):184–202.

Hedberg, D. "Om krav paa bedre lønsvilkaar ved lægeposter og vedkommende læges forhold til posten, da den overtoges." *Tidsskrift for Den norske lægeforening*, (1905):271

Hegbom, E. "De offentlige læger og dieten," *Tidsskrift for Den norske lægeforening*, (1932):1502–1506.

Hegbom, E. B. "Våre distriktslæger," *Tidsskrift for Den norske lægeforening*, (1932): 1498–1500.

Heiberg, C. "Udsigt over Christiania Lægeforenings Virksomhed i Aaret 1842," *Ugeskrift for Medicin og Pharmacie*, II (1843):29–30.

Heidenheimer, A. J. "Professional knowledge and state policy in comparative historical perspective: law and medicine in Britain, Germany and the United States," *International Social Science Journal*, 41(1989):529–553.

Heil, J. "Traces of things past," *Philosophy of Science*, 45(1978):60–72.

Helfer, O. and R. Winau. *Männer und Frauen der Medicin*. Berlin: 1986.

Helk, V. *Dansk-norske studierejser fra reformationen til enevældet 1536–1660: med en matrikel over studerende i udlandet*, Odense: Odense Universitetsforlag, 1987.

Helk, V. *Dansk-norske studierejser 1661–1813 bd I,* Odense: Odense Universitetsforlag, 1991.

Helk, V. *Dansk-norske studierejser 1661–1813 II. Matrikkel over studerende i udlandet*. Odense: Odense Universitetsforlag, 1991.

Helland, A. *Topografisk-Statistisk beskrivelse af Hedemarkens Amt*. Kristiania: Aschehoug, 1902.

Helland, A. *Norges land og folk, bind 9 (del 1 og 2)*. Kristiania: – Nedenes amt: H. Aschehoug & co (W. Nygaard), 1903.

Helland, A. *Norges land og folk, bind 10 (del 1 og 2)*. Kristiania: – Lister og Mandals amt: H. Aschehoug & co (W. Nygaard), 1904.

Hellberg, I. "Könsutjämning och könspolarisering inom professionerna på dagens svenska arbetsmarknad," in *Kampen om yrkesutövning, status och kunskap*, ed. Selander, S. Lund: Studentlitteratur, 1989.

Heller, R. "Officiers de Santé: the second-class doctors of nineteenth-century France," *Medical History*, 22(1978): 25–43.

Hellström, M. and G. Westlander. *Läkares arbetsvillkor inom olika specialiteter*. Solna: Arbetsmiljöinstitutet, 1993.

Helman, C. G. *Culture, Health and Illness*. London: Wright, 1990.

Helman, C. G. "Limits of biomedical explanation," *Lancet*, 337(1991):1080–1083.

Hennum, J. O. "Embedslægernes lønningsforhold," *Tidsskrift for Den norske lægeforening*, (1902):1061–1064.

Herzlich, C. "Sociology of health and illness in France, retrospectively and prospectively," *Social Science and Medicine*, 20 (1985):121–122.

Herzlich, C. "Professionals, intellectuals, visible practitioners? The case of 'medical humanitarism'." *Social Science and Medicine* 41 (1995): 1617–1619.

Herzlich, C. and J. Pierret. "The social construction of the patient: Patients and illnesses in other ages," *Social Science and Medicine*, 20(1985):145–151.

Herzlich, C. "The evolution of relations between French physicians and the state from 1880 to 1980," *Sociology of Health & Illness*, 4(1982):241–253.

Hessel, S. T. *Medicine: The Gundersen Experience 1891–1991*. La Crosse, Wis. Gundersen Clinic, 1991.

Heurtin-Roberts, S. and E. Reisin. "The relation of culturally influenced lay models of hypertension to compliance with treatment," *American Journal of Hypertension*, 5(1992):787–792.

Hill, T.P. "The cultural and philosophical foundations of normative medical ethics." *Social Science and Medicine*, 39 (1994):1149–1154.

Hjort, P. F. "Primary health care in Sweden and Norway," *Läkartidningen*, 90(1993): 3101–3102.

Hjort, P. F. "Gode leger – hvordan blir studentene det?" *Tidsskrift for Den norske lægeforening, III (1991):3700–3702..*

Hjort, E. F. "Rekruttering av Norges leger på 1800-tallet," *Tidsskrift for Den norske lægeforening*, (1983):1149–1154.

Hjortdahl, P. *Continuity of care in general practice, Thesis.* Oslo: Department of General practice, University of Oslo, 1992.

Hobsbawm, E. "Introduction: Inventing Traditions," in *The Invention of Tradition*, eds. Hobsbawm, E. and T. Ranger. Cambridge: Cambridge University Press, 1983.

Hobsbawm, E. and T. Ranger. eds. *The Invention of Tradition*. Cambridge: Cambridge University Press, 1983.

Hodne, B. "Autobiografier som folkloristisk kilde: Et forsøk på en avklaring," *Norveg*, 26(1983):5–40.

Hodne, F. *An economic history of Norway 1815–1970.* Bergen: Tapir, 1975.

Hodne, F. *Norges økonomiske historie 1815–1970*. Oslo: J.W. Cappelens forlag, 1981.

Hodne, F. "Medisin og miljø – nye synspunkter," in *Legene og samfunnet*, eds. Larsen, Ø. O. Berg, and F. Hodne. Oslo: Seksjon for medisinsk historie, Universitetet i Oslo og Den norske lægeforening, 1986.

Hodne, F. "Økonomisk vekst og helse," in *Legene og samfunnet*, eds. Larsen, Ø. O. Berg, and F. Hodne. Oslo: Seksjon for medisinsk historie, Universitetet i Oslo og Den norske lægeforening, 1986.

Hodne, F., and O. Honningdal Grytten. *Norsk Økonomi 1900–1990.* Oslo: TANO, 1992.

Hoesch, K. "Die Bemühungen in Deutschland tätiger Ärztinnen um die Approbation von 1877–1900," *Medizinhistorisches Journal. Internationale Vierteljahresschrift för Wissenschaftsgeschichte*, 30(1995): 353–376.

Hoffmaster, B. "The forms and limits of

medical ethics." *Social Science and Medicine*, 39(1994):1155–1164.

Hofoss, D. *Spesialisering av helsepersonell – hvorfor og hvordan?* Oslo: Norges almenvitenskaplige forskningsråds gruppe for helsetjenesteforskning, 1980.

Holck, P. "Leger og sykdommer i 1600-årene," *St Hallvard*, (1976):130–136.

Holck, P. "En Finnmarks–lege," *Tidsskrift for Den norske lægeforening*, 107(1987): 3006–3012.

Holloway, S. W. F. "Medical education in England, 1830–1858: A sociological analysis," *History*, (1964):299–324.

Holm, A. "Løst og fast fra Medorg," *Æsculap*, 3(1966):14–15.

Holmen, J., K. Midthjell, K. Bjartveit, P.F. Hjort, P.G. Lund–Larsen, T.Moum, S. Næss and H.T. Waaler. *The Nord-Trøndelag Health Survey 1984–1986.* Verdal: Folkehelsa (SIFF), 1990.

Holst, A. "Om arbeiderhygienen i England," *Tidsskrift for Den norske lægeforening*, 6(1892):225–240.

Holst, J. M. "Kirurgiens stilling til den øvrige medisin og til samfundet," *Norsk Magazin for Lægevidenskaben*, (1930): 1241–1252.

Holst, J. F. *Levemaaden og hygiæniske Forhold i Sortlands Distrikt.* Beretning om Sundhedstilstanden m.m. i Norge, 1878.

Holst, J. M. "Om organisasjonen av vårt offentlige sykehusvesen." *Tidsskrift for Den norske lægeforening*, 55(1935):302–311.

Holst, P.M. *Våre akutte folkesykdommers epidemiologi og klinikk.* Oslo: H. Aschehoug & co, 1954.

Holst, P.M. "Helseforholdene i Norge omkring 1880", *Tidsskrift for Den norske lægeforening,* Jubileumsnummer, 1955.

Hoolihan, C. "Health and Travel in Nineteenth-Century Rome," *The Journal of the History of Medicine and Allied Sciences*, 44 (1989):462–485.

Hopstock, H. *Det anatomiske institutt, 1815–1915*. Oslo: Aschehougs Boghandel, 1915.

Horobin, G. "Professional Mystery: the Maintenance of Charisma in General Medical Practice," in *The Sociology of the Professions: Lawyers, Doctors and Others*, eds. Dingwall, R. and P. Lewis. London: Macmillan, 1983. pp. 84–105.

Hovdhaugen, E. *Husmannstida*. Oslo: Det Norske Samlaget, 1976.

Howarth, D. *The Shetland Bus (new edition)*. Glasgow: The Grafton Books, 1991.

Hughes, E. C. "Professions," *Dædalus*, 92 (1963):655–668.

Hughes, E. *Men and Their Work*. Illinois: Free Press of Glencoe, 1958.

Hughes, E. C. *The Sociological Eye: Selected Papers*. New Brunswick NJ: Transaction Books, 1984.

Humphreys, R. S. "The historian, his documents, and the elementary modes of historical thought," *History and Theory*, 19 (1980):1–20.

Hunstadbråten, K. *Tannleger i trekvart århundre. Norsk odontologi 1800–1875*. Lic. avh. Vikersund: 1970.

Hunstadbråten, K. *Odontologiens utvikling*. Oslo: Folkets brevskole, Norsk kommuneforbund, Universitetsforlaget, 1979.

Hunstadbråten, K. "Fra våre kollegers praksis for 100 år siden," *Norsk Tannlegeforenings Tidsskrift*, 100(1990):596–599.

Hunt, L. M. and C. H. Browner. "Hypoglycemia: Portrait of an illness construct in everyday use," *Medical Anthropology Quarterly*, 4(1990): 191–210.

Hustad, O. R. *Verandagutar. Frå livet til verandagutane på Kysthospitalet i Hagevik.* Bergen: GeoGrafisk A.S.

Hylland Eriksen, T. and T. Sørheim Arntsen. *Kulturforskjeller i praksis. Perspektiver på det flerkulturelle Norge.* Oslo: ad Notam Gyldendal, 1994.

Høegh, S. "Iagttagelser under en Epidemie af Diphteritis faucium", *Norsk Magazin for Lægevidenskaben,* (1864):120–149.

Høidahl, O. *Quisling – a study in treason.* Oslo: Universitetforlaget, 1988.

Høyer, S. *Pressen mellom teknologi og samfunn. Norske og internasjonale perspektiver på pressehistorien fra Gutenberg til vår tid.* Oslo: Universitetsforlaget, 1995.

Ibsen, H. *Mellom profitt og moral.* Oslo: Tano, Aschehoug, 1996.

Illich, I. "The Professions as a Form of Imperialism," *New Society*, 25(1973):633–635.

Illich, I. *Medical Nemesis: the Exprопriatation of Health.* New York: Pantheon, 1974.

Illich, I. ed. *Disabling Professions.* London: Marion Boyars, 1977.

Illich, I. *Toward a history of needs.* New York: Bantam, 1980.

Illich, I. "Pathogenesis, immunity and the quality of public health," *Qualtitive Health Research*, 5(1995):7–14.

Imhof, A. E. "The implications of increased life expectancy for family and social life," in *Medicine in society. Historical essays*, ed. Wear, A. Cambridge: Cambridge University Press, 1992.

Imhof, A. E., and Ø. Larsen. *Sozialgeschichte und Medizin. Probleme der quantifizierenden Quellenbearbeitung in der Sozial- und Medizingeschichte.* Oslo: Universitetsforlaget, 1975 and Stuttgart: Gustav Fischer Verlag, 1975.

Innstilling om legetjenesten og tannlegetjenesten. Innstilling I fra komiteen til utredning av spørsmålet om tilstrekkelig tilgang på og spredning av helsepersonell (Helsepesonellkomiteen) oppnevnt ved kongelig resolusjon av 22. november 1963. Avgitt i juni 1967. Ibid.

Innstilling om PET. Oslo: Rikshospitalet, 1994.

Innstilling fra Den kongelige lægelovkommission. Kristiania:1908.

International Committee of Medical Journal Editors. "Guidelines on authorship," *BMJ,* 291(1985):722.

Irgens, L. M. "Leprosy in Norway. An epidemological study based on national patient registry," *Leprosy Review*, 51 (1980) Suppl. 1. 1–130..

Iversen, O. H., and P. F. Marton (red). *Den norske Patologforenings 50 års jubileum 1923–1973.* Sarpsborg: Frank Vardings Trykkeri, 1973.

Jackowski, A. and V. L. Smith. "Polish Pilgrim-Tourists," *Annals of Tourism Research*, 19(1992):92–106.

Jackson, J. A. ed. *Professions and Professionalization.* Cambridge: Cambridge University Press, 1970.

Jackson, S. W. "Melancholia and Mechanical Explanations in Eighteenth-Century Medicine," *Journal of the History of Medicine and Allied Sciences*, 38(1983):298–319.

Jacobsen, K. D. *Teknisk hjelp og politisk struktur.* Oslo: Universitetsforlaget, 1964.

Jacobson, P. "Medical malpractice and the tort system," *Journal of the American Medical Association*, 262(1989):3320–3327.

Jacobsson, N. "Magister Andreæ Hesselii anmärkningar om hans resa till Amerika och vistande där 1711–1724: *Ett Delawareminne*," *Linnesällskapets årsskrift*, (1938):95–140.

Jarcho, S. "Auenbruger, Laennec and John Keats: Some notes on the early history of percussion and auscultation," *Medical History*, 5(1961):167–172.

Jefferys, M. "Social science and medical education in Britain: a sociologic analysis of their relationship," *International Journal of Health Services*, 4(1974)

Jenkinson, J. "The Role of Medical Societies in the Rise of the Scottish Medical Profession 1730–1939," *Social History of Medicine*, 4(1991):253–275.

Jenswold, J. R. ""I live well, but..."; Letters from Norwegians in industrial America," *Norwegian–American Studies*, 31(1986): 113–129.

Jerome, J. K. *Three men in a boat.* New York: Viking Penguin, 1978.

Jervell, A., K. Meyer and K. Westlund.

"Coronary heart disease and serum cholestrol in males in different parts of Norway," *Acta Med Scand*, 177(1965):13–23.

Jewson, N. D. "Medical Knowledge and the Patronage System in 18th Century England," *Sociology*, 8(1974):369–385.

Jewson, N. D. "The disappearance of the sick man from medical cosmology," *Sociology*, 10(1976):225–244.

Jobe, T. H. "Medical Teories of Melancholia in the Seventeenth and Early Eighteenth Centuries," *Clio Medica*, 11(1976):217–231.

Johannessen, F.E., and J. Skeie. *Bitre piller og sterke dråper. Norske apotek gjennom 400 år 1595–1995,* Oslo: Norsk farmasihistorisk museum, 1995.

Johannesen, T. *Controlled trials in single subjects: a comparison of the symptomatic effect of cimetidine versus placebo in single patients with dyspepsia.* Trondheim: Faculty of Medicine, University of Trondheim, 1992.

Johannison, K. *Medicinens öga*. Stockholm: Norstedts, 1990.

Johanson, M., U. S. Larsson, R. Säljö, and K. Svärdsudd. "Lifestyle in primary health care discourse," *Social Science and Medicine*, 40(1995):339–348.

Johnsen, E. B. ed. *Virkelighetens forvaltere*. Oslo: Universitetsforlaget, 1995.

Johnsen, E. B. *Den andre litteraturen. Hva sakprosa er*. Oslo: Cappelen, 1995.

Johnsen, T. "Fra mine distriktslægeår," in *Kvinnelige studenter 1882–1932*, Oslo: Gyldendal, 1932.

Johnson, A. "Medisinsk studium i utlandet og Licentia practicandi i Norge for Læger med medisinsk eksamen fra utenlandsk universitet," *Tidsskrift for Den norske lægeforening,* 74(1954):661–662.

Johnson, M. "Medical sociology and sociological theory," *Social Science and Medicine*, 9(1975):227–232.

Johnson, M. "Professional Careers and Biographies," in *The Sociology of the Professions: Lawyers, Doctors and Others*, eds. Dingwall, R. and P. Lewis. London: Macmillan, 1983.

Johnson, T. *Profession and Power*. London: Macmillan, 1967.

Johnson, T. "Imperialism and the Professions: Notes on the Development of Professional Occupations in Britain's Colonies and the New States," *Sociological Review Monograph*, 20(1973):281–309.

Johnson, T., G. Larkin, and M. Saks. "Introduction," in *Health professions and the state in Europe*, eds. Johnson, T. G. Larkin, and M. Saks. London: Routledge, 1995.

Johnson, T. "Governmentality and the institutionalization of expertice," in *Health professions and the state in Europe*, eds. Johnson, T. G. Larkin, and M. Saks. London: Routledge, 1995.

Jones, C. "Montpellier Medical Students and the Medicalisation of 18th-Century France," in *Problems and Methods in the History of Medicine*, eds. Porter, R. and A. Wear. Beckenham: Croom Helm Ltd, 1987.

Jones, F. E. "Social Origins in Four Professions: a Comparative Study," *International Journal of Comparative Sociology*, 3–4 17 (1976):143–163.

Jones, K. and G. Moon. *Health, Disease and Society: An introduction to medical geography*. London: Routledge & Kegan Paul, 1987.

Jones, R. M. "American doctors in Paris 1820–1861: A Statistical Profile," *Journal of the History of Medicine*, 25(1970): 143–157.

Jones, R. M. "American doctors and the Parisian medical world, 1830–1840," *Bulletin of the History of Medicine*, 47 (1973):40–65.

Kaada, B. ed. *Norges leger 1976*. Oslo: Den norske lægeforening 1978.

Kahrs, C. "122 Trakeotomier i Difterit", *Norsk Magazin for Lægevidenskaben,* (1888):441–462.

Kaisen, A., G. A. Kjetså, R. K. Lie, R. Hjetland, P. T. Haaland, P. Møller, H. E. Oulie,

T. Tveit, and J. G. Mæland. "Intern's evaluation of their preparation for general practice: a comparison between the University of Tromsø and the University of Bergen," *Medical Education*, 18(1984): 349–354.

Kallevik, S. A. "Ønsker medisinske fagbøker på norsk", Tidsskrift for Den norske lægeforening, 113(1993):2454.

Kallevik, S. A. "Utenlandske bøker foretrekkes," *Tidsskrift for Den norske lægeforening*, 113 30(1993):2455.

Kancelli-innlegg av 3. desember 1803.

Karasek, R. "Job demands, job decision latitude, and mental strain: Implications for job redesign," *Administrative Science Quarterly*, 24(1979):285–308.

Karasek, R. and T. Theorell. *Healthy work. Stress, productivity, and reconstruction of working life*. BasicBooks/ A division of Harper Collins Publishers, 1990.

Kasl, S. V. "An epidemiological perspective on the role of control in health," in *Job control and worker health*, eds. Sauter, S. L. J. J. Hurrell, and C. C. Cooper. London: Wiley, 1989.

Katz, M. B. "Occupational Classification in History," *The Journal of Interdisciplinary History*, 3(1972):63–88.

Kauppinen-Toropainen, K., I. Kandolin, and P. Mutanen. "Job dissatisfaction and work-related exhaustion in male and female work," *Journal of Occupational Behaviour*, 4(1983):193–207.

Kaurin, E. "Sygepleiesagen," *Tidsskrift for Den norske lægeforening*, (1905):291–293.

Kehoe, J. "Representation and resistance: British medical discourses surrounding veneral disease and the shaping of sociosexual relations in New Zealand 1769–1870," *Revue Internationale de Sociologie*, 3(1993):117–143.

Kellermann, P. "Professions and Expert Labor," *Innovation*, 3(1990):185–194.

Kemper, T. D. "The division of labour: a post-Durkheimian analytical view," *American Sociological Review*, 37(1972): 739–753.

Kestner, C. W. *Medicinisches Gelehrten-Lexicon*. Hildesheim: 1971.

Kevan, S. M. "Quests for cures: a history of tourism for climate and health," *International Journal of Biometeorology*, 37(1993): 113–124.

Kevan, S. M. "In search of health and pleasure," *Geoscope*, 18(1984):47–53.

Kierulf, C.T. "Indberetning om en med Stipendium foretagen videnskabelig Reise i Udlandet," *Norsk Magazin for Lægevidenskaben*, (1853):361–401.

Kimball, B. A. *The "True Professional Ideal" in America*. Cambridge: Blackwell, 1992.

King, L. S. "Theory and practice in eighteenth century medicine," *Studies on Voltaire and the Eighteenth Century*, 153(1976): 1201–1218.

King, L. S. *Medical Thinking*. Princeton: 1982.

King, L. S. "Some problems of causality in eighteenth century medicine," *Bulletin of the History of Medicine*, 38(1963):15–24.

King, L. S. "What Is a Diagnosis?" *Journal of the American Medical Association*, 202 (1967):714–717.

King, L.S. "Medicine – Trade or profession?" *The Journal of the American Medical Association* 253 (1985): 2709–2710.

King, L. S. ed. *A history of medicine*. Harmondsworth: Penguin, 1971.

King, L. S. *Medical World of the Eighteenth Century*. Chicago: The University of Chicago Press, 1958.

Kirk, K. W. "Women in male-dominated professions," *Journal of Hospital Pharmacy*, 39(1982):2089–2093.

Kiær, F.C. *Norges Læger i det nittende Aarhundrede (1800–1871)*, Christiania: A Cammermeyer, 1873.

Kiær, F.C. *Norges Læger i det nittende Aarhundrede (1800–1886) Anden betydeligt forøgede Udgave bd I*, Christiania: A Cammermeyer, 1888.

Kiær, F.C. *Norges Læger i det nittende Aarhundrede (1800–1886) Anden betydeligt forøgede Udgave bd II*, Christiania: A Cammermeyer, 1890.

Kiær, F.C. "Opfordring til Kolleger i Anledning af en ny Udgave af 'Norges Læger'", *Norsk Magazin for Lægevidenskaben,* April Heftet(1886):303–306.

Kiær, F.C. "Opfordring til Landets Læger," *Norsk Magazin for Lægevidenskaben*, (1871):271–272.

Kjelland, A. *Bygdebok for Lesja. Bind 1&2.* Lesja: Lesja kommune, 1987 and 1992.

Kjelstadli, S. *Hjemmestyrkene Bs. I Hovedtrekk av den militære motstanden under okkupasjonen.* Oslo: Aschehoug, 1959.

Kjær, A-Th. *Akershus amt 1814–1914.* Christiania: Steenske boktrykkeri Johannes Bjørnstad, 1921.

Kjærheim, K. *Mellom kloke koner og hvitkledte menn.* Oslo: Seksjon for medisinsk historie, 1978 and Oslo: Samlaget, 1987.

Kjærheim, K. *Alcohol and Cancer in the Restaurant Business.* Oslo: The Cancer Registry of Norway, Institute of Epidemiological Cancer Research. Institute of General Practice and Community Medicine. The Faculty of Medicine, University of Oslo, 1996.

Kjølstad, S. "Omkring det offentlige lægevesen," *Tidsskrift for Den norske lægeforening*, (1932):355–364.

Kjølstad, S. Article in Aftenposten, Wednesday afternoon 11. april 1934.

Klave, K. *Soll ich Medizin studieren?* Leipzig: 1941.

Klaveness, E. *Norske Læger i Amerika 1840–1942.* St.Paul, Minn. 1943.

Klaveness, S. T. *Oslo kommunale sykehus i krigens tegn.* Oslo: Cammermeyer, 1947.

Klaveness.""Elida"'s vintertogt 1900/1901," *Norsk Magazin for Lægevidenskaben*, (1901): 236–241.

Klegon, D. "The Sociology of Professions: An Emerging Perspective," *Sociology of Work and Occupations*, 5(1978):259–283.

Kleinman, A. *Patients and healers in the context of culture.* Berkeley: University of California Press, 1980.

Kluge, E.H. "The physician as entrepreneur." *Canadian Medical Association Journal*, 149(1993):204–205.

Kluge, E.H. "Codes of ethics and other illusions." *Canadian Medical Association Journal*, 146(1992):1234–1235.

Klyve, P., J.Ø. Ihler jr., and J. P. Torgersen. *Håndbok for norske Oftalmologer 1994.* Asker: Stikka Trykk Asker og Bærums Budstikke AS, 1994.

Kobro, I. ed. *Norges Læger 1800–1908. Bind 1(Aa-K) og 2(L-Ø).* Kristiania: H. Aschehoug & Co (W. Nygaard), 1908–1912 and 1915.

Kobro, I. ed. *Norges Læger 1909–1915.* Kristiania: A. Cammermeyer – Lars Swanstrøm, 1916.

Kobro, I. ed. *Norges Læger 1909–1925.* Oslo: H. Aschehoug & co. (W. Nygaard), 1927.

Kobro, I. ed. *Norges Læger 1926–1936.* Oslo: H. Aschehoug & co. (W. Nygaard), 1938.

Kobro, I. ed. *Tillegg til Norges læger 1800–1908.* Oslo: H. Aschehoug & Co (W. Nygaard), 1944.

Kobro, I. ed. *Norges Læger 1937–1946.* Oslo: H. Aschehoug & co. (W. Nygaard), 1951.

Koch, E. *Ärzte, die Geschichte machten.* Augsburg: 1982.

Kolsrud, O. ed. *Oslo kapitels forhandlinger 1609–1616.* Kristiania/Oslo: 1913–49.

Kolstad, A. "Korrespondance," *Norsk Magazin for Lægevidenskaben*, (1898):800–805.

Koren, A. "Nogle Optegnelser fra en Udenlandsreise væsentlig vedkommende veneriske Sygdomme," *Norsk Magazin for Lægevidenskaben*, (1875):273–283.

Kosa, J. "Entrepreneurship and charisma in the medical profession," *Social Science and Medicine*, 4(1970):25–40.

Kosthold og helse. Oslo:Landsforeningen for kosthold og helse, 1956.

Kracauer, S. "Time and History," *History and Theory*, Beheift 6(1966):65–78.

Krau, A. M. "Healers and strangers. Immigrant attitudes toward the physician in America – A relationship in historical perspective," *Journal of the American Medical Association*, 263(1990): 1807–1811.

Kreyberg, H. J. A. "A study of tobacco smoking in Norway," *British Journal of Cancer*, (1954):8–13.

Kreyberg, L. *Etter ordre eller uten.* Oslo: Gyldendal, 1976.

Kreyberg, L. *Kast ikke kortene.* Oslo: Gyldendal, 1978.

Kringlen, E. *Medisin og samfunn*. Oslo: Universitetsforlaget, 1986. 2. utg. 1996.

Kristiansen, A. *Bygd og by i Norge – Agder.* Oslo: Gyldendal norsk forlag, 1977.

Kristiansen, I. S. and O. H. Førde. "Medical specialists' choice of location: The role of geographical attachment in Norway," *Social Science and Medicine*, 34(1992): 57–62.

Kristiansen, K. and Ø. Larsen. *Ullevål sykehus i hundre år*. Oslo: Oslo kommune, Ullevål sykehus, 1989.

Kristiansen, K. and Ø. Larsen. "Surgical science, general surgery and superspesialization. The development of surgery in Norway in the 20th Century," *Acta Chirurgica European Journal of Surgery*, Suppl. 565 (1991).

Krohn, C. "Har de norske læger liten økonomisk ansvarsfølelse?" *Tidsskrift for Den norske lægeforening*, (1930):1037–1038.

Kronus, C. L. "The evolution of occupational power," *Sociology of Work and Occupations*, 3(1976):3–37.

Kuhn, T. S. "Scientific Growth: Reflections on Ben-David's "Scientific Role"," *Minerva*, 10(1972):166–178.

Kumpusalo, E., K. Mattila, I. Virjo, L. Neittaanmäki, S. Kataje, M. Jääskeläinen, R. Luhtata and M. Isokoski. "Medical education and the corresponding professional needs of young doctors: the Finnish Junior Physician 88 Study," *Medical Education*, 25(1991):71–77.

Kunitz, S. J. "Professionalism and Social Control in the Progressive Era: The Case of the Flexner Report," *Social Problems*, 22 (1974):16–27.

Kushner, H. I. "Social, gender, and the fear of modernity in nineteenth-century medical and social thought," *Journal for Social History*, 26(1993):461–490.

Kvittingen, J. "Norsk helsetjeneste i London mai 1940 til mai 1941", *Norsk Bedriftshelsetjeneste,* 1984:62–78.

Kvittingen, J. "Fra den kongelege norske marines sanitetsteneste i Storbritannia under krigen. 1940–1945", *Tidsskrift for Den norske lægeforening,* 107(1987): 1688–89.

Kyvik, S. *Productivity in science. Scientific publishing at Norwegian Universities*. Oslo: Norwegian University Press, 1991.

Laache, S. B. *Norsk medicin i hundrede aar.* Kristiania: Steenske Bogtrykkeri, 1911.

La Berge, A. and M. Feingold. ed. *French medical culture in the 19th century*. 1994.

Lamberts, H. and M. Wood. *ICPC – International classification of primary care.* Oxford: Oxford University Press, 1987.

Lane, J. "The medical practitioners of provincial England," *Medical History*, 28 (1984):353–371.

Lange, B. "Bemerkninger til lovforslaget ang. foranstaltninger mod tuberkulosen," *Tidsskrift for Den norske lægeforening*, (1896):176–181.

Lange, B. "Sundhedsloven paragraf 15," *Tidsskrift for Den norske lægeforening*, (1903):430

Lange, B. "Den nye lægeordning," *Tidsskrift for Den norske lægeforening*, (1900):379–381.

Lange, B. "Lægeforholdene i Nordre Aurdal," *Tidsskrift for Den norske lægeforening*, (1903):837–838.

Lange, M. I. ed. *Konfrontasjon. Striden om Kunstforeningen* 1875–1885. Oslo: Oslo Kunstforening, 1986.

Lange, O. J. "Legebemanningen ved våre indremedisinske avdelinger," *Tidsskrift for Den norske lægeforening*, 109(1989):3489–3495.

Langsley, D. "Foreword," in *The Impaired Physican*, eds. Scheiber and Doyle. New York and London: Plenum Medical Book Company, 1983.

Lansbury, R. "Careers, work and leisure among the new professionals," *Sociological Review*, 22(1974):385–400.

LaPorte, R. E., E. Marler, S. Akazawa, F. Sauer, C. Gamboa, and C. E. Shenton. "The death of biomedical journals," *British Medical Journal*, 310(1995):1387–1390.

Larsen, C. F. "Om forekomst av Tyfoidfeber i Norge indtil 1876," *Norsk Magazin for Lægevidenskaben*, 9(1879):1–123.

Larsen, C. F. "Hvorfor tiltager Utbredningen af Lungetuberkulose i Norge?" *Norsk Magazin for Lægevidenskaben*, 4(1889): 229–263.

Larsen, I. M. *Norske universitetsforskere – kosmopolitter i forskningen?* Rapport 11/92. Oslo: NAVF utredningsinstitutt, 1992.

Larsen, Ø. "Legesøkning i et distrikt i Trønderlag," *Tidsskrift for Den norske lægeforening*, 85(1965):1770–1772.

Larsen, Ø. "Urtebøkene," *Liv og Helse*, 33(1966):181–184.

Larsen, Ø. "Gamle trykk, Legebøker i Danmark og Norge," *Liv og Helse*, 33(1966): 231–4,237.

Larsen, Ø. "Legen, hans profesjon og verden omkring," *Kirke og Kultur*,79(1975): 227–236.

Larsen, Ø. "Å være lege," in *Legene og samfunnet*, eds. Larsen, Ø. O. Berg, and F. Hodne. Oslo: Seksjon for medisinsk historie, Universitetet i Oslo og Den norske lægeforening, 1986.

Larsen, Ø. *Mangfoldig medisin*. Oslo: Det medisinske fakultet, Universitet i Oslo, 1989. (The history of the medical faculty in Oslo).

Larsen, Ø. "Arbeidsmedisinens utvikling i Norge". *Norsk bedriftshelsetjeneste* 11(1990):140–152.

Larsen, Ø. "Vekst i byen og helse på landet – noen trekk ved folkehelse og befolkningsutvikling på slutten av 1800–tallet", *Jord og Gjerning*,5(1991):66–78.

Larsen, Ø. (ed.) *Forebyggende medisin.* Oslo, Bergen, Tromsø: Universitetsforlaget, 1975.

Larsen, Ø., H. Haugtomt and W. Platou. *Sykdomsoppfatning og epidemiologi 1860–1900. Epidemiske sykdommer i Norge og helsemyndighetenes vurdering av folkehelsen – presentasjon av data.* Oslo: Seksjon for medisinsk historie, Universitetet i Oslo, 1980.

Larsen, Ø. and A. Heiberg (eds.). *Medisinske fag i velferds-Norge.* Oslo: Seksjon for medisinsk historie, Universitetet i Oslo, 1983.

Larsen, Ø., O. Berg and F. Hodne. eds. *Legene og samfunnet.* Oslo: Seksjon for medisinsk historie, Universitetet i Oslo og Den norske lægeforening, 1986.

Larsen, Ø. ed. *Norges leger 1986.* Oslo: Den norske lægeforening, 1986.

Larsen, Ø. and F. Hodne. "Health Conditions, Population and Physicians in Norway 1814–1986. Notes on the Development of a Profession," in *Society, Health and Population during the Demographic Transition*, eds. Brändström, A. and L. Tedebrand. Stockholm: Almqvist and Wiksell International, 1988.

Larsen, Ø. and B. I. Lindskog. *Sundhedstidende 1778–1781. Johann Clemens Tode.* Oslo: Seksjon for medisinsk historie, Universitetet i Oslo, 1991.

Larsen, Ø. et al. eds. *Samfunnsmedisin i Norge – teori og anvendelse.* Oslo: Universitetsforlaget, 1992.

Larsen, Ø. ed. *Berglege Henrik Rosted og levekårene på Kongsberg på slutten av 1700-tallet.* Konsberg: Sølvverkets venner, 1994.

Larsen, Ø. ed. *Norges leger I–V.* Oslo: Den norske lægeforening, 1996.

Larson, M. S. *The Rise of Professionalism: A Sociological Analysis*. Berkeley, Los Angeles and London: University of California Press, 1977.

Larson, M. S. "Proletarianization and educated labor," *Theory and Society*, 9(1980): 131–175.

Lawrence, B. "The Fifth Dimension – Gender and General Practice," in *In a Man's World: Essays on Women in Male–dominated Professions*, eds. Spencer, A. and D. Podmore. London: Tavistock, 1987.

Lawrence, C. "Incommunicable Knowledge: Science, Technology and the Clinical Art in Britain 1850–1914," *Journal of Contemporary History*, 20(1985):503–520.

Lawrence, C. *Medicine in the Making of Modern Britain, 1700–1920*. London: Routledge, 1994.

Lawrence, S. C. "Entrepreneurs and private enterprice: The development of medical lecturing in London, 1775–1820," *Bulletin of the History of Medicine*, 62(1988): 171–192.

Lazarus, R. S. and S. Folkman. *Stress, appraisal, and coping*. New York: Springer Publishing Company, 1984.

Le Fanu, W. R. "The lost half-century in English medicine, 1700–1750," *Bulletin of the History of Medicine*, XLVI(1972): 319–348.

Leavitt, J. W. "Medicine in Context: A Review Essay of the History of Medicine," *The American Historical Review*, 95(1990):1471–1484.

Lee, K. L., E. Scwarz, and K. Y. K. Mak. "Improving oral health through understanding the meaning of health and disease in a Chinese culture," *Int Dent J*, 43 (1993):2–8.

Leegaard, F. "Lægerne – alkoholspørsmaalet," *Medicinsk Revue*, (1903):5–11, 143–144.

Leegaard, F. "Lægernes livsbetingelser og arbeidsvilkaar," *Tidsskrift for Den norske lægeforening*, (1912):1063

Leegaard, F. "Centralstyrets forslag til endringer i "Regler for specialisters godkjennelse etc."," *Tidsskrift for Den norske lægeforening*, (1930):571–573.

Leegaard, F. "Fastlønnede læger," *Tidsskrift for Den norske lægeforening*, (1914):1044–1046.

Leenwenhost Working Party. *The general practitioner in Europe.* The Netherlands: Leenwenhost Group, 1974.

Leiper, N. "The Framework of Tourism: Towards a Definition of Tourism, Tourist, and the Tourist Industry," *Annals of Tourism Research*, 6(1979):390–407.

Leira, H. *Trøndelag Medisinske Selskap 150 år*. Trondheim: Tapir, 1993.

Lepovitz, H. W. "Pilgrims, Patients, and Painters: The Formation of a Tourist Culture in Bavaria," *Historical Reflections*, 18(1992):121–145.

Lesky, E. *Die Wiener medizinische Schule im 19.Jahrhundert*. Graz-Köln: Verlag Hermann Böhlaus Nachf. 1965.

Lethbridge, L. "The spa towns of Bohemia," *Contemporary Review*, 257(1990): 156–159.

Leufkens, H., F. Haaijer-Ruskamp, A. Bakker, and G. Dukes. "Scenario analysis of the future of medicine," *British Medical Journal*, 309(1994):1137–1140.

Levekårsundersøkelsen 1991. Oslo, Kongsvinger: SSB, 1991.

Lever, A. F. "Medicine under challenge," *Lancet*, 352(1977)

Lexchin, J. "The Medical Profession and the Pharmaceutical Industry: An Unhealthy Alliance," *International Journal of Health Services*, 18(1988):603–616.

Lie, S. O. "Asbjørn Føllings sykdom," *Tidsskrift for Den norske lægeforening,* 104 (1984):2381–2385.

Light, D. W. "Status, Purity, and Professional "Regression"," *American Journal of Sociology*, 90(1984):182–184.

Light, D. and S. Levine. "The Changing Character of the Medical Profession: A

Theoretical Overview," *The Milbank Quarterly*, 66(1988):10–32.

Lilleaas, U. *Før var jeg et arbeidsjern. Kvinner med muskelsmerter i et kjønnsrolleperspektiv*. Oslo: Institutt for forebyggende medisin , 1991.

Lindbekk, T. *Mobilitets- og stillingsstruktur innenfor tre akademiske profesjoner 1910–63*. Oslo: Universitetsforlaget, 1967.

Lindbekk, T. *Rekrutteringen av leger til de norske utkantområder (utvidet og revidert utgave)*. Oslo: Institutt for samfunnsforskning, 1967.

Lindbekk, T. *Betydning av det medisinske fakultet i Bergen for norske medisineres geografiske lokalisering*. Oslo: Institutt for samfunnsforskning.

Lindbekk, T. "Educational Systems and the Attainment Process: A reappraisal of mobility studies in educational research," *Det Kongelige Norske Videnskabers Selskab Skrifter*, 1–23.

Lindeboom, G. A. Herman Boerhaave: The Man and his Work. London: 1968.

Ljunggren, E. "Nordiskt Medicinskt Arkiv och dess båda Acta. Ett hundreårsminne. I. Kirurgi," in *Yearbook of the Museum of Medical History Stockholm*, Växjö: Smålandspostens Boktryckeri AB, 1970.

Lock, M. and D. Gordon. eds. *Biomedicine examined*. Dordrecht: Kluwer, 1988.

Lock, S. "As things really were?" in *The future of medical journals*, ed. Lock, S. London: BMJ, 1991.

Lock, S. *A difficult balance. Editorial peer review in medicine*. London: The Nuffield Provincial Hospitals Trust, 1985.

Lock, S. "The medical journal – how?" in *Kunnskap er makt – og bør deles med andre*, eds. Fugelli, P. and M. Nylenna. Oslo: Universitetsforlaget, 1987.

Lock, S. "One hand clapping," *British Medical Journal*, 301(1990):677–678.

Lock, S. ed. *The future of medical publishing*. London: BMJ, 1991.

Lock, S. "Journalology: evolution of medical journals and some current problems," *J Int Med*, 232(1992):199–205.

Loock, H. D. *Quisling, Rosenberg und Terboven. Zor Vorgeschichte und Geschichte der nationalsozialistischen Revolution in Norwegen*. Stuttgart: Deutsche Verlags Anstalt, 1970.

Lorber, J. "Women and medical sociology: Invisible professionals an ubiquitous patients," *Sociological Inquiry*, 45(1975): 75–105.

Lorber, J. "Why women physicians will never be true equals in the American medical profession," in *Gender, Work and Medicine: Women and the Medical Division of Labour*, eds. Riska, E. and K. Wegar. London: SAGE, 1993.

Lossius, K. H. H. "Den norske lægeforening og "Tidsskriftet"", *Tidsskrift for Den norske lægeforening*, (1935):277–278.

Loudon, I. "Two Thousand Medical Men in 1847," *Society for the Social History of Medicine Bulletin*, 33(1983):4–8.

Loudon, I. "Medical practitioners 1750–1850 and the period of medical reform in Britain," in *Medicine in society. Historical essays*, ed. Wear, A. Cambridge: Cambridge University Press, 1992.

Lov av 1. april 1960 om endring av paragraf 22. 3. ledd, i lov om Universitetet i Bergen av 9. juli 1948.

Lov av 2. juni 1960.

Lovoll, O. S. A *Century of Urban Life – The Norwegians in Chicago before 1930*. Champaign, Ill. The Norwegian-American Historical Association, University of Illinois Press, 1988.

Lowell, B. L. "Sociological Theories and the Great Emigration", *Norwegian–American Studies* 32(1989):53–69.

Lund, O. *Som lege bak Lofotveggen*. Oslo: Gyldendal, 1975.

Lundberg, G. D. "Medicine – a profession in trouble?" *Journal of the American Medical Association*, 253(1985):2879–2880.

Lundberg, G. D. "Countdown to millennium – balancing the professionalism and business of medicine," *Journal of the American Medical Association*, 263(1990):86

Lunde, Aa. *Sandsværs historie, bind 1.* Sandsvær bygdebokkomite, 1973.

Lynn, K. S. "Introduction to the Issue "The Professions"", *Dædalus*, 92(1963):649–654.

Lyons, A. S. and R. J. Petrucelli. *Medicine, An Illustrated History*, Gyldendal Norsk Forlag, 1987.

Lærum, E. *Studies on urolithiasis in general practice. Thesis.* Oslo: Departement of General Practice, University of Oslo, 1983.

Lærum, F. and A. Stordahl. *Intervensjons-klinikk.* Oslo: Aker Sykehus, 1991.

Lærum, F. "Magnetic resonance imaging in Norway. Government policies," *Invest Radiol*, 28(1993): Suppl B, 46–47.

Løken, K. *Karjoldokt'ern.* Oslo: Cappelen, 1974.

Lønnum, A. *Helsevikt – en senfølge av krig og katastrofe.* Oslo: Gyldendal, 1969.

MacCannel, D. *The Tourist. A New Theory of the Leisure Class*, New York: Schocken Books, 1989.

MacCormack, C. "Ethnological studies of medical sciences." *Social Science and Medicine*, 39(1994):1229–1235.

MacDonald, K. M. "Social Closure and Occupational Registration," *Sociology*, 19(1985):541–556.

Macintyre, S. "Childbirth: the myth of the Golden Age," *Wld Med*, 71(1977)

MacLelland, C. E. *State, Society and University in Germany, 1700–1914.* Cambridge: 1980.

Madsen, S. T. "Medicinsk sprog og stil," *Medicinsk Revue*, (1918):204–205.

Makin, P. J., U. Rout, and C. L. Cooper. "Job satisfaction and occupational stress among general practitioners – a pilot study," *Journal of the Royal College of General Practitioners*, 38(1988):303–306.

Malm, O. J. "Polititroppene og sanitet i Sverige", in *Forsvarets sanitet: 50 år under felles ledelse 1941–1991,* ed. O. J. Malm (Oslo: Forsvarets Overkommando, 1991): 29–33.

Malterud, K. *Allmennpraktikerens møte med kvinnelige pasienter.* Oslo: TANO, 1990.

Malterud, K. "Medisinens hjelpeløshet I. Allmektige ambisjoner," *Nordisk Medicin*, 105(1990):27–29.

Mann, G. "Institutional Dynamics of Scientific Change: Ben-David's Legacy," *Social Studies of Science*, 23(1993):757–763.

Maretzki, T. W. "The *Kur* in West Germany as an Interface Between Neuropathic and Allopathic Ideologies," *Social Science and Medicine*, 24(1987):1061–1068.

Markowitz, G. E. and D. Rosner. "Doctors in Crisis: Medical Education and Medical Reform During the Propressive Era, 1895–1915," in *Health Care in America. Essays in Social History*, eds. Reverby, S. and D. Rosner. Philadelphia: Temple University Press, 1979. pp. 185–205.

Marland, H. and R. Richardson. "Medicine Comes to Town. Medicine and Social Structure in Urban Britain, 1780–1870," *Journal of Urban History*, 17 (1990):79–87.

Marshall, T. H. "The Recent History of Professionalism in Relation to Social Structure and Social Policy," *Canadian Journal of Economics and Political Science*, 5(1939): 325–340.

Martens, D.G. "Tracheotomie mod Croup foretaget med heldigt Udfald", *Norsk Magazin for Lægevidenskaben,* (1858): 560–568.

Martin, S. C., R. M. Arnold, and R. M. Parker. "Gender and medical socialization," *Journal of Health and Social Behavior*, 29 (1988):333–343.

Martinsen, K. "Legers interesse for svangerskapet – en del av den perinatale omsorg. Tidsrommet ca. 1890–1940," *Historisk Tidsskrift*, 3(1987):373–389.

Marzuk, P. M. "Sounding board. When the

patient is a physician," *The New England Journal of Medicine*, 317(1987):1409–1411.

Mathias, P. ed. *Science and Society*. Cambridge: Cambridge University Press, 1972.

Mathisen, C. "Inntrykk fra distiktslægedager nordenfor polarcirkelen," in *Kvinnelige studenter 1882–1932*, Oslo: Gyldendal, 1932.

Maulitz, R. C. "Channel crossing: the lure of French pathology for English medical students, 1816–1836," *Bulletin of the History of Medicine*, 55(1982):475–496.

Maurice, M. "Propos sur la sociologie des professions," *Sociologie du Travail*, 13 (1972):213–225.

Mayer, J. D. "Challenges to understanding spatial patterns of disease: Philosophical alternatives to logical positivism," *Social Science and Medicine*, 35(1992):579–587.

Mc Gregor Hellstedt, L. *Women Physicians of the World*. New York: 197.

McCarthy, D. J. "Why are today's medical students choosing high-technology specialities over internal medicine?" *New England Journal of Medicine*, 317(1991): 25–33.

McClelland, C. E. *State, society, and university in Germany, 1700–1914*. Cambridge: Cambridge University Press, 1980.

McClelland, C. E. *The German Experience of Professionalization: Modern Learned Professions and Their Organization from the Early Nineteenth Century to the Hitler Era*. Cambridge: Cambridge University Press, 1991.

McGlashan, N. "Towards the geography of health," *Progress in Human Geography*, 2(1978):532–536.

McGrew, R. E. *Encyclopedia of Medical History*. New York: McGraw-Hill, 1985.

McKeown, T. "A sociological approach to the history of medicine," *Medical History*, 14(1970):342–351.

McKeown, T. *The Role of Medicine: Dean, Mirage or Nemesis*. London: The Nuffield Provincial Hospitals Trust, 1976.

McKeown, T. *The Origins of Human Disease*. Oxford: Basil Blackwell, 1988.

McKeown, T. *The Modern Rise of Population*. London: Arnold, 1976.

McKibben, B. *The end of nature*. London: Viking, 1990.

McKinlay, J. B. "On the professional regulation of change," *Sociological Review Monograph*, 20(1973):61–84.

McKinlay, J. B. "The Business of Good Doctoring or Doctoring as Good Business: Reflections on Freidsons View of the Medical Game," *International Journal of Health Services*, 7(1977):459–487.

McKinlay, J. B. "The Changing Character of the Medical Profession: Introduction," *Milbank Quarterly*, 66(1988):1–9.

McKinlay, J.B. and J. Arches. "Towards the proletarianization of physicians." *International Journal of Health Services* 15 (1985): 161–195.

McKinlay, J. B. and J. Arches. "Historical Changes in Doctoring: A Reply to Milton Roemer," *International Journal of Health Services*, 16(1986):473–477.

McKinlay, J.B., and J.D. Stoeckle. "Corporatization and the social transformation of doctoring." *Sosiaalilääketieteellinen Aikakauslehti* (Sosialmedisinsk tidsskrift), 24 (1987):73–84.

McKinlay, J. B. and J. D. Stoeckle. "Corporatization and the social transformation of doctoring," *International Journal of Health Services*, 18(1988):191–205.

McKinlay, J.B., D. Light, S. Levine, et al. "The changing character of the medical profession. (Volume 66, Supplement 2):" *The Milbank Quarterly* 66 (1988): 1–225.

McMichael, A. J. *Planetary overload. Global environmental change and the health of the human species*. Cambridge: Cambridge University Press, 1994.

McWhinney, I. R. *A textbook of family medicine*. Oxford: Oxford University Press, 1989.

Mechanic, D. "General medical practice in England and Wales; its organization and future," *New England Journal of Medicine*, 279(1968):680–689.

Medicinalberetningene. *Avlevering fra medisinaldirektoratet 1932. Medicinalberetningen og innberetninger om epidemiske sykdommer, kolera etc. 1835–1921*. Riksarkivet i Oslo.

Medisinerforeningens historie. Kristiania: Det Mallingske Boktrykkeri, 1883.

Meland, E. and P. Fugelli. "Perestrojka – i medisinen også," *Tidsskrift for Den norske lægeforening*, 111(1991):354–356.

Melbye, H. "Diagnosis of pneumonia in adults in general practice". Tromsø: *ISM skriftserie 24*. Institute of Community Medicine, University of Tromsø, 1992.

Mellbye, F. "Sunnhetsloven av 1860 og de menn som skapte den," *Liv og Helse*, 5 (1960).

Mellbye, F. *Slit med helsa. Bilder fra medisinsk samtid*. Oslo: Gyldendal, 1989.

Mellbye, P. A. M. *Norges kursteder og deres kurmidler*. Kristiania: Alb. Cammermeyers forlag, 1903.

Melville, A. "Job satisfaction in general practice: Implications for prescribing," *Social Science and Medicine*, 14A(1980): 495–499.

Menzel, H. "Innovation, Integration, and Marginality: A Survey of Physicians," *American Sociological Review*, XXV(1960): 704–713.

Merton, R. K. "Priorities in scientific discovery: A chapter in the sociology of science," *American Sociological Review*, 22 (1957):635–659.

Merton, R. K. "The Unanticipated Consequences of Purposive Social Action," *American Sociological Review*, 1(1936): 894–904.

Merton, R. K. "The role set: Problems in sociological theory," *British Journal of Sociology*, 8(1957):106–120.

Merton, R. K. "Social structure and anomie," *American Sociological Review*, 3 (1939):672–682.

Metzger, W. P. "A specter is haunting American scholars: the specter of "professionalism"," *Educational Researcher*, 16 (1987):10–19.

Midre, G. *Bot, bedring eller brød*. Oslo: Universitetsforlaget, 1990.

Miké, V. "American Medicine Today: Values in Conflict," *Bull Sci Tech Soc*, 8 (1988):374–377.

Miller, L. G. "Pain, Parturition, and the Profession: Twilight Sleep in America," in *Health Care in America. Essays in Social History*, eds. Reverby, S. and D. Rosner. Philadelphia: Temple University Press, 1979.

Minkowski, W. L. "Physician Motives in Banning Medieval Traditional Healers," *Women Health*, 21(1994):83–96.

Minkowski, W. L. "Women healers of the middle ages: selected aspects of their history." *American Journal of Public Health*, 82(1992):288–295.

Minute Book of the Health Commission of the Municipality of Ringsaker 1861–1942.

Mitchell, W. J. T. ed. *On Narrative*. University of Chicago Press, 1981.

Moe, E. *Den siste distriktslege*. Stord: 1994.

Moen, E. *Rift om brødet? Thesis in history.* University of Oslo, 1984.

Moen, E. *Modum – ei bygd, tre elver.* Caspersens trykkeri, 1993.

Molland, E. *Fra Hans Nielsen Hauge til Eivind Berggrav. Hovedlinjer i Norges kirkehistorie i det 19. og 20. århundre*. Oslo: Gyldendal, 1968.

Monro, T. K. *The Physician. As man of letters, science and action*. Edinburgh: 1951.

Montagna, P. "Professionalization and bureaucratization in large professional organizations," *American Journal of Sociology*, 74 (1968):138–145.

Montgomery, K. "Professional dominance and the threat of corporatization," *Current Research on Occupations and Professions*, 7(1992):221–240.

Montgomery, K. "A Prospective Look at the

Speciality of Medical Management," *Work and Occupations*, 17(1990):178–198.

Morantz, R. M. and S. Zschoche. "Professionalism, Feminism, and Gender Roles: A Comparative Study of Nineteenth-Century Medical Therapeutics," *The Journal of American History*, 67(1980):568–588.

Moritz, M. S. *Deutsche Kliniker Am die Jahrundertwende.* Köln: 1958.

Morrison, I. and R. Smith. "The future of medicine," *British Medical Journal*, 309(1994):1099–1100.

Morton, L. T. *A Medical Bibliography (Garrison and Morton): an Annotated Checklist of Texts Illustrating the History of Medicine.* 1983.

Moum, T., T. Sørensen, S. Næss and J. Holmen. "Gir diagnosen høyt blodtrykk endret livskvalitet? Resultater fra en medisinsk masseundersøkelse i Nord-Trøndelag", *Tidsskrift for Den norske lægeforening*, 112(1992):18–23.

Mull, D. J. "Cross-cultural communication in the physician's office," *West Journal of Medicine*, 159 (1993):609–613.

Munthe, E. and Ø. Larsen. *Revmatisme – gamle plager – ny viten.* Oslo: Tano, 1987.

Murphy, T. D. "The French medical profession's perception of its social function between 1776 and 1830," *Medical History*, 23(1979):259–278.

Murphy, R. "The Struggle for Scholarly Recognition. The Development of the Closure Problematic in Sociology," *Theory and Society*, 12(1983):631–658.

Murphy, R. "Power and Autonomy in the Sociology of Education," *Theory and Society*, 11(1982):179–203.

Murphy, R. *Social Closure: The Theory of Monopolization and Exclusion.* Oxford: Clarendon Press, 1988.

Murphy, R. "Explotation or exclusion," *Sociology*, 19(1985):225–243.

Murphy, R. "The structure of closure: a critique and development of the theories of Weber, Collins, and Parkin," *The British Journal of Sociology*, 35(1984):547–567.

Murphy, R. "Weberian closure theory: a contribution to the ongoing assessement," *The British Journal of Sociology*, 1 37 (1986):21–41.

Murray, R. M. "The health of Doctors. A review," *Journal of the Royal College of Physicians*, 12(1978):403–415.

Mustelin, O. "Vetenskapliga studieresor från Finland til kontinenten under 1800–tallet," *Finsk tidskrift*, 3(1970): 146–158.

Muzzin, L. J., G. P. Brown, and R. W. Hornosty. "Consequences of Feminization of a Profession: The Case of Canadian Pharmacy," *Women & Health*, 21(1994): 39–56.

Myren, J. and C.W. Janssen. *Fra gastroenterologiens historie i Norge.* Oslo: Norsk Gastroenterologisk Forening, 1995.

Myhre, JE. *Oslo bys historie, bind 3*. Oslo: 1990.

Myklebost, H. *Norges tettbygde steder 1875–1950*. Oslo, Bergen: Universitetsforlaget, 1960.

Møller, D. J. *Studentene fra 1943.* Oslo: Oscar Andersens Boktrykkeri, 1968.

Møller, K. O. *Udkast til Oppraab til danske Læger om økonomisk Støtte til norske Medisinerstudenter,* 1945.

Måseide, P. "Possibly abusive, often benign, and always necessary. On power and domination in medical practice," *Sociology of Health & Illness*, 13(1991):545–561.

Måseide, P. "Health and Social Inequity in Norway," *Social Science and Medicine*, 31 (1990):331–342.

Naisbitt, J. and P. Aburdene. *Megatrends 2000.* London: Pan books, 1990.

Nash, D. "The Rise and Fall of an Aristocratic Tourist Culture, Nice: 1763–1936," *Annals of Tourism Research*, 6(1979): 61–75.

National Archives (Riksarkivet), (Ministry of Health and Social Affairs, Directorate of Medicine, Doctor's Office), The boxes

1, 147, 148, 151, 154, 156, 158, 168, 197, 202.

Natvig, H. *Lærebok i hygiene.* Oslo: Liv og helses forlag, 1958.

Natvig, H. "Blaafarveverket på Modum. Kosthold og leveforhold i en arbeiderfamilie på Modum i 1845", *Liv og Helse*, 1963.

Natvig, H. "Refleksjoner ved opphøret av Nordisk Hygiensk Tidsskrift", *Nordisk Hygienisk Tidsskrift,* 55(1974):129–37.

Natvig, H. "Kosthold, levevilkår og arbeidsforhold blant arbeidere ved Modum Blaafarveværk i 1845", *Norsk bedriftshelsetjeneste*, 6(1985):292–302.

Natvig, H. and E. Thiis-Evensen sen. "Arbeidsmiljø og helse", *Norsk bedriftshelsetjeneste*, 4(1983): 1–333.

Navarro, V. *Medicine under Capitalism.* London: Croom Helm, 1977.

Navarro, V. "Health and the Corporate Society," *Social Policy*, 5(1979):41–49.

Navarro, V. *Crisis, Health, and Medicine: A Social Critique.* New York: Tavistock, 1986.

Navarro, V. "Professional Dominance or Proletarianization?: Neither", *Milbank Quarterly*, 66(1988):57–75.

Neittaanmäki, L., R. Luhtala, I. Virjo, E. Kumpusalo, K. Mattila, M. Jääskeläinen, S. Kujala and M. Isokoski. "More women enter medicine; young doctors' family origin and career choice." *Medical Education*, 27(1993):440–445.

NEM (Den internasjonale forskningsetiske komiteen for medisin). *Etiske sider ved prioritering og ressursfordeling i medisinsk forskning*. Oslo: 1995.

Nerbøvik, J. *Norsk Historie 1870 – 1905.* Oslo: Det Norske Samlaget, 1986.

Nerheim, H. *Vitenskap og kommunikasjon. Paradigmer, modeller og kommunikative strategier i helsefagenes vitenskapsteori*. Oslo: Universitetsforlaget, 1995.

Neumann, D. *Studentinnen aus dem Russichen Reich in der Schweiz (1867–1914)*. Zürich: 1987.

Newman, C. "The Rise of Specialism and Postgraduate Education," in *The Evolution of Medical Education in Britain*, ed. Poynter, F. N. L. London: Pitman Medical Publishing Company Ltd, 1966.

Nichter, M. and N. Vuckovic. "Agenda for an anthropology of pharmaceutical practice," *Social Science and Medicine*, 39(1994): 1509–1525.

Nicolaysen, J. "Om reservelægernes forandrede økonomiske stilling ved Rigshospitalet," *Tidsskrift for Den norske lægeforening*, (1894):104–113, 162–164, 183

Nicolaysen, K. G. "Er egne medlemsblad løsningen?" *Tidsskrift for Den norske lægeforening,* 114(1994):2176–7, 2304–5, 2432–3.

Nicolson, M. and C. McLaughlin. "Social constructionism and medical sociology: a reply to M. R. Bury," *Sociology of Health & Illness*, 9(1987):107–126.

Nicolson, M. "The introduction of percussion and stethoscopy to early nineteenth-century Edinburgh," in *Medicine and the five senses*, eds. Bynum, W. F. and R. Porter. Cambridge: Cambridge University Press, 1993.

Nielsen, J. (ed) *Social Security in the Nordic Countries. Scope, expenditure and financing.* Köbenhavn: Nordic Social-Statistical Committee, 1995.

Nilsson P. and B. Persson. "Dödsorsaker bland svenska provinsläkare 1840–1879", *Allmänmedicin*, 1(1995): 30–31.

Nilsson, H. *Mot bättre hälsa. Dödlighet och hälsoarbete i Linköping 1860–1894*. Linköping: Linköping Studies in Arts and Science, 1994.

Nissen-Lie, H. S. *Noen tanker ved Norsk Ortopedisk Forenings 25-års jubileum.* November 1972.

Nordang, J. A. "Lægeforholdene paa Vardø," *Tidsskrift for Den norske lægeforening* (1891):427–431.

Nordang, J. A. "Lægeforholdene paa Vardø," *Tidsskrift for Den norske lægeforening*, (1892):391.

Nordby, T. *Karl Evang*. Oslo: Aschehoug, 1989.

Nordby, T. ed . *Arbeiderpartiet og planstyret 1945–1965*. Oslo: Universitetsforlaget, 1994.

Nordby, T. "Profesjokratiets periode innen norsk helsevesen – institusjoner, politikk og konfliktemner," *Historisk Tidsskrift*, 3 (1987):301–323.

Nordenfelt, L. and P.A. Tengland (eds). *The Goals and Limits of Medicine.* Stockholm: Almquist & Wiksell International, 1996.

Nordhagen, R. "Fra legekvinne til lege, og litt om det som har hendt siden Livius Smitt talte det Medisinske fakultet midt imot og skaffet kvinnen adgang," in *Kvinner på Universitet 100 år*, Oslo: Likestillingsutvalget Universitetet i Oslo, 1984, p. 69–97.

Nordhagen, R. "Akademiske grader og skiftende sans for seremonier", *Tidsskrift for Den norske lægeforening*,115(1995):3753–6.

Nordisk Medicinhistorisk Årbok 1968. Yearbook of the Museum of Medical History, Stockholm.

Norge vårt land. Den vide bygd – der fjerne åser blåner. Oslo: Gyldendal Norsk Forlag, 1984.

Norman, J. M. ed. *Morton's medical bibliography*. 5th ed. Aldershot: Scolar Press, 1991.

Norsk Etnografisk samlings spørreskjemaer: "Folkemedisin". (Emnenr. 80, 1960) Questionnaires.

Norske elever og studenter i utlandet. Oslo: Statens lånekasse for utdanning, several years.

Norske militærleger 1882–1932. *Oslo 1932.*

"Notes on health resorts. Nauheim," Editorial, *The British Medical Journal,* 7(1904): 1203–1204.

Nuland, S. B. *Doctors: The Biography of Medicine*. New York: 1989.

Nylenna, M. "Det nasjonale medisinske tidsskrift – hvorfor?" *Ugeskrift for læger*, 152(1990):3761–3765.

Nylenna, M. "Tidsskriftets leserundersøkelse 1990", Tidsskrift for *Den norske lægeforening,* 110(1990):3912–3913.

Nylenna, M. "Norske legers lesevaner," *Nordisk Medicin*, 106(1991):53–55.

Nylenna, M. *Cancer – A challenge to the general practitioner. Thesis.* Oslo: The Norwegian Cancer Society, Department of General Practice, University of Oslo, 1992.

Nylenna, M. "The future of medical journals: An editor's view," *Croatian Medical Journal*, 35(1994):195–198.

Nylenna, M. "Så mye å lese, så liten tid å gjøre det på," *Tidsskrift for Den norske lægeforening*, 115(1995):2043

Nylenna, M., "Norway's Decentralized, Single-Payer Health System Faces Great Challenges". 274,*JAMA* (1995):120–124.

Nylenna, M., O. G. Aasland, and E. Falkum. "Keeping professionally updated: Perceived coping and CME-profiles among physicians," *(Submitted)*.

Nylenna, M. and H.M. Svabø. "Tidsskriftets målsetting," *Tidsskrift for Den norske lægeforening,* 107(1987):3003.

Nylenna, M. and R. Smith, "American retreat on SI units", *British Medical Journal,* 305(1992):268.

O'Brien, P. "Transport and Economic Development in Europe, 1789–1914," in *Railways and the Economic Development of Western Europe, 1830–1914*, ed. O'Brien, P. London: Macmillan, 1983.

O'Neill, J. "The medicalization of social control," *Canadian Review of Sociology and Anthropology*, 23(1986):350–364.

Odelstingsproposisjon nr. 28, 1924.

Odelstingsprorosisjon nr. 29, 1934.

Odelstingsprorosisjon nr. 34, 1859–1860.

Odelstingsprorosisjon nr. 46, 1938.

Odelstingsproposisjon nr. 76, 1949.

Oehri, A. *Kurzbiographien amerikanicher Ärzte und Naturwissenchaftler die zwischen 1930 und 1940 verstorben sind.* 1987.

Ofstad, H. *Vår forakt for svakhet*. Oslo: Pax Forlag, 1991.

Oldershaw, J. "Accessing the literature," *British Journal of Hospital Medicine*, 47

(1992):433–437.

Olsen, T. B., *Forskning ved norske sykehus. Rapport 5/91*. Oslo: NAVFs utredningsinstitutt, 1991.

Olsen, T. B., *Norske doktorgrader i tall – med særlig vekt på tiårsperioden 1984–93*. Rapport 9/94. Oslo: Utredningsinstituttet for forskning og høyere utdanning, 1994.

Olsen, T. B. and H. Skoie. eds. *Noen forskningspolitiske spørsmål i norsk medisin*. Rapport 19/91. Oslo: NAVFs utredningsinstitutt, 1991.

Olsen, T. B., H. F. Hansen, T. Luukonen, O. Persson, and G. Sivertsen. *Nordisk forskning i internasjonal sammenheng – en bibliometrisk beskrivelse av publisering og siteringer i naturvitenskaplig og medisinsk forskning*. Copenhagen: Nordisk Ministerråd, 1994.

Oppenheimer, M. "The proletarianization of the professional," *Sociological Review Monograph*, 20(1973):213–227.

Ore, O. "Norwegian emigrants with university training 1830–1880," *Norwegian-American Studies and Records,* Vol. XIX, pp. 168–88. Northfield, Minn: Norwegian-American Historical Association, 1956.

"Orker vi å være sykehusleger lenger?" *Tidsskrift for Den norske lægeforening*, 115 (1995):3315.

Orzack, L. H. "Work as a "central life interest" of professionals," *Social Problems*, 7 (1959):125–132.

Osborne, T. "Medicine and epistemology: Michel Foucault and the liberality of clinical reason," *History of the Human Sciences*, 5(1992):63–93.

Osborne, T. "On liberalism, neo-liberalism and the "liberal profession" of medicine," *Economy and Society*, 22(1993):345–356.

Oseid, S. *Norsk Idrettsmedisinske Forening 25 år 1966–1991*. Grøset: Grafisk Senter, 1991.

Osmond, H. and M. Siegler. "Doctors as patients," *The Practitioner*, 218(1977): 834–839.

Ottesen, H. "Litt om lægeforhold i Finnmarken," *Tidsskrift for Den norske lægeforening*, (1916):207–209.

Oversigt over Det norske Civile Lægevæsens historiske Udvikling og nuværende Ordning. (Report from the Royal Commission for Doctors 1898). Supplements to the proposals of the Public Medical Services Act (1912).

Pachter, L. M. "Culture and clinical care. Folk illness beliefs and behaviors and their implications for health care delivery," *Journal of the American Medical Association*, 271(1994):690

Palmstrøm, H. "Om en befolkningsgruppes utvikling gjennom de siste 100 år", *Statsøkonomisk tidsskrift, 49(1935):161–370.*

Parks, G. B. "The turn to the romantic in travel literature of the eighteenth century," *Modern Language Quarterly*, 25(1964): 22–33.

Parsons, T. "Remarks on Education and the Profession," *The International Journal of Ethics*, 47(1937):365–381.

Parsons, T. "The professions and social structure," *Social Forces*, 17(1939):457–467.

Parsons, T. *The Social System*. New York: Free Press, 1951.

Parsons, T. "Illness and the role of the physician: A sociological perspective," *American Journal of Orthopsychiatry*, 121 (1951):452–460.

Parsons, T. and R. Fox. "Illness, Therapy, and the Modern Urban American Family," *Journal of Social Issues*, 8(1952): 31–44.

Parsons, T. "The Superego and the Theory of Social Systems," *Psychiatry*, 15(1952): 15–25.

Parsons, T. "Social Change and Medical Organization in the United States: A Sociological Perspective," *The Annals of The American Academy of Political and Social Science: Medicine and Society*, 346(1963): 21–33.

Parsons, T. "The Sick Role and the Role of

the Physician Reconsidered," *Milbank Memorial Fund Quarterly: Health and Society*, 53(1975):257–278.

Parssinen, T. M. "Professional deviants and the history of medicine: Medical mesmerists in Victorian Britain," *Sociological Review Monograph*, (1979):103–120.

Paterson, A. "Becoming a Judge," in *The Sociology of the Professions: Lawyers, Doctors and Others*, eds. Dingwall, R. and P. Lewis. London: Macmillan, 1983.

Pavalko, R. M. *Sociology of Occupations and Professions*. Itasca, IL: F. E. Peacock, 1971.

Pavalko, R. M. ed. *Sociological Perspectives on Occupations*. Itasca, Ill. F. E. Peacock, 1972.

Payer, L. *Medicine and Culture: Varieties of Treatment in the United States, England, West Germany and France*. New York: Henry Holt and Company, 1988.

Payne, R. and J. Firth-Cozens. *Stress in health professionals* New York: John Wiley & Son, 1987.

Pedersen, P., T.Risør, T.R.Eriksen, et al. "Den sociale rekruttering af lægestuderende i 1992/1993 ved Københavns Universitet." *Ugeskrift for læger* 156 (1994): 7372–7376.

Perkin, H. *The rise of professional society: England since 1880*. London: Routledge, 1989.

Pflanz, M. "Relations between social scientists, physicians and medical organizations in health research," *Social Science and Medicine*, 9(1975)

Phillips, D. P., E. J. Kanter, B. Bednarczyk, and P. L. Tastad. "Importance of the lay press in the transmission of medical knowledge to the scientific community," *New England Journal of Medicine*, 325 (1991):1180–1183.

Pierach, C. A., S. D. Wangensteen, and H. B. Burchell. "Spa Theraphy for Heart Disease Bad Nauheim (circa 1900)," *The American Journal of Cardiology*, 72(1993): 336–342.

Pill, R. and N. Stott. "Concepts of Illnesses, Causation and Responsibility," *Social Science and Medicine*, 16(1982):43–52.

Pines, A., K. Skulkebo, E. Pollak, E. Peritz and J. Steif. "Rates of sickness absenteeism among employees of a modern hospital: the role of demographic and occupational factors," *British Journal of Industrial Medicine,* 42(1985):326–335.

Pingitore, D. "Family Medicine: American Culture in American Medicine," *Science as Culture*, 4:167–211.

Pinner, M. and B. F. Miller. eds. *When doctors are patients*. New York: Norton & Comp, 1952.

Porter, D. "Public Health", in *The Companion Encyclopaedia of the History of Medicine Vol 2*, eds. Bynum, WF and R. Porter. London: Routledge, 1993.

Porter, R. "Lay medical knowledge in the eighteenth century: The evidence of the Gentleman's magazine," *Medical History*, 29(1985):138–168.

Porter, R. "Introduction," *Medical History*, (1990):7–12.

Porter, R. "Madness and its institutions," in *Medicine in society. Historical essays*, ed. Wear, A. Cambridge: Cambridge University Press, 1992. 277–301.

Porter, R. "The patient in England, c. 1660–c. 1800," in *Medicine in society. Historical essays*, ed. Wear, A. Cambridge: Cambridge University Press, 1992.

Porter, R. "The rise of physical examination," in *Medicine and the five senses*, eds. Bynum, W. F. and R. Porter. Cambridge: Cambridge University Press, 1993.

Porter, R. *Health for Sale: Quackery in England, 1660–1850*. 1989.

Porter, R. ed. *The Popularization of Medicine*. London: 1992.

Porter, R. and A. Wear. eds *Problems and Methods in the History of Medicine*. Beckenham: Croom Helm Ltd, 1987.

Porter, R. ed. *Patients and practitioners*. Cambridge: Cambridge University Press, 1985.

Portwood, D. and A. Fielding. "Privilege and the Professions," *Sociological Review*, 29(1981):749–773.

Posen, S. "The portrayal of the physician in non-medical literature – the physician and his colleages." *Journal of the Royal Society of Medicine*, 85(1993):410–412.

Posen, S. "The portrayal of the physician in non-medical literature – the physician and his family (editoral)." *Journal of the Royal Society of Medicine*, 85(1992): 314–317.

Posen, S. "The portrayal of the physician in non-medical literature-resentment, confrontation, litigation." *Journal of the Royal Society Medicine*, 85(1992):520–523.

Posen, S. "The portrayal of the physician in non-medical literature – the one-track mind (editorial)." *Journal of the Royal Society of Medicine*, 85(1992):66–68.

Posen, S. "The portrayal of the physician in non-medical literature: career choises." *Journal og the Royal Society of Medicine*, 87 (1994):675–680.

Posen, S. "The portrayal of the physician in non-medicine literature – the physician and politics." *Journal of the Royal Society of Medicine,* 87(1994):237.241.

Posen, S. "The postrayal of the physician in non-medical literature – versatile scholar or ignorant boor?" *Journal of the Royal Society of Medicine*, 87(1994):104–106.

Posen, S. "The portrayal of the physician in non-medical literature – the physician who dislikes his trade." *Journal of the Royal Society of Medicine*, 86(1993):67–68.

Posen, S. "The portrayal of the physician in non-medical literature – favourable portrayals." *Journal of the Royal Society of Medicine*, 86(1993):724–728.

Posen, S. "The portrayal of the physician in non-medical literature – the physician and religion." *Journal of the Royal Society of Mesicine*, 85(1992):659–662.

Posen, S. "The portrayal of the physician in non-medical literature – the female physician." *Journal of the Royal Society of Medicine*, 86(1993):345–348.

Posen, S. "The portrayal of the physician in non-medical literature – the bedside manner." *Journal of the Royal Society of Medicine*, 86(1993):582–586.

Posen, S. "The portrayal of the physician in non-medical literature – sexual fantasies and encounters (editorial)." *Journal of the Royal Society of Medicine*, 86(1993):128–129.

Powles, J. "On the limitations of modern medicine," *Sci Med Man*, 1(1973)

Poynter, F. N. L. ed. *The Evolution of Medical Education in Britain*. London: Pitman Medical Publishing Company Ltd, 1966.

Preus, J.K.K. "Indberetning til Kirke-Undervisnings-Departementet om en med Stipendium foretagen videnskabelig Reise i Udlandet," *Norsk Magazin for Lægevidenskaben*, (1847):434–451.

Price, R. "Hydropathy in England 1840–70," *Medical History*, 25(1981):269–280.

Pryser, T. *Norsk historie 1800–1870. Frå standssamfunn mot klassesamfunn*. Oslo: Det Norske Samlaget, 1993.

Puschmann, T. *A History of Medical Education*. New York: 1965.

Rabin, D. and P. Bush. "The use of medicine: historical trends and international comparisons," *International Journal of Health Services*, 4(1974)

Ramsey, M. "Review essay: History of a profession, Annales style: The work of Jacques Leonard," *Journal of Social History*, 17(1983):319–338.

Rasmussen, E. "Legen i norsk litteratur," *Tidsskrift for Den norske lægeforening*, 11(1961):701–705.

Rasmussen, S. *Barnhjertighetsfronten. Norsk Røde Kors 1940–45*. Oslo: Halvorsen og Larsen forl., 1950.

Reader, W. J. *Professional Men – The Rise of the Professional Classes in Nineteenth-Century England*. London: Weidenfield & Nicholson, 1966.

Reed, R. R. and D. Evans. "The deprofessionalization of medicine. Causes, effects, and responses." *The Journal of the Royal American Medical Association*, 258(1987): 3279–3282.

Reichborn-Kjennerud, I. "Medicinske forhold i Norge i 1300-aarene," *Norsk Magazin for Lægevidenskaben*, 86(1925): 637–653.

Reichborn-Kjennerud, I. "En oversigt over og karakteristik av de gamle nordiske lægebøker," *Tidsskrift for Den norske lægeforening*, 44(1924):381–386, 424–429.

Reichborn-Kjennerud, I., F. Grøn and I. Kobro. *Medisinens historie i Norge*. Oslo: Grøndahl & Søns forlag, 1936.

Relman, A. R. "The purpose and prospects of the general medical journal," *Bull NY Acad Med*, 64(1988):875–880.

Relman, A. S. "The new medical-industrial complex," *New England Journal of Medicine*, 303(1980):963–970.

Renaud, M. "On the constraints to state intervention in health," *International Journal of Health Services*, 5(1975)

Reports on the Public Health in Norway 1853, 1860 & 1900. Department of the Interior (1856 & 1863) & The Director of Medicine(1902).

Reverby, S. and D. Rosner. *Health Care in America. Essays in Social History*. Philadelphia: Temple University Press, 1979.

Reverby, S. and D. Rosner. "Beyond "the Great Doctors"," in *Health Care in America. Essays in Social History*, eds. Reverby, S. and D. Rosner. Philadelphia: Temple University Press, 1979.

Rheinberger, R. *Liechtensteiner Ärzte des 19. Jahrhunderts*. 1991.

Richards, C. *The health of doctors*. KF project paper nr. 78. King Edvard's Hospital Fund for London, 1989.

Richards, R. K. "Physicians' self-directed learning. A new perspective for continuing medical education. I. Reading," *Möbius*, 6(1986):1–13.

Riis, P. "New paradigms in journalology," *J Int Med*, 232(1992):207–213.

Rikstrygdeverket. *Trygdestatistisk årbok 1994*. Oslo: Utredningsavdelingen Rikstrygdeverket, 1994.

Riksaasen, R. "Påkjenninger i legeyrket," *Tidsskrift for Den norske lægeforening*, 109 16(1989):1798–1799.

Rimpelä, A. H., N. M. Nurminen, P.O. Pulkkinen, M.K. Rimpelä and T. Valkonen. "Mortality of doctors: do doctors benefit from their medical knowledge?" *Lancet*, 1(1987):84–86.

Ringdal, J. R. "Borte bra – men hjemme best," *Dagbladet*,(1959): 27th of January.

Riska, E. and K. Wegar. *Gender, Work and Medicine: Women and the Medical Divisions of Labour*. London: SAGE, 1993.

Riska, E. and K. Wegar. "The medical profession in the Nordic countries: medical uncertainty and gender-based work," in *Health professions and the state in Europe*, eds. Johnson, T. G. Larkin, and M. Saks. London: Routledge, 1995.

Riska, E. "The Professional Status of Physicians in the Nordic Countries," *The Milbank Quarterly*, 66(1988):133–147.

Riska, E. and K. Wegar. "Women physicians: a new force in medicine," in *Gender, Work an Medicine: Women and the Medical Divisions of Labour*, eds. Riska, E. and K. Wegar. London: SAGE, 1993.

Riska, E. Läkarprofessionens förandrade ställning: En fallstudie av kvinnelige läkare i Finland." *Sosiaalilääketieteellinen Aikakauslehti (Socialmedicinsk tidsskrift), 24(1987):105–115.*

Riska, E. "Läkarprofessionens utveckling i olika länder." *Sosiaalilääketieteellinen Aikakauslehti (Sosialmedisinsk tidsskrift), 25(1988):27–37.*

Risse, G. B., J. W. Leavitt, and R. L. Numbers. *Medicine without Doctors*. New York: Science History Publications, 1977.

Riste, O. *Londonregjeringa Vol II*. Oslo: Det norske samlaget, 1979.

Röber, F.A. *Von der Sorge des Staats für die*

Gesundheit seiner Bürger. Dresden: Carl Gottlob Gärtner, 1805.

Roberts, K., F. G. Cook, S. C. Clark, and E. Semenoff. "The family life-cycle, domestic roles and the meaning of leisure," *Society and Leisure*, 8(1976):7–20.

Roemer, M. I. "Proletarianization of Physicians or Organization of Health Services?" *International Journal of Health Services*, 16(1986):469–472.

Rogers, E.M. "Diffusion of innovations." 3rd ed. New York: The Free Press, 1983.

Roness, A. *Utbrent? Arbeidspress og psykiske lidelser hos mennesker i utsatte yrker*. Oslo: Universitetsforlaget, 1995.

Rosen, G. "An eighteenth-century plan for a national health service," *Bulletin of the History of Medicine*, 16(1944):429–436.

Rosen, G. and B. Caspari-Rosen. *400 Years of a Doctors life*. New York: 1947.

Rosen, G. and Rosenberg. eds. *The Structure of American Medical Practice 1875–1940*. Philadelphia: 1983.

Rosen, G. "Cameralism and the concept of medical police," *Bulletin of the History of Medicine*, 27(1952):21–42.

Rosen, G. "Medical care and social policy in seventeenth century England," *New York Academy of Medicine Bulletin*, 29(1953): 420–437.

Rosen, G. *A History of Public Health*. New York: 1958.

Rosen, G. "Mercantilism and health policy in eighteenth century French thought," *Medical History*, 3(1959):259–275.

Rosenberg, C. E. "The therapeutic revolution: Medicine, meaning, and social change in nineteenth-century America," *Perspectives in Biology and Medicine*, 20 (1977):485–506.

Rosenkrantz, B. G. "Cart before Horse: Theory, Practice, and Professional Image in American Public Health 1870–1920," *Journal of the History of Medicine and Allied Sciences*, 29(1974):55–73.

Rosenstein, A. H. "Consumerism and health care," *Postgraduate Medicine*, 79 (1986):13–18.

Rosvold, E.O. and Ø. Larsen. "Krankheiten im Arztberuf. Die Gesundheit norwegischer Ärzte und ihrer Angehörigen im ausgehenden 19. Jahrhundert", *Medizinhistorisches Journal,* 1–2(1996):167–180.

Roth, J. A. "Professionalism: The sociologists decoy," *Sociology of Work and Occupations*, 1(1974):6–23.

Roth, M. S. "The Time of Nostalgia: Medicine, history and normality in 19th-century France," *Time & Society*, 1(1992): 271–286.

Rousseau, G. S. and R. Porter. eds. *The ferment of knowledge. Studies in the Historiography of Eighteenth-Century Science*. Cambridge: Cambridge University Press, 1980.

Rueschemeyer, D. "Doctors and lawyers: a comment on the theory of professions," *Canadian Journal of Sociology and Anthropology*, 1(1964):17

Rueschemeyer, D. "Professional Autonomy and the Social Control of Expertise," in *The Sociology of the Professions: Lawyers, Doctors and Others*, eds. Dingwall, R. and P. Lewis. London: Macmillan, 1983.

Rueschemeyer, D. "Comparing Legal Professions Cross-nationally: From a Professions-centered to a State-centered Approach," *American Bar Foundation Research Journal*, (1986):415–446.

Rutle, O. et al. "Den oppbrukte legen," *Tidsskrift for Den norske lægeforening*, 108 23(1988):1819–1824.

Rydberg, S. *Svenska studieresor till England under frihetstiden*. Uppsala: Almqvist & Wiksells Boctryckeri AB, 1951.

Rådet for medisinsk forskning. *Medisinsk forskning og teknologi. Utvikling og konsekvenser (Del 1)*. Oslo: Norges allmennvitenskapelige forskningsråd, 1986.

Saint-Léger, A.de and F. Le Play. "Fondeur des usines à cobalt du Buskerud". *In: Ouvriers Européens. Etudes sur les Travaux.*

La vie domestique, et la Condition Morale de Populations Ouvriers de l'Europe, 2. éditition. Tome 13, Les Ouvriers du Nord. Paris, Marne: chapter II, 1877.

Sakula, A. "European Medicine: A Historical Perspective," *British Journal of Rheumatology*, 32(1993):2–4.

Saltonstall, R. "Healthy bodies, social bodies: Men's and women's concepts and practices of health in everyday life," *Social Science and Medicine*, 36(1993): 7–14.

Samra, R. J. "The Image of the Physician: A Rhetorical Perspective," *Public Relations Review*, 19(1993):341–348.

Sandberg, O. "Indberetning til Kirke- og Underviisnings-Departementet om en med Stipendium foretagen videnskabelig Reise i Udlandet," *Norsk Magazin for Lægevidenskaben*, (1851):613–663.

Sandvik, E. "Medisinstudentene får landsomfattende organisasjon," *Æsculap*, 2 (1981):6–12.

Sandvik, H. "Psykiatriske pasienter i privat pleie. Historisk analyse fra en Vestlandskommune," *Tidsskrift for Den norske lægeforening*, 110(1990):1666–1668.

Sandvik, H. "Ingen sammenheng mellom skarlagensfeber og giktfeber. Historisk analyse fra Ytre Nordhordland 1862–84," *Tidsskrift for Den norske lægeforening*, 112(1992):3803–3805.

Sandvik, H. "Spedalskhet og arv. En distriktsleges betraktninger fra 1884," *Tidsskrift for Den norske lægeforening*, 112(1992): 3799–3801.

Sandvik, H. "De siste dødsfall av kopper i Ytre Nordhordland. En distriktleges erfaringer," *Tidsskrift for Den norske lægeforening*, 113 16(1993):2096–2098.

Sandvik, H. "Tyfoidfeber i Ytre Nordhordland legedistrikt. Smitteveier, insidens og letalitet i perioden 1854–83," *Tidsskrift for Den norske lægeforening*, 113(1993): 1990–1993.

Sandvik, H. ""Dei Vise forvilde Væræ!!. En distriktsleges kamp mot overtro og troldom på 1800-tallet," *Tidsskrift for Den norske lægeforening*, 113(1993):3572–3574.

Sandvik, H. "Bekjempelse av skabb i Ytre Nordhordland legedistrikt. Et samfunnsmedisinsk eksperiment i 1860-årene," *Tidsskrift for Den norske lægeforening*, 113(1993):40–43.

Sandvik, P. T. *Fabrikken ved Nidelven*. Thesis in history, University of Trondheim, 1993.

Sargent, D. A. e. a. "Preventing physician suicide. The role of family, colleagues, and organized medicine," *Journal of the American Medical Association*, 237 (1977):143–145.

Sarton, G. "The History of Science versus the History of Medicine," *Isis*, 23(1935): 319–320.

Sauter, S. L., J. J. Hurrell, and C. C. Cooper. eds. *Job control and worker health*. New York: Wiley, 1989.

Schaffer, S. "Natural philosophy," in *The ferment of knowledge. Studies in the Historiography of Eighteenth-Century Science*, eds. Rousseau, G. S. and R. Porter. Cambridge: Cambridge University Press, 1980.

Scharffenberg, J. "Havde de priviligerede Kirurger Eneret til at utøve Kirurgi?" *Ugeskrift for læger*, 31(1902):721–723.

Scharffenberg, J. "Bidrag til de norske lægestillingers historie før 1800. I. Bergens stadsfysikat," *Norsk Magazin for Lægevidenskaben*, 65(1904):225–295.

Scharffenberg, J. "Bidrag til de norske lægestillingers historie før 1800. II. Kristianias stadsfysikat," *Norsk Magazin for Lægevidenskaben*, 65(1904):1329–1384.

Scharffenberg, J. "Bidrag til de norske lægestillingers historie før 1800. III. Kristianias stadsfysikat," *Norsk Magazin for Lægevidenskaben*, 66(1905):825–872.

Schei, B., G. Botten, and J. Sundby. eds. *Kvinnemedisin*. Oslo: ad Notam Gyldendal, 1993.

Scheiber, S. C. and B. B. Doyle. eds. *The Impaired Physician*. New York and London:

Plenum Medical Book Company, 1983.

Schicke, R. K. "Socio-economic systems of medicaments," *Social Science and Medicine*, 10(1976):277–281.

Schiøtt, C.T. and C.A. Egeberg, "Beretning om en ifølge Kgl. Befaling foretagen Reise til Leirsamlingen ved Stockholm i 1843". *Norsk Magasin for Lægevidenskaben,* 8 (1844) 1–16.

Schiøtz, A. and R. Nordhagen. "Om å sette sin kvinnelighet på spill. Kvinners adgang til det medisinske studium; Marie Spångberg og andre pionerer." *Tidsskrift for Den norske lægeforening* 112 (1992): 3784–3790.

Schiøtz, A. "De offentlige legene – fra krigen og rettsoppgjøret." *Tidsskrift for Den norske lægeforening* 115 (1995): 3757–3764.

Schiøtz, A. ""Hvor vi har ventet paa hende!"," in *Kvinnemedisin*, eds. Schei, B. G. Botten, and J. Sundby. Oslo: ad Notam Gyldendal, 1993.

Schjønsby, H. P. *Helserådet*. MPH thesis. Göteborg: Nordiska Hälsovårdshögskolan, 1985.

Schrader-Frechette, K. S. "Comparative risk assessement and the naturalistic fallacy," *Tree*, 10(1995):50

Schreiner, A. "Infeksjonssykdommer", *Tidsskrift for Den norske lægeforening*, 23 110 (1990):3045–3047.

Schrøder, K. A. Letter to his friend Dr. Hans Krag Sandberg, Kjøllefjord 1936. Owned by the Schrøder family.

Schytte, T. *Vägledning för emigranter. En kort framställning av utvandringarnes svårigheter och fördelar, jemte en skildring af de skandinaviska koloniernas ekonomiska, politiska och religiösa tillstånd i Nordamerika. Med ett bihang om de år 1847 utvandrade Erik Janssons anhängares sorglige öde*. Stockholm: Joh. Beckman, 1849. (Reprint: Stockholm: Bokförlaget Rediviva, 1970.)

Schønberg, E. "Medicin," in *Illustrert Norsk Literaturhistorie*, ed. Jæger, H. Kristiania: Hjalmar Bieglers forlag, 1896.

Scull, A. T. "From madness to mental illness: medical men as moral entrepreneurs," *European Journal of Sociology*, 16(1975):218–261.

Sedelow, W. A., jr. and S. Y. Sedelow. "The history of science as discourse, the strucutre of scientific and literary texts: Part II. Some issues posed by computational methodology," *Journal of the History of Behavioral Sciences*, 15(1979):63–72.

Seglen, P. "Bruk av siteringsanalyse og andre bibliometriske metoder i evaluering av forskningskvalitet," *Tidsskrift for Den norske lægeforening*, 109(1989): 3229–3234.

Seidler, E. *Medizinhistoriche Reisen. 1: Paris*. Stuttgart: 1971.

Seip, A. L. "Fattiglov og fattigvesen i mellomkrigstiden – et forsørgelsessystem under krise," *Historisk Tidsskrift*, 3(1987): 276–300.

Seip, A. L. *Sosialhjelpstaten blir til. Norsk sosialpolitikk 1740–1920*. Oslo: Gyldendal, 1984. 2. ed., 1994.

Seip, A. L. *Veien til velferdsstaten. Norsk sosialpolitikk 1920–75*. Oslo: Gyldendal, 1994.

Seip, J. A. "Flerpartistaten i perspektiv," *Nytt norsk tidsskrift*, (1994):203–220.

Seip, J. A. *Utsikt over Norges historie. Første del*. Oslo: Gyldendal, 1974.

Seip, M. Articles in *Dagbladet,*(1959): 10th of January and 12th of February.

Selander, S. ed. *Kampen om yrkesutövning, status och kunskap*. Lund: Studentlitteratur, 1989.

Selye, H. *The stress of life*. New York: McGraw-Hill, 1976.

Semb, C. "Den militære sanitets organisasjon", *Sanitetsnytt,* 11(1965):3–25.

Semb, G. *In interview with Bertelsen*, T. 16. november 1995.

Semmingsen, I. *Veien mot vest. Utvandringen fra Norge til Amerika 1825–1865*. Oslo: Aschehoug, 1941.

Semmingsen, I. *Veien mot vest. Utvandringen*

fra Norge til Amerika 1865–1915. Oslo: Aschehoug, 1950.

Semmingsen, I. "Det første halve århundre – hvor langt nådde vi?" in *Kvinner på Universitetet 100 år*, Oslo: Likestillingsutvalget Universitetet i Oslo, 1984.

Shafer, H. B. *The American Medical Profession, 1783–1850*. New York: Columbia University Press, 1936.

Shapin, S. "Property, patronage, and the politics of science: The founding of the Royal Society of Edinburgh," *The British Journal for the History of Science*, 7 (1974): 1–41.

Shapin, S. "The audience for science in eighteenth century Edinburgh," *History of Science*, (1974):95–121.

Shapin, S. "Phrenological Knowledge and the Social Structure of Early Nineteenth-Century Edinburgh," *Annals of Science*, 32 (1975):219–243.

Shapin, S. "Social uses of science," in *The ferment of knowledge. Studies in the Historiography of Eighteenth-Century Science*, eds. Rousseau, G. S. and R. Porter. Cambridge: Cambridge University Press, 1980.

Sharlin, A. "From the study of social mobility to the study of society," *American Journal of Sociology*, 85(1979):338–360.

Shils, E. "Charisma, order, and status," *American Sociological Review*, 30(1965): 199–213.

Shils, E. "Intellectuals, Tradition, and the Traditions of Intellectuals: Some Preliminary Considerations," *Dædalus*, 101 (1972):21–34.

Shorter, E. "Private clinics in central Europe 1850–1933," *The Society for the Social History of Medicine*, 3(1990):159–195.

Shortt, S. E. D. "Clinical Practice and the Social History of Medicine: A Theoretical Accord," *Bulletin of the History of Medicine*, 55(1981):533–542.

Shortt, S. E. D. "Physicians, science and status: Issues in the professionalization of anglo-american medicine in the nineteenth century," *Medical History*, 27(1983): 51–68.

Shyrock, R. H. ""The Historian Looks at Medicine"," *Bulletin of the History of Medicine*, 5(1937):887–894.

Shryock, R. H. *The Development of Modern Medicine – an Interpretation of the Social and Scientific Factors Involved.* New York: Knoph, 1947.

Shryock, R. H. "The Interplay of Social and Internal Factors in Modern Medicine, an Historical Analysis," *Centaurus*, 3(1953): 107–125.

Shyrock, R. H. *Medical Licensing in America 1650–1965*. Baltimore: Johns Hopkins University Press, 1967.

Shyrock, R. H. "The History of Quantification in Medical Science," *Isis*, 52(1961): 215–237.

Siem, H. *Choices for health.* Oslo: Universitetsforlaget, 1986.

Sigerist, H. E. "The history of medical licensure." *Journal of the American Medical Association*, 10(1935):1057–1060.

Sigerist, H. E. "The History of medicine *and* the History of Medicine," *Bulletin of the Institute of the History of Medicine*, 4(1936):6

Sigerist, H. E. *Grosse Ärzte*. München: 1931.

Sigsworth, E. M. "Gateways to death? Medicine, hospitals and mortality, 1700-1850," in *Science and Society*, ed. Mathias, P. Cambridge: Cambridge University Press, 1972.

Silver, G. A. "Virchow, The Heroic Model in Medicine: Health Policy by Accolade," *American Journal of Public Health*, 77 (1987):82–88.

Silverstein, A. M. and T. Söderqvist. "History of Immunology, The structure and Dynamics of Immunology, 1951–1972: A Peosopographical Study of International Meetings." *Cellular Immunology*, 158 (1994):1–28.

Sivertsen, G. *Norsk forskning på den internasjonale arenaen*. Rapport 1/91. Oslo:

NAVFs utredningsinstitutt, 1991.

Sivertsen, G. *Internationalization via Journals – scientific and scholarly journals edited in the Nordic countries*. NORD 1991:49. Copenhagen: Nordic Council of Ministers, 1991.

Sjurseth, K. *Hordaland fylke 1837–1937*. Bergen: Hordaland fylke, 1937.

Skappel, S. *Hedemarkens Amt 1814–1914*. Kristiania: Grøndahl & Søn, 1914.

Skodvin, O. *Forskerrekruttering til det medisinske fagområdet. Status og perspektiver mot år 2010*. Rapport 6/91. Oslo: NAVFs utredningsinstitutt, 1991.

Skoglund, E. "Legers videre- og etterutdannelse," *Tidsskrift for Den norske lægeforening*, 106(1986):1220-1226.

Skolbekken, J. A. "The risk epidemic in medical journals," *Social Science and Medicine*, 40(1995):291–305.

Skre, B.G. "Garden Havrå på Osterøy", *Jord og Gjerning*, 5(1991):88-105.

Skre, R. K. *Bjørn West i aktiv innsats*. Oslo: Gyldendal, 1946.

Skaare, D., G. Jacobsen, "Leger i gapestokk? Om legetabber og tabbeleger i norsk tabloidpresse". *Tidsskrift for Den norske lægeforening*, 116(1996):265–269.

Slagstad, R. "Den annen front – i går og i dag," *Nytt norsk tidsskrift*, 1(1995):12-24.

Slocum, W. L. *Occupational Careers*. Chicago: Aldine, 1966.

Smith, A. "Distriktslægernes boliger – bolig for Surendalens distriktslæge," *Tidsskrift for Den norske lægeforening* (1912):88

Smith, G. D., M. Bartley, and D. Blande. "The Black report on socioeconomical inequalities in health 10 years on," *British Medical Journal*, 301(1990):373-377.

Smith, G. D., and M. Egger. "Socioeconomic differentials in wealth and health", *British Medical Journal*, 307(1993):1085–1086.

Smith, H. *Lægebog, inholdenis Mange skøne oc utvalde Lægedoms stycker1577*. København, Rosenkilde og Bagger: Faksimileutgave, 1976.

Smith, R. "Through the crystal ball darkly," in *The future of medical journals*, ed. Lock, S. London: BMJ, 1991.

Söderqvist, T. and A. M. Silverstein. "Participation in Scientific Meetings: A New Prosopographical Approach to the Disciplinary History of Science – The Case of Immunology, 1951-72," *Social Studies of Science*, 24(1994):513-548.

Sontag, S. *Illness as Metaphor*. London: Allen Lane, 1979.

Sosialdepartementet, Helsedirektoratet: "Redegjørelse for studenter, som akter å studere medisin i utlandet," 23. Juli 1953.

Sosialdepartementet, Medisinaldirektoratet, Legekontoret. (Ministry of Health and Social Affairs, Directorate of Medicine, Doctor's Office) The boxes 1, 147, 148, 151, 154, 156, 158, 168, 197, 202.

Spence, G. E. "Towards a theory of work," *Philosophical Forum*, 10(1979):306-320.

Spencer, A. and D. Podmore. eds. *In a Man's World: Essays on Women in Male-dominated Professions*. London: Tavistock, 1987.

Spicker, S. F. "An Introduction to the Medical Epistemology of Georges Canguilhem: Moving Beyond Michel Foucault," *The Journal of Medicine and Philosophy*, 12 (1987):397-411.

SSB. *Statistisk Årbok 1995/Statistical Yearbook 1995*. Oslo/Kongsvinger: Statistisk Sentralbyrå, 1995.

SSB. *Historisk Statistikk 1968/Historical Statistics 1968*. Oslo: Statistisk Sentralbyrå, 1969.

SSB. *Historisk Statistikk/Historical Statistics*, Oslo: Statistisk Sentralbyrå, 1978.

SSB. *Historisk Statistikk 1994/Historical Statistics 1994*. Oslo/Kongsvinger: Statistisk sentralbyrå, 1995.

SSB. *Helseundersøkelsen 1985*. Oslo: Statistisk Sentralbyrå, 1985.

SSB. *Flyttingene i Norge 1971 og 1949–1973*.

Rapport nr. 3 fra Flyttemotivundersøkelsen 1972. Oslo: Statistisk Sentralbyrå, 1975.

St.meld. nr. 18–1926, Innst. nr. 2.

St.meld.45. *Om behovet for akademisk arbeidskraft,* 1950.

St.meld. nr. 85 /1970–71) Om helsetjeneste utenfor sykehus.

St.meld.9. *Sykehusutbygging m.v. i et regionalisert helsevesen.* 1975.

St.meld. 37 *Utfordringer i helsefremmende og forebyggende arbeid.* 1992.

St.prop.no.108, 1937.

Stacey, M. and H. Homans. "The Sociology of Health and Illness: its present state, future prospects and potential for health research," *Sociology*, 12(1978):281-307.

Stahl, S. K. D. "The Personal Narrative as Folklore," *Journal of the Folklore Institute*, 14(1977):9-30.

Stang, J. "Indberetning til det akademiske Kollegium om en med offentligt Stipendium i 1871 foretagen Udenlandsreise," *Norsk Magazin for Lægevidenskaben*, (1872) 422-440, 3 (1873):171-197, and 6 (1876) 836–851,

Starr, P. "Medicine and the Waning of Professional Sovereignty," *Dædalus*, 107 (1978):175-193.

Stearns, P. N. *European Society in Upheaval. Social History Since 1750.* New York: Macmillan Publishing Co, 1975 and London: Collier Macmillan Publishers, 1975.

Stebbins, R. A. *Amateurs, Professionals, and Serious Leisure.* Montreal: McGill-Queen's University Press, 1992.

Steen, S. *Ferd og fest.* Oslo: Aschehoug, 1942.

Stevens, M. L. "Wistful thinking: the effect of nostalgia on interpretation," *History News*, 36(1981):10–13.

Stevensen, J. "Observations on illness from the inside," in *When doctors are patients*, eds. Pinner, M. and B. F. Miller. New York: Norton & Comp, 1952.

Stevenson, L. G. "A second opinion," *Bulletin of the History of Medicine*, 54(1980): 134–140.

Stinson, E. R. and D. A. Mueller. "Survey of health professionals' information habits and needs," *Journal of the American Medical Association*, 243(1980):140–143.

Stoltenberg, C. *Doktorhistorier*. Kristiania: 1912.

Storm-Mathisen, H. "Hvilken betydning har "Tidsskriftet" hatt for den praktiserende lege og for sykehuslegen?" *Tidsskrift for Den norske lægeforening*, 101 (1981):43–46.

Stortingsforhandlinger nr. 90, 1917, 30. mars.

Stortingstidende. Spørretime 26. mars 1958.

Stoye, J. "Reisende Engländer in Europa des 17. Jahrhunderts und ihre Reisemotive," in *Reiseberichte als Quellen europäischer Kulturgeschichte. Aufgaben und Möglichkeiten der historischen Reiseforschung*, eds. Maczak, A. and H. J. Teuteberg. Herzog August Bibliothek Wolfenbüttel, 1982.

Strand, S. "Utenfor kirken – ingen frelse?" *Tidsskrift for Den norske lægeforening*, 115 (1995):2698–2702.

Strandberg, M. and B. Arentz. "Kvinnliga läkare mår sämre än sina manliga kolleger," *Läkartidningen*, 86(1989):4402–4405.

Strong, P. M. "The Rivals: an Essay on the Sociological Trades," in *The Sociology of the Professions: Lawyers, Doctors and Others*, eds. Dingwall, R. and P. Lewis. London: Macmillan, 1983.

Strong, P. M. "Sociological imperialism and the profession of medicine. A critical examination of the thesis of medical imperialism," *Social Science and Medicine*, 13A (1979):199–215.

Strøm, A. *Velferdssamfunn og helse. Et 60-årig tilbakeblikk.* Oslo: Gyldendal Norsk Forlag, 1980.

Strøm, A. "Licentia practicandi i Norge for læger med medisinsk eksamen fra utenlandske universitet," *Tidsskrift for Den norske lægeforening,*74(1954b):503–505.

Strøm, A. "Lægebehovet i Norge," *Tidsskrift for Den norske lægeforening,* 72(1952): 325–328.

Strøm, A. "Tilsvar til Anton Johnson," *Tidsskrift for Den norske lægeforening,* 74 (1954c):662–663.

Strøm, A. "Medisinsk studium i utlandet," *Tidsskrift for Den norske lægeforening,* 74 (1954b):476.

Strøm, A. "Lægeforeningen under okkupasjonen", *Tidsskrift for Den norske lægeforening,* 81(1961):674–7.

Studenterne fra 1890. Kristiania: Grøndahl og Søns boktrykkeri, 1915.

Studenterne fra 1891. Kristiania: Grøndahl og Søns boktrykkeri, 1916.

Studenterne fra 1892. Kristiania: Grøndahl og Søns boktrykkeri, 1917.

Studenterne fra 1893. Kristiania: Grøndahl og Søns boktrykkeri, 1918.

Studenterne fra 1894. Kristiania: Grøndahl og Søns boktrykkeri, 1919.

Sundin, J. *Fræmmande studenter vid Uppsala universitetet före andra verdenskriget.* Uppsala: 1973.

Sundt, E. *Om dødeligheten i Norge.* Oslo: Gyldendal, 1975.

Sundt, E. *Om Renligheds-Stellet i Norge.* Christiania: Chr. Abelsted, 1869, Gyldendal norsk forlag, 1975.

Sunnanå, L. S. "Orker vi å være sykehusleger lenger?" *Tidsskrift for Den norske lægeforening,* 115(1995):3315.

Susser, M. "Introduction to the theme: a critical review of sociology in health," *International Journal of Health Services,* 4(1974).

Sussman, G. D. "The Glut of Doctors in Mid-Nineteenth-Century France," *Comparative Studies in Society and History,* 19 (1977):287–304.

Sutherland, V. J. and C. L. Cooper. "Job stress, satisfaction, and mental health among general practitioners before and after introduction of new contract," *British Journal of Medicine,* 304(1992): 1545–1548.

Svalestuen, A. "Medisinalvesenets sentraladministrasjon 1809–1940," in *Norsk Arkivforum. Administrasjonshistoriske oversikter,* Oslo: Arkivarforeningen, 1988.

Sveriges läkarförbund. *Läkares arbetsmiljö – en rapport från Läkarforbundets arbetsmiljögrupp.* Stockholm: Sveriges läkarforbund, 1988.

Sverre, NA. *Et studium av farmasiens historie. 2.ed.* Oslo: Norges Apotekerforening, 1982.

Szasz, T. S. "Power and Psychiatry," *Society,* 18(1981):16–18.

Szreter, S. "The importance of Social Intervention in Britain's Mortality Decline c. 1850–1914: a Re-interpretation of the Role of Public Health," *The Society for the Social History of Medicine,* 1(1988):1–38.

Sæther, P. *Modum Blaafarveverk, et verkssamfunn i 1830 – 1840 årene.* Oslo: Thesis in ethnology, University of Oslo, 1976.

Søgnen, R. *Dynamisk treghet. Endringsprosesser i NAVFs råd for medisinsk forskning (RMF) 1975–1993. Rapport 12/94.* Oslo: Utredningsinstituttet, 1994.

Sørensen, Ø., ed. *Nordic paths to national identity in the nineteenth century.* KULTs skriftserie nr. 22. Oslo: The Research Council of Norway, 1994.

Taeusch, C. F. "Fees and charges as an index of professionalism," *International Journal of Ethics,* 35(1925):368–376.

Taubes, G. "Science journals go wired", *Science,* 271(1996):764–766.

Taylor, R. and A. Rieger. "Medicine as Social Science: Rudolf Virchow on the Typhus Epidemic in Upper Silesia," *International Journal of Health Services,* 15(1985): 547–559.

Temkin, O. "Therapeutic trends and the treatment of syphlis before 1900," *Bulletin of the History of Medicine,* 29(1955): 309–316.

Temkin, O. "The role of surgery in the rise of modern medical thought," *Bulletin of the History of Medicine*, 25(1951): 248–259.

Thacher, J. *American Medical Biography*. New York: 1967.

Thaulow, H. A. "Beretning om Reiser til tydske Bade, foretagne i Aarene 1863 og 65,"*Norsk Magazin for Lægevidenskaben*,(1866):312–330.

The Royal Norwegian Ministry of Health and Social Affairs. *Report on Public Health in Norway*. Statement of the Ministry of Health to the Storting 30. April 1996.

The Norwegian Ministry of Health and Social Affairs. "Welfare towards 2030," *Summary version of white paper*, 35 (1994–95).

The Ministry of Health and Social Affairs. *Health Policy towards year 2000*. A Survey Norway, 1990.

The Norwegian Medical Association, *Yearbook 1990–1991*.

The Norwegian Medical Association, *Yearbook 1995*.

Thiel, P. *Männer Gegen Tod und Teufel: Aus dem Leben Grosser Ärzte*. Berlin: 1943.

Thiis-Evensen, E. *Sånn var livet*. Skien: Arne Kunstforlag, 1992.

Thorleifsen, M. *Husmannskår i Gålåskroken og Vang ca. 1780–1903. Magistergradsavhandling i etnologi*. Oslo: Universitet i Oslo, 1991.

Thürmer, H., K. Bjartveit and A. Hauknes. "Norske legers røykevaner 1952–84," *Tidsskrift for Den norske lægeforening*, 106 19(1986):2961–2964.

Tidsskrift for den norske lægeforening, (1918):125, 190; (1928):75–77; (1933): 155; (1934):437; (1935):1381; (1942): 336; (1961):701–705; (1986):1221.

Titon, J. F. "The Life Story," *Journal of American Folklore*, 93(1980):276–292.

Tjomsland, A. ed. *The Saga of Hrafn Sveinbjarnarson*. Ithaca, New York: Cornell University Press, 1951.

Torgersen, U. *Profesjonssosiologi*. Oslo-Bergen-Tromsø: Universitetsforlaget, 1972.

Torgersen, U. "Profesjoner – verdigrunnlag, kunnskapsenhet og kompetanse," *Kirke og Kultur*, 79(1974):193–199.

Torgersen, U. "Profesjoner, markedskonjunkturer og markedspolitikk," *Sosiologi i dag*, 1(1981):5–19.

Torgersen, U. *Profesjoner og offentlig sektor*. Oslo: TANO, 1994.

Torstendahl, R. and M. Burrage. eds. *The Formation of Professions. Knowledge, State and Strategy*. London: SAGE, 1990.

Toulmin, S. "How Medicine Saved the Life of Ethics," *Perspectives in Biology and Medicine*, 25(1973):735–750.

Toulmin, S. "The Tyranny of Principles", *Hastings Center Report*, (December 1981): 31–39.

Toverud, K. U. "Helsearbeide for barn og mødre i praksis," *Tidsskrift for Den norske lægeforening*, (1937):323–331.

Toverud, K. U. "Organiseringen av forebyggende helsearbeide i svangerskapet og barnealderen i vårt land," *Tidsskrift for Den norske lægeforening*, (1936):1389–1396.

Towner, J. "The Grand Tour: A Key Phase in the History of Tourism," *Annals of Tourism Research*, 12(1985):297–333.

Towner, J. "Tourism History," *Annals of Tourism Research*, 17(1990):154–166.

Towner, J. "The Grand Tour: Sources and a methodology for an historical study of tourism," *Tourism Management*, 5(1984): 215–222.

Tranberg, A. "Korn og klasseskille," in *Bind 3. Bygdebok for Brøttum, Ringsaker & Veldre*, Moelv: Brøttum, Ringsaker & Veldre historielag, 1993.

Tranøy, K. E., and Sars, M. *Tysklandsstudentene*. Oslo: Cappelen, 1946.

Trenn, T. J. "Ludwik Fleck's "On the question of the foundations of medical knowledge"," *The Journal of Medicine and Philosophy*, 6(1981):237–256.

Try, H. "Yrkesstruktur og sosial struktur,"

in *Norges historie Bind 11*, Oslo: Cappelen, 1979.

Tschudi Madsen, S. and O. Sollied. *Medisinsk liv i Bergen*. Bergen: Det medisinske selskap, 1931.

Turner, B. S. *Medical Power and Social Knowledge*. Newbury Park, Calif: Sage, 1987.

Turner, B. S. *The body and society*. Oxford: Basil Blackwell, 1984.

Turner, B. S. "Talcot Parsons, Universalism and the Educational Revolution: Democracy versus Professionalism," *British Journal of Sociology*, 44(1993):1–24.

Turner, R. S. "The Growth of Professorial Research in Prussia, 1818 to 1848 –Causes and Context," *Historical Studies in the Physical Sciences*, 3(1971):137–182.

Tveiten, G. *Hole Herred Ringerike*. Kristiania: Centraltrykkeriet i Kristiania, 1914.

Tveterås, H. L. *Norske tidsskrifter. Bibliografi over periodiske skrifter i Norge inntil 1920*. Oslo: Universitetsforlaget, 1984.

Twain, M. T*he Innocents Abroad*. New York: 1966.

Uhlenberg, P. and T.M. Cooney. "Male and female physicians: family and career comparisons." *Social Science & Medicine* 30 (1990): 373–378.

Ullmann, D., R.L. Phillips, L. Beeson, H.G. Dewey, B.N. Brin, J.W. Kuzma, C.P. Mathews and A.E. Hirst. "Cause-specific mortality among physicians with differing life-style," *The Journal of the American Medical Association*, 265(1991):2352–2359. *Universitetet i Bergens historie I–II*. Bergen: Universitetet i Bergen, 1996.

Universitetet i Oslo 1911–1961. Bd I. Oslo: Universitetsforlaget, 1961.

Universitetet i Oslo 1911–1961. Bd II. Oslo: Universitetsforlaget, 1961.

Utredningsinstituttet. *FoU-statistikk og indikatorer. Forskning og utviklingsarbeid 1995 (R&D Statistics – Science and Technology Indicators)*. Oslo: Utredningsinstituttet, 1994.

Vaglum, P. "Legestudiet – fortsatt et menneskebehandlende studium?" *Tidsskrift for Den norske lægeforeningen*, 114(1994): 3171–3172.

Vald Directory of Medical Schools. Geneva: World Health Association, 1963.

Vallgårda, S. "The increased obstetric activity: a new meaning to induced labour?" *Journal of Epidemiology and Community Health* 43(1989):48–52.

Vallgårda, S. "The History of Medicine in Denmark," *The Society for the Social History of Medicine*, 8(1995):115–123.

van der Korst, J. K. *Om lijf en leven. Gezondheotszorg en geneeskunst in Nederland 1200–1960*. Utrecht: Boon, Scheltema & Holkema, 1988.

Vanebo, J. O. "Trøndersk industri i går, i dag og i morgen", in *Trøndelag -82*, Trønderlaget, Trondheim 1982.

Varmus, H. "Shattuck lecture – Biomedical research enters the steady state," *New England Journal of Medicine*, 333(1995): 811–815.

Vartiovaara, I. "Stress and burnout in the medical profession. (Burnout och läkarne)," *Suomen Lääkärilehti*, 43(1988): 1258–1259.

Vatten, I. Å. *Doktor'n vår*. Trondheim: Rune Forlag, 1978.

Veatch, R. *A Theory of Medical Ethics*. Basic books Inc Publishers, 1981.

Veblen, T. *The Theory of the Leisure Class* (1899). London: Unwin, 1970.

Velle, W. *Norges veterinærer 1988*. Bærum: Den norske veterinærforening, 1988.

Venanzoni, G. "The evolution and prospects of the National Health Service," *Revue Internationale de Sociologie*, 3(1993): 65–106.

Vikanes, Å., V. Akre, and P. Hjortdahl. "Medisinsk grunnutdanning i utakt," *Tidsskrift for Den norske lægeforening*, 112 19(1992):2541–2545.

Vinje, A. *Ferdaminne frå sumaren 1860*. Oslo: Gyldendal, 1967.

Virchow, R. and R. Leubuscher. *Die medizinische Reform. Eine Wochenschrift erschienen vom 10. Juli 1848 bis zum 29. Juni 1849.* Berlin: G. Reimer.

Vittaliano, Maiuro, Russo, Mitchell, Carr, and Van Citters. "A biopsychosocial model of medical school distress," *Journal of Behavioral Medicine*, 11(1988):311–331.

Vogel, M. J. "The Transformation of the American Hospital, 1850–1920," in *Health Care in America. Essays in Social History*, eds. Reverby, S. and D. Rosner. Philadelphia: Temple University Press, 1979.

Vollmer, H. M. and D. L. Mills. eds. *Professionalization*. Prentice-Hall: Englewood Cliffs, 1966.

Voss, J.A. "Indberetning til Kirke- og Underviisnings-Departementet om en med Stipendium foretagen videnskabelig reise i Udlandet," *Norsk Magazin for Lægevidenskaben*, (1851):566–585.

Voss, J.A. "Optegnelser fra en Reise i de forenede Stater i Nord-amerika i sommeren 1857," *Norsk Magazin for Lægevidenskaben*, (1858):834–854.

Waddington, I. "The development of medical ethics – A sociological analysis," *Medical History*, 19(1975):36–51.

Waddington, I. *The Medical Profession in the Industrial Revolution*. Dublin: Gill and Macmillan, 1985.

Waddington, I. "The movement towards the professionalisation of medicine," *British Medical Journal*, 301(1990):688–690.

Wagner, G. and G. Wessel. *Medizinprofessoren und ärztliche Ausbildung*. Jena: 1992.

Waitzkin, H. and B. Waterman. "Social Theory and Medicine," *International Journal of Health Services*, 6(1976):9–23.

Walby, S. "Theorising patriarchy," *Sociology*, 23(1989):213–234.

Walby, S. "From Private to Public Patriarchy: The Periodisation of British History," *Women's Studies International Forum*, 3(1990):91–104.

Walderhaug, E. "Faste kontordager – godtgjørelsen for dem," *Tidsskrift for Den norske lægeforening*, (1914):239–241.

Walderhaug, E. "Distriktslægenes boliger og bostedsspørsmaalet. Motorbåtreiser, honorartariffer," *Tidsskrift for Den norske lægeforening*, (1915):1234–1237.

Wang, C. "Culture, meaning and disability: injury prevention campaigns and the production of stigma," *Social Science and Medicine*, 35(1992):1093–1102.

Wangensteen, O. H., J. Smith, and S. D. Wangensteen. "Some highlights in the history of amputation reflecting lessons in wound healing," *Bulletin of the History of Medicine*, 41(1967):97–131.

Warner, J. H. "The selective transport of medical knowledge: Antebellum American physicians and Parisian medical therapeutics," *Bulletin of the History of Medicine*, 59(1985):213–231.

Warner, J. H. "Remembering Paris: Memory and the American disciples of French medicine in the nineteenth century," *Bulletin of the History of Medicine*, 65 (1991):301–325.

Warner, J. H. "Science in Medicine," *Osiris*, 1(1985):37–58.

Warr, P., J. Cook, and T. Wall. "Scales for the measurement of some work attitudes and aspects of psychological well-being," *Journal of Occupational Psychology*, 52 (1979):129–148.

Warren, K. S. "From papyrus to paper to pixels: information technology and the future of medical publishing," in *The future of medical journals*, ed. Lock, S. London: BMJ, 1991.

Washington, A. W. "Moving toward cultural competence in the transplant milieu," *Transplantation Proceedings* 25(1993): 2499–2501.

Waters, B. "The past and the historical past," *Journal of Philosophy*, 52(1955): 253–269.

Waters, M. "Collegiality, Bureaucratization, and Professionalization: A Weberian Analysis," *American Journal of Sociology*, 94(1989):945–972.

Wear, A. "The Selective Transport of Medical Knowledge," *Bulletin of the History of Medicine*, 59(1985):213–231.

Wear, A. *Medicine in Society. Historical essays.* Cambridge: Cambridge University Press, 1992.

Weber, M. *Makt og byråkrati.* Oslo: Gyldendal Norsk Forlag, 1971.

Wefring, K. W. *Vestfold Sentralsykehus Barneavdelingen 1959–1994.* Tønsberg: Cicero Grafisk AS, 1994.

Wegar, K. "Conclusions," in *Gender, Work and Medicine: Women and the Medical Divisions of Labour*, eds. Riska, E. and K. Wegar. London: SAGE, 1993. pp. 173–188.

Weindling, P. "Bourgeois values, doctors and the state: the professionalization of medicine in Germany 1848–1933," in *The German bourgeoisie*, eds. Blackbourne, D. and R. J. Evans. London: Routledge, 1991.

Weisz, G. "Water cures and science: The French Academy of Medicine and mineral waters in the nineteenth century," *Bulletin of the History of Medicine*, 64(1990):393–416.

Weisz, G. "The Development of Medical Spezialization in Nineteenth-Century Paris," *Clio Med*, 25(1994):149–188.

Wessel, A. B. "Epidemier og Lægeforhold i Finnmark i slutten av det 18de og begynnelsen av det 19. aarhundre," *Tidsskrift for Den norske lægeforening*, 48(1928):118–133.

Wessel, A.B. "Av Finmarks medicinalhistorie. Lægeforhold og jordmorvæsen i Finmark i eldre tider." *Tidsskrift for Den norske lægeforening.*

Wester, K. *Norsk Nevrokirurgisk Forening.* Bergen: 1994.

White, K. "Introduction," *Revue Internationale de Sociologie*, 3(1993):109–116.

White, K. "The sociology of health and illness." *Current Sociology* 39 (1991): 1–134.

Wickersheimer, E. *Dictionnaire Biographique des Médecins en France au moyen âge.* Genéve: 1979.

Wiench, P. *Die Großen Ärzte.* Zürich: 1982.

Wiers-Jensen, J., P. Vaglum, and Ø. Ekeberg. "On the doorstep of medical school: Sex segretation, motivation, professional aspirations and specialty preferences. A nation-wide study." *Medical Education* (1996) (In press).

Wiers-Jenssen, J. *Rekruttering til medisinstudiet. En studie av et årskull medisinerstudenter, med vekt på sosial bakgrunn, poengsamling, studiemotiver og ambisjonsnivå.* Hovedfagsoppgave i sosiologi. Oslo: Institutt for sosiologi, Universitetet i Oslo, 1994.

Wiers-Jenssen, J., P. Vaglum, and Ø. Ekeberg. "Repetisjon og privatisteksamener – veien til det medisinske studium," *Tidsskrift for Den norske lægeforening*, 115 21(1995):2659–2662.

Wilensky, H. L. "The Professionalization of Everyone?" *American Journal of Sociology*, LXX(1964):137–148.

Wilkin, D., P. Hodgkin, and D. Metcalfe. "Factors affecting workload: is received wisdom true?" in Gray, P. ed., *The medical annual, 1986. The yearbook of general practice*, Bristol: Wright, 1986.

Williams, R. "Concepts of health: an analysis of lay logic," *Sociology*, 17(1983): 185–205.

Willis, E. "Doctoring in Australia: A View at the Bicentenary," *The Milbank Quarterly*, 66(1989):167–181.

Wilson, L. "Medical History without Medicine," *Journal of the History of Medicine*, 35 (1980):5–7.

Wilson, R. N. "The Social Structure of a General Hospital," *The Annals of The American Academy of Political and Social Science: Medicine and Society*, 346(1963): 67–76.

Winge, P.E. "Beretning om en ved Stipendium foretagen Reise i Udlandet," *Norsk Magazin for Lægevidenskaben*, (1848):81–104.

Wise, T. N. "Depression and fatigue in the primary care physician," *Primary Care*, 18(1991):451–464.

Witz, A. *Professions and Patriarchy*. London: Routledge, 1992.

Wood, M. L. "Naming the illness: The power of words," *Family Medicine*, 23(1991): 534–538.

Worboys, M. "The Sanatorium Treatment for Consumption in Britain, 1890–1914," in Pickstone J. V. ed., *Medical Innovations in Historical Perspective*, London: Macmillan, 1992.

Wrangel, E. "Forskningar om svenskarnes universitetsstudier i Tyskland," *Samlaren*, 25(1904):1–6.

Wright, P. W. "A study in the legitimisation of knowledge: The "Success" of Medicine and the "Failure" of Astrology," *Sociological Review Monograph*, (1979): 85–101.

Wright, G. H. v. *Vetenskapen och förnuftet*. Stockholm: Bonnier, 1986.

Wyller, I. "Det 19. århundre", in *Sykepleiens historie i Norge*. Oslo: Gyldendal, 1990.

Wyller, T. *Nyordning og motstand.* Oslo: Universitetsforlaget, 1958.

Wyman, A. L. "The surgeoness: The female practitioner of surgery 1400–1800," *Medical History*, 28(1984):22–41.

Young, R. "Autonomous patients and medical professionalism." *Med J Aust* 160 (1994): 305–306.

Zimmermann, L. M. "Surgeons and the rise of clinical teaching in England," *Bulletin of the History of Medicine*, 37(1963): 167–177.

Zola, I. K. "Medicine as an institution of social control," *Sociological Review*, 60 (1972):487–503.

Zola, I. K. "In the name of health and illness: on some sociopolitical consequences of medical influence," *Social Science and Medicine*, 9(1975).

Ødegaard, Ø. "Emigration and Insanity. A study of mental disease among the norwegianborn population of Minnesota," in *Acta Psychiatrica et Neurologica Supplementum IV*. Köbenhavn: Levin & Munksgaard, 1932.

Ødegaard, N. *Kristians Amt 1814–1914*. Kristiania: Grøndahl & Søn, 1918.

Ørbeck, A. L. and T. Quelprud. *Setedalsrykkja (Chorea progressiva hereditaria)*. Oslo: J Dybwad, 1951.

Østby, L. *Geografisk mobilitet. En gjennomgåelse av dens teoretiske grunnlag, og behandling av flyttingene i Norge 1966–1967, 1–2,* Oslo: Meddelelser fra Geografisk Institutt, Universitetet i Oslo, Kulturgeografisk Serie nr. 4, 1970.

Østby, L.*Hvem flytter i Norge? Tendenser i flyttegruppenes sammensetning etter 1950.* Oslo: Statistisk Sentralbyrå, 1975.

Østerberg, D. "Byens form og materie," in *Kultur og Barbari. Essays om kunst- og samfunnskritikk*, ed. Østerberg, D. Oslo: Brutus Östlings Forlag Symposion, 1991.

Øyen, O. *Milorg D13 i kamp.* Oslo: Norsk kunstforlag, 1961.

Åquist, A. "Om patriarkatteori – en o-modern betraktelse," *Nordisk Samhällsgeografisk Tidsskrift*, 10(1989):37–48.

CHAPTER 34

Index

CHAPTER 35

Contributors

The team of authors behind this book included (in alphabetical order):

Abrahamsen, Ingvild Stokke, medical student, Oslo.

Austnes, Bård, medical student, Oslo.

Berg, Ole, professor, health administration, Oslo.

Bertelsen, Torstein, professor, opthalmology (retired), Bergen.

Christie, Vigdis Moe, social researcher, Oslo.

Engelskjøn, Naidi, philosopher and medical student, Oslo.

Evensen, Stein A., professor, internal medicine, Oslo.

Falkum, Erik, psychiatrist, researcher, Oslo.

Forsdahl, Anders, professor, family medicine, Tromsø.

Frich, Jan Christian, medical student, Oslo.

Fugelli, Per, professor, social medicine, Oslo.

Gogstad, Anders C., professor, social medicine (Bergen) (retired), Helle.

Hagesveen, Arild, medical student, Oslo.

Hjortdahl, Per, professor, family medicine, Oslo.

Holck, Per, professor, anatomy, Oslo.

Hunstadbråten, Kai, dentist, Åmot.

Høeg, Anna Victoria, medical student, Oslo.

Ingstad, Benedicte, professor, medical anthropology, Oslo.

Kvarenes, Hanne Winge, medical student, Oslo.

Larsen, Anne Sofie Frøyshov, medical doctor, Sandnessjøen.

Larsen, Øivind, professor, medical history, Oslo.

Leira, Håkon Lasse, chief physician, occupational medicine, Trondheim.

Lærum, Even, professor, family medicine, Oslo.

Lærum, Frode, professor, radiology, Oslo.

Lærum, Ole Didrik, professor, pathology, Bergen.

Nyborg, Gunhild, medical student, Oslo.

Nylenna, Magne, medical doctor, editor of The Journal of the Norwegian Medical Association, Oslo.

Olsen, Bent Olav, researcher, human geography, Sandnessjøen.

Rosvold, Elin Olaug, researcher, medical history, Oslo.

Sandvik, Hogne, research fellow, Bergen.

Schiøtz, Aina, historian, Oslo.

Schjønsby, Hans Petter, chief county physician, Brummunddal.

Stene-Larsen, Geir, project coordinator, Ministry of Health and Social Affairs, Oslo.

Storesund, Asbjørn, associate professor, natural sciences, Bø.

Aasland, Olaf Gjerløw, professor, health administration, Oslo.